Development
of the
Human Spinal Cord

DEVELOPMENT
of the
HUMAN SPINAL CORD

An Interpretation Based on
Experimental Studies
in Animals

JOSEPH ALTMAN

SHIRLEY A. BAYER

OXFORD
UNIVERSITY PRESS
2001

OXFORD
UNIVERSITY PRESS

Oxford   New York
Athens   Auckland   Bangkok   Bogotá   Buenos Aires   Calcutta
Cape Town   Chennai   Dar es Salaam   Delhi   Florence   Hong Kong   Istanbul
Karachi   Kuala Lumpur   Madrid   Melbourne   Mexico City   Mumbai
Nairobi   Paris   São Paulo   Shanghai   Singapore   Taipei   Tokyo   Toronto   Warsaw

and associated companies in
Berlin   Ibadan

Published by Oxford University Press Inc.,
198 Madison Avenue, New York, New York 10016
http://www.oup-usa.org

Oxford is a registered trademark of Oxford University Press.

Library of Congress Cataloging-in-Publication Data
Altman, Joseph, 1925–
Development of the human spinal cord: an interpretation based on
experimental studies in animals/
Joseph Altman, Shirley A. Bayer
p.; cm. Includes bibliographical references and index.
ISBN 0-19-514427-9
1. Spinal cord—Growth. 2. Developmental neurobiology.
I. Bayer, Shirley A. (Shirley Ann), 1940–
II. Title
DNLM: 1. Spinal Cord—growth & development. 2. Models, Animal.
3. Spinal Cord—embryology.
WL 400 A445da 2001] QP371 .A45 2001 612.6′ 40182—dc21 2001021135

We would like to thank the authors, journals, and publishers for their permission
to reprint the following figures in this text:

From Wiley for figures reproduced from the *Journal of Comparative Neurology (JCN):*

W. Willis et al. *JCN*, 1979, vol.188, p. 543.
S. A. Keirstad and P. K. Rose. *JCN*, 1983, vol. 219, p. 273.
K. E. McKenna. *JCN*, 1986, vol. 248, p. 532.
P. Shortland et al. *JCN*, 1989, vol. 289, p. 416.
P. E. Phelps. *JCN*, 1990, vol. 291, p. 9.
E. A. J. F. Lakke. *JCN*, 1991, vol. 314, p. 67.
Y. Shinoda. *JCN*, 1992, vol. 316, p. 151.

From Elsevier for figures reproduced from *Brain Research (BR)*:

L. J. Stensaas. *BR*, 1971, vol. 31, p. 67.
J. Rastad. *BR*, 1977, vol. 135:1.
T. M. Jessell. *BR*, 1978, vol. 152, p. 183.

From Wolters Kluwer for a figure reproduced from M. E. Schwab.
Journal of Neurocytology, 1989,
vol. 18, p. 161.

From Mosby for a figure reproduced from:
K. F. Swaiman and S. Ashwal (eds.), "Pediatric Neurology: Principles and
Practice," 1999, p. 39.

2 4 6 8 9 7 5 3 1

Printed in Hong Kong on acid-free paper.

PREFACE

The central nervous system is a unitary organ whose primary function is integration. Nevertheless, the common distinction of two divisions within the unitary central nervous system – the brain and the spinal cord – is justified. This is so not only because the two look very different and are situated in different parts of the body, one in the cranium and the other in the vertebral canal, but also because the two perform different functions in the integration of organic activities and in the coordination of the individual's transactions with the environment. The brain's immediate relationship, with regard to sensory functions, is with the special senses of the head that scan the external world – especially, the organs of vision, audition and olfaction. These sense organs provide the brain with information about the properties of distant objects and the features of distant events. In contrast, the spinal cord's immediate relationship is with some of the less specialized sense organs distributed over the rest of the body that convey information about the properties of objects that come in direct contact with the body and events that transpire within the body. Sensors scattered in the skin convey information about the mechanical, thermal and noxious properties of stimuli that affect the body exterior; sensors embedded in muscles and joints provide feedback about the status of the motor apparatus and the position of body parts in relation to one another; and sensors attached to the internal organs send messages to the spinal cord about the condition of the viscera. With regard to motor functions, it is the spinal cord that, by way of the motor nerves that innervate the skeletal muscles, enables the organism to change its posture, move from place to place, and grasp and handle objects. With the exception of motor functions controlled by the cranial nerves, the spinal cord is responsible for the execution of all overt behavior.

But even though the brain and the spinal cord have different functions, they operate in complete unison under normal conditions. This integration is brought about by massive communication lines that interconnect the two. Information reaching and processed by the spinal cord is concurrently communicated to higher brain stations by ascending channels for further processing and multisensory integration. Similarly, descending channels from the brain carry feedback signals and motor commands to the spinal cord, thereby modulating its reflexes and automatisms, and enabling it to execute voluntary acts. The great importance of these communication lines between brain and spinal cord is dramatically brought home by accidents and diseases that sever connections between the two. Depending on the exact location and extent of the damage, the body may become paralyzed on one side (hemiplegia), or the paralysis may affect the lower body (paraplegia). In the most severe cases, the entire body and all four of the extremities may become paralyzed (quadriplegia). In other forms of spinal cord injury or disease, skin sensitivity may be reduced (analgesia) or heightened (hyperalgesia), or motor performance may be degraded by muscular rigidity (spasticity), muscular weakness (flaccidity), tremor, and other movement disorders.

Since the mature spinal cord is the end-product of its ontogenetic history, familiarity with the time course, sequential steps, and interactive mechanisms of spinal cord development is bound to contribute to a better understanding of its normal organization and operation. Just as importantly, any realistic hope to promote recovery from spinal cord disease or damage, and devise procedures to remedy or repair that insult, must be based on an understanding of the normal course of spinal cord development. Fortunately, there is a vast corpus of data, based both on normative descriptions and experimental manipulations, on spinal cord development in lower vertebrates and mammals. Regrettably, there is much less descriptive information currently available about the course of spinal cord development in man and, due to ethical and legal considerations, virtually no experimental data. The purpose of this study is to fill this gap by presenting a comprehensive account of the normal course of spinal cord development in man – beginning with the earliest stages of its embryonic development, through the fetal period, up to the second year of postnatal life – and interpret this descriptive evidence in light of currently available experimental data and theories in lower vertebrates and mammals.

The first part of the book (Chapters 1-4) deals with descriptive and experimental studies of spinal cord development in animals. Chapter 1 is an introduction to our current understanding of the structural and functional organization of the spinal cord in mammals, including man. Special attention is paid to the following: the laminar organization of the dorsal horn; the segregation of afferents reaching the spinal cord; the columnar organization of motoneurons with different peripheral targets; and the functions of the major ascending and descending tracts that interconnect the spinal cord with the brain. Chapter 2 is a comparative (phylogenetic) review of spinal cord organization that ranges from the lowest extant vertebrates to primates. This review is an essential part of this study because our interpretation of spinal cord organization is explicitly an evolutionary one. We distinguish within the mammalian and human spinal cord between paleospinal (phylogenetically old) and neospinal (phylogenetically new) sensory mechanisms, and paleospinal and neospinal motor mechanisms. Chapters 3 and 4 provide a detailed account of our experimental studies of spinal cord development in the rat, with special reference to an autoradiographic analysis of spinal cord neurogenesis and a histological analysis of its differentiation. Three major divisions of spinal cord neuroepithelium (the embryonic source of all neurons of the spinal cord) are distinguished: those that sequentially produce the motoneurons of the ventral horn, the interneurons of the intermediate gray, and the microneurons of the ventral horn. A detailed account is also given of the maturation of spinal cord neurons, the growth of the ascending pathways to supraspinal structures, and the growth of descending pathways to the spinal cord. These two chapters represent a revision and substantial extension of data we presented earlier in a monograph, entitled *The Development of the Rat Spinal Cord*, published as volume 85 in the *Advances in Anatomy, Embryology and Cell Biology* by the Springer-Verlag (Berlin, 1984). Much of this experimental evidence is the basis of our interpretation of the early events in the development of the human spinal cord.

The second part of the book (Chapters 5-9) deals specifically with the development of the human spinal cord. Chapter 5 describes spinal cord development during the embryonic period (about gestational weeks 3-13 during the first trimester). Three epochs (with 10 stages) are distinguished during this period: the production of neuroepithelial stem cells (NEP cells); the successive exodus of different classes of spinal cord neurons from the neuroepithelium; and the stage of the neuroepithelial production of satellite cells (neuroglia and ependymal cells). Chapter 6 describes some of the major events in spinal cord development during the fetal period, encompassing the second trimester (about gestational weeks 14-26) and the third trimester (about gestational week 27-39). In this chapter, the emphasis is on the overall maturation of the gray matter, including the growth of motoneurons and the segregation of motor columns, the growth of some of the larger ascending and descending fiber tracts of the white matter, and the onset of myelination in some of these fiber tracts. Chapter 7 deals specifically with the growth of the great corticofugal tract, and the descent of the corticospinal tract through the length of the spinal cord during the second and third trimesters. This subject is continued in Chapter 8, which deals with the successive steps in the progressive myelination (proliferative gliosis, reactive gliosis, and myelination proper) of the corticospinal tract during the first year of postnatal life. Finally, Chapter 9 is devoted to an attempt to correlate the development of motor behavior with the different stages of spinal cord development through the embryonic and fetal periods, and the first year of postnatal life. The early absence of motility is correlated with the neuroepithelial stage of spinal cord development. The transition from the gross (holokinetic) spontaneous motility to the more discrete (ideokinetic) movements of the fetus are tentatively correlated with the successive development of intraspinal and supraspinal connections. Finally, the transition from the involuntary reflexes and automatisms of the fetal and early infantile period to the voluntary activites that develop, in a rostral-to-caudal and a proximal-to-distal order, during late infancy and early childhood, is correlated with the myelination of the corticospinal tract during that period in the same orthograde direction.

Most specimens of the developing human spinal cord reproduced and analyzed in this book have come from three sources – the Carnegie Collection, the Yakovlev Collection, and the Minot Collection – all of them currently housed at the National Museum of Health and Medicine, Armed Forces Institute of Pathology, Washington D. C. The *Carnegie Collection* originated in the Department of Embryology of the Carnegie Institution of Washington, under the leadership of Franklin P. Mall (1862-1917), George L. Streeter (1873-1948), and George W. Corner (1889-1981). Initial descriptions and analyses of this material in relation to spinal cord development (most of them in the context of other facets of embryonic development) were published in the early 1900s in the *Contributions to Embryology, The Carnegie Institution of Washington*. The *Yakovlev Collection* is a product of the labor of love of a single individual, Paul I. Yakovlev (1894-1983). Over a period of more than 40 years, Dr. Yakovlev assembled and organized the preparation of over 1500 normal and pathological human specimens, ranging in age from the fetal period through old age. Unfortunately, Dr. Yakovlev and his associates published only a few papers of human brain development based on this collection and no report, to our knowledge, has ever appeared in print on spinal cord development. Finally, the *Minot Collection* consists of about 100 beautifully prepared, serially sectioned human embryos. According to the biographical reference books we have consulted, Dr. Charles S. Minot (1852-1914), was an embryologist at Harvard University and is credited with the invention of the automatic rotary microtome. The author of several books and articles on various biological subjects (including *Human Embryology*, published in 1892), Dr. Minot collected by the end of the nineteenth century over 1900 embryos of a variety of animal species and summarized many of his observations in his *Laboratory Text-Book of Embryology* in 1903. Some time during this period Minot must have turned his attention to the collection of human embryos. The accession numbers assigned to these specimens suggest that most of them were collected in the first decade of the twentieth century. A note found in one of the slide trays and signed by Dr. Minot is dated December 10, 1913. Dr. Minot died the next year. We have found no reference to this collection in the biographical entries of the period or in the embryological literature. Judging by the accumulated grime that had to be removed from the slides, they were probably not looked at with a microscope for decades.

During 1996 and 1997, we surveyed all three of these collections and took photomicrographs of the best preserved normal specimens using 35 mm Kodak Technical Pan film. Low magnification photos where taken either with a Wild macroscope or with a close-up lens mounted on a Nikkormat 35 mm camera. Medium magnification pictures were taken with an Olympus photomicroscope. The thick sections of most of the fetal material were not suitable for high magnification photomicrographs. The rest of the work that went into producing this book was carried out in our private laboratory. All negatives were digitized at 2,700 dots/inch resolution using a Nikon LS-1000 scanner and Adobe Photoshop (version 5.5) software. Extensis intellihance (version 4.0) was used to adjust tonal imbalances in the negatives due to uneven staining and/or fading in the old preparations. These files were stored on CDs and became the database on human spinal cord development that we then correlated with our own, similarly processed database on rat spinal cord development. For the preparation of the text and the art work, and the completion of this camera-ready copy we have used Microsoft Word (version 6.0), Adobe Illustrator (version 8), and Adobe InDesign (version 1.5).

We thank Dr. Adrianne Noe, the Director of the National Museum of Medicine, and Col. Michael Dickerson, the Director of the Armed Forces Institute of Pathology, for permission to use the facilities. The late Mohamad Haleem, Curator of the Yakovlev Collection, was especially helpful in familiarizing us with that collection. We also thank Mr. Archibald J. Fobbs, the current Curator of the Yakovlev Collection, and Ms. Elizabeth C. Lockett and Mr. Bill Discher for their help with the Carnegie and Minot Collections. We are most grateful to Dr. James M. Petras at the Walter Reed Institute of Research who made his dark room facilities available to us. That enabled us to develop all the photomicrographs on location and thereby greatly facilitated our work. We take this opportunity to express our gratitude to the technicians who helped us over many years to assemble our extensive rat nervous system collection. Sharon Evander, Peggy Cleary, Paul Lyons, and Carol Landon provided excellent histological and autoradiographic work, while Donna Whitehurst and Julie Henderson did exceptional photographic work.

Indianapolis, Indiana
December 11, 2000

Joseph Altman
Shirley A. Bayer

CONTENTS

Development

of the

Human Spinal Cord

1 AN OVERVIEW OF SPINAL CORD ORGANIZATION

1.1 The Spinal Cord as a Whole

1.1.1 Macroscopic Features. The spinal cord is the elongated, bilaterally symmetrical, cylindrical portion of the central nervous system that extends from the medulla caudally within the vertebral canal (Figure 1-1A). Like the brain, the spinal cord is richly supplied with blood vessels, is covered by a protective meningeal coating, and is bathed in cerebrospinal fluid, exteriorly in the subarachnoid space and interiorly in the central canal. The human spinal cord is connected by way of 31 pairs of spinal nerves (Figure 1-1B) with most of the body, including the posterior skull, the neck, the trunk, and the upper and lower extremities (Figure 1-2). The face and its specialized organs are innervated by cranial nerves. The spinal cord is shorter than the vertebral column; it tapers off at the level of the lower thoracic or upper lumbar vertebrae and ends by forming the conus medullaris and the meningeal filum terminale (Figures 1-1A). Beyond this level, the only neural elements inside the vertebral canal are the vertically oriented lumbar, sacral and coccygeal nerves, collectively known as the cauda equina (Figures 1-1A). Because of the disparity between the length of the spinal cord and the length of the vertebral column, there is a mismatch between the position of segmental levels in the vertebral foramina and the exit of spinal nerves from the bony vertebrae (Figure 1-2).

The 31 pairs of spinal nerves are traditionally divided into 8 cervical (C1-C8), 12 thoracic (T1-T12), 5 lumbar (L1-L5) and 5 sacral (S1-S5) nerves, and 1 coccygeal nerve (Figure 1-2). The discrete spinal nerves divide the longitudinally continuos spinal cord into separate spinal segments (Figure 1-2, left). The segmental spinal nerves divide the body into sensory and motor segments, sometimes referred to as dermatomes and myotomes, respectively. The segmental course of sensory and motor nerves is relatively straightforward at thoracic levels (T2-T12), but is more difficult to follow at cervical and lumbosacral

levels where several spinal nerves intermingle (or anastomose) to form complex plexuses (Keegan and Garrett, 1948; Figure 1-2, right). Spinal nerves C1-C4 fuse (anastomose) to form the cervical plexus. The cervical plexus contains the sensory and motor fibers that innervate the posterior head and the neck. Spinal nerves C5-T1 form the brachial plexus, which innervates the neck, the shoulder, and the upper extremities. Spinal nerves T2-T12 innervate the trunk and the abdominal region. Spinal nerves L1-L5 form the lumbar plexus and innervate the pelvis, the thigh, and parts of the lower extremities. Spinal nerves S1-S5 form the sacral plexus and innervate other segments of the limbs and some organs of the urogenital system. Spinal nerves S3-S5 (forming the pudendal plexus; not shown), innervate the reproductive organs (Clark, 1984). There may be individual variability in the organization of plexuses.

Quantitative data about the length, weight, and volume of the spinal cord indicate some variability that may reflect individual differences, population differences, and measurement errors. The length of the vertebral column averages about 70 cm, while the length of the spinal cord, according to Elliott (1945), ranges between 40 and 45 cm or, according to Perese and Fracasso (1959), between 36.2 and 45.7 cm. According to Cayaffa (1981), the average length of the spinal cord is 42 cm in women and 45 cm in men. Of the total length, the cervical segments occupy about 13 cm, the thoracic segments 26 cm, and the lumbosacral segments 5 cm (Cayaffa, 1981). The length of the spinal cord in proportion to the length of the body is 26.4% in men and 26.2% in women (McCotter, 1916). The length of the conus medullaris is about 24 cm (quoted by Blinkov and Glezer, 1969). The weight of the spinal cord ranges from 34 to 38 g (Blinkov and Glezer (1968). The volume of the spinal cord is 28.14 cm^3 (Lassek and Rasmussen, 1938). Of this total, the cervical segments account for 9.29 cm^3, the thoracic segments for

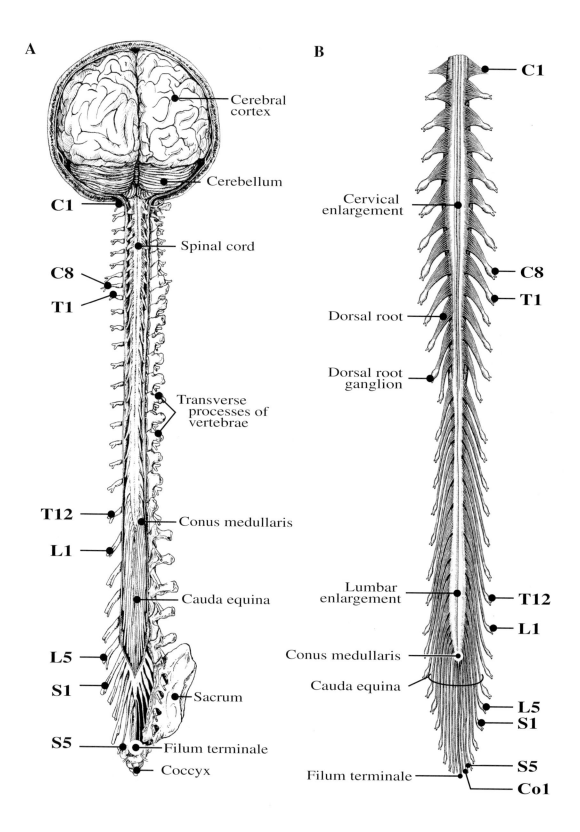

Figure 1-1. A. Dorsal (posterior) view of the human central nervous system. The vertebrae were removed on the top and on the left to expose the spinal cord and the dorsal root ganglia. After Clark (1984). **B.** Dorsal view of the human spinal cord. Note the lengthening of the dorsal roots from rostral to caudal, and the gradual downward shift of the dorsal root ganglia. After Crosby et al. (1962).

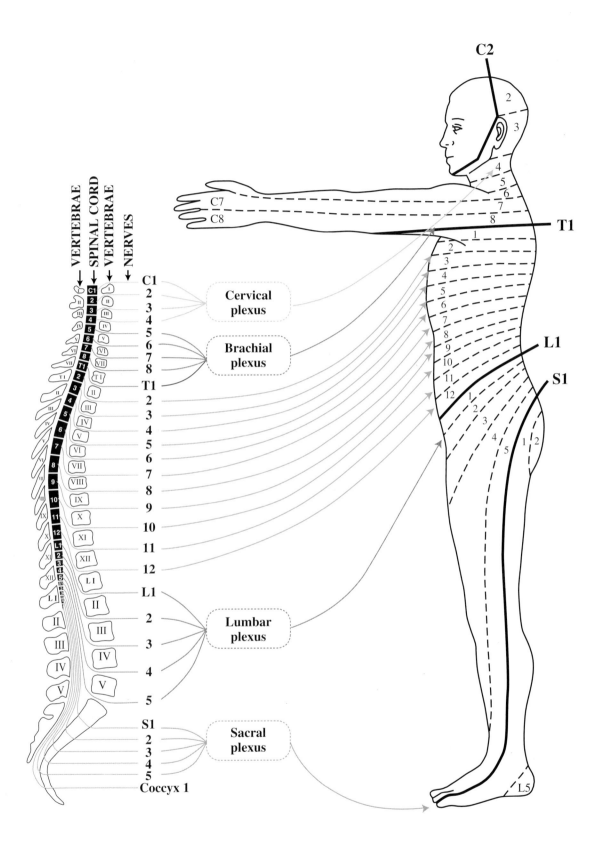

Figure 1-2. Diagram showing the relationship between the bony vertebrae, spinal cord segments and spinal nerves (**left**), and the segmental sensory innervation (dermatomes) of the skin (**right**). The complex arrangement of spinal nerves within the cervical, brachial, lumbar, and sacral plexuses is not shown. Based on illustrations by Haymaker and Woodhall (1953), and Gardner (1968).

14.32 cm³, the lumbar segments for 3.33 cm³, and the sacral segments for 1.20 cm³.

1.1.2 Microscopic Features. The spinal nerves, near their attachement to the cord, are composed of sensory (or afferent) nerves that form the dorsal root, and motor (or efferent) nerves that form the ventral root (Figure 1-3A). The pseudounipolar cell bodies of the sensory nerves, the spinal ganglion cells, reside within the dorsal root ganglia (Figure 1-3B). The spinal ganglia are situated outside the lumen of the vertebral column in the intervertebral foramina. The axon of each ganglion cell has a distal (or peripheral) branch and a proximal (or central) branch. The distal branch, which may be very long, reaches sensors embedded in skin (exteroceptors, or somesthetic receptors), in muscle and joints (propriceptors, or kinesthetic receptors), and the viscera (interoceptors, or visceroceptors). The proximal branch of the axon enters the spinal cord through the dorsal root (Figure 1-3A). The dorsal root breaks up into several rootlets before it penetrates the spinal cord from its dorsal aspect (Figure 1-3A). In the human spinal cord the number of dorsal rootlets varies from 3 to 15, with an average of 6, and the

diameter of the rootlets varies from 0.25 to 1.5 mm (Sindou et al., 1974). The ganglion cell and its axon is the primary afferent neuron of the spinal cord and the sole source of sensory input from the body (the special senses of the head excepted) to the central nervous system.

All spinal nerves have dorsal root ganglia, with the exception of C1 (which may share its ganglion with the spinal accessory nerve) and perhaps the coccygeal nerve (Figure 1-1B). Because the dorsal root ganglia are situated outside the vertebrae, the proximal branch of the ganglion cell axon (which forms peripherally the dorsal root) is quite short in the cervical spinal cord but lengthens through the thoracic, lumbar and sacral levels (Figure 1-1B). Agduhr (1934) counted the total number of dorsal root fibers (both myelinated and unmyelinated) in a 30-year-old man and found over 925,000 on the left side, and 1,142,000 on the right side. According to Davenport and Bothe (1934), there are about 49,000 ganglion cells at C2 level, 60,000 at C6, 24,000 at T4, 59,000 at L3, and 3,400 at S5. Davenport and Bothe found a close match between the number of ganglion cells and the number of dorsal root fibers within the same seg-

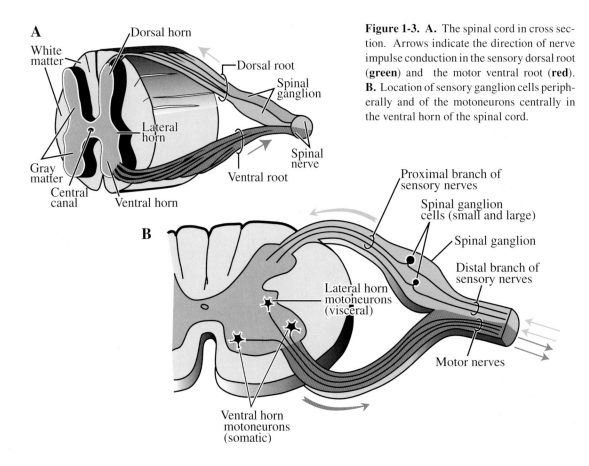

Figure 1-3. A. The spinal cord in cross section. Arrows indicate the direction of nerve impulse conduction in the sensory dorsal root (**green**) and the motor ventral root (**red**). **B.** Location of sensory ganglion cells peripherally and of the motoneurons centrally in the ventral horn of the spinal cord.

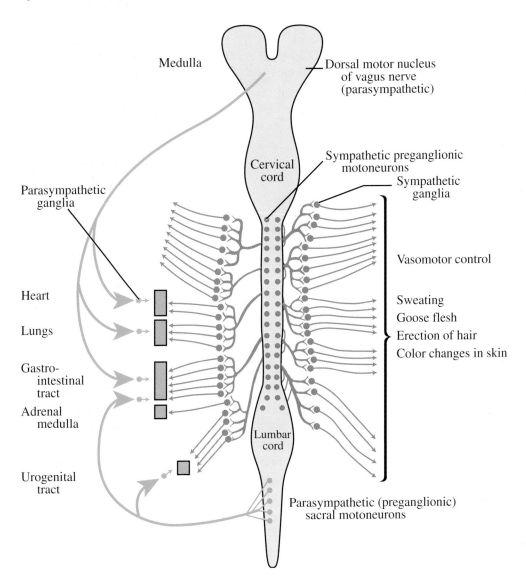

Medulla

Dorsal motor nucleus
of vagus nerve
(parasympathetic)

Cervical
cord

Sympathetic preganglionic
motoneurons

Sympathetic
ganglia

Parasympathetic
ganglia

Vasomotor control

Heart

Sweating
Goose flesh
Erection of hair
Color changes in skin

Lungs

Gastro-
intestinal
tract

Adrenal
medulla

Lumbar
cord

Urogenital
tract

Parasympathetic (preganglionic)
sacral motoneurons

Figure 1-4. Illustration of the location of preganglionic motoneurons that innervate the sympathetic ganglia in the thoracic cord (red), and the location of the preganglionic motoneurons that innervate the parasympathetic ganglia in the medulla and the sacral cord (blue). The targets of the postganglionic efferents are shown schematically. The axons of preganglionic motoneurons that synapse with the sympathetic ganglia are short, whereas the axons of preganglionic motoneurons that synapse with the parasympathetic ganglia are long. After Pick (1970).

ment. The ratio of myelinated to unmyelinated fibers in the dorsal root was 0.52 at the C2 level and 1.22 at the S3 level.

The motor fibers of the ventral roots are the axons of somatic and visceral motoneurons situated in the gray matter of the spinal cord (Figure 1-3B). The somatic motoneurons are situated in the ventral horn and their terminals (the end plates) synapse peripherally with skeletal muscle. The visceral (autonomic, preganglionic) motoneurons are situated in the lateral horn (and some other locations), but their axons exit jointly with the axons of somatic motoneurons in the ventral roots. The axons of preganglionic motoneurons of the thoracic and upper lumbar spinal cord synapse with postganglionic neurons in the sympathetic chain of ganglia, whereas the axons of the preganglionic motoneurons of the sacral spinal cord synapse with postganglionic neurons in the parasympathetic ganglia (Figure 1-4). The number of ven-

tral root motor fibers is much lower than the number of dorsal root sensory fibers; in some segments the ratio is as low as 1:10 (Agduhr, 1934). Table 1-1 (next page) summarizes the breakdown of the number of dorsal root and ventral root fibers at three levels of the human spinal cord.

The spinal nerves have two somatic branches peripherally, known as the dorsal ramus and the ventral ramus. The dorsal ramus innervates the skin and muscles of the neck and the back, whereas the ventral ramus innervates the skin and muscles of the chest, trunk, and limbs. Both the dorsal ramus and the ventral ramus divide into superficial (skin) and deep (muscle) nerves, and these split further as they approach their peripheral targets. The third branch, the ramus communicans, contains visceral fibers and consists, at thoracic levels, of a white and a gray portion. The white ramus communicans contains the myelinated preganglionic fibers that terminate in the sympathetic chain of ganglia; the gray ramus communicans is composed of unmyelinated postganglionic sympathetic axons.

The tissue of the spinal cord is composed of a central core of gray matter and a surrounding shell of white matter (Figure 1-5). The gray matter has a distinctive H-shape in cross sections. This shape is due to two pairs of wings, the dorsal (posterior) horn and the ventral (anterior) horn, that are linked to one another by the intermediate gray and by the central gray across the midline. In general, the gray matter is composed of the cell bodies (somata or perikarya) of neurons, their input and output extensions (dendrites and axons), and a network of incoming and outgoing axons (afferents and efferents), their collaterals, and terminals. A major component of the dorsal horn are small neurons that are the targets of the sensory fibers of the dorsal root. These small cells are the local receiving neurons of the spinal cord. The ventral horn contains many very large and some smaller multipolar neurons, the motoneurons. The axons of the larger motoneurons, often referred to as alpha motoneurons, innervate the skeletal muscles. The smaller multipolar cells, the gamma motoneurons, innervate the intrafusal muscle fibers of the muscle spindles, the specialized proprioceptors that are embedded in the skeletal muscles. There are also many small and medium-sized interneurons in both the dorsal horn and the ventral horn. These interneurons are responsible for intra- and intersegmental connections within the spinal cord, for relaying sensory information to supraspinal levels of the nervous system and, last but not least, they are constituents of the local operating circuitry of the spinal cord. The third component of the gray matter, the intermediate gray, is interposed between the dorsal horn and the ventral horn. It is composed of a heterogeneous population of dispersed interneurons, and also some distinctive cell aggregates, including the large neurons of Clarke's column and the central cervical nucleus dorsally, and the preganglionic, visceral motoneurons laterally.

The massive white matter, which wraps around the gray matter, is composed of myelinated and unmyelinated fibers. The larger subdivisions of the white matter are known as funiculi or columns. These include the dorsal funiculus (posterior white column), the ventral funiculus (anterior white column), and a pair of lateral funiculi (lateral white

Table 1-1

Number of Dorsal Root and Ventral Root Fibers in the Spinal Cord of a Man, on the Left and Right Side, at Three Spinal Cord Levels.

After Agduhr (1934)

Spinal Cord Levels	Dorsal Root		Ventral Root	
	Left	Right	Left	Right
Cervical enlargement (C4 - T1)	283,398	301,262	40,667	57,922
Thoracic segments (T2 - T12)	205,691	221,902	73,426	95,959
Lumbar enlargement (L1 - S3)	389,631	463,514	52,734	60,988

columns). The funiculi are composed of small and large fasciculi and tracts. These tracts include (i) intrasegmental and intersegmental intraspinal (propriospinal) fibers; (ii) ascending fibers that terminate in the medulla, pons, midbrain and diencephalon; and (iii) descending fibers from all levels of the suprasegmental nervous system, including the cerebral cortex. The high proportion of myelinated fibers gives the white matter its distinctive pale appearance in fresh tissue, and its opacity in tissue processed with sudanophilic myelin stains (Figure 1-5).

The gray matter is most extensive in two regions, the cervical and lumbar enlargements that innervate the forelimbs and hind limbs, respectively. The bulk of the white matter, with some regional variations, increases from sacral to cervical levels because of the accretion of ascending supraspinal fibers (particularly in the dorsal funiculus) from caudal to rostral, and the dwindling of descending supraspinal fibers from rostral to caudal. Regional differences in the cross-sectional configuration of the human spinal cord are illustrated in Figure 1-6 at all segmental levels from C2 to S3 (Kameyama et al., 1996). Quantitative areal differences in the gray and white matter at these levels are summarized in Figure 1-7. Kameyama et al (1996) found that in spite of individual variability in the absolute size of the spinal cord, the relative differences in cross sectional areas were quite similar in all the specimens examined.

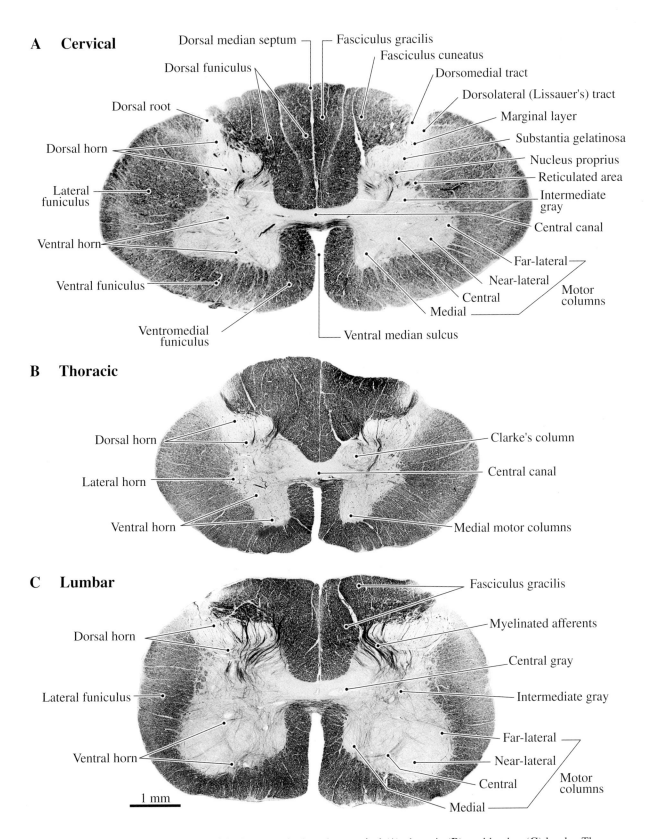

Figure 1-5. Coronal sections of the human spinal cord at cervical (**A**), thoracic (**B**), and lumbar (**C**) levels. The gray matter is pale, and the white matter is opaque in these myelin-stained sections. Note the different configuration of the gray and white matter at different levels of the spinal cord. Specimen # Y132-61; 11 month-old child. Loyez stain.

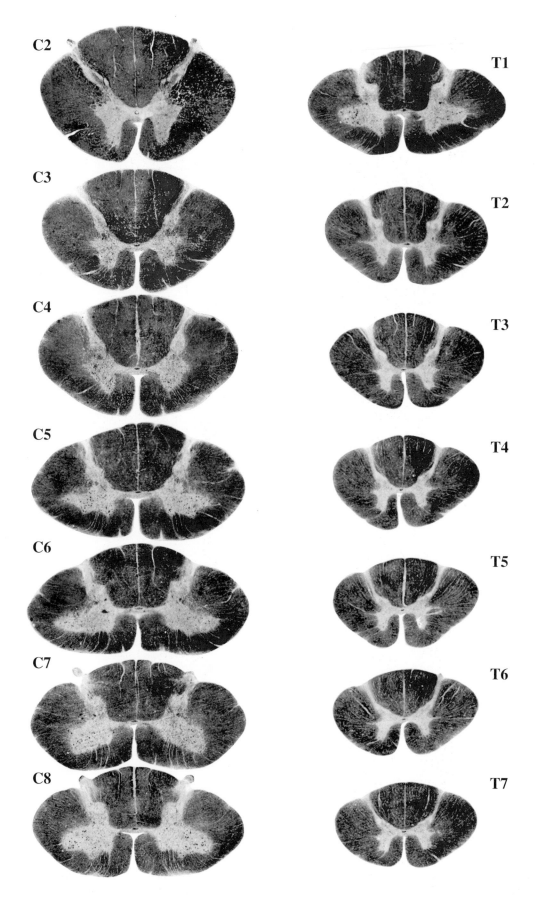

Figure 1-6 *(continued on the next page).*

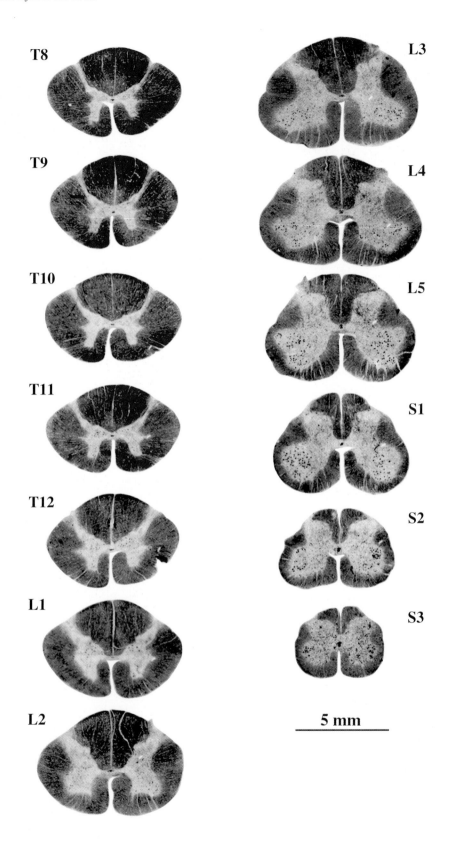

Figure 1-6 (**continued**). Distinctive configuration of the adult human spinal cord in coronal sections, at successive segmental levels from C2 to S3. Klüver-Barrera stain. After Kameyama et al. (1996); electronically reprocessed.

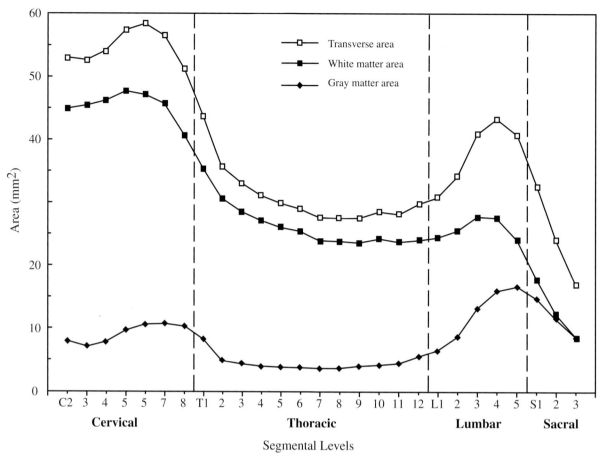

Figure 1-7. The averaged (n=12) total transverse area, white matter area, and gray matter area in coronal sections of the human spinal cord at successive segmental levels from C2 to S3. After Kameyama et al. (1996).

1.2 The Spinal Ganglia and the Dorsal Root

1.2.1   Spinal Ganglion Cells. The spinal ganglion cells are unique among neurons in having a configuration that is referred to as pseudounipolar (Figures 1-3B, 1-8A). The single, often convoluted axon that issues from the cell body bifurcates and one branch proceeds peripherally towards the body, the other centrally towards the spinal cord. Light microscopic (Hatai, 1901; Andres, 1961) and electron microscopic (Yamadori, 1971; Lawson et al., 1974; Duce and Keen, 1977) observations established that there are two types of spinal ganglion cells: one lightly staining and larger, the other darkly staining and smaller (Figure 1-8B). The large, pale ganglion cell contains clumps of endoplasmic reticulum (Nissl substance), many microtubules, and neurofilaments. The endoplasmic reticulum is more evenly distributed in the small, dark ganglion cell, and it contains few or no neurofilaments but many Golgi bodies. A monoclonal antibody against neurofilament protein was found to label in mouse spinal ganglia

the larger light cells but not the smaller dark cells (Lawson, 1979). Larger ganglion cells are reported to display carbonic anhydrase activity (Wong et al., 1983). Finally, immunohistochemical studies have shown that the small ganglion cells, but not the large ones, stain for substance P (Hökfelt et al., 1975; Persson et al., 1995) and for nitric oxide (Zhang et al., 1993). The large ganglion cells have myelinated axons (Figure 1-8 A/b), while the axons of many of the small ganglion cells are unmyelinated (Figure 1-8A/a). Correspondingly, the dorsal roots and the spinal nerves (Figure 1-9) contain large caliber myelinated fibers and small caliber unmyelinated axons.

Classical psychological studies suggested that there are discrete "sensory spots" in the skin (Blix, 1884; von Frey, 1897; Dallenbach, 1927) for the different somesthetic modalities (pain, light touch, pressure, warmth, and cold). However, the association of these different sensory spots with discrete cutaneous receptors (Pacinian corpuscles, Krause end bulbs, Merkel corpuscles, Ruffini endings, etc.) remains controversial (Nafe, 1929; Geldard, 1972; Sinclair, 1981).

A

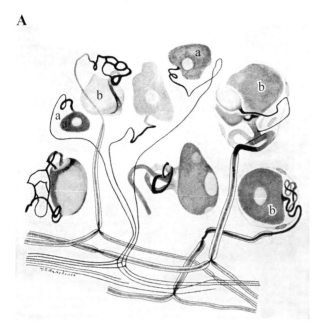

B

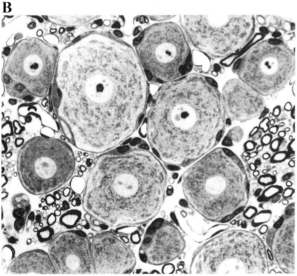

Figure 1-8. A. Drawings of small ganglion cells with unmyelinated axons (**a**) and large ganglion cells with myelinated axons (**b**). Dog; pyridine silver stain. From Ranson and Clark (1959). **B.** Photomicrograph of large light, and small dark ganglion cells. Rabbit; toluidine stain. From Lieberman (1976).

The same applies to the exact relationship between different sensory modalities and different types of ganglion cells. A preliminary electrophysiological study in the rat indicated that the large and small ganglion cells have axons with different conduction velocities (Lawson and Harper, 1985). There is also accumulating evidence, as we shall see later, that the smaller ganglion cells have short axons that terminate in the dorsal horn and mediate responses to nociceptive (pain-evoking) stimuli; in contrast, many of the larger ganglion cells have long axons that ascend

uninterruptedly in the dorsal funiculus to terminate in the dorsal column nuclei of the medulla. These axons convey primarily (though not exclusively) exteroceptive (tactile) messages from cutaneous sensors that respond to innocuous mechanical stimuli.

1.2.2   The Primary Sensory Fibers. Electrophysiological studies have established that spinal nerves contain sensory fibers with different properties. Erlanger and Gasser (1937) showed that the "compound action potential" recorded in peripheral nerves to stimuli applied to the skin (Figure 1-10) is a composite of a series of waves with different conduction velocities, stimulus thresholds, and response latencies (Figure 1-11). Erlanger and Gasser called the low threshold, fast, and short latency electrical potential the α wave, or A wave, and associated it with large caliber axons. The slowly propagating, high threshold, and long latency C wave, was related to smaller caliber axons. Subsequent research distinguished a larger spectrum of sensory fibers on the basis of their physiological properties, including the additional feature of slow or fast adaptation to sustained stimulation (Adrian and Zotterman, 1926; Hunt and McIntyre, 1960;). In addition to the fast adapting cutaneous afferents, there are also slow adapting afferents from muscle sensors (B. H. C. Matthews, 1933; P. B. C. Matthews, 1972), and visceral sensors. This physiological research has led to an unwieldy subdivision of A fibers with several Greek

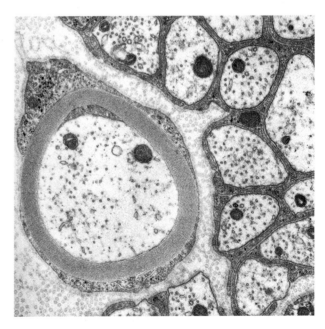

Figure 1-9. Transverse section of the sciatic nerve with a myelinated axon (**left**) and several unmyelinated axons. Electron micrograph. From Webster (1974).

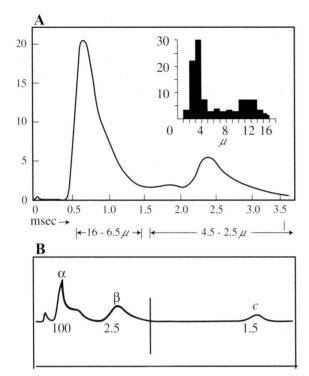

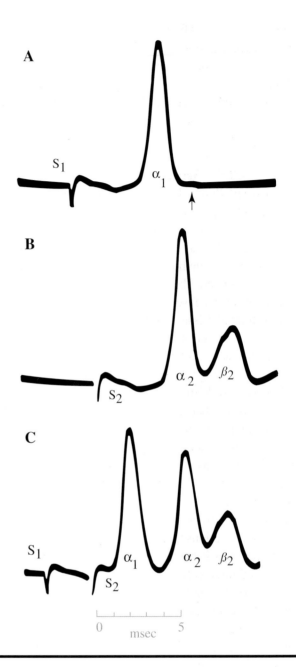

Figure 1-10. **A.** Compound action potential of a frog nerve composed of fibers of different diameters and conduction velocities. Insert shows the distribution of fibers of different diameter (μ) in the nerve. From Gasser (1943). **B.** Compound action potential of a human cutaneous nerve. The three peaks (α, β, c) indicate that the nerve is composed of three major groups (conduction velocities indicated below the tracing in meters/second). After Heinbecker et al. (1933); from Ottoson (1983).

Figure 1-11. Latencies and amplitudes of components of a compound action potential of the frog sciatic nerve to a weak electric shock (S_1 in **A**), a stronger shock (S_2 in **B**), and to two successive shocks (S_1 and S_2 in **C**). From Erlanger and Gasser (1937); after Brinley (1974).

Table 1-2
Two Classifications of Sensory Axons (Modified after Ottoson, 1983)

Fiber type	Fiber type	Function	Innervation or Sensory Modality	Diameter mµ	Speed (m/sec)
Aα	Ia	proprioceptive	muscle spindle (primaries)	15-20	70-120
Aα	Ib	proprioceptive	tendon organs	15-20	70-120
Aβ	II	exteroceptive	touch, pressure	5-10	30-70
Aβ	II	proprioceptive	muscle spindle (secondaries)	5-10	30-70
A∂	III	exteroceptive	heat, cold, pain	2-5	12-30
C	IV	nociceptive	pain	0.5-1	0.5-2

subscripts (Aα, Aß, Aγ, A∂) and, in addition, to an alternative classification of group I, II, III and IV fibers, with added subscripts (reviewed by Ottoson, 1983, and Perl, 1992). A simplified classification of sensory fibers is given in Table 1-2. (A corresponding classification of motor fibers is presented in Table 1-3 on page 40.)

1.2.3 Segregation of Sensory Fibers in the Dorsal Root.
Lissauer (1885) noted some time ago the segregation of small caliber and large caliber fibers in the dorsal root near their site of entry into the spinal cord; he called the former the lateral bundle, the latter the medial bundle. The lateral bundle of unmyelinated fibers has since become known as the dorsolateral fasciculus, or Lissauer's tract. The unmyelinated Lissauer's tract is easy to distinguish in myelin-stained sections from the adjacent dorsal funiculus, as the latter is composed mostly of myelinated fibers (Figure 1-12B). Subsequent research (Ranson and Billingsly, 1916; Spivy and Metcalf, 1959) showed that severance of the unmyelinated lateral bundle, but not of the myelinated medial bundle, blocked vasomotor and respiratory reactions when the spinal nerve was stimulated. This finding, in combination with clinical reports, supported the idea (to be discussed in greater detail below) that the fibers of Lissauer's tract mediate nociceptive and related affective sensations (Earle, 1952; Szentágothai, 1964). More recently it has been claimed that, in man, the small and large caliber fibers are intermingled in the distal part of spinal nerves but become gradually segregated near the vicinity of the spinal cord entry zone (Sindou et al. 1974). It has also been argued that there may be species differences in this regard, with the segregation of fine and coarse afferents holding for the macaque monkey but not for the squirrel monkey and the cat (Snyder, 1977).

A representative illustration from a 2-month old human child (Figure 1-12B) indicates that the distribution of unmyelinated and myelinated fiber bundles is more complicated than it is usually described. Instead of a single unmyelinated bundle, there are two of them at the dorsal root entry zone. One fascicle of unmyelinated fibers is situated *medially*, adjacent to the myelinated dorsal funiculus. This we identify as the unmyelinated component of the dorsal root entry zone. Another fascicle of unmyelinated fibers is situ-

ated *lateral* to the myelinated fibers of the dorsal root entry zone and above the lateral aspect of the dorsal horn. This is the dorsolateral fasciculus, or Lissauer's tract. In addition to the nociceptive fibers (or collaterals) of the dorsal root, Lissauer's tract also contains small caliber higher-order afferents that originate in interneurons (Cervero et al., 1979; Chung et al. 1979c).

1.3 Laminar Organization of the Dorsal Horn

1.3.1 Structure of the Dorsal Horn.
The early anatomists distinguished four regions in coronal sections of the dorsal horn: (1) a thin cap, or apex; (2) a large head, or caput, (3) a narrower neck, the cervix; and (4) the base of the dorsal horn (Figure 1-12). The cap of the dorsal horn has also been called the marginal zone, the zona spongiosa, nucleus posteromarginalis, or, because it contains some large neurons, the nucleus magnocellularis pericornualis (Clarke, 1859; Waldeyer, 1888; Jacobsohn, 1908; Massazza, 1922; Bok, 1928). The head of the dorsal horn has at least two parts: an upper, small-celled and translucent region, named the substantia gelatinosa by Rolando in 1824 (Gobel et al., 1980), and a more compact lower portion, the nucleus proprius dorsalis, or nucleus magnocellularis centralis. Recognizing the fact that these bands constitute dorsoventrally stacked continuous sheets along the entire spinal cord, and taking into account their different cellular composition, Rexed (1952, 1964) introduced the now widely accepted laminar subdivision of the dorsal horn (Figure 1-12). Below we present some of the details of the cellular organization of the dorsal horn within the framework of Rexed's nomenclature.

1.3.2 The Marginal Zone or Lamina I.
The marginal zone, or lamina I, is a thin sheet of gray matter that caps the surface of the dorsal horn. It contains the cell bodies of the large marginal cells, first identified by Waldeyer (1888), and named after him. The spindle-shaped Waldeyer cells have disc-shaped dendrites that spread some distance horizontally within lamina I (Figure 1-13); some of the dendrites dip into the lower-lying layers of the dorsal horn (Ramón y Cajal, 1909; Scheibel and Scheibel, 1968; Szentágothai, 1964; Beal and Cooper, 1978; Light et al., 1979; Price et al., 1979; Bennett et al.,

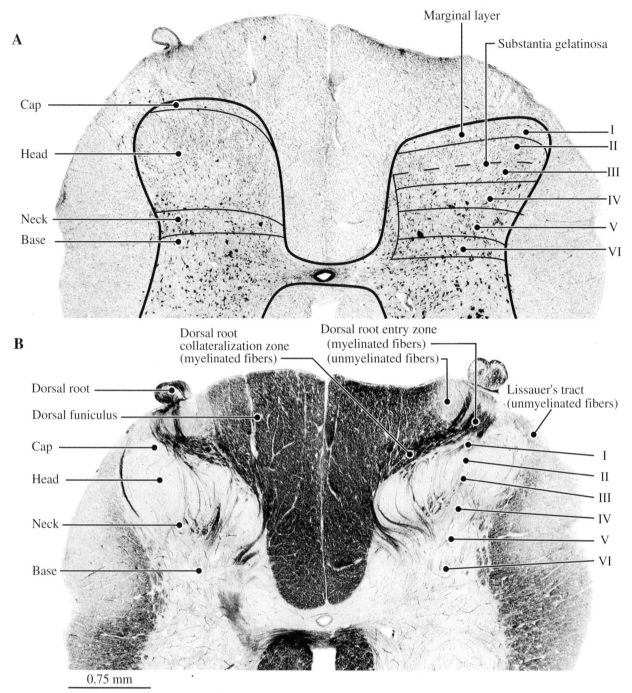

Figure 1-12.   A. Dorsal region of the lumbar spinal cord of a 2-month-old human infant stained for cell bodies with hematoxylin-eosin.   Traditional subdivisions (**left**) and Rexed's laminar scheme (**right**). **B.** Nearby section stained for myelinated fibers with the Loyez technique.   Specimen # Y130-61.

1981). In the monkey, the perikarya of Waldeyer cells are 10-15 μm in diameter, some exceeding 20 μm (Ralston, 1979). In man, the tangential spread of dendrites of Waldeyer cells average 800 μm (Schoenen, 1982). Recent studies (Beal, et al., 1981; Lima and Coimbra, 1986) have distinguished as many as four different cell types in lamina I: fusiform spiny neurons, multipolar neurons, flattened aspiny neurons, and pyramidal neurons. Physiological studies indi-

cate that most marginal cells are selectively excited by painful mechanical and/or thermal stimuli (Christensen and Perl, 1970; Willis et al., 1974; Menétrey et al., 1977; Cervero et al., 1979; Light et al., 1979; Price et al., 1979; Bennett et al., 1981; Miletic, et al., 1984; Hylden et al., 1986). Anatomical studies with the retrograde labeling technique have established that these nociceptive marginal cells have extensive connections. Intraspinal (propriospinal) fibers terminate

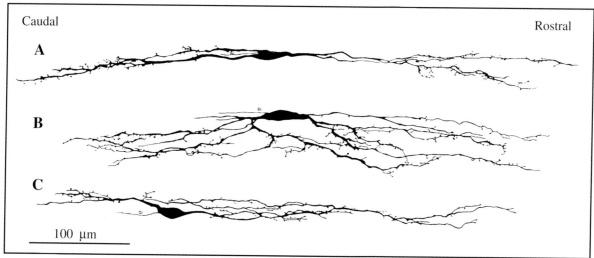

Figure 1-13. Types of fusiform spiny neurons (**A**, **B**, **C**) in the marginal zone (lamina I) of the dorsal horn. Rat; Golgi technique. After Lima and Coimbra (1986).

in nearby or distant spinal cord segments (Burton and Loewy, 1976; Matsushita et al. 1979; Molenaar and Kuypers, 1978; Skinner et al., 1979) while ascending supraspinal fibers project to the cerebellum (Snyder et al., 1978) as well as midbrain regions implicated in pain, particularly the periaqueductal gray and cuneiform nucleus (Menétrey et al, 1982; Wiberg and Blomquist, 1984; Hylden et al., 1986; Craig, 1995). The marginal cells also project to select regions of the somatosensory thalamus (Trevino and Carstens, 1975; Carstens and Trevino, 1978; Willis et al., 1979; see Figure 1-14). The ascending fibers of lamina I course towards their targets principally in the dorsolateral funiculus (Apkarian et al., 1985; Jones et al., 1985).

The foregoing findings suggest that the marginal (Waldeyer) cells of lamina I play an important role in the mediation of painful sensations. Pharmacological and immunohistochemical findings support this inference. The somata of marginal cells are immunoreactive to the opioid peptide, leucine-enkephalin (Glazer and Basbaum, 1981; Hunt, 1983), and analgesic opioids, such as morphine and naloxone, inhibit spinal nociceptive neurons (Calvillo et al., 1974; Duggan et al., 1976). Moreover, there is some evidence that the analgesia produced by electrical stimulation of the midbrain periaqueductal gray region or by injection of opiates into this site (Mayer and Price, 1976) results from inhibition of spinal nociceptive neurons whose afferents ascend in Lissauer's tract (Basbaum and Fields, 1978). In addition to nociceptive fibers, there is evidence of the presence in Lissauer's tract in the sacral cord of

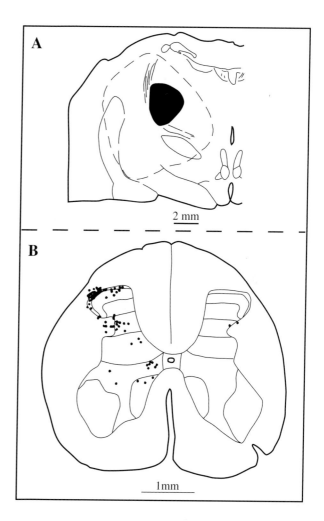

Figure 1-14. Distribution of retrogradely labeled spinothalamic tract interneurons in the spinal cord of a monkey (black dots in **B**) following injection of HRP into the medial thalamus (opaque area in **A**). From Willis et al. (1979).

interoceptive (visceral) fibers from the pelvic and pudendal nerves(Morgan et al., 1981; Roppolo et. al., 1985; McKenna and Nadelhaft, 1986; Kawatani et al., 1986). Conceivably, these afferents mediate not only pain but also the comforting or pleasurable sensations (the sense of relief) associated with micturition, defecation, erectile functions, and orgasmic sensations. If both painful and pleasurable sensations are mediated by small caliber fibers, a reconsideration of Head's (1920) broader concept of "protopathic" (primordial affective) sensations for this system may be warranted.

1.3.3   The Substantia Gelatinosa or Laminae II-III.

Laminae II and III roughly correspond to the substantia gelatinosa of the traditional literature. The majority, and perhaps principal neurons of the substantia gelatinosa are small, short-axoned Golgi type II cells or microneurons that Ramón y Cajal (1909) called central cells. The perikaryon of the central cells consists of a small nucleus surrounded by a thin rim of cytoplasm, with a diameter in the range of 8-10 μm (Ralston, 1979). In Golgi-impregnated coronal sections, the vertically distributed dendrites of central cells form narrow tufts that traverse perpendicularly much of the width of the substantia gelatinosa (Figure 1-15A; two cells on the-left). Depending on the perikaryon's location, the tufts point either dorsally or ventrally, or in both directions. Scheibel and Scheibel (1968), who also examined these cells in sagittal sections, discovered that the "tufts" of these small neurons form planar sheets extending some distance in the rostrocaudal plane (Figure 1-15A; right). En masse, as seen in horizontal sections (Figure 1-15B; left)), the planar dendrites of gelatinosal central cells form thin slabs aligned parallel to the long axis of the spinal cord Afferent axons that end in this region form complementary terminal arbors (Figure 1-15B; right). We shall return to this spatial organization in greater detail in Chapter 2.

In addition to the abundant central cells, Ramón y Cajal (1909) also described two larger cell types in the substantia gelatinosa, the stalked cells and the islet cells. Gobel et al. (1980) and Bennett et al. (1980) have recently analyzed these two cell types in the cat spinal cord. Stalked cell perikarya are abundant in the superficial part of lamina II. The stalk-like branches and cone-shaped dendritic arbor of these neurons are compressed mediolaterally and,

fan out about 500 μm in the rostrocaudal direction through the width of lamina II (Figure 1-16A). The axons of stalked cells are directed dorsally and form an umbrella-like dense canopy in lamina I. Thus, the principal target of stalked cells is lamina I, presumably the Waldeyer cells. The islet cell perikarya are concentrated mostly in the middle of lamina II. The large dendritic arbor of islet cells extends some distance rostrocaudally but is more restricted mediolaterally and dorsoventrally. Their axons, like the dendrites, terminate within lamina II (Figure 1-16B). Hence, the islet cells are aptly characterized as local interneurons. In a physiological analysis, Bennett et al. (1980) distinguished three classes of islet cells and stalked cells: (1) high threshold neurons that respond only to painful stimuli; (2) neurons that respond to both painful and innocuous mechanical stimuli; and (3) low threshold neurons that respond to gentle touch. It has been suggested that islet cells, whose transmitter may be GABA (McLaughlin et al., 1975),

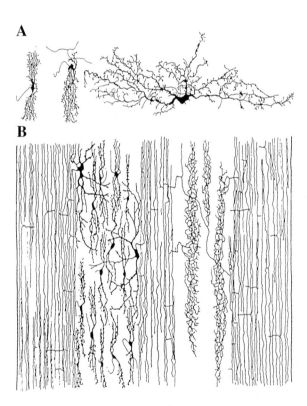

Figure 1-15. A. Gelatinosal central cells in coronal (**left and middle**) and sagittal (**right**) sections of the dorsal horn. **B.** Orientation of central cells and their dendrites (**left half**) and matching dorsal root terminals (**right half**) in a horizontal section of the dorsal horn. Cat; Golgi technique. After Scheibel and Scheibel (1968).

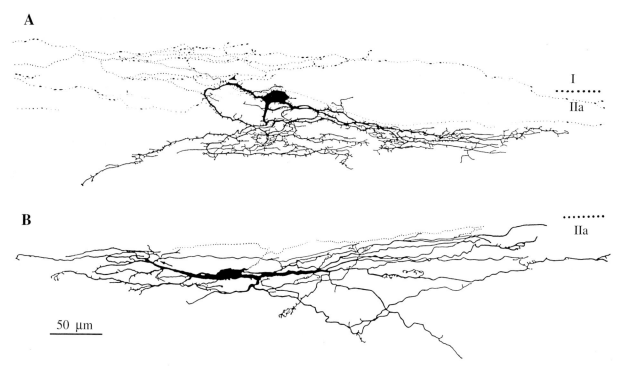

Figure 1-16. A. Identified nociceptive stalked cell, with dendrites in lamina IIa and axon collaterals (fine dots) in lamina I. **B.** Nociceptive islet cell with dendrites and axon in lamina IIa. Intracellular HRP technique. After Bennett et al. (1980).

according to physiological evidence, are inhibitory interneurons whereas the stalked cells are excitatory interneurons (Gobel et al., 1980).

In lamina II of the human spinal cord, Schoenen (1982) distinguished four cell types oriented in the sagittal plane. (1) Islet cells (about 30% of the total) have a flattened cylindrical dendritic arbor that extends about 600 μm rostrocaudally. The axons of islet cells are confined to the territory of the dendritic arbor. (2) Filamentous cells (so called because of their multiple, filiform dendrites) have a trapezoid dendritic arbor with a spread of about 280 μm. The axons of filamentous cells penetrate lamina I and Lissauer's tract. Filamentous cells constitute about 20% of the total population. (3) Curly cells (about 10%) have complex, twisted, spine-rich dendritic arbors about 200 μm in diameter. The axons of curly cells, too, enter lamina I and Lissauer's tract. The perikarya of these three cell types are most frequent in outer lamina II. (4) Stellate cells (about 40% of the total) are concentrated in inner lamina II. The spine-poor dendrites cover a large elliptical territory (longest diameter about 500 μm). The axons of stellate cells proceed ventrally and penetrate laminae III and IV. Schoenen concludes that the cytoarchitecton-

ics of the human dorsal horn differs in some details from that found in other mammals.

Typical ultrastructural components of the substantia gelatinosa are the synaptic glomeruli. These are complex structures where gelatinosal neurons make synaptic contact with the terminals of peripheral afferents and local (propriospinal) fibers (Réthelyi and Szentágothai, 1969; Ralston, 1979; Gobel et al., 1980; Knyihar-Csillik et al., 1982). Ribeiro-da-Silva and Coimbra (1982) distinguished two types of synaptic glomeruli in the middle and lower portions of lamina II. (Glomeruli are rare in the upper part of lamina II and virtually absent in lamina I.) In the middle of lamina II, type I glomeruli are predominant (about 79% of the total). The core of type I glomerulus consists of a small, electron-dense axonal terminal that has a corrugated contour and is filled with densely packed spherical vesicles. Abutting this ending are some presynaptic dendritic spines and axon terminals rich in discoid synaptic vesicles. In the ventral portion of lamina II, type II glomeruli are predominant (about 66%). The core of this glomerulus has an electron-lucent terminal with a regular contour, and it contains fewer synaptic vesicles.

Although the cells of lamina III are similar to those of lamina II (Scheibel and Scheibel, 1968), lamina III is distinguished from lamina II by several features. First, lamina III is characterized by a dense meshwork of fine as well as coarse myelinated axons that are absent or rare in lamina II. This suggests that lamina III is the target of large caliber fibers that reach the dorsal horn by way of the dorsal funiculus. Second, whereas synapses with round vesicles (presumably with excitatory action) predominate in lamina II, synapses with flat vesicles (presumably with inhibitory action) are more numerous in lamina III (Ralston (1979). Third, in contrast to lamina II, where type I glomeruli are most common (see above), type II glomeruli are present exclusively in lamina III (Bennett et al., 1980). The presence of glomeruli may account for the gelatinous appearance of laminae II and III in some histological preparations. Indeed, in spite of some differences in the structure of lamina II and lamina III, some investigators have questioned the validity of this subdivision of the substantia gelatinosa. Beal and Cooper (1978) proposed instead a subdivision of the substantia gelatinosa into an outer, middle, and inner region, based on the preferred orientation of dendrites in the outer region ventrally, in the middle region longitudinally, and in the inner region dorsally. In the human spinal cord, Schoenen (1982) described two cell types in the substantia gelatinosa: antenna-like neurons and radiate cells. The antenna-like neurons have a vertical, cone-shaped dendritic domain, whereas radiate cells have a smaller spherical dendritic territory.

1.3.4   The Nucleus Proprius Dorsalis or Laminae IV-V.

The cytoarchitecture of lamina IV is distinguished from the overlying substantia gelatinosa by several features: (1) the presence of a fair concentration of medium-sized neurons and of a larger, pyramidal type neuron (Ramón y Cajal, 1909; Scheibel and Scheibel, 1968; Réthelyi, 1984); (2) synaptic profiles containing neurofilaments; (3) the absence of glomeruli (Ralston, 1968); and, finally, (4) the fact that the dendrites of typical lamina IV neurons radiate in all planes rather than sagittally (Scheibel and Scheibel, 1968), with a preferential spread in the lateral direction (Proshansky and Egger, 1977). The dendrites of lamina IV neurons penetrate the overlying laminae III and II, and their axons have two components, a rich local plexus in lamina V (Rastad et al. 1977; Brown et al., 1977) and a main branch that proceeds towards the lateral funiculus.

The main branch, which gives off numerous collaterals along its course (Maxwell and Koerber, 1986), has been traced to the spinocervical tract (Brodal and Rexed, 1953; Craig, 1978; Rastad et al., 1977), the dorsal funiculus (Brown, 1981), the spinothalamic tract (Willis et al., 1979) and the spinohypothalamic tract (Burstein et al., 1990b). This indicates that the large lamina IV neurons are long-distance relay (or projection) neurons. In the human spinal cord, all lamina IV neurons have an antenna-like dendritic domain that is oriented laterally and may reach a dorsal height of 1 mm (Schoenen, 1982).

The spinocervical neurons of lamina IV (Figure 1-17) are distributed through the length of the spinal cord and their axons terminate in the lateral cervical nucleus (Brodal and Rexed, 1953; Rastad et al., 1977; Craig, 1978) located within and lateral to the dorsal horn in the upper segments of the spinal cord (Craig, 1976; Brown 1981). This nucleus has been identified in several mammalian species, including the rat (Giesler et al., 1979), cat and dog (Brodal and Rexed, 1953; Morin and Catalano, 1955; Kitai et al., 1965; Craig, 1976, 1978), and monkey (Mizuno et al., 1967; Ha, 1971; Boivie, 1980). However, the lateral cervical nucleus is poorly developed in man;

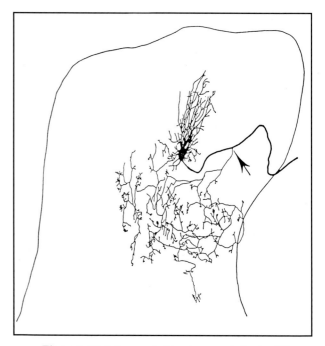

Figure 1-17. Spinocervical tract neuron in lamina IV of the cat dorsal horn. The dendrites arborize in the substantia gelatinosa dorsally, and the axon (arrow) gives off a rich local plexus of collaterals ventrally, then leaves the dorsal horn. Intracellular HRP technique. From Rastad et al. (1977).

its cells are thought to be scattered in the dorsolateral reticulated substance (Kircher and Ha, 1968; Truex et al., 1968). Input to the lateral cervical nucleus is mainly from low threshold (exteroceptive) receptors (Morin et al., 1963; Oswaldo-Cruz and Kidd 1964; Kitai et al., 1965; Landgren et al., 1965; Andersen et al., 1966; Brown, 1981). But there is also converging input from nociceptors (Brown and Franz, 1969; Cervero et al., 1977; Giesler et al., 1979) and proprioceptors (Hamann et al., 1978; Hong et al. 1979; Hammar et al., 1994). The axons of the lateral cervical nucleus cross the midline in the dorsal spinal commissure (Boivie and Perl, 1975), join the medial lemniscus, and then proceed to the ventrobasal complex and the posterior nuclei of the thalamus (Morin, 1955; Landgren et al., 1965; Boivie, 1970; Ha, 1971; Boivie, 1970; 1980). Recent physiological studies indicate that the local axonal plexus of spinocervical neurons (Figure 1-17) may be responsible for the intersegmental influence exerted by spinocervical neurons on spinal reflexes (Djouhri and Jankowska, 1998). In turn, the widely distributed local collaterals of the lateral cervical neurons may be responsible for influences on impulse transmission in the dorsal funiculus (Jankowska et al., 1979; Brown et al., 1986; Enevoldson and Gordon, 1989), the spinomesencephalic tract (Djouhri et al., 1997), and the spinothalamic tract (Djouhry et al., 1995). The distribution of retro-

gradely labeled spinocervical neurons, and their partial overlap in lamina IV with neurons of the spinothalamic and spinohypothalamic tracts, is illustrated in Figure 1-18. Whereas the spinocervical neurons are limited to and are distributed throughout the entire width of lamina IV, the spinothalamic and spinohypothalamic neurons appear to be concentrated laterally in lamina IV.

Laminae V and VI constitute the base of the dorsal horn. The dendrites of lamina V neurons, in contrast to those of lamina IV, are planar, extending mediolaterally and dorsoventrally but not sagittally (Scheibel and Scheibel, 1968). Their dendritic arbor thus forms stacked discs lined up transversely along the length of the cord. The dendrites of lamina VI neurons are less regular (Scheibel and Scheibel, 1968). Whereas the targets of laminae I-IV neurons are cutaneous afferents, lamina V neurons, as we shall see later (Section 1.8.2), are targets of descending corticospinal and rubrospinal tract fibers.

1.3.5 Lamination of the Dorsal Horn in the Human Spinal Cord. We summarize our current understanding of the laminar organization of the dorsal horn by using silver-impregnated coronal sections from the spinal cord of an adult human male. As seen at low magnification (Figure 1-19), this metallic

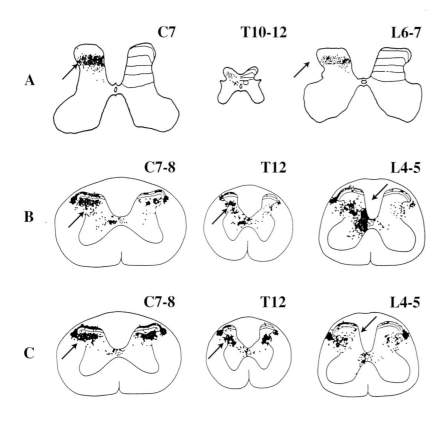

Figure 1-18. A. Retrogradely labeled *spinocervical* tract neurons in lamina IV of the cat spinal cord at cervical (C), thoracic (T), and lumbar (L) levels. After Craig (1978). **B.** Retrogradely labeled *spinothalamic* neurons at three corresponding levels in the rat spinal cord. After Burstein et al. (1990). **C.** Retrogradely labeled *spinohypothalamic* neurons at three levels of the rat spinal cord. After Burstein et al. (1987). The dorsal horn distribution of spinothalamic and spinohypothalamic relay neurons differs from that of the spinocervical relay neurons. Arrows point to highest concentration of labeled projection neurons. HRP technique.

stain reacts not only with axons (note that the perpendicularly cut longitudinal fibers appear as fine dots in the white matter and as threads of various lengths in the gray matter) but also with the perikarya of neurons (note the staining of motoneurons in the ventral horn). Particularly striking are the dozen or so vertically oriented, oval bushy structures lined up in a single band in the upper dorsal horn. We interpret these to be vertically oriented, central cells with bushy dendrites (Figure 1-15A) together with flame-shaped terminals of a similar configuration and orientation of some dorsal root collaterals (to be described later). As seen at higher magnification (Figure 1-20), these darkly staining bushy profiles are probably located in lamina III. In this illustration, the demarcation of lamina I (the cap of the dorsal horn) is based on the presence of many horizontally oriented, spindle shaped neurons, the classical Waldeyer cells, with similarly oriented processes (compare with Figure 1-13). Lamina II is devoid of these horizontal cells but seems to contain superficially a few less precisely oriented larger neurons; these may be stalked cells

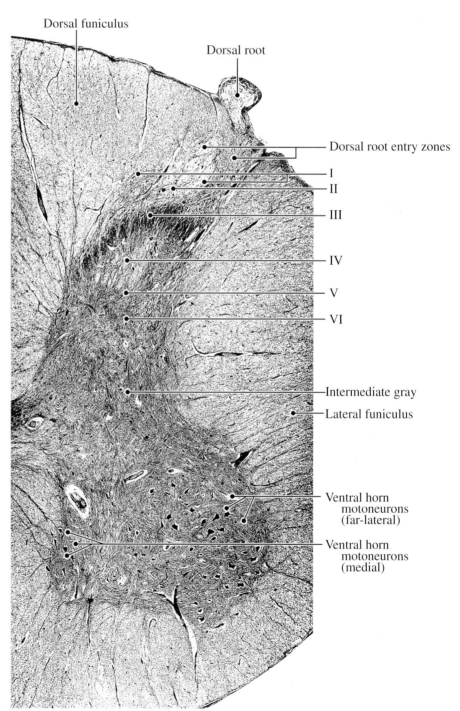

Figure 1-19. Coronal section of the cervical spinal cord of a 37-year-old man, with Rexed's subdivision of the dorsal horn (**right**). The silver stain used has affinity for the membranes of neuronal perikarya (e.g., motoneurons in the ventral horn), dendrites and axons (note that the transected myelinated axons in the white matter appear as fine dots). The central cells with their bushy dendrites (and possibly the flame terminals that contact them) are conspicuous in the upper dorsal horn. Photomicrograph of material kindly supplied by Dr. William DeMyer.

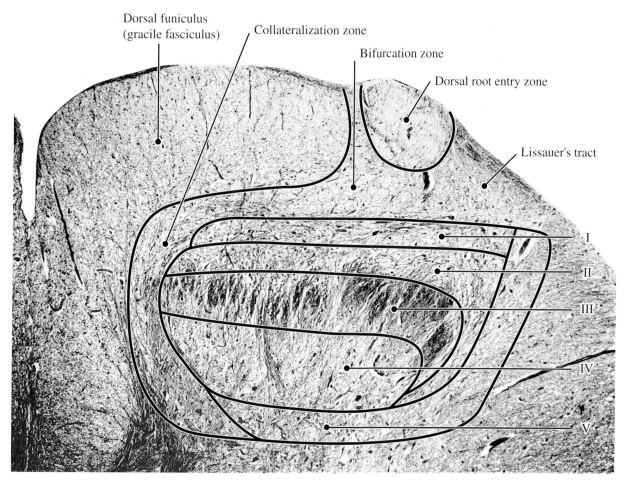

Figure 1-20. Coronal section of the dorsal horn in the lumbar spinal cord of the same human specimen shown in Figure 1-19. Lamina I contains horizontal cells, whereas lamina III is distinguished by bushy entities, presumably the dendrites of central cells and associated axon terminals. Lamina V may be club-shaped at this level of the spinal cord.

and/or islet cells. The rest of lamina II may contain smaller neurons but they are indistinct. In these silver-stained preparations of the human spinal cord, lamina II and lamina III appear to have a different cytoarchitectonic organization. Lamina IV contains medium-sized cells of various orientations; which agrees with earlier descriptions of cell types in this layer. Lamina V seems to be club-shaped at this level of the human spinal cord.

1.4 Segregation of Sensory Fibers in the Dorsal Horn

1.4.1 Varieties of Nerve Fibers that Terminate in the Dorsal Horn. The fibers that terminate in the dorsal horn come from three sources: (1) peripheral sensory fibers from the body, including its internal organs; (2) descending fibers from the brain stem and the forebrain; and (3) intrinsic (propriospi-

nal) fibers from within the spinal cord. We begin with a consideration of the termination pattern of the the primary dorsal root afferents from the periphery. It has been known for some time that upon entering the white matter of the spinal cord, the dorsal root sensory fibers bifurcate into ascending and descending branches (Figure 1-21A). These branches give off local collaterals that penetrate the gray matter and, after extensive ramification, terminate there (Figure 1-21B). The primary sensory fibers that enter the dorsal horn differ in terms of (i) their peripheral origins (skin, muscle, tendon, or viscera); (ii) whether of small or large caliber; (iii) whether myelinated or unmyelinated; (iv) their sensory modality (pain, cold, warmth, touch, pressure, stretch, etc.); (iv) topographic origin (somatotopy); and some additional properties, such as (v) threshold of excitation, (vi) size of their receptive field, and (vii) slow or fast adaptation to stimuli. It has been suspected for some time that the laminar organization of the dorsal horn that we have discussed in the preceding section is related to the selective termination of different kinds of sensory fibers in the spinal cord.

To distinguish the different classes of sensory fibers that reach the spinal cord, we adopt here Sherrington's (1906) terminology of four classes of peripheral sense organs: nociceptors, exteroceptors, proprioceptors, and interoceptors. (The special senses of the head – of sight, hearing, and smell – classified by Sherrington as teleceptors, will not be discussed here.)

The prototypical function of nociceptors is the mediation of pain. Exteroceptors are epitomized by the cutaneous sense of touch. Proprioceptors are

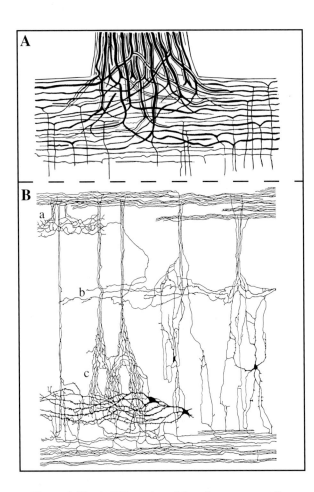

Figure 1-21. A. Bifurcation of dorsal root sensory fibers (top center) into ascending and descending branches and some perpendicularly oriented collaterals. After Edinger; from Ranson and Clark (1959). **B.** Sagittal section through the lumbosacral spinal cord of a cat, showing the termination of collaterals in the dorsal horn (**a**), the intermediate gray (**b**), and the ventral horn (**c**). After Scheibel (1984). Golgi technique.

the mechanical sensors of muscle, joints and tendons. Interoceptors convey information from the the internal organs, especially the viscera. A variety of anatomical and physiological research methods have been used in the last century to unravel the relationship between the sensory function of dorsal root fibers and their mode of termination in the spinal cord. We begin this review with the evidence that the small caliber nociceptive fibers and the large caliber exteroceptive fibers have different laminar targets in the dorsal horn.

1.4.2 Termination Sites of Small Caliber Nociceptive Fibers. Histological studies begun early in the twentieth century (Ramón y Cajal, 1909; Ranson, 1913a) and pursued later (Earle, 1952; Pearson, 1952; Szentágothai, 1964; Réthelyi, 1977; LaMotte, 1977; Light and Perl, 1979a; Ralston and Ralston, 1979; Grant et al., 1981) have established that the collaterals of the small caliber fibers of the dorsal root penetrate the dorsal horn from its surface (Figure 1-22A) and terminate preferentially (though not exclusively) in the marginal layer (lamina I) and the substantia gelatinosa (laminae II-III). Correlated clinical evidence (Pearson, 1952; White and Sweet, 1969), together with physiological and behavioral studies (reviewed by Willis, 1985; Besson and Chaouch, 1987; Willis and Westlund, 1997) linked these small caliber sensory fibers to the transmission of high threshold, tissue-damaging stimuli, the kind that often trigger painful (nociceptive) sensations.

Ramón y Cajal (1909) identified the "marginal plexus of collaterals" as the site where fibers of Lissauer's tract enter the dorsal horn (Figure 1-22b), and Szentágothai (1964) described two termination sites and patterns of arborization of small caliber fibers in the upper laminae of the dorsal horn. In lamina I, these axons arborize as a tangential plexus, and make synaptic contacts with the horizontal Waldeyer cells. In lamina II the terminal arbors are smaller and more discrete. Ralston and Ralston (1979) distinguished two classes of synaptic endings at the latter sites. Electron-lucent terminals with dense core vesicles predominate in lamina I and in the outer part of lamina II (IIo), whereas in the inner part of lamina II (IIi) electron-dense terminals are more common. These two types of sensory terminals may correspond to the physiologically identified high threshold, slow conducting A∂ and C fibers, respectively. The A∂ fibers preferentially terminate

A Dorsal funiculus Dorsal root Lissauer's tract

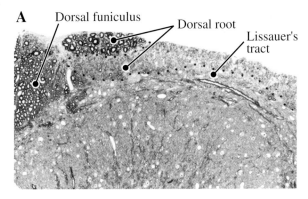

B Dorsal funiculus Dorsal root Lissauer's tract

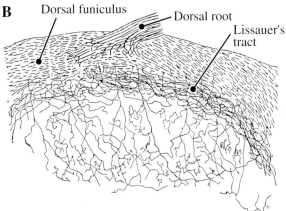

Figure 1-22. A. Myelinated and unmyelinated fibers of the dorsal root, and unmyelinated fibers of Lissauer's tract in a cat. After Chung and Coggeshall (1987). **B.** Collaterals of dorsal root fibers in Lissauer's tract and their terminals in the substantia gelatinosa of a kitten. After Ramón y Cajal (1911).

in lamina I and in lamina IIo, while C fibers preferentially terminate in lamina IIi (Brown, 1981). On the basis of this sort of evidence, it has been hypothesized that the small caliber, myelinated A∂ fibers convey heat and cold (thermal) sensations, whereas the finest, unmyelinated C fibers mediate pain (see Table 1-2). The possibility that there are two different classes of C fibers is currently being investigated (Snider and McMahon, 1998).

That the superficial laminae of the dorsal horn, the targets of the small caliber nociceptive fibers, have some unique molecular properties was first suggested by the localization of substance P, a peptide, in the dorsal roots (Lembeck, 1953). Subsequent biochemical (Takahashi and Otsuka, 1975) and histochemical (Hökfelt et al., 1975; Cuello, et al., 1976; Chan-Palay and Palay, 1977; Pickel et al., 1977) studies have established that substance P is concentrated in laminae I and II (Figure 1-23), and that there ensues a precipitous drop in the concentration

of substance P following transection of the dorsal roots (Hökfelt et al., 1975; Takahashi and Otsuka, 1975). (We may recall that a class of small ganglion cells reacts positively with antibodies for substance P.) Correlated physiological studies showed that substance P has an excitatory influence on those dorsal horn neurons that preferentially respond to noxious stimuli (Henry et al., 1976; Randic and Miletic, 1977), and that this peptide is released in the spinal cord in response to dorsal root stimulation (Otsuka and Konishi, 1976). Moreover, the analgesic effect of opiates has been related to the high concentration of opiate receptors in laminae I-III (Pert et al., 1975; LaMotte et al., 1976).

Further support for this relationship between substance P release and excitation in the nociceptive pathway was received by an analysis of the pain-modulating action of capsaicin. This pungent ingredient of red pepper and other hot spices first stimulates peripheral nociceptors but then causes a long-

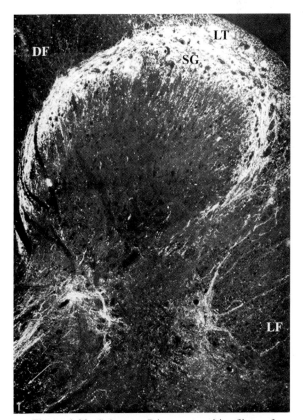

Figure 1-23. Substance P immunopositive fibers of Lissauer's tract (LT) and the superficial substantia gelatinosa (SG) in the dorsal horn of a cat. The dorsal funiculus (DF), the lateral funiculus (LF), and the core of the dorsal horn contain few fluorescent fibers. After Hökfelt et al. (1975). Fluorescent technique.

lasting insensitivity to chemically elicited pain (Jancsó and Jancsó-Gábor, 1959). Capsaicin was found to produce a calcium-dependent release of substance P from the spinal cord (Theriault et al., 1979) and a subsequent depletion of substance P in the substantia gelatinosa (Jessell et al., 1978; Figure 1-24). A behavioral study in rats indicates that this capsaicin-induced inhibition of pain is exerted only on chemically or mechanically produced nociception but not on nociception produced by thermal stimulation (Hayes and Tyers, 1980). Since capsaicin had no effect on the density of opiate receptor binding sites in the dorsal horn (Jessell, et al. 1978), it is thought that its action is due to a metabolic disturbance of the nociceptive transmitter system.

Another chemical implicated in nociception is nitric oxide, a substance formed from arginine by nitric oxide synthase. Nitric oxide synthase has been located in spinal ganglion cells and small neurons of the dorsal horn, in particular those in lamina IIi and the central gray surrounding the spinal canal (Zhang et al., 1993). Physiological studies suggest that nitric

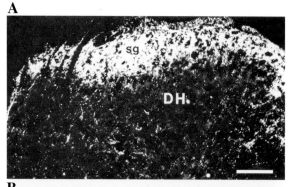

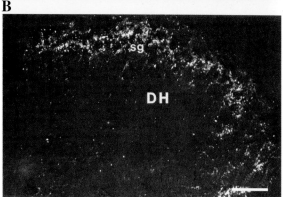

Figure 1-24. A. Substance P fluorescence in the superficial substantia gelatinosa (sg) in an untreated rat. The core of the dorsal horn (DH) contains few fluorescent fibers. **B.** Reduction in substance P fluorescence in the substantia gelatinosa following treatment with capsaicin. From Jessell et al. (1978). Scales: 100 μm.

oxide may stimulate the discharge of nociceptive spinal cord neurons (Pehl and Schmid, 1997; Rivot et al., 1997; Gao and Qiao, 1998). The concentration of nicotinamide adenine dinucleotide phosphate diaphorase (NADPH; which may be identical with nitric oxide synthase) was found to be high in the superficial laminae of the dorsal horn and in the gray matter surrounding the central canal (Spike et al., 1993). Finally, another substance, calcitonin gene-related peptide, has been co-localized with nitric oxide synthase (Zhang et al., 1993) and substance P (Wiesenfeld-Hallin et al., 1984; Gamse and Saria, 1984), and implicated in nociception. This peptide enhances the release of endogenous glutamate and aspartate (Kangrga and Randic, 1990). Glutamate (Weinberg et al., 1987; Miller et al., 1988; De Biasi and Rustioni, 1988; Young et al., 1997) and aspartate (Rustioni and Cuénod, 1982; Tracey et al., 1991), neurotransmitters with a wide distribution in the spinal cord, may exert an excitatory effect on nociception.

While pain is produced by the excitatory action of peripheral signals of tissue damage, it is also attenuated by central inhibitory processes. Interneurons of the superficial laminae of the dorsal horn have a high concentration of both gamma amino butyric acid (GABA), a putative inhibitory transmitter, and its synthesizing enzyme, glutamate decarboxylase (Albers and Brady, 1959; Miyata and Otsuka, 1972; Ljungdahl and Hökfelt, 1973; Kelly et al., 1973; McLaughlin et al., 1975; Ribeiro-da-Silva and Coimbra, 1980). Thus it has been hypothesized that GABA is the transmitter of local inhibitory influences exerted on neurons of the substantia gelatinosa. The phenomenon of endogenous analgesia suggests that inhibitory influences may be exerted on nociception by supraspinal mechanisms. Thus the attenuation or abolition of pain responses to injury during intense behavioral arousal has been attributed to descending supraspinal effects upon opiate receptors in the superficial laminae of the dorsal horn (Mayer and Price, 1976; Basbaum and Fields, 1978; Ma et al., 1997). Some of these descending actions are mediated by serotonergic fibers that originate in the brain stem raphe nuclei (Dahlström and Fuxe, 1965; Bowker et al., 1981; Nicholas et al., 1992). Indeed, the evidence for the role of monoamines in the modulation of nociception is quite compelling. First, electrical stimulation in the region of the raphe magnus nucleus produces behavioral analgesia (Oliveras et al., 1975) and, second, inhibits the discharge of dorsal horn nociceptive neurons (Beall et al., 1976; Fields et al., 1977; Belcher et al., 1978). Third, direct injection of serotonin into the dorsal horn mimics the effect of nucleus magnus stimulation (Yaksh and Wilson, 1979). Fourth, some of the synapses that contact dendrites in laminae I and II bind tritiated serotonin (Ruda and Gobel, 1980). Fifth, the neurons inhibited by raphe magnus stimulation were identified directly as lamina I marginal cells and lamina II stalked cells (Miletic et al., 1984). Finally, sixth, the concentration of serotonin immunoreactive terminals was found to be higher in laminae I and II neurons that were suppressed by raphe magnus stimulation than in unaffected lamina II neurons (Miletic et al., 1984). Analgesic effects have also been obtained by stimulation of several mesencephalic and diencephalic structures, in particular the midbrain periaqueductal gray (Liebeskind et al., 1973) and the periventricular thalamus and hypothalamus (Oliveras et al., 1974; Akil and Liebeskind, 1975).

1.4.3 Termination Sites of Large Caliber Exteroceptive Fibers. Two morphological features distinguish the trajectory of large caliber exteroceptive fibers from the trajectory of small caliber nociceptive fibers. First, whereas the thin nociceptive fibers penetrate the dorsal horn from its surface, the thick exteroceptive fibers enter it from beneath. This is illustrated in Figure 1-25 in a myelin stained section from the lumbar spinal cord of a human child. Note that the bundle of myelinated semicircular fibers that pass along the wall or within the dorsal funiculus, enter the gray matter underneath the substantia gelatinosa and then turn upward. Some of the recurving fibers enter the substantia gelatinosa and a few may move upward between its "slabs." Second, as originally shown with the Golgi technique by Ramón y Cajal (1909), the recurving collaterals terminate in the substantia gelatinosa with a distinctive upright arbor (Figure 1-26A). These "flame-shaped" terminals, according to Scheibel and Scheibel (1968), have

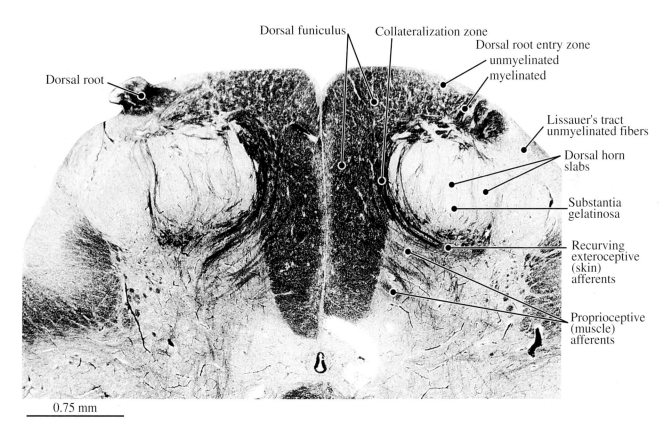

0.75 mm

Figure 1-25. Myelin-stained section of the upper half of the lumbar spinal cord of a 6-week-old child. Some of the myelinated dorsal root collaterals course along the lateral wall of the dorsal funiculus, turn medially underneath the substantia gelatinosa, then curve upward to enter it from underneath. Other myelinated collaterals turn downward. The former will be identified as exteroceptive collaterals, the latter as proprioceptive collaterals. The nociceptve fibers of Lissauer's tract are unmyelinated. Specimen # Y152-61; Loyez stain.

a planar configuration, about 20 μm wide in the coronal plane and up to several hundred micrometers in the sagittal plane. The matching shape of flame terminals and the dendritic arbor of central cells, as drawn by Ramón y Cajal, is illustrated in Figure 1-26B. The sagittal spread of these flame terminals complements the dendritic arbor of central cells (Figure 1-15), and stalked cells and islet cells (Figure 1-16) of the substantia gelatinosa.

Recent physiological tracers studies (Brown, 1981; Shortland et al., 1989) showed that the low threshold hair-follicle (exteroceptive) afferents have recurving collaterals with flame-like endings that terminate in lamina III (Figure 1-27). In an ultrastructural study, Ralston and Ralston (1979) observed that

lamina III contains an abundance of terminals with large synaptic profiles; these may be the synapses of flame terminals. The flame terminals are particularly dense and regularly aligned in the cervical and lumbar enlargements of the cat spinal cord, with an average of 15 "flames" in cross sections (Scheibel and Scheibel, 1968). (Compare that with the illustration of the human spinal cord in Figures 1-19 and 1-20.) The orientation of the flame arbors is less regular or dense in the thoracic spinal cord. The high concentration of flame terminals in the cervical and lumbar enlargement may be related to the circumstance that tactile receptors and touch spots are most numerous, and their receptive fields the smallest, in the hand and foot (Sinclair 1981).

Physiological studies indicate that the large caliber, myelinated dorsal root collaterals that end in the substantia gelatinosa are low threshold, fast conducting Aß afferents that selectively respond to innocuous mechanical stimuli (Light and Perl 1979a; Brown, 1981; Price, 1984). They do not respond to thermal stimuli and do not discharge at a higher rate in response to noxious mechanical stimulation. Therefore, this input line is well suited to convey information about the texture, size, shape and other objective properties of things touched, grasped or palpated. This is in contrast to the nociceptive input that provides subjective information about harm or damage done to the tissues of the body. Of significance in this context is the observation that, in addi-

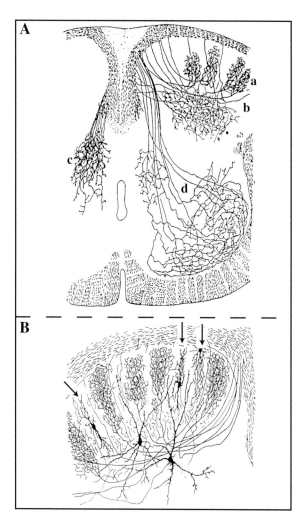

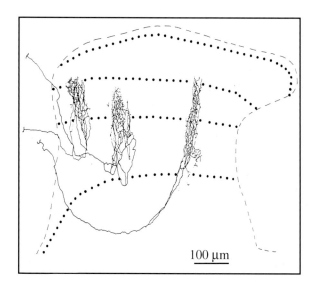

Figure 1-26. A. Flame terminals of the recurving dorsal root collaterals in the substantia gelatinosa (**a**). Other collaterals form terminal plexuses at the base of the dorsal horn (**b**), in the intermediate gray (**c**), and the ventral horn (**d**). **B.** The complementary configuration of the recurving flame terminals and the dendritic arbor of central cells (arrows). After Ramón y Cajal (1911). Golgi technique.

Figure 1-27. Physiologically identified low threshold hair follicle afferents with recurving collaterals and flame terminals in the rat dorsal horn. From Shortland et al. (1989). Intracellular HRP staining.

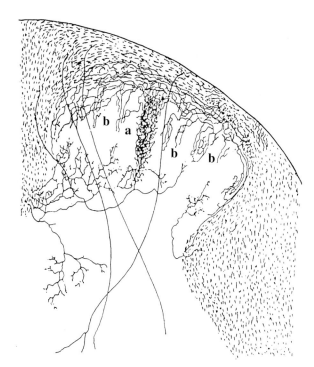

Figure 1-28. A flame terminal (**a**) and cap terminals (**b**) in the cat dorsal horn. The flame terminals are the arbors of recurving large caliber exteroceptive collaterals that enter the dorsal horn from below. The cap terminals are the endings of small caliber nociceptive fibers that enter the dorsal horn from above. We propose that the two synapse in the substantia gelatinosa with the ventral and the dorsal dendritic tufts of central cells, respectively. After Scheibel and Scheibel (1968). Golgi technique.

tion to the upward spreading "flame" terminals of the large caliber exteroceptive collaterals, the substantia gelatinosa also receives shorter downward spreading "cap" terminals from the small caliber nociceptive afferents (Figure 1-28). As we shall discuss this in some detail later (Section 2.2.2), the flame terminals and cap terminals may be forming synapses with the basal and apical dendritic tufts of central cells, respectively. If so, the central cells would be in a position to integrate exteroceptive and nociceptive afferent input and then, through relays, pass on these integrated messages to the brain.

We noted earlier, the pivotal role played by substance P in synaptic transmission in the nociceptive pathway. The identity of neurotransmitters mediating impulse transmission in the large caliber exteroceptive dorsal root afferents remains to be determined. Evidence has been available for some time that glutamate serves as an excitatory neurotransmit-

ter in the spinal cord (Curtis and Watkins, 1960), and that the concentration of glutamate is much higher in the dorsal root than in the ventral root (Curtis and Johnston, 1974). Moreover, immunocytochemical studies have shown that there is a high concentration of glutamate in the dorsal horn (Broman et al., 1993). However, to what extent glutamate is specifically involved in impulse transmission in the large caliber exteroceptive pathway is unclear because, as we have seen earlier, glutamate also plays a role in nociceptive transmission.

1.4.4 Termination Sites of Proprioceptive Fibers. When a skeletal muscle is stretched, the muscle spindle receptors embedded in the muscle are stimulated and that results in the contraction of the lengthened muscle. This proprioceptive response, known as the myotatic or stretch reflex (Sherrington, 1906), is mediated by the primary (annnulospiral) afferents of the muscle spindle (Lloyd, 1944). Input from the muscle spindle secondary (flower spray) afferents, and from tendon and joint receptors, trigger disynaptic or multisynaptic reflexes of a more complex nature (Matthews, 1972). The muscle spindle primary afferents, and afferents from tendons and joints, are classified as Aα fibers (Table 1-2 on page 14). They are large caliber (15-20 μm) myelinated fibers that conduct impulses at a high velocity (70-120 m/sec). The muscle spindle secondary afferents are classified as Aβ fibers; they are thinner (5-10 μm) myelinated fibers that conduct impulses at a lower speed (30-70 m/sec). The bifurcating ascending and descending branches of these dorsal root fibers (see Figure 1-21) travel a long distance rostrally and caudally in the lateral aspect of the dorsal funiculus, and give off collaterals, on the average at 1 mm intervals (range 0.1-2.6 mm). These collaterals penetrate the gray matter from its dorsomedial or medial aspect (Scheibel and Scheibel, 1969; Scheibel, 1984). In contrast, to the myelinated collaterals of exteroceptive afferents, which curve dorsally upon entering the gray matter, the proprioceptive collaterals turn ventrally (Figure 1-25). Then, after a short downward course, these collaterals terminate and form discrete plexuses at three locations: (i) the base of the dorsal horn laterally; (ii) Clarke's column medially; and (iii) the vicinity of the motor nuclei ventrally (Figures 1-26A, 1-29, 1-30). The terminals of these proprioceptive collaterals have the ultrastructural features of excitatory synapses (Conradi et al., 1983). The proprioceptive fibers that terminate in Clarke's column

synapse with neurons that are the source of the spinocerebellar tract, whereas those that proceed to the
ventral horn make synaptic contacts either directly
with motoneurons or with interneurons that surround
the motor columns. Arborization of proprioceptive
collaterals is particularly abundant in the ventral
horn (Figure 1-30). Direct contact with motoneurons
is responsible for the monosynaptic stretch reflex.
According to Scheibel and Scheibel (1969), the proprioceptive collaterals do not descend individually but
in tight fascicles of thick and thin fibers, what they
called microbundles (Figure 1-30). Importantly, the
terminal arbors of proprioceptive afferents – unlike
the arbors of exteroceptive afferents – have a limited
rostrocaudal spread (in the range of 10-30 μm) and
extend mostly mediolaterally (Brown, 1981).

The findings of the Scheibels in Golgi material were confirmed and extended by Ishizuka et al.
(1979) who made three-dimensional reconstructions
of the trajectory of 23 physiologically identified Ia
afferents from several hindlimb muscles of the cat.
Using intracellularly injected HRP, the trajectory of
these fibers was traced in the lumbar spinal cord from

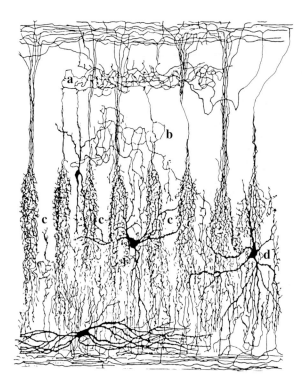

Figure 1-30. The lumbosacral spinal cord of the cat in
sagittal plane, showing the distribution of proprioceptive
collaterals in the dorsal horn (**a**), Clarke's column (**b**), the
intermediate gray (**c**), and the ventral horn (**d**). The "microbundles" form a rich terminal plexus in the ventral horn.
After Scheibel and Scheibel (1969). Golgi technique.

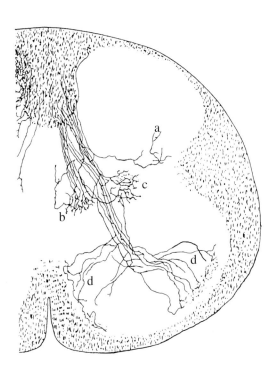

Figure 1-29. Termination pattern of putative proprioceptive dorsal root collaterals in the cat spinal cord
at the base of the dorsal horn (**a**), in Clarke's column
(**b**), the intermediate gray (**c**), and the ventral horn (**d**).
After Scheibel and Scheibel (1969). Golgi technique.

5.8 to 15.7 mm rostrocaudally. Over these lengths,
5-11 collaterals were given off from the ascending
and descending branches. Typically, these collaterals passed along the medial aspect of the dorsal horn
and gave off terminal arbors in the regions of the gray
matter previously described. The number of terminals issuing from one collateral ranged from 136 to
725. This investigation also revealed that proprioceptive collaterals from different muscles had a different
trajectory and termination pattern (Figure 1-31). Terminals from the hamstrings (which act on hip and
knee joints) were sparse in the dorsal horn and the
intermediate gray, and profuse at the base of the
ventral horn. Terminals from the medial gastrocnemius (an ankle flexor) were concentrated in Clarke's
column and the dorsal aspect of the ventral horn. It
was estimated that one axon from the medial gastrocnemius (which had an average of 216 terminals at a
single coronal level) had 2160 terminals over its 10
mm spread in the spinal cord. Finally, proprioceptive
terminals from the flexor digitorum hallucis longus
(a great toe flexor) were most numerous in Clarke's
column and the dorsal horn, and had sparse endings
in the ventral horn dorsolaterally. About 10% of Ia

COLLATERALS   TERMINALS

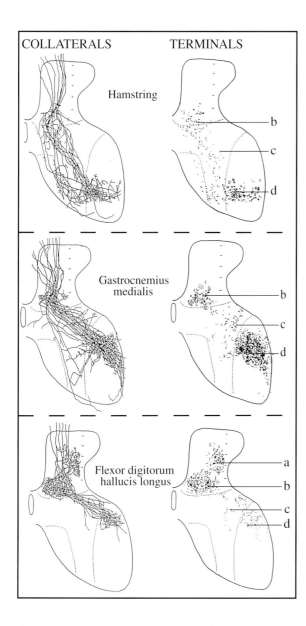

Figure 1-31. Trajectory of physiologically identified proprioceptive collaterals (**left**) from three hindlimb muscles of the cat, and the distribution of their terminal boutons (**right**) in the following regions: the dorsal horn (**a**), Clarke's column (**b**), the intermediate gray (**c**), and the ventral horn (**d**). Terminal boutons from the hamstring muscles are concentrated in the ventral horn; those from the gastrocnemius are concentrated in Clarke's column and the far-lateral ventral horn. Flexor digitorum boutons are concentrated in the lower laminae of the dorsal horn and Clarke's column, with sparse termination in the retrodorsal ventral horn. This pattern indicates, first, that proprioceptive fibers from specific skeletal muscles terminate in the vicinity of the motor columns that innervate those muscles. Second, that only proprioceptive afferents from prehensile distal muscles (flexor digitorum longus) but not those from ballistic proximal muscles (hamstrings) have an extensive feedback projection to the dorsal horn. After Ishizuka et al. (1979). Intracellular HRP technique.

terminals that reach the motor nuclei contact the perikarya of motoneurons; the rest is believed to terminate on motoneuron dendrites (Ishizuka et al., 1979; Brown, 1981). Synaptic contacts may be made with motoneuron dendrites 0.8 mm away from the perikaryon (Brown, 1981).

1.4.5 Termination Sites of Interoceptive Fibers. The distribution of interoceptive (including the visceral sensory) fibers in the gray matter of the spinal cord is poorly understood. Three visceral nerves have received some attention recently, the pelvic nerve, the splanchnic nerve, and the pudendal nerve.

The Pelvic Nerve. According to Langley and Anderson (1986), the pelvic nerve, which innervates the bladder and colon, is composed almost entirely of small caliber axons less than 4-5 μm in diameter. In a tracer study in which HRP was applied to the cut pelvic nerve, Morgan et al. (1981) found that the ganglion cells of the pelvic nerve, which are concentrated in S1-S3, are among the smallest neurons of the sacral dorsal root ganglia. At the dorsal root entry zone, most pelvic nerve afferents join Lissauer's tract (Figure 1-32) and are distributed over several segments of the lumbosacral cord; some of the fibers enter the dorsal funiculus. Some axon collaterals are concentrated superficially in lamina I, others (the fibers of the so-called lateral collateral pathway) end laterally in the intermediate gray, and may reach the preganglionic neurons of the sacral parasympathetic columns in the lateral horn. Still others (the fibers of the medial collateral pathway) terminate in the central gray above the central canal. Significantly, the pelvic fibers avoid laminae II-IV. As seen in coronal sections (Figure 1-32), the labeled pelvic fibers form a semicircle around the walls and base of the dorsal horn. (Compare this with the semicircular lamina V outlined in Figure 1-20.)

The Splanchnic Nerve. The splanchnic nerve innervates the abdominal organs. There is clinical and experimental evidence that splanchnic sensory fibers play an important role in the mediation of abdominal pain (Sheehan, 1933; Bain et al., 1935; Moore, 1938; Gross, 1974; White, 1974). A recent tracer study (Kuo and De Groat, 1985) showed that HRP applied to the cut end of the major splanchnic nerve of the cat labels fibers along the entire length of the thoracic cord in Lissauer's tract and in the dorsal

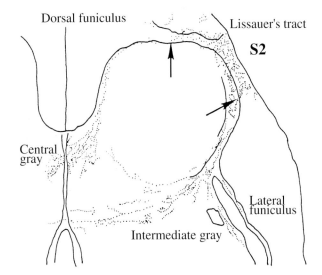

Figure 1-32. Distribution of pelvic nerve afferent collaterals in the sacral spinal cord of the cat. Arrows point to the lateral boundaries of Lissauer's tract. The collaterals of this visceral nerve course over the lateral and medial walls of the dorsal horn, and terminate beneath the dorsal horn in the intermediate gray and in the dorsal part of the central gray (central autonomic area). After Morgan et al. (1981). HRP technique.

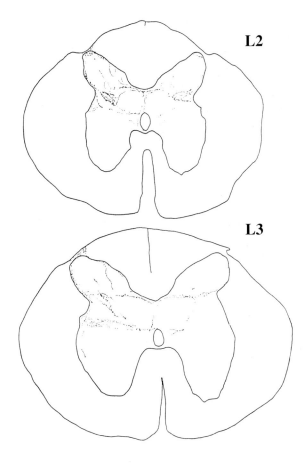

Figure 1-33. Distribution of renal afferents in the lumbar spinal cord of the cat. The fibers of this visceral nerve are distributed in Lissauer's tract (**left**), and terminate bilaterally in the intermediate gray and the dorsal gray (central autonomic area) but avoid Clarke's column. From Kuo et al (1983). HRP technique.

funiculus. Although neuronal responses to splanchnic nerve stimulation can be recorded from the gracilis nucleus (Aidar et al., 1952; Rigamonti and Hancock, 1974), that excitatory effect is attributed to the action of postsynaptic fibers rather than primary dorsal root afferents (Al-Chaer et al., 1996). The termination pattern of splanchnic afferents in the spinal cord resembles that seen in the pelvic nerve, with a loop around the external border of the dorsal horn.

HRP applied to the renal nerve, labeled ganglion cells from T2 to L6, and renal afferents from T11 to L6, with greatest concentration between L1 and L3 (Kuo et al., 1983). The intraspinal distribution of these sensory fibers to the kidney (which course in the minor splanchnic nerve) is similar to that seen in the major splanchnic nerve. The fibers of the medial collateral pathway avoid Clarke's column as they cross to the opposite side (Figure 1-33).

The Pudendal Nerve. The sensory fibers of the pudendal nerve convey messages from the skin and mucous membranes of the anal canal and urogenital system. A tracer study showed that, in the monkey, the ganglion cells of the pudendal nerve are located at level S1 or S2, and the fibers that enter Lissauer's tract and the dorsal funiculus extend as far as L1 and S3 (Roppolo et al., 1985). In the cat, the intra-

spinal distribution of afferents extends from L7 to S3 (Ueyama et al., 1984). The semicircular termination pattern of these afferents resembles that of other visceral afferents (Figure 1-34). In the rat, the labeled ganglion cells of the pudendal nerve are located at L6 and S1 levels, and display a sexual dimorphism in the sense that they are larger in males than in females (McKenna and Nadelhaft, 1986).

Interoceptive fibers are of two kinds: those that respond to innocuous mechanical stimuli and those that respond to noxious chemical or mechanical stimuli. The former may bring messages about the stretching of anal and urethral sphincter muscles, as conveyed by muscle spindle receptors that are embedded in them (Evans, 1963; Todd, 1964); the latter are probably involved in the mediation of visceral pain. In a recent study (Laird et al., 1996), recordings were made of the response of dorsal horn neurons to light

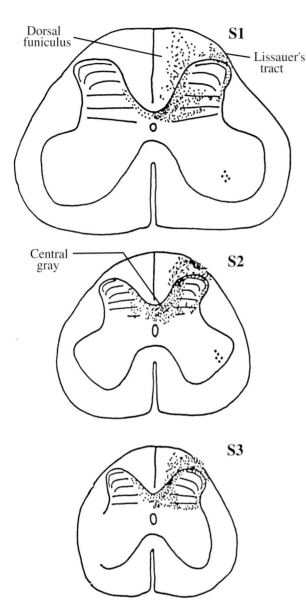

Figure 1-34. Distribution of pudendal nerve afferents in the sacral spinal cord of the cat. The afferents coursing in Lissauer's tract and the dorsal funiculus avoid the core of the dorsal horn and seem to terminate at its base, in the intermediate gray and the central gray (central autonomic area). After Ueayama et al. (1984). HRP technique.

and heavy pressure applied to the ureter in the rat. The results indicate that the majority of these neurons respond to the kind of stimuli that produce urethral pain in man.

1.4.6 Topographical Distribution of Dorsal Root Sensory Fibers.

The exteroceptive large caliber afferents terminate in the dorsal horn in a precise topographic order (Szentágothai and Kiss, 1949; Brown and Culberson, 1981; Koerber and Brown, 1982; Shortland et al., 1989; Brown et al., 1991). The

fibers of the dorsal ramus (which, at thoracic levels, innervate the skin and muscles of the back) and the fibers of the ventral ramus (which innervate the skin and muscles of the thorax) terminate at different sites in the dorsal horn. This was demonstrated in a degeneration study by Grant and Ygge (1981) who found that dorsal ramus axons terminate laterally in the rat dorsal horn, whereas ventral ramus axons terminate medially (Figure 1-35). This was confirmed in a tracer study by Smith (1983) in which HRP was applied in the rat to both the ventral and dorsal rami or, selectively, either to the ventral ramus or the dorsal ramus (Figure 1-36). Another facet of this topographic distribution is the observation that afferents coursing in different spinal nerves or subdivisions of a larger nerve terminate in different locations. This was shown by Swett and Woolf (1985) in the lumbar spinal cord where subdivisions of the sciatic nerve (the sural, lateral sural, superficial peroneal, and tibial nerves) project to different regions of the dorsal horn, extending from L2 to L5 (Figure 1-37). Rivero-Mélian and Grant (1990), who traced the termination

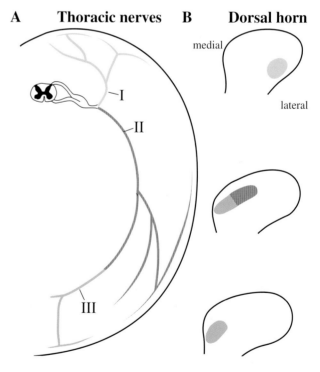

Figure 1-35. The effects of severing different branches of thoracic nerves (**A**) on the distribution of degenerating terminals in the dorsal horn of the rat (**B**). Severing the dorsal ramus (I) produced degeneration laterally (green). Severing the ventral ramus (II) produced degeneration in both the intermediate (red) and medial (blue) dorsal horn Severing the distal intercostal nerve (III) produced degeneration limited to the medial dorsal horn (blue). After Grant and Ygge (1981). Fink-Heimer technique.

A

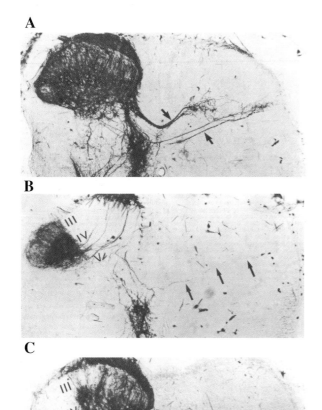

B

C

Figure 1-36. Topographic distribution of dorsal root afferents in the dorsal horn of the rat. **A.** Administration of HRP to both the dorsal and ventral rami labels afferents through the entire width of the rat dorsal horn. **B.** The tracer confined to the dorsal ramus labels afferents terminating in the lateral dorsal horn. **C.** The tracer confined to the ventral ramus labels afferents terminating in the medial dorsal horn. Arrows point to a few contralaterally projecting fibers. After Smith (1983).

pattern of the saphenous, anterior femoral, and lateral femoral cutaneous nerves made similar observations. This topographic projection represents, at least to a certain degree, a somatotopic map of the body surface. Thus, Nyberg and Blomqvist (1985) found that, in the cat, cutaneous fibers from the back, arm, forearm, the dorsum of the paw, the wrist, the digits, and the palm occupy discrete lateral-to-medial bands in the lower cervical dorsal horn (Figure 1-38). Sensory fibers from the paw occupy the largest area in the dorsal horn, with digits 2-5 arranged sequentially in a rostrocaudal sequence. A similar pattern was reported in the cat, squirrel monkey, and macaque

by Florence et al. (1989, 1991). The rostrocaudal sequence in the representation of digits 1-5, and the large area of the dorsal horn dedicated to the overall representation of the digits in the macaque monkey, is illustrated in Figure 1-39.

The observation that cutaneous representation in the dorsal horn is somatotopic (Figures 1-38,

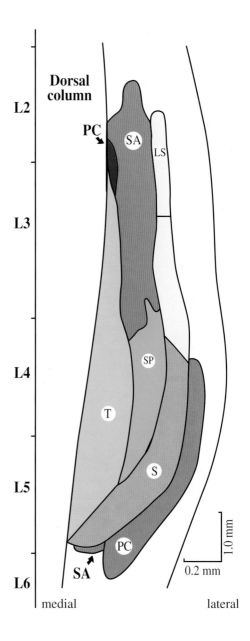

Figure 1-37. Reconstruction (in the horizontal plane) of the topographic distribution of afferents that course in different nerves in the rat dorsal horn. Abbreviations: tibial (T), sural (S), lateral sural (LS), saphenous (SA), superficial peroneal (SP), and posterior cutaneous (PC). After Swett and Woolf (1985). HRP technique.

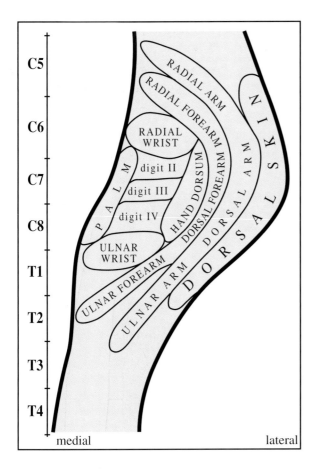

Figure 1-38. Somatotopic organization of cutaneous afferents in laminae II-III of the cervical and upper thoracic (brachial) spinal cord of the cat. Sensory fibers from the dorsal skin, arm, forearm, and hand are arranged in a lateral-to-medial order. Digits II, III, and IV are represented in a rostral-to-caudal order. After Nyberg and Blomquist (1985). HRP technique.

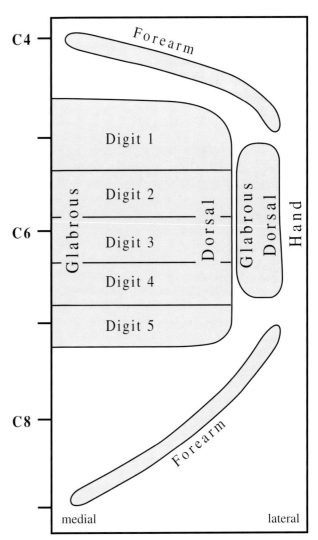

Figure 1-39. Topographic representation of the hand in the dorsal horn of the brachial spinal cord of a macaque monkey. In this map, width is exeggerated relative to the length of the cord. After Florence et al. (1991). HRP technique.

1-39) rather than dermatomal (compare with Figure 1-2, right), implies that the fiber-sorting that has been described as a topograhic feature in the dorsal funiculi and the dorsal column nuclei (Whitsel, et al., 1970; Brown and Fuchs, 1975) is also charactreristic of the termination of exteroceptive collaterals in the dorsal horn. It is of some significance that the topographic distribution of high threshold nociceptive (C) afferents, which terminate superficially in the dorsal horn, is very similar to the low threshold exteroceptive (Aß) fibers (Woolf and Fitzgerald, 1986). However, it has been claimed that the topographic organization of the small caliber nociceptive fiber terminals is less distinct in lamina I than the topographic arrangement of the large caliber exteroceptive fiber terminals in laminae II-III (Rivero-Mélian and Grant, 1990).

1. 5 Motoneurons of the Ventral Horn

1.5.1 Types of Neurons in the Ventral Horn.
The ventral horn contains three major classes of neurons with different connections and functions. (1) Large multipolar motoneurons, sometimes referred to as alpha motoneurons, innervate skeletal muscles and other striated muscles. The alpha motoneurons are typically aggregated in nuclei or columns (Figure 1-40A). (2) Similar but smaller gamma motoneurons, which innervate the intrafusal muscle fibers of muscle spindle sensors, are scattered among the alpha motoneurons (Figure 1-40B). (3) Excitatory and inhibitory interneurons of varying sizes and shapes are dis-

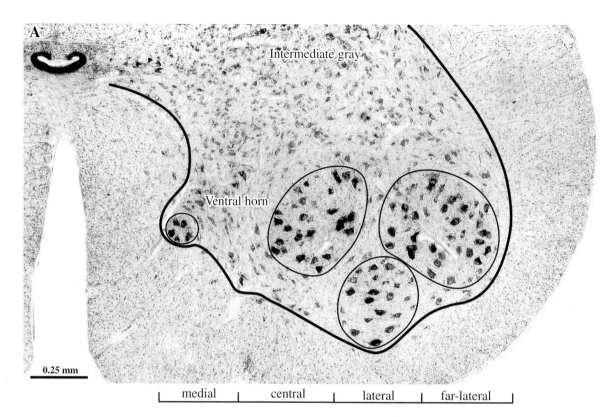

medial | central | lateral | far-lateral

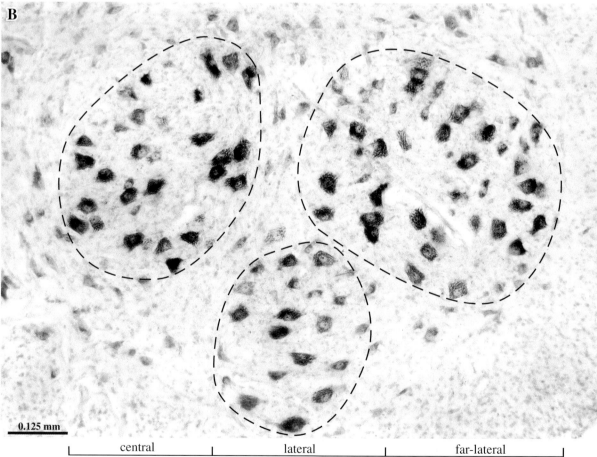

central | lateral | far-lateral

Figure 1-40. Motoneuron columns (with approximate panel markers) in the lumbar ventral horn of a human fetus at lower (**A**) and higher (**B**) magnification. Scattered among the large alpha motoneurons are a few smaller gamma motoneurons. Note also the presence of still smaller interneurons in the ventral horn Specimen # Y162-61; gestational age: 31 weeks. Cresyl violet.

tributed in the ventral horn above and around the motor nuclei (Figure 1-40A). The ventral horn inter-neurons, together with the interneurons of the inter-mediate gray, are responsible for the organization of intra- and intersegmental reflexes (Jankowska and Lindström, 1972) and are believed to function as cen-tral pattern generators (Grillner, 1975; Stein et al., 1984). They are sometimes called premotor neurons or last-order premotor neurons (Hongo, et al., 1989; Puskár and Antal, 1997). These interneurons (includ-ing those in the intermediate gray) are said to out-number motoneurons by a ratio of 30:1 (Gelfan et al., 1970). We briefly review below some of the structural and functional properties of alpha motoneurons.

1.5.2 The Cytology of Motoneurons.

Alpha motoneurons have multipolar perikarya (Figure 1-41), with a diameter (in the cat) of 30-70 μm and a surface area of up to 25,600 μm² (Aitken and Bridger, 1961; Gelfan et al. 1970). Each pole of the moto-neuron perikaryon is the site where a primary den-drite originates. An investigation based on the Golgi method indicates that a large motoneuron may have as many as 11 primary dendrites, with a median of 5 (Gelfan et al., 1970). According to that study, the primary dendrites may be 1.0-1.5 mm long, and the dendritic surface area may reach up to 87,000 μm². Another study employing a different staining technique (intracellular staining with a Procion dye) showed that a motoneuron may have as many as 22 primary dendrites and a surface area of up to 250,000 μm² (Barrett and Crill, 1974). The primary dendrites give off a large number of secondary and higher order dendritic branches. The dendritic expanse of a moto-neuron may spread in the coronal plane across the entire ventral horn (Figure 1-42) and the intermedi-ate gray. In some regions, motoneuron dendrites pen-etrate the white matter ipsilaterally or cross into the contralateral gray matter. (We shall return to the subject of motoneuron dendritic bundles in Section 1.6.8.)

The cytoplasm of the motoneuron perikaryon (soma) is filled with clumps of Nissl substance (Figure 1-43A). The Nissl substance, as seen with electron microscopy, is composed of a ribosome-studded endo-plasmic reticulum (Figure 1-44), a system of organ-elles involved in protein synthesis. The cytoplasm is also rich in mitochondria, and cisterns and vesicles of the Golgi apparatus, organelles involved in energy metabolism and membrane production, respectively. The powerful metabolic machinery of the motoneu-

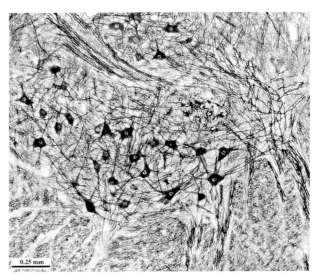

Figure 1-41. Multipolar motoneurons in the ventral horn of the lumbar cord of a human neonate. Speci-men # Y23-60. Bielschovsky's silver stain.

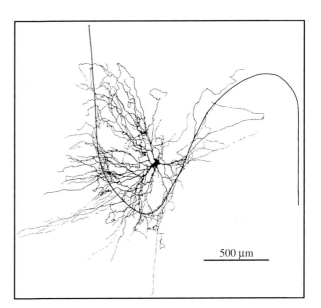

Figure 1-42. Dendritic spread of an identified splenius motoneuron in the upper cervical cord of a cat. The den-dritic arbor was reconstructed from 30 serially cut 100 μm coronal sections. From Keirstead and Rose (1983). Intracellular HRP technique.

ron perikaryon is responsible for the maintenance of its extensive surface membrane and its very long axon. The surface of the perikaryon and dendrites is studded with axon terminals, or boutons, of other neurons (Figure 1-43B). Terminals on the dendrites and the soma are distinguished as axodendritic and axosomatic synapses, respectively (Figure 1-44).

A

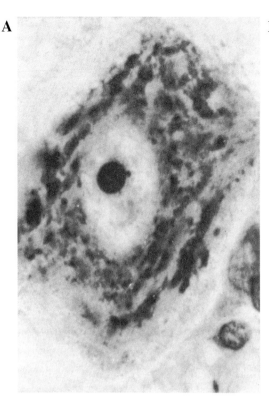

B

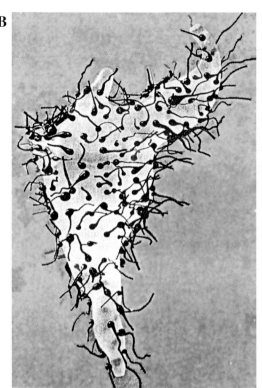

Figure 1-43. A. An alpha motoneuron in the cat ventral horn. The cytoplasm is filled with darkly staining clumps of Nissl substance. From Barr et al. (1950). **B.** Model of a cat motoneuron with small and large synaptic boutons on its surface. Reconstruction from serial sections. From Haggar and Barr (1950).

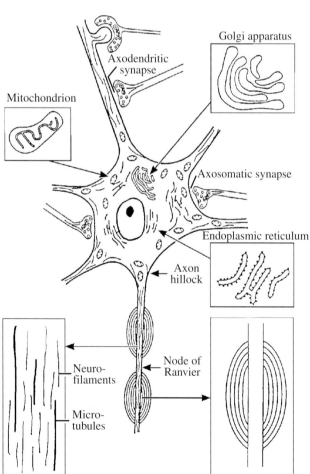

Figure 1-44. Schematic illustration of the organelles and inclusions of a neuron, as revealed by electron microscopy.

The axon of the motoneuron differs from the perikaryon by the presence of a cytoskeleton of neurofilaments and microtubules (Figure 1-44). The axon sometimes follows a circuitous course within the ventral horn and then joins other axons to form the fascicles (Figure 1-45) that exit the ventral horn as rootlets. Jointly the ventral rootlets form a discrete segmental ventral root. Different types of motoneurons have axons of different caliber and conduction velocity (Table 1-3). The long axon conducts action potentials (motor commands) that reach skeletal muscles and autonomic ganglia, many of which are located at a considerable distance from the spinal cord. All components of somatic and visceral motoneurons – the perikaryon, dendrites, and axon – contain the neurotransmitter, acetylcholine (Silver and Wolstencroft, 1971; Barber et al., 1984). Continuous anterograde and retrograde axoplasmic flow ensures the metabolic integrity of the axon and the cycling and recycling of its synaptic vesicles and neurotransmitter at the axon terminal.

1.5.3 The Synaptology of Motoneurons.

It has been calculated that the surface of the perikaryon and dendrites of a motoneuron is covered by at least 50,000 (Ulfhake and Cullheim, 1988), and up to 140,000 (Örnung et al., 1998) boutons or synapses. Some boutons make contact with the smooth surface of the soma or dendrites of the motoneuron, others

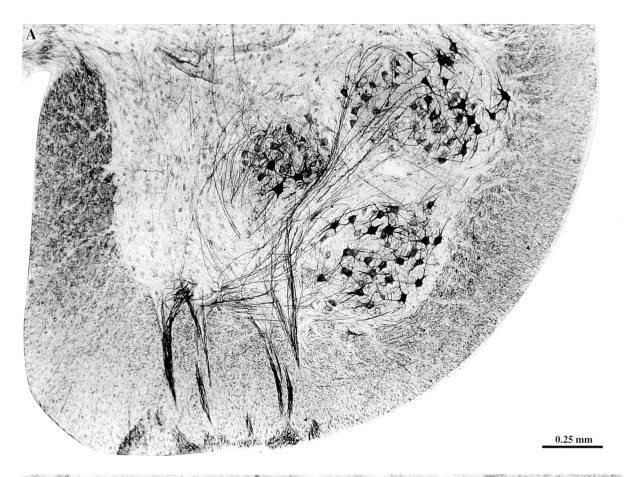

0.25 mm

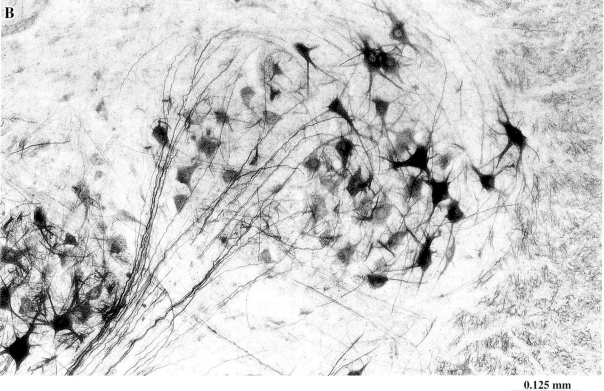

0.125 mm

Figure 1-45. Motoneuron axons in the ventral horn of the lumbar cord of a preterm human neonate, at lower (**A**) and higher (**B**) magnification. Some axons take a straight course to the ventral rootlets, others follow a more roundabout route. Specimen# Y76-60. Bielschowsky's silver stain.

Table 1-3 Varieties of Motor Nerve Fibers (Modified after Ottoson, 1983)				
Fiber type	Function	Innervation	Diameter (μm)	Speed (m/sec)
Aα	somatic	skeletal muscle	70-120	15-20
Aγ	somatic	intrafusal muscle	70-120	15-20
B	visceral	preganglionic	3-15	3
C	visceral	postganglionic	0.5-2	0.5-1

A   Axodendritic Synapses

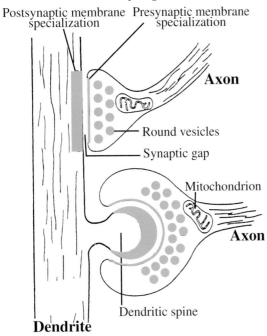

B   Axosomatic Synapses

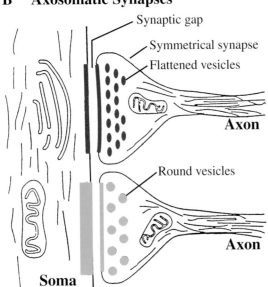

form a cap over the dendritic spines (Figures 1-44, 1-46). Some boutons are filled with round synaptic vesicles and are contiguous with a thick postsynaptic membrane; other boutons contain flattened synaptic vesicles and are associated with a thin postsynaptic membrane (Figure 1-46). Uchizono (1966) hypothesized that boutons containing round vesicles are excitatory, whereas boutons containing flat vesicles are inhibitory. Others (e.g., Bodian, 1966; Gray, 1969) have questioned this generalization. Boutons with round and flat synaptic vesicles intermingle on the surface of motoneurons in a seemingly irregular manner (Figure 1-47a). However, McLaughlin (1972) found that synapses with spherical vesicles are more frequent on the distal dendrites of motoneurons, and synapses with flattened vesicles on the soma and proximal dendrites. Conradi (1969) distinguished six morphological classes of synapses, using such added features as bouton size and complexity of the pre- and postsynaptic membrane. McLaughlin (1972) made a similar classification.

There is biochemical evidence that the principal excitatory transmitter of the efferents that contact motoneurons is glutamate and/or aspartate (Curtis and Watkins, 1960; Engberg et al., 1979; Jessell et al., 1986), and the principal inhibitory transmitter is glycine (Werman et al., 1967) and GABA (Eccles et al., 1963). Immunohistochemical studies have sought

Figure 1-46. A. Asymmetrical axodendritic synapses (green) with round vesicles on a dendrite (**top**) and its spine (**bottom**). In asymmetrical synapses the postsynaptic membrane is thicker than the presynaptic membrane. **B.** A symmetrical axosomatic synapse (red) with flat vesicles (**top**), and an asymmetrical axosomatic synapse with round vesicles (green). In symmetrical synapses the thickness of the postsynaptic is similar to that of the presynaptic membrane. Synapses with round vesicles are probably excitatory (green, "go") while synapses with flat vesicles are inhibitory (red, "stop").

to locate in situ these excitatory and inhibitory synapses (Ljungdahl and Hökfelt, 1973; McLaughlin et al., 1975; Holstege, 1991). Örnung et al. (1998), analyzing nearly 800 boutons on motoneurons, found that 94% were immunoreactive to glutamate, glycine, and/or GABA, supporting the idea that these amino acids are the principal neurotransmitters acting upon motoneurons. Of this total, 35% of the boutons were immunopositive for glutamate, and 59% for glycine and/or GABA (glycine and GABA are frequently co-localized). According to this study, the proportion of glutamate terminals (the putative excitatory transmitters) is higher in distal dendrites than in proximal dendrites, while glycine and/or GABA terminals (the putative inhibitory transmitters) predominate in the proximal dendrites and soma. All boutons immunoreactive to glutamate, contained spherical synaptic vesicles, and all boutons immunoreactive to glycine and GABA had flattened synaptic vesicles. This supports Uchizono's hypothesis (Figure 1-47A). In addition to these amino acid transmitters, several other putative neurotransmitters and neuromodulators have been identified, including noradrenaline, acetylcholine, and several peptides (Shupliakov et al., 1993).

1.5.4 The Electrophysiology of Motoneurons.
Early physiological studies showed that, as judged by the contraction or relaxation of skeletal muscles, the stimulation of dorsal root fibers may either excite or inhibit motoneurons (Sherrington, 1906). This dual excitatory and inhibitory action within the spinal cord, according to Sherrington, is responsible for the reciprocal action of agonistic and antagonistic muscles (e.g., extensors and flexors) when a limb is induced to extend or flex. Later research with the intracellular microelectrode recording technique (Eccles, 1964) established that stimulation of different afferents that synapse with a motoneuron may produce either an excitatory (depolarizing) or an inhibitory (hyperpolarizing) postsynaptic generator potential (EPSP or IPSP) of variable magnitudes (Figure 1-47B). The features of motoneuron excitation and inhibition have been most intensively studied by stimulating Ia muscle spindle fibers that produce the monosynaptic stretch reflex (e.g., Edwards et al., 1976; Sypert and Munson, 1984; Carlen et al., 1984). The results indicate that the amplitude of EPSPs and IPSPs is affected by many variables. These include the number of synapses activated, the amount of transmitter released at a synaptic site, the distance of active synapses from the motoneuron perikaryon, and the duration of synaptic action. The generator poten-

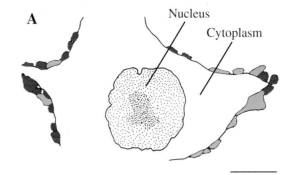

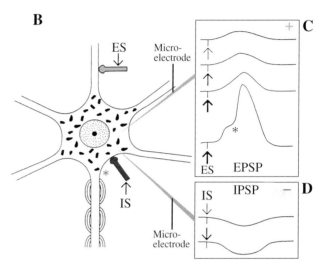

Figure 1-47. A. Excitatory (green) and inhibitory (red) synapses on the soma of a motoneuron in the cat spinal cord. After Uchizono (1966). **B.** Intracellular recording with microelectrodes of electric potentials generated in response to stimulation (arrows) of an excitatory synapse (ES) or an inhibitory synapse (IS). **C.** Stimulation of the excitatory synapse produces a graded EPSP. If the magnitude of the EPSP reaches a critical level, an all-or-none action potential is fired at the axon hillock (asterisk). **D.** Stimulation of the inhibitory synapse produces a graded IPSP that reduces the probability of motoneuron firing. After Eccles (1964).

tials spread decrementally toward the trigger zone of the axon hillock and the integrated sum total of EPSPs and IPSPs determines whether or not a postsynaptic potential of sufficient amplitude reaches the trigger zone to produce an all-or-none action potential. Once an action potential is triggered, it is propagated nondecrementally to its peripheral target, irrespective of the length of the axon, and causes the release of synaptic transmitter, acetylcholine, at the myoneural junction or the autonomic ganglion. There is good evidence that the reciprocal inhibitory influence on antagonistic muscles is mediated by intercalated interneurons (Eccles, 1964; Jankowska and Roberts, 1972). These interneurons are stimulated by Ia afferents and their action produces the inhibition of the motoneuron. Importantly, these interneurons are under the influence not only of Ia afferents but also some efferents, including the collaterals of other motoneurons (Hultborn and Udo, 1972). Like the motoneurons, so also the interneurons integrate excitatory and inhibitory influences acting upon them to produce their particular action.

The axons of motoneuron branch peripherally and their endplates may synapse with a variable number of muscle fibers (Eccles and Sherrington, 1930; Clark, 1931). Because the nondecrementally conducted action potential of the axon mandates the contraction of all muscle fibers that it contacts, and because most muscle fibers are innervated only by a single axon, a motoneuron and its affiliated muscle fibers constitute a tightly-knit functional entity, the motor unit (Liddell and Sherrington, 1925). The number of muscle fibers innervated by a single motoneuron axon (the size of the motor unit) varies in different types of muscle. For instance, in man, the ratio is 1:100 in the intrinsic muscles of the hand but 1:2000 in the gastrocnemius muscle of the leg (Feinstein et al., 1955). Differences in the precision of action and, alternatively, the force produced by different muscles depend on the size of their motor units. Motor units also vary in terms of the type of muscles they innervate, such as fast contracting and easily fatiguing white muscle or slowly contracting and fatigue-resistant red muscle. These two classes have been distinguished as phasic and tonic motor units (Granit et al., 1956). These investigators proposed that motoneurons innervating phasic and tonic muscles have matching properties: phasic motoneurons conduct action potentials faster and at a higher frequency than do tonic motoneurons. This idea received subsequent experimental support (Eccles et al., 1958; Kuno, 1959). Importantly, motor units (and, by implication, the motoneurons) do not act in isolation from one another but are linked together into dynamic motor pools to produce weaker or stronger, and shorter or longer contractions. This is the phenomenon of recruitment (Eccles and Sherrington, 1930). The more motor units are activated simultaneously or successively within a muscle or a group of synergistic muscles, the more powerful and enduring that contraction becomes (Milner-Brown et al., 1973; Desmedt and Godaux, 1977).

1.6   Motoneuron Columns and Subcolumns

1.6.1   Descriptive Studies of Motoneuron Columns. It was known for a long time that motoneurons are not distributed evenly in the ventral horn but form more or less distinct aggregates called motor nuclei. The nuclear organization of motoneurons is typical of all vertebrates: frog, lizard, pigeon, chick, rat, rabbit, guinea pig, cat, dog, and primates (for references see, VanderHorst and Holstege, 1997), including man (Onuf, 1900; Van Gehuchten and de Neef, 1900; Bruce, 1901; Jacobsohn, 1908; Massazza, 1922; Bok, 1928; Elliott, 1942). Although it was recognized by the end of the nineteenth century that the motor nuclei form longitudinal columns (Waldeyer, 1888; Kaiser, 1891) many anatomists referred to them as nuclei. This practice prevails to this day and is justified by the fact that in order to delineate the length of the columns (indeed, their identity) requires laborious reconstruction from serially cut spinal cord sections.

The early terminologies of spinal cord motor nuclei were based on a combination of topographic location and assumed function. Thus, Jacobsohn (1908) distinguished a mediodorsal nucleus with visceromotor (sympathetic) functions, and medioventral nucleus with somatomotor functions in the medial portion of the lumbar enlargement of the human spinal cord (Figure 1-48). In the lateral ventral horn,

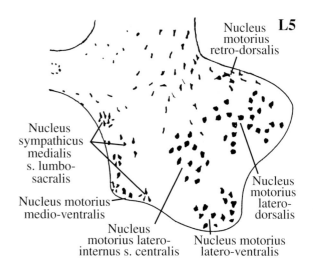

Figure 1-48. Jacobsohn's (1908) terminology applied to the motor nuclei of the lumbar spinal cord (L5) in man. The nomenclature is partly based on presumed function (e.g., sympathicus vs. motorius) and partly on location.

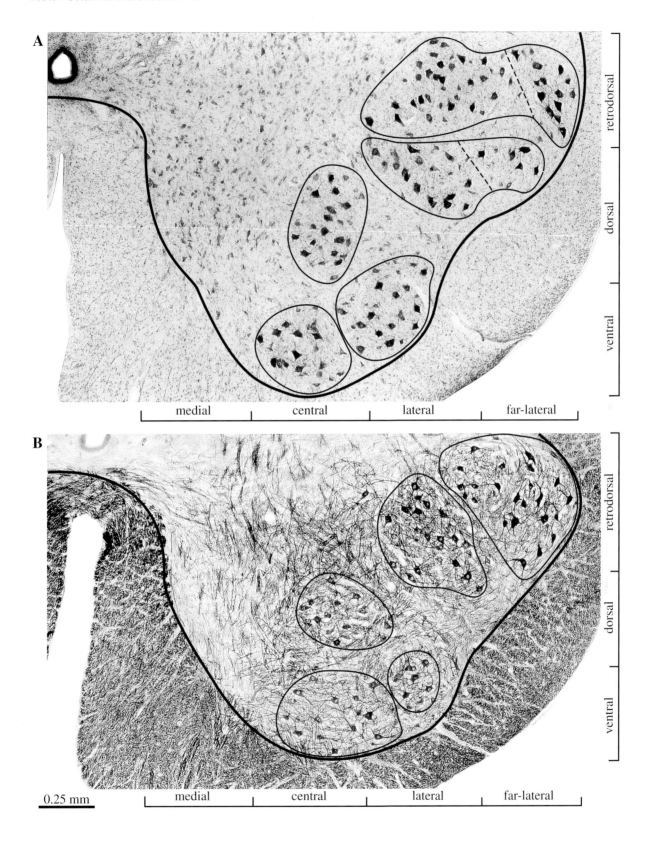

Figure 1-49. Motor nuclei in the lumbar spinal cord of a human neonate, processesd with two different techniques. **A.** In the perikaryon-stained (hematoxylin-eosin) section, the cell-free areas between aggregates of motoneurons provide the basis for drawing the uncertain boundaries of motor nuclei. **B.** In the silver-stained (Bielschowsky) section, regional differences in dendritic architecture and neuropil density provide additional clues. Specimen # Y23-60. The rationale for the vertical and horizontal subdivisons is described in the following pages.

he distinguished four additional sets of motor nuclei with somatomotor functions: (iii) the laterocentral, (iv) the lateroventral, (v) the laterodorsal, and (vi) the retrodorsal. Bruce (1901) proposed a similar subdivision for both the lumbar and cervical enlargement. (The lateral motor columns are absent at thoracic levels.) It was also recognized by the turn of the nineteenth century that there are considerable regional differences in the size and distribution of motor nuclei. In our illustration of the lumbar spinal cord of a human child (Figure 1-49), the medial nuclei appear to be absent, and at least five (rather than four) lateral nuclei can be distinguished in terms of cell clustering in a perikaryon-stained section (Figure 1-49A) and in terms of dendritic architecture in a nearby silver-stained section (Figure 1-49B).

Bruce's (1901) illustration of motoneuron columns at selected spinal cord segments from C1 to S4 has been repeatedly reproduced. The illustration and nomenclature in Figure 1-50 is an adaptation of that from a popular mid-twentieth century textbook of neuroanatomy (Ranson and Clark, 1959). In addition to the naming of motor nuclei in terms of their location, two nuclei (the accessory and the phrenic) are identified in terms of their nerve outflow. Because the medial motor nuclei are present throughout much of the spinal cord, they are generally assumed to be innervating axial (neck, trunk, and tail) muscles. In contrast, the lateral motor nuclei, whose presence creates the cervical and lumbosacral enlargements, has been assumed to supply motor fibers to the brachial and lumbosacral plexuses that innervate the appendicular muscles of the forelimb and hind limb, respectively. Since the lateral motor nuclei are absent at thoracic levels, it is evident that the similarly named nuclei at cervical and lumbar levels do not form a continuous column. This was recognized by Elliott (1944) who, in a comparative study of the motor columns in cat, dog and man, described a total of 21 columns: 8 of them in the cervical cord and 7 at lumbosacral levels.

In most illustrations of the ventral horn (as in Figure 1-50), the successive cord segments are realistically aligned from rostral to caudal in relation to the central canal. In Figures 1-51 and 1-52 we modified this by aligning six selected segments with reference to the medial wall of the gray matter. Doing this permits us to divide the ventral horn into a maximum of four vertical *panels* – the medial, central, lateral,

and far-lateral – and a maximum of three horizontal *tiers* – the ventral, dorsal, and retrodorsal. Within this idealized 3x4 grid we can roughly assign a motor column at any level of the spinal cord to one or more of a maximum of 12 "sectors." (We shall return later to the possible functional significance of these "sectors.")

Examining the six selected sections in Figure 1-51, it appears that the slender ventral horn at C1 has only two panels (medial, central) and two tiers (ventral, dorsal), and all four sectors (medial ventral, medial dorsal, central ventral, central dorsal) are occupied by a variable number of motoneurons. The expanding ventral horn at C4 has an additional panel, the lateral, and the greatly expanded ventral horn at C8 has an additional panel, the far-lateral, and an additional tier, the retrodorsal. Not all potential sectors are actually present at C8 (note the narrow ventral tier) and not all existing sectors (note the central panel) are occupied by motor columns. Turning to the selected thoracic and lumbar segments in Figure 1-52, motoneurons are present at T2 in the two existing panels (medial, central) and two tiers (ventral, dorsal). At L2, motoneurons are also present in the lateral panel and the retrodorsal tier. At L4, the far-lateral panel has sectors only in the dorsal and retrodorsal tiers. In Figure 1-53 we offer a revised motor column nomenclature for the 11 segments previously shown in Figure 1-50. The assigned names are based on the location of the motor column within the idealized 3x4 grid. (We replaced the directional terms *anterior* with *ventral*, and *posterior* with *dorsal*.)

1.6.2   *Experimental Studies of Motoneuron Subcolumns.*

The task of determining what muscles or muscle groups are innervated by motoneurons of a specific column, referred to by earlier investigators as the problem of motor localization, had to await the introduction of reliable experimental techniques. Earlier experimenters used the retrograde degeneration (chromatolysis) of motoneurons with some success following transection of portions of the cervical or lumbosacral plexus, or of an individual nerve root (e.g., Marinesco, 1898; Bikeles, 1905; Knape, 1901; Goering, 1928; Sprague, 1948). In a landmark study, Romanes (1951) described chromatolytic changes in discrete motor columns following stimulation of selected ventral roots with electric pulses for up to 10.5 hours. Romanes distinguished 8 different columns in the lumbosacral enlargement (L4 and S2)

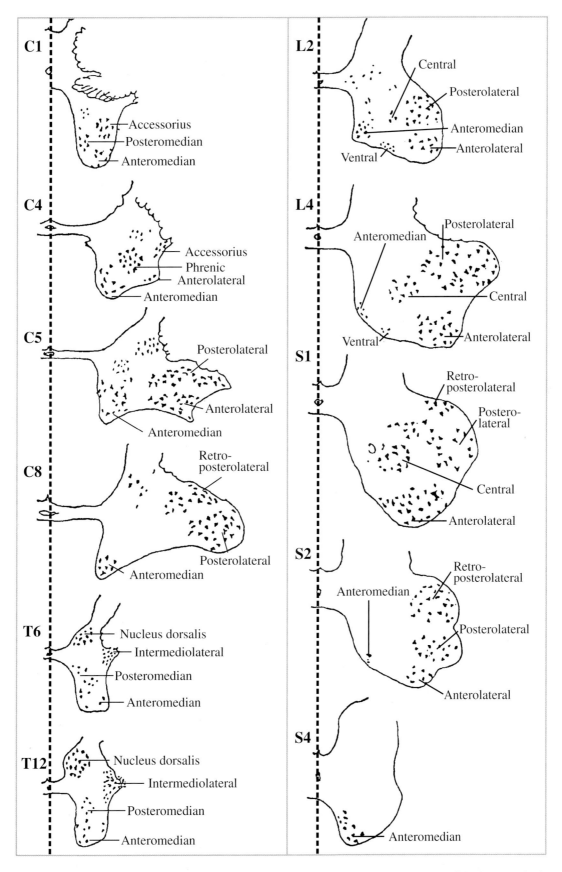

Figure 1-50. Motor column nomenclature applied to 11 selected segments (C1–S4) of the human spinal cord by Bruce (1901), and Ranson and Clark (1959). The original illustration was modified by aligning the cord segments with reference to the central canal (broken vertical lines).

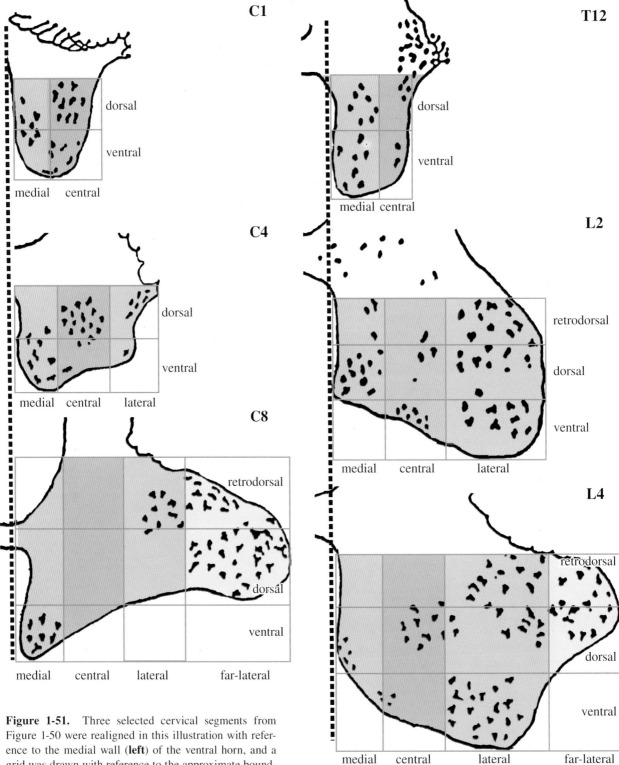

Figure 1-51. Three selected cervical segments from Figure 1-50 were realigned in this illustration with reference to the medial wall (**left**) of the ventral horn, and a grid was drawn with reference to the approximate boundaries of the different motor columns. The vertical lines delineate up to four potential *panels*, and the horizontal lines up to three potential *tiers* in the ventral horn at different segmental levels. The 3x4 grid provides a maximum of 12 ventral cord *sectors*. The number of actual sectors varies at different segmental levels and, even where present, the sector may be devoid of motor columns (e.g., the central panel in C8). There are only 4 sectors in C1, 6 sectors in C4, and 10 occupied sectors in C8.

Figure 1-52. Application of the 3x4 grid to the ventral horn of one thoracic and two lumbar segments selected from Figure 1-50. At T12, there are only 4 sectors present, at L2, there are 8 occupied sectors, and at L4, as many as 11 occupied sectors. The concentration of motoneurons varies in different sectors, not all existing sectors are occupied by motoneurons, and some motor columns may occupy more than one sector.

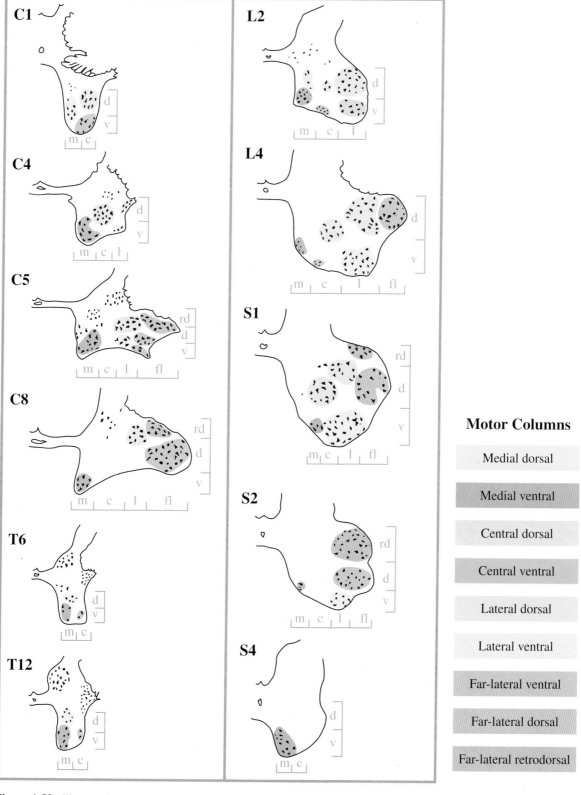

Figure 1-53. Motor column nomenclature based on the 3x4 grid system and applied to all cord segments illustrated in Figure 1-50. (Posterior was replaced by *dorsal*, and anterior by *ventral*.) Each column (see color code) is identified by its grid location: the first term indicates its panel coordinate (m, c, l, fl). the second term its tier coordinate (v, d, rd). In some cases a column identified in one segment can be traced through many segments of the spinal cord (e.g., medial ventral from C4 to S4). In other cases a column of the same name (e.g., far-lateral retrodorsal) is present only at select levels. That discontinuity indicates that the two are discrete columns and, therefore, have to be distinguished by their specific location (cervical or lumbar).

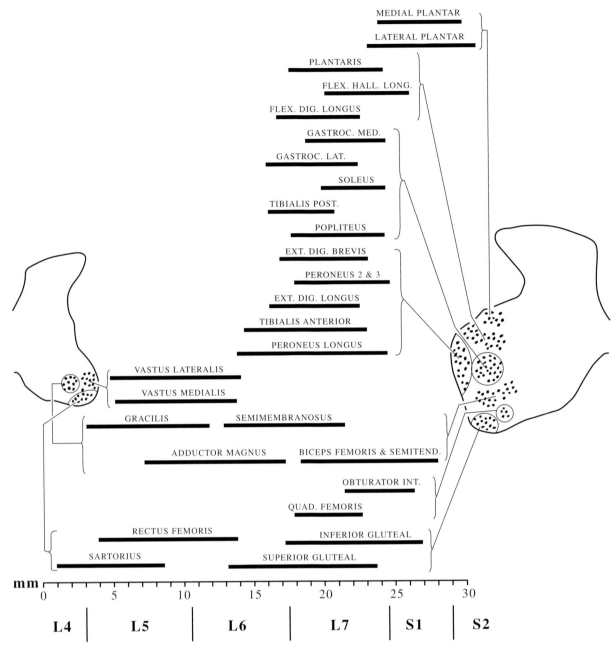

Figure 1-54. Location of motor columns (heavy horizontal lines) between L4 and S2 in the lumbosacral spinal cord of the cat in relation to the muscles they innervate. The experimental technique involved the prolonged and intense stimulation of a select muscle with electric current and the subsequent localization of degenerating (chromatolytic) motoneurons in the spinal cord. After Romanes (1951).

and concluded that, with considerable overlap, there is a rostral-to-caudal and medial-to-lateral shift in the location of motoneurons in relation to the proximodistal order of the muscle groups they innervate (Figure 1-54). Romanes' results were summarized in functional terms by Rustioni et al. (1971), and are shown in modified form in Figure 1-55. Motoneurons that innervate the proximal hip muscles are located medially from L4 to L7. Motoneurons that act on the knee muscles are located more laterally and dorsally

from L5 to L7. Motoneurons that act on distal ankle and toe joints are located still more caudally (L6 to L7, and L7 to S2, respectively), and farther dorsally and laterally.

The newer technique of applying tracers to discrete motor nerves or isolated muscles has made the experimental analysis of motoneuron localization much easier and far more reliable. Among the tracers used for this purpose are the retrogradely transported

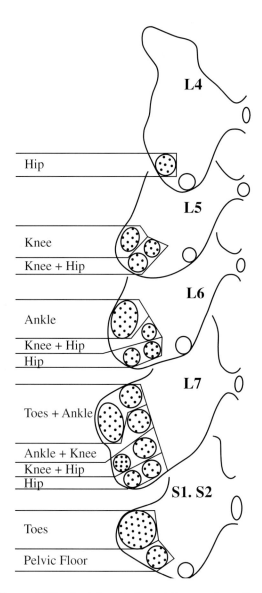

Figure 1-55. An interpretation of Romanes' results in terms of the functions of the muscles innervated by the different motor columns. Motoneurons that control the proximal hip muscles are located more medially and ventrally than those that control the muscles of the extremities. Motoneurons that control the muscles of the knee, ankle, and toes are located more laterally, and in a rostral-to-caudal sequence After Rustioni et al. (1971).

enzyme horseradish peroxidase (HRP), various conjugates of HRP, several fluorescent dyes, and viral cell markers. With a few exceptions noted below, most of these studies were limited to a few nerves or muscles, and differed in experimental methodology. in particular, whether the tracer was applied to a nerve or injected into a muscle. Indeed, there is currently no report available from a single laboratory that has examined the innervation of the principal muscles of the entire body in a single species.

We review below the localization of motoneurons at upper cervical, lower cervical, thoracic, lumbosacral, and sacrocaudal levels of the spinal cord, with particular reference to the innervation of the muscles of the neck, shoulder, arm, wrist, and hand; the thorax and abdomen; and the hip, thigh, leg, foot, and toes. In most of these experiments the location of the retrogradely labeled motoneurons has not been correlated with the nuclei or columns of descriptive histology. We will, therefore, refer to the motoneuron cell groups identified with the tracer technique as "subcolumns" and will reserve the term "columns" for the cell aggregates of descriptive histology.

1.6.3 Motoneuron Subcolumns in the Upper Cervical Cord. We begin with a review of current physiological tracer studies that have dealt with muscle groups that act on: (i) the head and neck, (ii) the diaphragm, (iii) the shoulder joints, and (iv) the joints of the forearm, wrist and hand. We will deal with the relevant muscles or muscle groups in a rostrocaudal order and, in the case of limb muscles, in a proximodistal sequence.

Most studies concerned with the localization of motoneurons of neck muscles that move the head or stabilize its position were carried out in the cat (Figure 1-56). According to Kitamura and Richmond (1994), the retrogradely labeled motoneurons that supply the ventral and lateral suboccipital muscles (rectus capitis anterior and rectus capitis lateralis) are clustered medially in the ventral horn. Of these, the motoneurons supplying the rectus capitis lateralis are confined to the C1 segment, those supplying rectus capitis anterior are distributed from C1 to C4. The motoneurons innervating the dorsal suboccipital muscles have a separate distribution more ventrally. The motoneurons of rectus capitis posterior are clustered mostly in the ventromedial nucleus, whereas the motoneurons innervating complexus and obliquus capitis superior are clustered dorsomedial to the rectus capitis posterior motoneurons. The motoneurons that supply the rectus capitis major and rectus capitis minor are interdigitated in this location (Gordon and Richmond, 1991).

Rapoport et al. (1978) investigated the localization of motoneurons of two neck muscles, the sternocleidomastoid and trapezius. The motoneurons of the sternocleidomastoid (a ventral muscle that acts as a head flexor and rotator) were located at C1 and C2

A. SHOULDER, ARM   **B. ARM, WRIST, DIGITS**

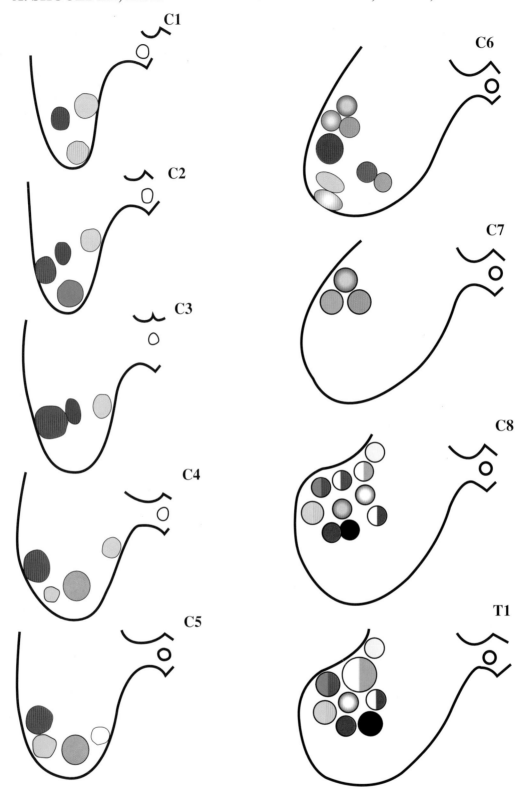

Figure 1-56. Localization of motoneuron subcolumns in the upper cervical (**A**) and brachial (**B**) spinal cord of the cat. Selected data from experimental work by different investigators with different techniques (HRP, flourescent dyes, and other tracers). The location and size of the subcolumns are schematic. The muscles or muscle groups innervated by the color-coded subcolumns, and source references, are given in the Table on the next page.

Table for Figure 1-56

Code	Segment	Muscle	Investigators
◐	C1	Oblique capitis internus	Kitamura and Richmond (1994)
		Rectus capitis posterior	Kitamura and Richmond (1994)
●	C1-C3	Sternomastoid; Cleidomastoid	Rapaport (1978); Liinamaa et al.(1997)
○	C1-C4	Rectus capitis anterior lateralis	Kitamura and Richmond (1994)
◉	C2	Semispinalis cervici; Spinalis dorsalis	Gordon and Richmond (1991)
◍	C2-C6	Trapezius	Rapaport (1978); Vanner and Rose (1984)
			Liinamaa et al. (1997)
◉	C4-C6	Diaphragm	Webber et al. (1997); and others.
○	C4-C6	Rhomboideus minor and major	Liinamaa et al. (1997)
◕	C6	Deltoid	Liinamaa et al. (1997)
○	C6	Radialis	Liinamaa et al. (1997)
○	C4-C6	Levator scapula	Fritz et al. (1986a)
○	C6-C7	Extensor carpi radialis (Brachioradialis)	Fritz et al. (1986a)
◍	C6-C7	Supinator	Fritz et al. (1986b)
○	C7	Flexor carpi radialis, Pronator teres	Fritz et al. (1986a)
◑	C8-T1	Extensor digitorum communis,	Fritz et al. (1986a)
		Extensor digitorum lateralis	Fritz et al. (1986a)
●	C8-T1	Extensor carpi ulnaris	Fritz et al. (1986a)
○	C8-T1	Abductor pollicis longus	Fritz et al. (1986a)
○	C8-T1	Extensor indicis proprius	Fritz et al. (1986b)
◐	C8-T1	Flexor digitorum profundus (1-5)	Fritz et al. (1986b)
○	C8-T1	Median hand	Fritz et al. (1986b)
●	C8-T1	Flexor carpi ulnaris	Fritz et al. (1986b)
◖	C8-T1	Ulnar hand (Ramis palmaris profundus)	Fritz et al. (1986b)
◑	C8-T1	Palmaris longus	Fritz et al. (1986b)

in the mediodorsal sector. The highest concentration of trapezius motoneurons (the trapezius acts as a head extensor and rotator, and as an elevator of the scapula) was seen more caudally and ventrally at C2-C4. Vanner and Rose (1984), in a more detailed study, obtained somewhat different results. The trapezius muscle in the cat is composed of three heads that insert into the clavicle and the scapula. Vanner and Rose found that HRP injected into the clavotrapezius labeled motoneurons mainly in C2 and C3, most acromiotrapezius motoneurons were located in C3-C5, whereas the spinotrapezius motoneurons were distributed in C4-C6. The motoneurons of the trapezius muscle as a whole formed a single straight subcolumn from C2 to C6. Similar results were obtained by Liinamaa et al. (1997). They located the motoneurons of trapezius, sternomastoid, and cleidomastoid muscles within a single motor column that stretched from the spinomedullary junction to the middle of C6. Within this column, the motoneurons of sternomastoid, cleidomastoid, and trapezius formed subcolumns that were aligned in a medial-to-lateral order. The sternomastoid and cleidomastoid motoneurons were confined to the upper cervical segments, whereas the trapezius motoneurons, as previously reported by Vanner and Rose (1984), extended to C6. Richmond et al. (1978) and Keirstead and Rose (1983) studied the distribution of motoneurons of splenius. They found that different subunits of this complex muscle supplied by C2, C3 and C4 nerves are arranged in discrete subcolumns.

Several studies have dealt with the localization of motoneurons of the phrenic nerve, which innervates the muscles of the diaphragm. Webber et al. (1979) reported that, following intradiaphragmatic injection of HRP, the labeled phrenic motoneurons formed a compact, 17-21 mm long medioventral sub-

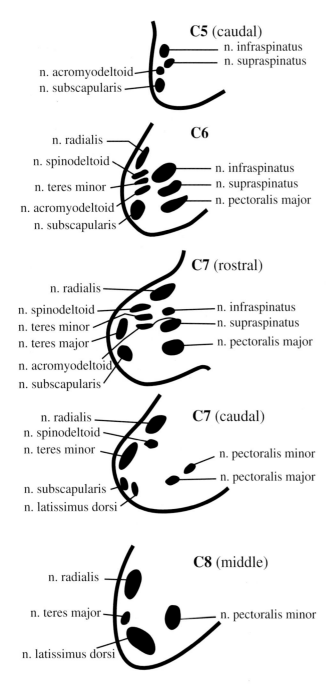

Figure 1-57. Motoneuron subcolumns of 11 motor nerves that innervate the muscles of the arm. The motoneurons are distributed between C5 and C8. After Hörner and Kümmel (1993). Monkey; fluorochrome tracer technique.

column from C4 to C6. The concentration of motoneurons was highest at the junction of C5 and C6, with cell concentration tapering off symmetrically in both rostral and caudal directions. This localization in the cat was confirmed by others (e.g., Rikard-Bell and Bystrzycka, 1980; Cameron et al., 1983).

1.6.4   Motoneuron Subcolumns in the Lower Cervical (Brachial) Cord.

In the cat, the motoneurons of the rhomboid nerve, which innervate the shoulder muscles of rhomboid minor and rhomboid major, form a single slender subcolumn between C4 to C6 in the cervical enlargement (Liinamaa et al., 1997; Figure 1-56). These motoneurons are situated lateral to the motoneurons that innervate the deep neck muscles. By using different tracers to distinguish motoneurons that are the source of specific bundles of the rhomboid nerve, discrete subcolumns could be identified that are arranged in a rostrocaudal sequence in register with the rostrocaudal order of the nerve bundles. In the rat, the motoneurons of the acromiodeltoid and spinodeltoid muscles, two prime movers of the shoulder joint, are located laterally in the ventral horn at C5-C7 (Choi and Hoover, 1996). The motoneurons of the acromiodeltoid are located rostral and medial to the motoneurons of the spinodeltoid.

Hörner and Kümmel (1993) injected fluorochrome tracers into 11 spinal nerves that innervate the shoulder muscles in monkeys. Their results indicate that the motor fibers in each of these nerves originates in discrete subcolumns at C5 to T1, some extending over two segments, others occupying several segments (Figure 1-57; T1 is not shown). The motor subcolumns of the nerves that innervate the infraspinatus and supraspinatus muscles (which abduct and rotate the arm laterally) are distributed more medially from C5, C6 and C7 in two adjacent subcolumns. The motoneurons of the nerves that innervate the spinodeltoid, acromiodeltoid, and teres minor muscles (which likewise abduct and rotate the arm laterally) form short subcolumns through C6 and C7 in a more lateral position. The subcolumns of three other shoulder muscles, subscapularis, pectoralis major, and teres major (which rotate the arm medially) are also short (from C6 to C7). Situated more ventrally and caudally are the motoneuron subcolumns of lattisimus dorsi (between C7 to C8) and pectoralis minor (between C7 to T1). Most extensive is the subcolumn of the radial nerve, which occupies a retrodorsal position and extends all the way from C6 to T1. This subcolumn may be made up of two components, one rostral and the other caudal. The latter may innervate the more distal muscles of the forearm and hand.

The tracer studies of Fritz et al. (1986a, b), in the cat, supplement the localizations of Liinamaa and associates in the cat and Hörner and Kümmel's in the monkey. Fritz et al. (1986a) found that the motoneurons of the extensor carpi radialis and brachioradialis form a far-lateral subcolumn from rostral C6 to caudal C7. The motoneurons of supinator are lined up more medially. More caudally and dorsolaterally, extending from rostral C8 to the middle of T1, discrete subcolumns are formed by motoneurons of the extensor carpi ulnaris and abductor pollicis longus (ventrally), of the extensor indicis proprius (in an intermediate position), and of the extensor digitorum communis and extensor digitorum longus (dorsally). The motoneurons of the median nerve (Fritz et al., 1986b) extend from the middle of C7 to the middle of T1. The motoneurons of flexor carpi radialis and pronator teres are located in C7. Farther caudally, extending from C8 to T1, are the subcolumns of pronator quadratus (ventrally), palmaris longus (in intermediate position), and the motoneurons of flexor digitorum profundus 3,4, and 5 (dorsally). Farther dorsally (perhaps situated in the far-lateral retrodorsal sector) in C8 and T1 are the motoneurons of the median hand. The motoneurons of the ulnar nerve (Fritz et al., 1986b) extend from the middle of C8 to the middle of T1. Farthest ventrally are the motoneurons of flexor carpi ulnaris, and farthest laterally are the motoneurons of flexor digitorum profundus. The motoneurons of the ulnar hand (ramus palmaris profundus) are situated retrodorsally.

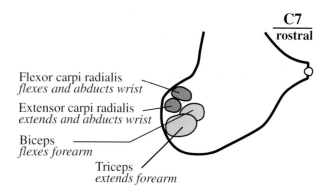

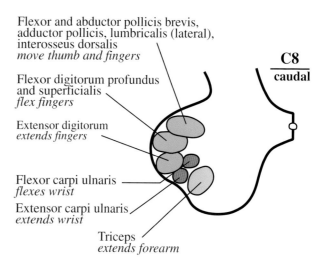

Figure 1-58. Motoneuron subcolumns that innervate the muscles of the forearm, wrist, and hand in the monkey. After Jenny and Inukei (1983).

In the monkey, Jenny and Inukei (1983) sought to determine the segmental location and columnar organization of motoneurons innervating 18 selected muscles of the forearm and hand. They found that the subcolumn of the biceps brachii (which acts on the elbow joint to flex and supinate the forearm) is distributed from C5 to C7, while that of the triceps brachii (which extends the forearm) is between C6 and C8 (Figure 1-58). The biceps motoneurons are located dorsal to the triceps motoneurons. Both subcolumns are located near the border of the white matter rostrally but as the gray matter expands more caudally, the subcolumns become displaced medially by other subcolumns occupying that position near the white matter. The motoneurons of the flexor carpi radialis (the muscle that flexes and abducts the hand) are located dorsolaterally in C6 and C7, while the motoneurons of extensor carpi radialis (which extends the hand) are located more ventrally in C7 and C8. The motoneurons of the flexor carpi ulnaris (which bends the wrist) and the extensor carpi ulnaris (which

steadies the wrist) are located in C8 and T1 ventrally, and the motoneurons that supply the intrinsic hand muscles are located in the same segments dorsally and retrodorsally. In general, the subcolumns of motoneurons that innervate forearm muscles are longer and begin more rostrally than those thta innervate wrist muscles. The motoneurons that innervate the forearm and the wrist shift ventromedially as the motoneurons innervating the digits emerge in the caudal segments. The motoneurons that innervate the digits are located retrodorsally and far-laterally in the most caudal segments of the cervical enlargement. Finally, the extensor subcolumns tend to be situated ventrolateral to flexor subcolumns.

1.6.5 Motoneuron Subclumns in the Thoracic Cord.
The slender thoracic cord differs from the lower cervical cord by the absence of lateral, far-lateral and retrodorsal motor columns. A study in the rat by Smith and Hollyday (1983) showed that the

motoneurons of the thoracic cord whose axons course in the dorsal ramus and the ventral ramus form separate subcolumns. Those motoneurons whose axons course in the dorsal ramus (which innervate muscles like the longissimus, levator costae, and transversospinalis) form subcolumns ventromedially, whereas the motoneurons whose axons course in the ventral ramus (which innervate muscles like the external and internal intercostal, and external oblique) form subcolumns ventrolaterally. More so than in other regions of the spinal cord, the motoneurons of the thoracic cord tend to be restricted to the segments from which their axons exit via the ventral roots (Tsering, 1992).

1.6.6   Motoneuron Subcolumns in the Lumbosacral Cord.

The motoneuron localization in the lumbosacral spinal cord has been studied with modern tracer techniques more extensively than any other region of the spinal cord. Some of these investigations were limited to the location of motoneurons of a single muscle or a few muscles, others dealt more comprehensively with many muscle groups. We start this review with studies that deal with motoneurons of select muscles, and will consider them in a proximodistal order, beginning with those that act upon the joints of the hip, knee and ankle, and ending with the intrinsic muscles of the foot and toes.

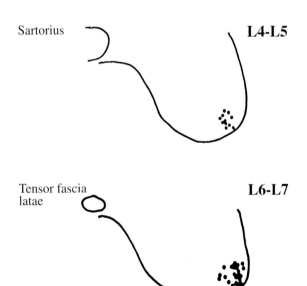

Figure 1-59. Distribution of motoneurons of sartorius and tensor fascia latae (two thigh muscles) in the lumbar spinal cord of the cat. These subcolumns may be located within a single column (lateral ventral?) in a rostrocaudal sequence. After Gordon et al. (1991).

Gordon et al. (1991) studied the topographic distribution of motoneurons that innervate two thigh muscles in the cat, the sartorius and tensor fasciae latae (Figure 1-59). Motoneurons that supply different parts of sartorius muscle and produce different mechanical actions were found to be intermingled in a single subcolumn ventrolaterally that stretches between L4 and L5. Motoneurons that supply different parts of the tensor fasciae latae were intermingled in the same subcolumn between L6 and L7. Apparently, the functional specialization within these thigh muscles is not correlated with an obvious segregation of their motoneurons. Brown et al. (1998) studied the distribution of motoneurons of caudofemoralis and gluteus maximus by applying different tracers to the two muscles. They found that the caudofemoralis motoneurons were distributed between L7 and S1 and overlapped extensively with the motoneurons of gluteus maximus. In coronal sections of the spinal cord the two appeared to be situated in the same motor column. The location and length of the subcolumns was bilaterally symmetrical within an animal but varied between animals. The typical length of the gluteus maximus subcolumn was about 1–1.5 segments. Burke et al (1977) investigated the distribution of motoneurons of gastrocnemius (which flexes the knee and ankle) and soleus (an ankle flexor). The motoneurons of these two muscles overlapped in a single dorsolateral subcolumn in segments L7 and S1, with the soleus motoneurons being distributed somewhat rostral to the gastrocnemius motoneurons (Figure 1-60). According to Weeks and English (1987), the motoneurons of the cat lateral gastrocnemius that innervate proximal muscle compartments are situated rostral to those motoneurons that innervate more distal compartments. A similar distribution of gastrocnemius motoneurons was reported by other investigators in the rat spinal cord (Rotto-Percelay et al., 1992; Hirakawa et al., 1992).

The localization of motoneurons of different components of the peroneal muscles has been studied in the cat by Horcholle-Bossavit et al. (1988). The largest of them, peroneus longus, is an ankle dorsiflexor, the peroneus brevis is an ankle extensor, and the small peronius tertius extends and abducts the fifth digit. The motoneurons of these foot muscles occupied thin subcolumns ventrolaterally in segments L6–S1 (Figure 1-61). The peroneus tertius motoneurons were situated dorsolaterally, those of the peroneus longus ventromedially, and the motoneurons

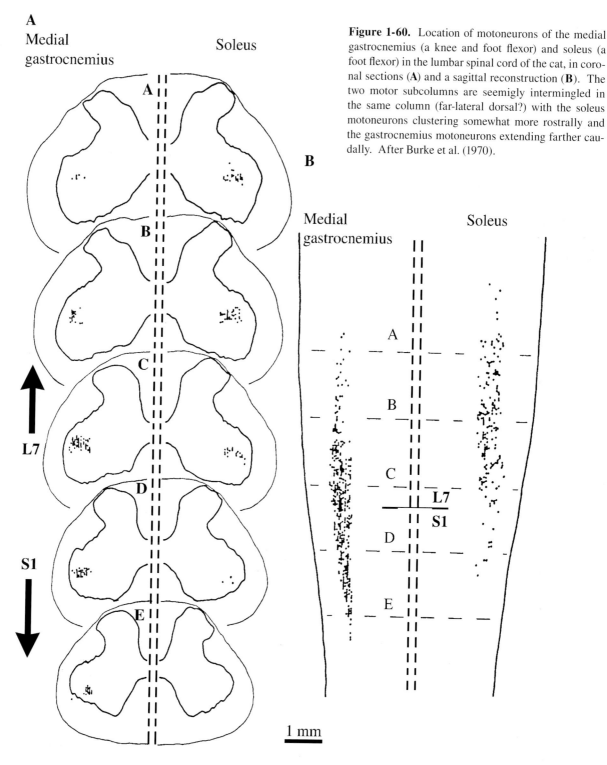

A
Medial
gastrocnemius   Soleus

B

Figure 1-60. Location of motoneurons of the medial gastrocnemius (a knee and foot flexor) and soleus (a foot flexor) in the lumbar spinal cord of the cat, in coronal sections (**A**) and a sagittal reconstruction (**B**). The two motor subcolumns are seemigly intermingled in the same column (far-lateral dorsal?) with the soleus motoneurons clustering somewhat more rostrally and the gastrocnemius motoneurons extending farther caudally. After Burke et al. (1970).

Medial
gastrocnemius   Soleus

1 mm

of peroneus brevis were in an intermediate position and overlapped with the other two subcolumns. Similar localizations were reported in other species (e.g., (McHanwell and Biscoe, 1981; Nicolopoulos-Stournaras and Iles, 1983). Hoover and Durkovic (1991) compared the distribution of motoneurons of two distally acting muscles, extensor digitorum longus (which extends digits II-V) and tibialis anterior (which dorsiflexes the ankle) with the distribution of motoneurons of semitendinosus, a proximal muscle that flexes the knee (Figure 1-62). The motoneurons of tibialis anterior occupied a dorsolateral position in L7 while the motoneurons of extensor digitorum longus occupied a retrodorsal position; the motoneurons of semitendinosus were distributed from L6 to S1 in a more ventral and medial position.

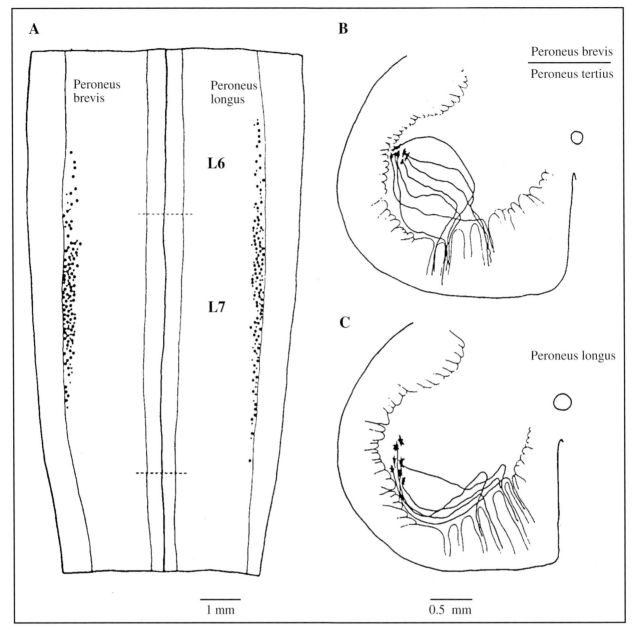

Figure 1-61. A. Location of the motor subcolumns of two components of the peroneal muscle in the cat, peroneus brevis (an ankle extensor) and peroneus longus (an ankle dorsiflexor). **B.** The axon trajectory of peroneus brevis and peroneus tertius motoneurons. **C.** The different axon trajectory of peroneus longus motoneurons. After Horcholle-Bossavit et al. (1988).

The most extensive study of motoneuronal localization of the lumbosacral cord was carried out recently by Vanderhorst and Holstege (1997) who injected HRP into 50 different muscles, or muscle compartments of the lower back, pelvic floor and hindlimb in the cat. Vanderhorst and Holstege classified these muscles into 10 groups: I, sartorius and iliopsoas; II, quadriceps; III, adductors; IV, hamstrings; V, gluteal and other proximal muscles of the hip; VI, posterior compartment of the distal hindlimb; VII, anterior compartment of the distal hindlimb; VIII, long flexors and intrinsic muscles of the foot; IX, pelvic floor muscles; and X, extensors of the lower

back and tail. Their results indicated that in spite of individual variability in the size and segmental organization of the different subcolumns, the spatial relationship among them was constant. We summarize schematically some of Vanderhorst and Holstege's findings in Figure 1-63. Their findings confirm (in broad outline, though not in all details) the earlier results of Romanes, and support four traditional generalizations. First, the motoneurons of the axial musculature are located medially. Second, the motoneurons that innervate proximal muscles (with the exception of two thigh muscles, tensor fascia latae and gluteus medius) are located in rostral segments of

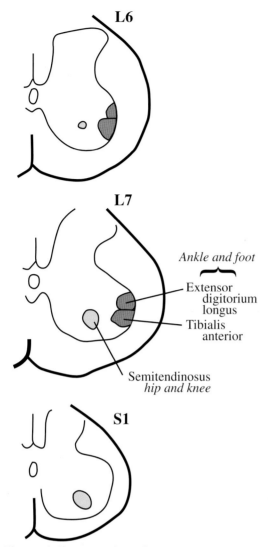

Figure 1-62. Location of motoneurons of three hindlimb muscles in the cat lumbosacral spinal cord. The semitendinosus (green) is situated in the lateral panel. The tibialis anterior (red) is situated in the far-lateral panel. The distal extensor digitorum longus (red) is situated in the same panel retrodorsally. After Hoover and Durkovic (1991). Fluoresent tracer technique.

CODE	MUSCLE OR MUSCLE GROUP	NERVE	TARGET
1 red	Iliopsoas	Femoral	hip
1' blue	Sartorius	Femoral	hip and knee
2 green	Quadriceps	Femoral	hip and knee
3 purple	Adductors	Obturator	hip and knee
4 pink	Hamstrings	Tibial	hip and knee
5 black	Proximal hip	Gluteal	hip
6 blue	Posterior hind limb	Tibial	Ankle
7 green	Anterior hind limb	Peroneal	foot
8 purple	Intrinsic foot	Tibial	foot
10 brown	Axial muscles	Vertebral	

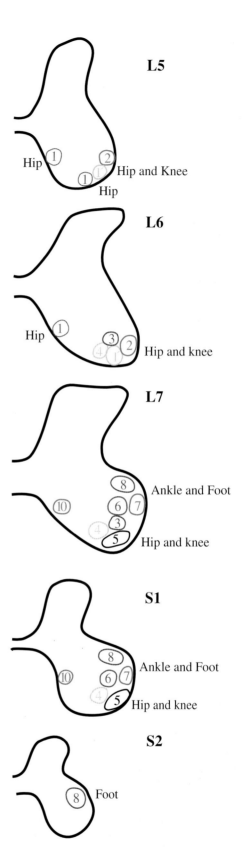

Figure 1-63. Approximate location of 10 groups of motor subcolumns that innervate different hindlimb muscle groups in the lumbosacral spinal cord of the cat. Group 9 moto-neurons, which innervate the urogenital system by the way of the pudendal nerve, is not shown. Schematic rendering, after Vanderholst and Holstege (1997). HRP technique.

the lumbosacral enlargement and those that inner-vate distal muscles are situated more caudally. Third, motoneurons of proximal muscles tend to be located ventrally within a segment, and those of distal mus-cles progressively more dorsally and laterally. Fourth, the motoneurons of the ankle and foot muscles are located retrodorsally and far-laterally in caudal seg-ments of the lumbosacral spinal cord.

1.6.7   Motoneuron Subcolumns in the Sacrocaudal Cord.

Distinct from the ventrolateral motoneurons of the lumbosacral enlargement that innervate the skeletal muscles of the hip and lower extremities, are the motoneurons of the lower sacral spinal cord that innervate the striated muscles of the anal and urogenital systems. Some of these moto-neurons innervate striated muscles responsible for the voluntary control of micturition and defecation (continence); others are parasympathetic pregangli-onic neurons that regulate the autonomic functions of these systems. The smooth muscles include the anal and urethral sphincter muscles, and the ischio-cavernosus and bulbospongiosus. The axons of these somatic and visceral motoneurons reach their targets by way of the pelvic (Kawatani et al., 1986) and the pudendal (Roppolo et al., 1985) nerves.

According to traditional accounts, the motor fibers of the pudendal nerve originate in Onuf's nucleus (Onuf, 1900; Schrøder, 1981; Figure 1-64). In man, Onuf's nucleus is located, with some individ-ual variability, in S1, S2 and S3 (Schrøder, 1981) or it may be limited to S1 (Pullen et al., 1997). The length of the nucleus is 4-7 mm, and it contains an average of 625 motoneurons (Pullen et al., 1997). Tracers applied to the pudendal nerve in the rat label moto-neurons located at L6 and L7 in a dorsomedial and ventrolateral position (Schrøder, 1980; McKenna and Nadelhaft, 1986; Collins, et al. 1992; Peshori et al., 1995). A similar localization has been obtained fol-lowing the application of a tracer to the bladder or the external urethral sphincter muscle (Marson, 1997). In the cat and dog, labeled motoneurons were located more caudally in L7, S1 and S2 (De Groat et al., 1978; Sato et al., 1978; Kuzuhara et al., 1980; Ueyama, et al., 1984); and in the monkey at L7 and S1 (Roppolo et al., 1985) or S1 and S2 (Rajaofetra et al., 1992). It appears that in the rat, motoneurons of the dorsome-dial subcolumn innervate the external anal sphinc-ter, and motoneurons of the ventrolateral subcolumn innervate the external urethral sphincter and the

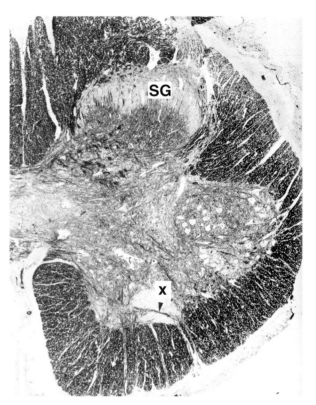

Figure 1-64. Location of Onuf's nucleus (x, pale region) in the central ventral sector of S2 in the human spinal cord. SG, substantia gelatinosa. From Schrøder (1981). Mahon myelin stain.

ischiocavernosus. In the cat, the dorsomedial subcol-umn is retrogradely labeled following application of the tracer to the external anal sphincter, and the ven-tromedial subcolumn is labeled following application of the tracer to the ischiocavernosus (Figure 1-65). At present it is not clear which subcolumns of the sacro-caudal cord innervate striated muscles and which innervate the pelvic viscera. (We shall deal in Sec-tion 1.7.2 with some fragmentary data relating to the columnar organization of the sacral parasympathetic motoneurons.)

The nuclei of the lumbar spinal cord that innervate the muscles involved in copulation are sexu-ally dimorphic in the rat: they contain far more moto-neurons in the male than in the female (Breedlove and Arnold, 1981; McKenna and Nadelhaft, 1986; Figure 1-66). This numerical difference, and the dimorphism in the size and dendritic complexity of motoneurons, is under hormonal control (Jordan et al., 1982; Breedlove and Arnold, 1983; Sengelaub and Arnold, 1989; Goldstein and Sengelaub, 1993; Hodges et al. 1993; Matsumoto, 1997). The sexually dimorphic pudendal motoneurons are distinguished by a high concentration of vasopressin receptor sites

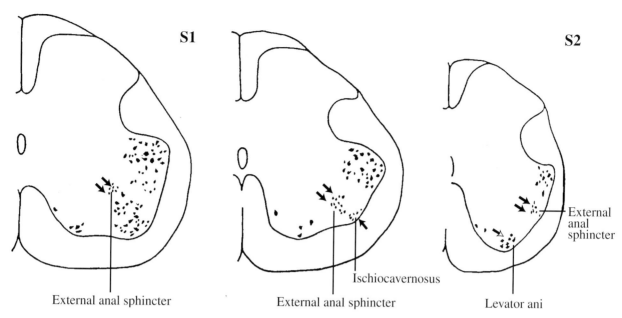

Figure 1-65. Labeled motoneurons in the sacral spinal cord of the cat following application of HRP to the the external anal sphincter (double arrow through S1 and S2), the ischiocavernosus (single arrow in caudal S1), and the levator ani muscle (open arrow in S2). After Sato et al. (1978).

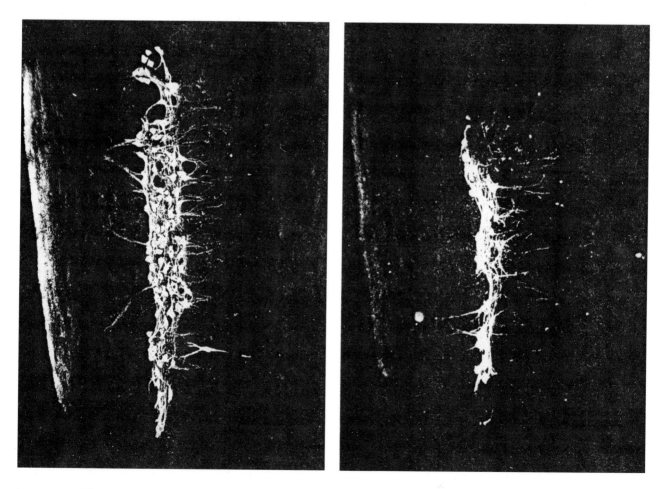

Figure 1-66. Labeled motoneurons in the sacral spinal cord in a male rat (**left**) and a female rat (**right**) following application of HRP to the pudendal nerve. From McKenna and Nadelhaft (1986).

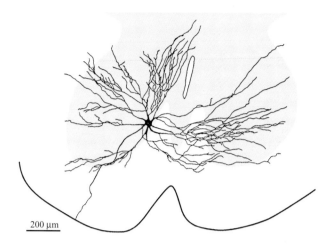

Figure 1-67. The dendritic spread of a sacrocaudal moto-neuron across the ipsilateral and contralateral gray matter in the cat. From Ritz et al. (1992). HRP technique.

(Tribollet, et al., 1997), and the areal extent and inten-sity of the vasopressin marker is higher in males than in females. However, in a small sample of human spinal cords no differences were found in the number of Onuf's nucleus neurons in males and females (Pullen et al. 1997). In the rat, there is no difference between males and females in the number of motoneurons that innervate the external anal or urethral sphincter muscles (McKenna and Nadelhaft, 1986; Collins et al., 1992).

Except in tailless species (apes and man), sacrocaudal motoneurons innervate the tail muscles. According to Ritz et al. (1992), the motoneurons that innervate different tail muscles of the cat are located in different columns. The dorsomedial tail muscle is innervated by nucleus commissuralis motoneurons whereas the dorsolateral and intertransversarius mus-cles by both ventromedial and commissural moto-neurons. The dendritic branches of the large moto-neurons extended as far dorsally as the base of the dorsal horn and spread throughout the contralateral ventral horn (Figure 1-67). The authors speculated that the contralateral dendrites are involved in the synchronization of co-contraction of medial muscles on two sides of the tail.

1.6.8 Motoneuron Dendritic Bundles. An interesting and as yet not fully understood feature of the columnar organization of motoneuron perikarya is the arrangement of their dendrites into regularly oriented bundles. Laruelle (1937, 1948), using the Bielschowsky staining method in longitudinally cut

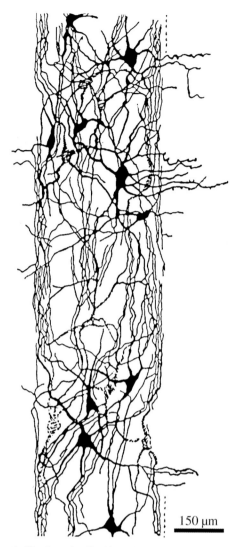

Figure 1-68. Longitudinally oriented dendritic bundles of sacral motoneurons in the cat spinal cord in horizontal sec-tion. From Scheibel and Scheibel (1970a). Golgi technique.

sections of the spinal cord in several species, was the first to note that the dendrites of motoneurons form extensive longitudinal bundles. This was sub-sequently confirmed by Scheibel and Scheibel (1970; Figure 1-68) and by Dekker et al. (1973). Later observers modified the generalization that the den-dritic bundles are always longitudinally oriented. To begin with, it was observed in rat, cat, monkey, and man (e.g., Anderson et al., 1976, 1988; Rose, 1981; Schoenen, 1982; Cameron et al., 1983; Keirstead and Rose, 1983; Vanner and Rose, 1984; Furicchia and Goshgarian, 1987; Beattie et al., 1990; Westerga and Gramsbergen, 1992) that the orientation of den-dritic bundles varies in different motoneuron col-umns. Thus, Anderson et al. (1976, 1988) described two discrete dendritic bundles in the lumbar enlarge-ment of the rat: a lateral bundle ventrolaterally and

A Phrenic
Sagittal

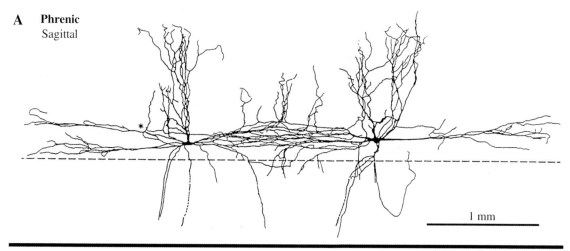

1 mm

B Trapezius
Horizontal

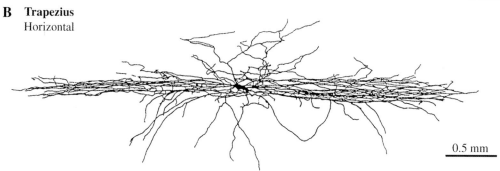

0.5 mm

Figure 1-69. A. Reconstruction of two phrenic motoneurons in the sagittal plane. In addition to their overlapping longitudinal dendritic bundles, these motoneurons also have dorsally and ventrally oriented dendritic branches. After Cameron et al. (1983). **B.** Reconstruction of a trapezius motoneuron in the horizontal plane. This cell with its longitudinal dendritic bundles also has medially and laterally oriented dendrites. From Vanner and Rose (1984). Intracellular HRP staining.

a medial bundle ventrally. The lateral bundle contained as many as 1,200-1,600 closely packed dendrites that spread over a distance of up to 2.4 mm. The medial bundle contained fewer dendrites, some of which crossed to the opposite side. Dendritic bundles appear to be far more dense in the rat than in the cat or monkey. Electron microscopy revealed numerous dendrodendritic and dendrosomatic contacts of the desmosomal type in the rat dendritic bundles. Light and Metz (1978) applied HRP to the ventral roots of sacrocaudal and coccygeal spinal cord in cats to stain the dendrites of motoneurons. They found an extensive ipsilateral distribution of dendrites and considerable dendritic spread into the contralateral gray and white matter. Schoenen (1982), who studied the organization of dendritic bundles in the lumbosacral enlargement of the human spinal cord, found that the orientation of the dendritic bundles differs in each motor column. Ventromedial motoneurons have elongated dorsal branches that form thick bundles oriented toward the ventral gray commissure. The dendritic bundles of central motoneurons are predominantly longitudinally oriented, and so are the

dendritic bundles of ventrolateral motoneurons. Longitudinal bundling appeared to be the common characteristic of motor columns of axial and proximal muscles involved in the maintenance of body posture. The dorsolateral columns that innervate distal muscles involved in dexterous movements have a radial dendritic organization. According to Schoenen, the dendritic bundles are finer and contain fewer dendrites in man than in the cat, and he has, therefore, called them "microbundles." Finally, studies with intracellular staining (e.g., Cameron et al., 1983; Keirstead and Rose, 1983) showed that a single motoneuron may have dendritic bundles projecting in different directions (longitudinally, dorsomedially, dorsolaterally) and they may be overlapping with similarly or dissimilarly projecting dendritic bundles of other motoneurons (Figure 1-69).

The significance of the dendritic bundling of motoneurons is not currently understood. The idea that the uniquely oriented bundles play an important role in the organization of motoneurons into functional motor pools is an attractive one. As an extension of that idea, we propose that the "sectors" in the ventral horn that we have demarcated earlier for descriptive purposes (Section 1.6.2), represent distinct structural and functional entities composed of neuropils containing not only afferents and efferents of distinctive origins but also dendritic bundles with different geometries. If this is correct, the location of an aggregate of motoneurons in a specific motor column within a particular sector of the ventral horn may be an important feature of its intraspinal and supraspinal connections and its fine circuitry.

1.7   The Heterogeneous Intermediate Gray

While neurons of the dorsal horn are dedicated to the registering, processing, and relaying of sensory information, and the neurons of the ventral horn are dedicated to the patterning and execution of motor activities, the heterogeneous intermediate gray is involved in diverse functions. The intermediate gray has two large-celled components, the preganglionic motoneurons laterally (the lateral horn) and Clarke's column medially, and several other structures, including the central gray and a large field with

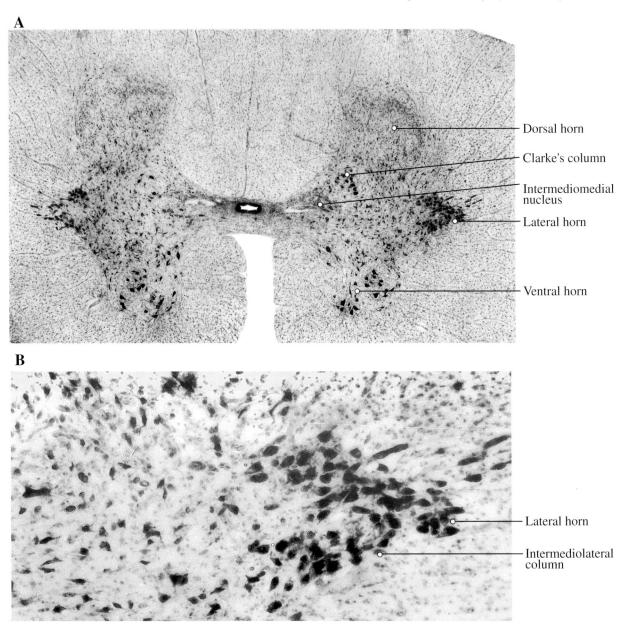

Figure 1-70. The lateral horn and the intermediolateral column of preganglionic motoneurons at lower (**A**) and higher (**B**) magnification in a newborn human. The intermediolateral column contains large neurons, the neurons of the intermediomedial nucleus are smaller. Specimen # Y23-60; cresyl violet stain.

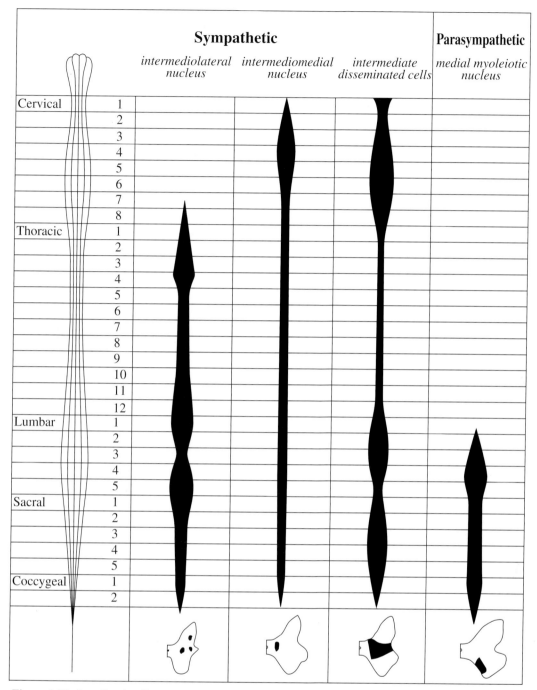

		Sympathetic			Parasympathetic
		intermediolateral nucleus	*intermediomedial nucleus*	*intermediate disseminated cells*	*medial myoleiotic nucleus*
Cervical	1				
	2				
	3				
	4				
	5				
	6				
	7				
	8				
Thoracic	1				
	2				
	3				
	4				
	5				
	6				
	7				
	8				
	9				
	10				
	11				
	12				
Lumbar	1				
	2				
	3				
	4				
	5				
Sacral	1				
	2				
	3				
	4				
	5				
Coccygeal	1				
	2				

Figure 1-71. Localization (**bottom**) and segmental distribution of the preganglionic motoneuron columns of the autonomic (sympathetic and parasympathetic) nervous system. After Massazza (1922) and Pick (1970).

interneurons of different sizes and orientation that extends between the dorsal and ventral horn.

1.7.1 The Sympathetic Preganglionic Motoneurons.
The intermediate gray contains a discrete region laterally, the intermediolateral column or lateral horn (Figure 1-70), composed of the preganglionic motoneurons of the autonomic nervous system (Gaskell, 1916; Poljak, 1924; Bok, 1928; Pick, 1970). The intermediolateral column is most conspicuous at thoracic and lumbosacral levels of the spinal cord.

In addition to the intermediolateral column, there are scattered preganglionic neurons and additional cell groups in the spinal cord (Jacobsohn, 1908; Massazza, 1924; Bok, 1928; Greving, 1928). Massazza referred to these as the intermediomedial nucleus and the intermediate disseminated cells (Figure 1-71). More recently, Petras and Cummings (1972) identified four major groups of preganglionic nuclei in the thoracic and lumbosacral cord of the monkey, called (i) the nucleus intermediolateralis pars principalis, (ii) the nucleus intermediolateralis pars funicularis, (iii)

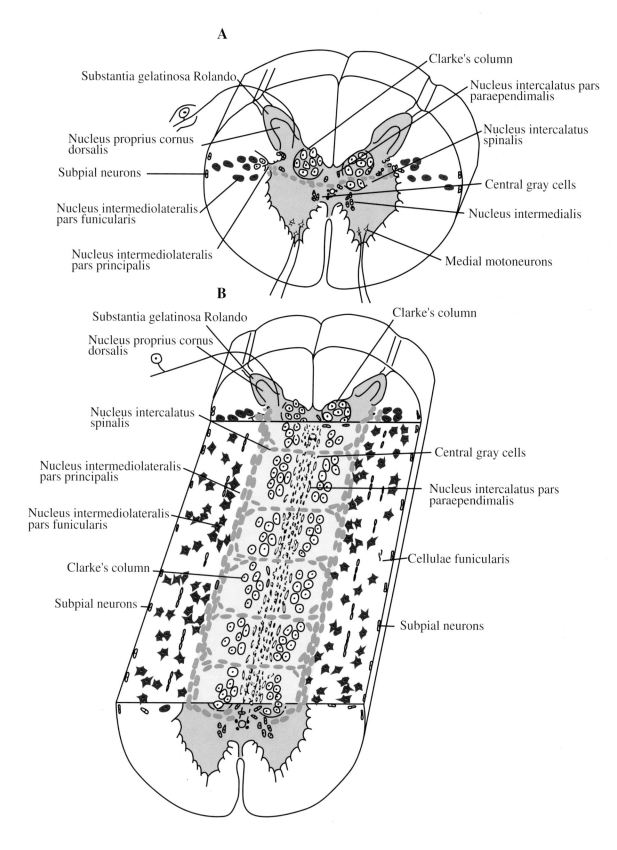

Figure 1-72. The preganglionic sympathetic motoneurons of the pars principalis (blue) and pars funicularis (red) of the intermediolateral column, and the rungs of intercalated cells (green) in a coronal section (**A**) and a horizontal reconstruction (**B**). After Petras and Cummings (1972). Retrograde degeneration technique.

the nucleus intermediomedialis, and (iv) the nucleus intercalatus spinalis (Figure 1-72). The neurons of the intermediolateralis pars principalis are spindle shaped cells that are aligned in the longitudinal plane and, between them, the neurons of the intercalatus spinalis are aligned transversely as rungs of a ladder. The neurons of the pars funicularis, which may be as large as somatic motoneurons, are scattered in the lateral funiculus. Finally, the neurons of the nucleus intermediomedialis surround the central canal. The latter may be identical with the thoracic central autonomic area of Chung et al. (1979b), or what Hancock and Peveto (1979) called in the lumbar spinal cord, the dorsal commissural nucleus.

Chung et al. (1979b) found that 78.2% of the labeled preganglionic neurons that project to the stellate ganglion are located in the intermediolateral cell column, 18.5% in the lateral funiculus, and 3.3% in the intercalated cell column and the central autonomic area. The labeled neurons extended from C8 to T8 ipsilaterally, with the highest concentration in T2. Oldfield and McLachlan (1981) reported an ipsilateral spread of stellate preganglionic motoneurons between T1 and T9. In a study of preganglionic motoneuron organization in the rat, Pyner and Coote (1994) applied different fluorescent dyes to the superior cervical ganglion, the stellate ganglion, and the adrenal medulla in the same animal. They could distinguish four subcolumns in the nucleus intermediolateralis (Figure 1-73). The preganglionic neurons of the adrenal medulla were situated ventrolaterally, those of the superior cervical ganglion dorsomedially, and those of the stellate ganglion (as well as those that projected to both the superior cervical ganglion and the stellate ganglion) were sandwiched between them. The spindle shaped neurons of the intermediolateral nucleus have longitudinally aligned dendrites with a spread of 1,500-2,540 µm (Oldfield and McLachlan, 1981). The dendrites overlap with one another and form longitudinally oriented dendritic bundles ((Dembowsky et al., 1985; Figure 1-74B). The dendritic orientation of the other sympathetic preganglionic motoneurons remains to be determined.

Although there is some degree of segmental order in the localization of preganglionic motoneurons that project to specific sympathetic ganglia, the longitudinal spread of preganglionic subcolumns over several segments is the rule rather than the excep-

tion. For instance, HRP injected into the superior cervical ganglion in the guinea pig, labeled preganglionic motoneurons from C8 to T7, with the majority of the motoneurons located in T1–T3 (Dalsgaard and Elfvin, 1979). Similar results were obtained by Rando et al. (1981) in the rat. These investigators found that the labeled preganglionic motoneurons were restricted ipsilaterally to segments T8–T5, with 90% of them concentrated in T1–T3. Labeled motoneurons were found in four areas: 75% in the intermediolateral nucleus; 23% in the lateral funiculus, 1% in the central autonomic area, and 1% in the intercalated region. The preganglionic motoneurons of the adrenal gland are spread between spinal segments T1 and L1, with approximately 50% of them located within segments T7 and T10 (Schramm et al., 1975). HRP injected into the inferior mesenteric ganglion labeled preganglionic motoneurons in segments T13–L4 bilaterally, with the majority of them concentrated in L2-L3 (Dalsgaard and Elfvin, 1979). Petras and Faden (1978) investigated the sympathetic innervation of the urinary bladder in the dog. They found that the bladder receives preganglionic sympathetic fibers principally from two lumbar nuclei (intermediolateralis pars principalis and nucleus intercalatus) that extend from C8 to L3

In addition to input from primary visceral sensory fibers (Section 1.4.4), the intermediolateral cell column also receives descending efferents from the medulla (Amendt et al., 1979; Loewy and Mc-Kellar, 1981; Ross et al., 1984), the pons (Loewy et al., 1979), the paraventricular and dorsomedial nuclei of the hypothalamus, and the lateral hypothalamic area (Saper et al., 1976; Buijs, 1978; Swanson and McKellar, 1979; Hosoya, 1980; Caverson, et al., 1984; Cechetto and Saper, 1988). Some of the medullary efferents are adrenergic, others serotonergic. The hypothalamic fibers from the paraventricular nucleus contain oxytocin, vasopressin, and neurophysin. Vasopressin receptors have been identified in the spinal cord; they are particularly dense in the vicinity of the sympathetic preganglionic neurons (Sermasi et al., 1998). There is also a dopaminergic projection to the sympathetic intermediolateral cell column (Holstege et al., 1996).

1.7.2 The Parasympathetic Preganglionic Motoneurons of the Sacral Cord. We have dealt earlier with the motoneurons of the sacrocaudal cord and pointed out that it is presently unclear which of

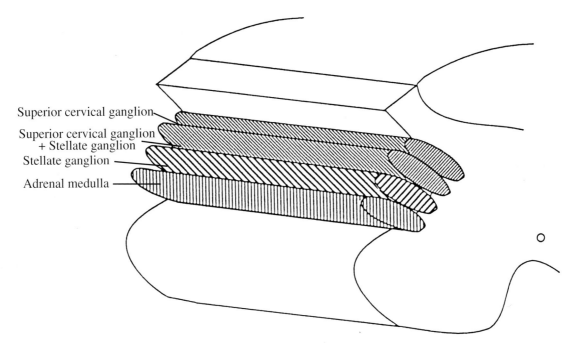

Figure 1-73. Subdivisions of the nucleus intermediolateralis in the thoracic spinal cord of the rat; based on labeling of the three target structures with different dyes. Preganglionic motoneurons that project to the adrenal medulla are situated ventrally, and those projecting to the superior cervical ganglion are situated dorsally. Sandwiched between them are the preganglionic motoneurons that project to the stellate ganglion or to both the superior cervical ganglion and the stellate ganglion. After Pyner and Coote (1994).

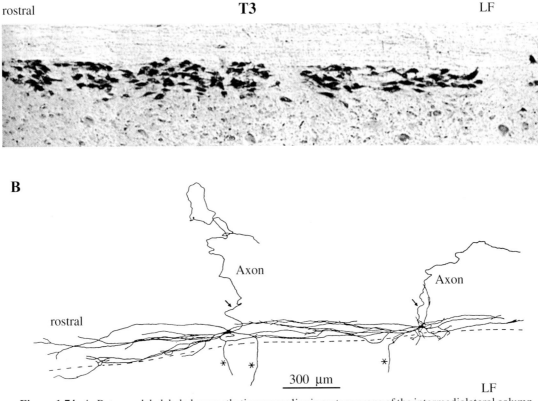

Figure 1-74. A. Retrogradely labeled sympathetic preganglionic motoneurons of the intermediolateral column in the upper thoracic cord of the cat. From Oldfield and McLachlan (1981). **B.** Longitudinal dendrites of two intracellularly stained preganglionic motoneurons in the cat thoracic spinal cord. Arrows point to the origin of the axons; asterisks mark the origin of medially oriented dendrites. After Dembowsky et al. (1985).

the motoneurons innervate the striated muscles, and which control the smooth muscles and glands of the anal and urogenital system (Section 1.6.7). Traditionally, the inferior intermediolateral nucleus at S2–S4 is believed to contain the preganglionic motoneurons of the pelvic viscera (Pick, 1970). Nadelhaft et al. (1980) and Morgan et al. (1981) investigated the distribution and morphology of parasympathetic preganglionic motoneurons of this system in the cat by applying HRP to the pelvic nerve. The labeled cells formed an ipsilateral subcolumn about 10 mm long, extending from S1–S3 but concentrated mainly in S2. These investigators distinguished two bands in this preganglionic column. The dorsal band (which con-

tained about one-third of the labeled motoneurons) is situated beneath the dorsal horn; the lateral band (with two-thirds of the labeled motoneurons) is situated in a region that may correspond to the intermediolateral column of the lateral horn. The motoneurons of the dorsal band innervate mainly the colon, whereas the motoneurons of the lateral band innervate mainly the bladder. The presumed parasympathetic preganglionic neurons were of medium size, oval or spindle-shaped, and transversely oriented. Lu et al. (1993) used a double-labeling technique to distinguish two parasympathetic preganglionic columns in the sacral intermediolateral column. Light and Metz (1978) illustrated presumed parasympathetic motoneurons whose dendrites reached the marginal layer of the dorsal horn and the central gray (Figure 1-75).

1.7.3 The Central Gray (Central Autonomic Area).

Known to earlier anatomists as the substantia grisea centralis, the central gray surrounds the central canal and provides a bridge between the two wings of the gray matter. The central gray is traversed by fibers of the dorsal and ventral gray commissures and contains a variable number of small- and medium-sized neurons. Rexed's (1952, 1964) designation of the central gray as lamina X has little merit since this region has none of the characteristics of a "layer," as that term can be applied to, say, the marginal zone or the substantia gelatinosa of the dorsal horn. The central gray is better thought of as a column that extends the entire length of the spinal cord and medulla, and continues into the midbrain as the periaqueductal gray.

Physiological recordings indicate that collaterals of high threshold dorsal root afferents project to the central gray (Light and Perl, 1979b) and that most central gray neurons are activated by nociceptive stimuli (Nahin et al., 1983). Many of the sensory fibers that terminate in the central gray come from visceral organs (Neuhuber, 1982; Ciriello and Calaresu, 1983; Nadelhaft and Booth, 1984). Histochemical studies indicate the presence in the central gray of compounds implicated in nociceptive functions, including substance P (Gibson et al., 1981; Ljungdahl et al. 1978), met-enkephalin (Hökfelt et al., 1977; Gibson et al., 1981), nitric oxide synthase (Zhang et al., 1993) and NADH diaphorase (Spike et al., 1993; Tang et al., 1995). Finally, labeling studies have shown that ascending axons of central gray neurons are widely distributed in the spinal cord in an

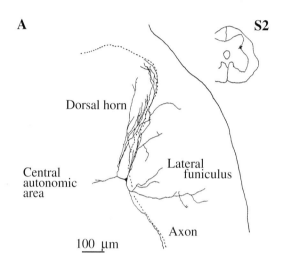

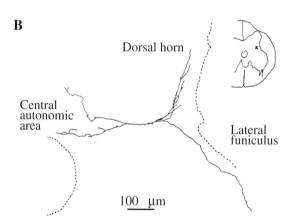

Figure 1-75. Two retrogradely labeled, putative parasympathetic preganglionic motoneurons in the intermediolateral nucleus of the sacral cord of the cat (**x** in insets shows their location). One of the motoneurons has dendrites along the lateral wall of the dorsal horn (**A**); the other also has dendrites reaching the central autonomic area (**B**). After Light and Metz (1978). Compare the distribution of these preganglionic motoneuron dendrites with the complimentary termination of visceral afferents, as seen in Figures 1-32, 1-33, and 1-34 (pages 32, 33).

area dorsal and lateral to the central canal (Matsushita, 1998), and many of them project to medial and lateral areas in the medullary and pontine reticular formation (Menétrey et al., 1983; Nahin et al., 1983; Nahin and Micevych, 1986; Chaouch et al., 1983; Villanueva et al., 1991). There is also a massive projection from the central gray to the periaqueductal gray of the mesencephalon (Mantyh, 1982; Menétrey et al, 1982; Liu, 1983), the thalamus (Burstein et al., 1990) and the hypothalamus (Burstein et al., 1987), and a small projection to the limbic forebrain (Burstein and Potrebic, 1993). The connection of the central gray with the hypothalamus is reciprocal, as axons from the hypothalamic paraventricular nucleus that transport oxytocin and neurophysin terminate here (Luiten et al., 1985). On the other hand, there is no evidence that central gray neurons contribute fibers to the spinocervical or spinothalamic tracts (reviewed by Nahin et al. 1983). These considerations justify the designation of the central gray as a visceral processing station, or "central autonomic area."

1.7.4 Clarke's Column. In the mid-nineteenth century, Clarke (1851, 1859) described the paired columns of large neurons dorsolateral to the central canal in the thoracic spinal cord of the ox that now bear his name (Figure 1-76). In addition to the large neurons of Clarke's column (also known as the dorsal nucleus), Lenhossék (1895) and Ramón y Cajal (1909) identified two additional types of nerve cells at this site, the small border cells and stellate cells. Boehme (1968) confirmed the existence of these cells in Clarke's column. Loewy (1970) distinguished the neurons of this column as class A, B, and C neurons. The smallest of them (the A cells) have a variable dendritic branching patterns. They account for 60% of the total population, outnumbering the large neurons 3:1. The medium-sized cells (the B cells) are either multipolar or fusiform in shape. The dendrites of the multipolar cells are radially oriented, whereas the dendrites of fusiform cells are perpendicularly oriented. The B cells account for 6%-16% of the total population. Finally, the large Clarke neurons (the C cells) have extensive longitudinally oriented dendrites that spread for over 1000 μm from the perikaryon. According to Randic et al. (1981), who used the intracellular staining technique in physiologically identified Clarke column neurons, the largest Clarke neurons may have dendrites extending to 2500 μm rostrocaudally but only 200-250 μm

mediolaterally. The cytology of Clarke's column in the human spinal cord is illustrated in Figure 1-77.

Clarke's column neurons receive monosynaptic input from proprioceptors in muscle, joint, and skin (Kuno et al. 1973; Randic et al., 1981). This input is by way of collaterals of primary afferents in the dorsal funiculus (Hogg, 1944; Liu, 1956) that terminate with large boutons on the dendrites of Clarke's column neurons (Boehme, 1968). These boutons may contain round vesicles that make repeated synaptic contacts with Clarke's column neurons (Réthelyi, 1970, 1984). In addition, collaterals of axons from the lateral funiculus have also been observed to terminate in Clarke's column; these synapse with smaller boutons on the dendrites of large neurons and the soma of small neurons (Boehme, 1968; Réthelyi, 1984). However, Clarke's column receives sensory fibers from much of the body (except the neck and head). The axons of the large Clarke neurons form the dorsal spinocerebellar tract and terminate in the ispilateral cerebellar vermis (Sherrington and Laslett, 1903; Strong, 1936; Yaginuma and Matsushita, 1987) as mossy fibers (Oscarsson, 1965). Collaterals of dorsal spinocerebellar fibers also reach the cerebellar deep nuclei (Matsushita and Gao, 1997). The dorsal spinocerebellar tract axons are among the fastest conducting ascending fibers of the spinal cord (Lloyd and McIntyre, 1950; Oscarsson, 1965).

1.7.5 The Intermediate Interneuronal Field. Much of the intermediate gray, except for the dis-

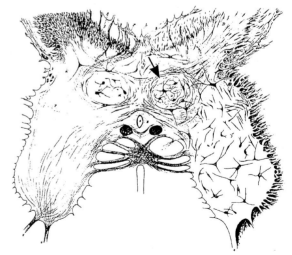

Figure 1-76. Clarke's (1859) drawing of the spinal cord of the ox, with a circular aggregate of large neurons dorsolateral to the central canal (arrow). Sometimes referred to as the dorsal nucleus, the nucleus is now known as Clarke's column.

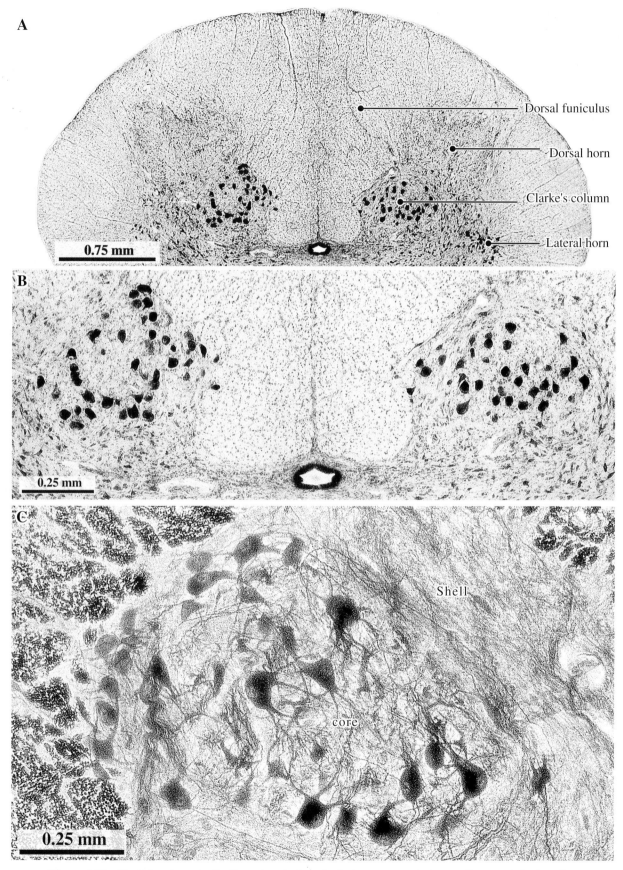

Figure 1-77. Clarke's column in the thoracic spinal cord of a human neonate in a perikaryon-stained section at lower (**A**) and higher (**B**) magnification. **C.** The dendritic configuration of the large Clarke neurons, and the fibrous shell of the column, in a fiber-stained section (Bielschowsky's technique). Specimen # Y23-60.

crete cell groups as Clarke's column and the intermediolateral nucleus, is composed of small- and mid-
sized interneurons. There is experimental evidence
that a high proportion of these interneurons are the
source of intraspinal (propriospinal) axons that terminate within the spinal cord (Sterling and Kuypers,
1968; Rustioni et al., 1971; Matsushita and Ikeda,
1973; Molenaar and Kuypers, 1978; Kitazawa et al.,
1993). Some of these are shorter axons that terminate within or adjacent to the segment of their origin;
others are longer that interconnect distant segments
of the cervical and lumbar spinal cord. The core of
the intermediate interneuronal field is Rexed's lamina
VII, but experimental data indicate that this field of
intraspinal interneurons extends to the base of the
dorsal horn and penetrates the interstices of the ven-

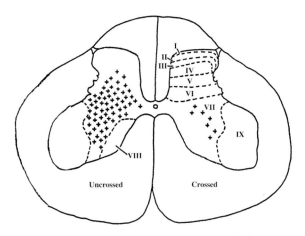

Figure 1-78. Location of interneurons of the extended
intermediate gray that are the source of short intraspinal (propriospinal) axons. Interneurons with uncrossed
fibers greatly exceed those with crossed fibers. After
Molenaar and Kuypers (1978). HRP technique.

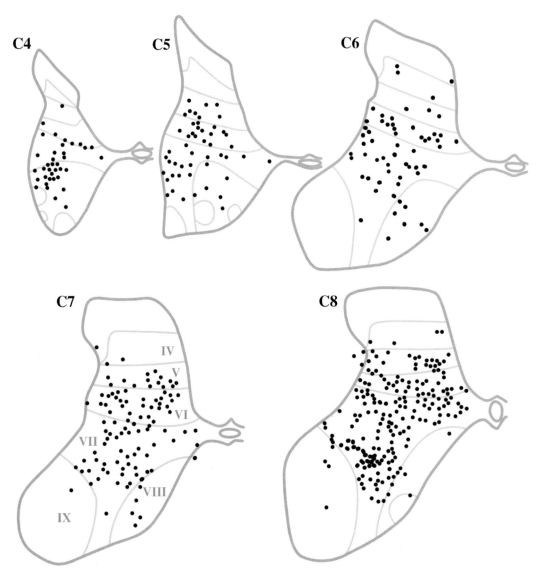

Figure 1-79. Retrograde labeling of intraspinal interneurons with HRP placed into the ulnar motor nucleus at T1.
The concentration of interneurons decreases with increasing distance from C8 to C4. After Kitazawa et al. (1993).

tral horn unoccupied by motoneurons (Figures 1-78, 1-79).

The interneurons of this extended intermediate field are targets of proprioceptive and exteroceptive fibers that, in turn, directly (monosynaptically) or indirectly (polysynaptically) regulate the excitability of ventral horn motoneurons (Jankowska et al., 1973, 1974; Lundberg, 1979). These interneurons are also targets of descending supraspinal efferents (e.g., Illert and Tanaka, 1978; Illert et al., 1978; Alstermark et al., 1984)). The bulk of intraspinal fibers course in the inferior lateral fasciculus of the lateral funiculus (to be described in the next Section).

There is a great diversity among interneurons. First, there are ipsilaterally projecting and contralaterally projecting interneurons; Ramón y Cajal (1911) distinguished the two as the funicular and commissural interneurons, respectively. Some commissural interneurons have recently been characterized in the lumbar spinal cord of the rat (Eide et al., 1999). Second, there are interneurons whose axons are confined to the spinal cord, while other interneurons have long axons that project to supraspinal brain regions (e.g., Grottel et al., 1999). Third, some interneurons have an excitatory action, others an inhibitory one (Hongo et al., 1966; Jankowska et al., 1973). The inhibitory interneurons are responsible for the reciprocal innervation of agonistic and antagonistic muscles, as originally postulated by Sherrington (1906). Finally, much attention has recently been paid to interneurons that have monosynaptic connections with motoneurons; these have been called last-order or premotor interneurons (Hongo et al., 1989; Puskár and Antal, 1997). These interneurons are assumed to be major constituents of the "central pattern generators" of the spinal cord.

The central pattern generators are hypothetical neural circuits responsible for the spatial ordering and temporal sequencing of discharges from different pools of motoneurons that produce reflexes, motor synergies and subroutines, and reiterated or cyclical automatisms. An example of the latter are the alternating limb movements during swimming or stepping. A technique used to study the spinal control of such automatisms is called fictive locomotion (Grillner, 1975; Shik and Orlovsky, 1976; Stein, 1984). In this procedure, a paralyzed or decapitated animal, or an isolated portion of the spinal cord is used from which to record the rhythmic electric discharge of motoneurons in the absence of exteroceptive input and/or proprioceptive feedback. Significantly, fictive locomotor discharge has been recorded not only from the ventral root or motoneurons but also from interneurons in vivo (Ritter et al., 1999) and in organotypic slice cultures in vitro (Ballerini et al., 1999).

1.8 Fiber Tracts of the White Matter

A massive envelope of white matter, made up of long ascending and descending supraspinal axons and shorter intraspinal axons, surrounds the gray matter of the spinal cord. The white matter is usually divided into four bilaterally symmetrical fiber columns or funiculi: (i) the dorsal (or posterior) funiculus between the two dorsal horns, (ii) the lateral funiculus between the dorsal horn and the ventral horn; (iii) the ventral (or anterior) funiculus between the two ventral horns, and (iv) the ventromedial funiculus abutting the ventral median sulcus (Figure 1-5). The clinical and experimental evidence of the existence of distinct fiber tracts within these funiculi (Figure 1-80; right side) justifies the subdivision of some of the funiculi into a variable number of smaller compartments, or fasciculi (Figure 1-80; left side). We describe below 10 compartments in the white matter of the cervical spinal cord that may qualify as its principal fasciculi.

The *dorsal funiculus* consists of two fasciculi: (1) the gracile fasciculus, composed principally of ascending dorsal root fibers from the lower body, and (2) the cuneate fasciculus, composed principally of ascending dorsal root fibers from the upper body. Because these ascending fibers terminate in the dorsal column nuclei, where they synapse with relay neurons whose axons form the medial lemniscus, we refer to these fasciculi as the lower and upper spinolemniscal tracts. Related to the dorsal funiculus is the smaller but functionally very important (3) dorsolateral fasciculus, better known as Lissauer's tract. The *lateral funiculus* contains at least five functionally distinct fasciculi. (4) The superior lateral fasciculus contains the descending corticospinal and rubrospinal tracts. (5) The marginal fasciculus is composed of the ascending dorsal and ventral spinocerebellar tracts. (6) The heterogeneous intermediate fasciculi contain the reticulospinal, tegmentospinal, and various visceral tracts. (7) The inferior lateral funiculus is com-

MORPHOLOGICAL SUBDIVISIONS (FASCICULI)

FUNCTIONAL SUBDIVISIONS (TRACTS)

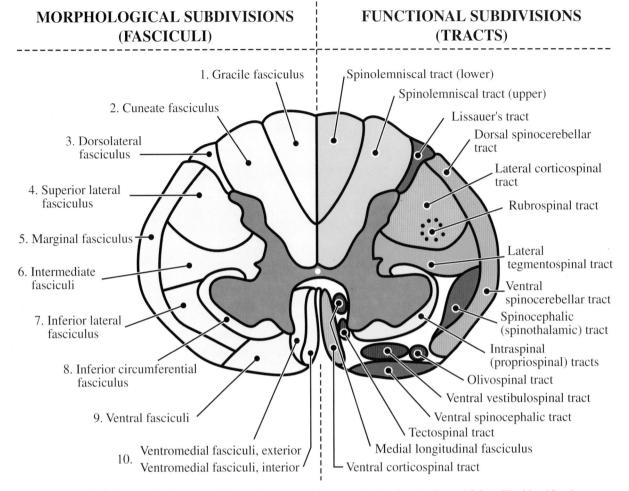

1. Gracile fasciculus
2. Cuneate fasciculus
3. Dorsolateral fasciculus
4. Superior lateral fasciculus
5. Marginal fasciculus
6. Intermediate fasciculi
7. Inferior lateral fasciculus
8. Inferior circumferential fasciculus
9. Ventral fasciculi
10. Ventromedial fasciculi, exterior
    Ventromedial fasciculi, interior

Spinolemniscal tract (lower)
Spinolemniscal tract (upper)
Lissauer's tract
Dorsal spinocerebellar tract
Lateral corticospinal tract
Rubrospinal tract
Lateral tegmentospinal tract
Ventral spinocerebellar tract
Spinocephalic (spinothalamic) tract
Intraspinal (propriospinal) tracts
Olivospinal tract
Ventral vestibulospinal tract
Ventral spinocephalic tract
Tectospinal tract
Medial longitudinal fasciculus
Ventral corticospinal tract

Figure 1-80. Principal fiber tracts of the white matter in the cervical spinal cord of man (**right**). The identifications are based on currently available clinical evidence and some experimental data. Proposed subdivision of the white matter into fasciculi that contain the identified ascending, descending, and intraspinal fiber tracts (**left**).

posed of the ascending spinocephalic (including the spinothalamic) tract. (8) The inferior circumferential fasciculus is composed of intraspinal (propriospinal) fibers that terminate in the ventral horn and the intermediate gray. The *ventral funiculus* (9) contains several tracts, including the descending vestibulospinal and the ascending ventral spinocephalic tracts. Finally, the *ventromedial funiculus* (10) has an exterior and interior part: the latter contains the medial longitudinal fasciculus and the tectospinal tract, the former the ventral corticospinal tract. Below we provide some of the details about the documentation undelying these identifications.

1.8.1 The Ascending Spinolemniscal Tracts of the Gracile and Cuneate Fasciculi. The major fiber constituents of the gracile and cuneate fasciculi of the dorsal funiculus are large caliber, myelinated dorsal root (i.e., presynaptic) axons that ascend all the way to the dorsal column nuclei of the lower medulla

and terminate there ipsilaterally. A high proportion of the ascending fibers of the dorsal funiculus come from the lumbar and cervical enlargements where sensory fibers from the hind limb and the forelimb, respectively, enter the spinal cord. However, the dorsal funiculus also contains a smaller complement of unmyelinated axons, as well as second- or higher-order (i.e., postsynaptic) axons (Keller and Hand, 1970; Millar and Basbaum, 1975; Florence et al., 1991; Giuffrida and Rustioni, 1992).

The dorsal funiculus is small at coccygeal and lower sacral levels but expands greatly in the lumbar spinal cord (Figure 1-6). Proceeding rostrally, more and more ascending dorsal root fibers join the dorsal funiculus and the caudal fibers are gradually displaced medially (Figure 1-81). At high thoracic levels and in the cervical cord, the caudal fibers form the gracile fasciculus and the rostral fibers the cuneate fasciculus (Figures 1-5A, 1-6). The gracile fasciculus contains the segmentally aligned fibers of the coccygeal, sacral and lower lumbar segments that convey sensory input from the lower body and the hind limb, while the fasciculus cuneatus contains fibers from the thoracic and cervical segments that bring sensory input from the trunk, the forelimb and the neck. There is some evidence (Uddenberg, 1968) for the segregation of afferents of different sensory modalities within the dorsal funiculus (Figure 1-82). Importantly, the segmentally arranged fibers are reorganized to form a somatotopic map of the body surface before they terminate in the dorsal column nuclei (Johnson et al., 1968; Whitsel et al., 1970; Hamilton

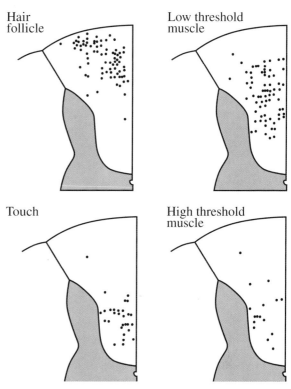

Figure 1-82. Localization of afferents of different sense modality in the dorsal funiculus of the cervical (C3) spinal cord of the cat. After Uddenberg (1968). Physiological recordings.

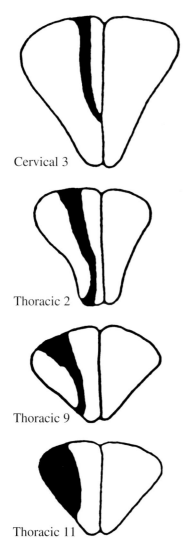

Figure 1-81. Location of degenerating ascending fibers in the dorsal funiculus (opaque area) in the human spinal cord, following severance of the dorsal roots at L1, T12, and T11. The dorsal root fibers that course laterally in T11 are gradually displaced medially by dorsal root fibers that enter at higher thoracic levels (T9, T2). At C3, the degenerating lumbar and low thoracic fibers are situated in the gracile fasciculus. After Foerster and Gagel (1932). Marchi stain.

and Johnson, 1973; Millar and Basbaum, 1975; Florence et al., 1991).

The major fiber constituents of the dorsal funiculus are large caliber, myelinated axons and, according to a recent estimate made in the fasciculus gracilis of the cervical cord, 80% of the myelinated fibers are ascending dorsal root axons (Patterson et al., 1989). But the dorsal funiculus also contains other classes of fibers. First, there are small caliber, unmyelinated dorsal root fibers with nociceptive properties (Patterson et al., 1989; Tamatani et al., 1989; Westman, 1989; Persson et al., 1995). Second, the dorsal funiculus also contains many postsynaptic (nonprimary) fibers that originate in interneurons located in the spinal gray matter and terminate in the dorsal column nuclei (Rothmann, 1899; Münzer and Wiener, 1910; Nathan and Smith, 1959; Uddenberg, 1968; Tomasulo and Emmers, 1972; Petit, 1972; Rustioni, 1973; Angaut-Petit, 1975; Rustioni and Kaufman, 1977; Giesler et al., 1984). According to Petit (1972), about 10% of the dorsal funiculus fibers in thoracic cord are postsynaptic axons. Some of these axons relay visceral input to the dorsal column nuclei (Berkley and Hubscher, 1995; Al-Chaer et al., 1996a). Finally, some of the primary and postsynaptic fibers course only for a short distance within the dorsal funiculus. Thus, according to Smith and Bennett (1987), only 15% of the fibers entering the dorsal columns in the lumbar cord of the rat reach the dorsal column nuclei. It is not currently known how these locally terminating fibers are related to some of the anatomically delineated subdivisions of the dorsal funiculus, namely: (i) the fasciculus interfascicularis (or comma tract of Schultze) in the cervical and thoracic cord; (ii) the septomarginal fasciculus (the oval area of Flechsig) at the same segmental levels (Figure 1-83); and (iii) the triangle of Gombault-Phillipe in the sacral cord (Ariens-Kappers et al., 1936; Scheibel, 1984).

Ascending fibers of the gracile fasciculus from the lower body terminate in the gracile nucleus of the medulla dorsomedially, whereas fibers of the cuneate fasciculus terminate in the cuneate nucleus dorsolaterally. Within the gracile and cuneate nuclei, different body regions are represented in sagittally arranged laminae (Ferraro and Barrera, 1935; Hamilton and Johnson, 1973; Millar and Basbaum, 1975). Topographic organization in the dorsal column nuclei is not segmental but somatotopic. Moreover, the somatotopic representation is "biased," with the disproportionately largest neuronal pools being assigned in all mammals, including man, to the digits of the hindlimb and the forelimb (Figure 1-84). The majority of dorsal funiculus fibers that reach the dorsal column nuclei convey exteroceptive information; the proprioceptive system is poorly represented at upper cervical levels in the dorsal column nuclei (Gordon and Paine, 1960; Whitsel et al., 1969; Boivie and Perl, 1975; Mense and Craig, 1988). In the nucleus gracilis no more than 10% of the neurons respond with tonic discharge to joint movements (Winter, 1965). There is also some evidence for the segregation of neurons in the dorsal column nuclei (as in the dorsal funiculus; Figure 1-82) in terms of sensory modality. In the cat, some gracile neurons are excited by hair follicle sensors, others by light touch sensors, still others by sensors responding to vibration (Perl et al., 1962; Gordon and Jukes, 1964).

The neurons of the dorsal column nuclei are the source of axons that form the medial lemniscus. The medial lemniscus is a massive fiber tract that crosses to the opposite side in the medulla (the

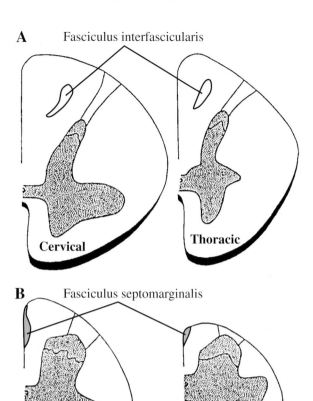

Figure 1-83. Location of the fasciculus interfascicularis in the cervical and thoracic cord (**A**), and of the fasciculus septomarginalis in the lumbar and sacral cord (**B**) in the human dorsal funiculus. After Crosby et al. (1962).

arcuate decussation) and terminates in the ventrobasal nucleus of the thalamus. The ventrobasal nucleus, in turn, is the principal exteroceptive (somesthetic) relay station to the cerebral cortex (Mountcastle and Henneman, 1952; Rose and Mountcastle, 1959). Physiological studies indicate that the majority of ventrobasal nucleus neurons respond to low threshold (i.e., innocuous) mechanical stimuli (Gaze and Gordon, 1954; Boivie and Perl, 1975). The nociceptive system is poorly represented in the medial lemniscus.

1.8.2   The Descending Corticospinal and Rubrospinal Tracts of the Superior Lateral Fasciculus.

The white matter lateral to the dorsal horn is composed in the human spinal cord of two major descending tracts of supraspinal origin, the massive lateral corticospinal tract and the much smaller rubrospinal tract.

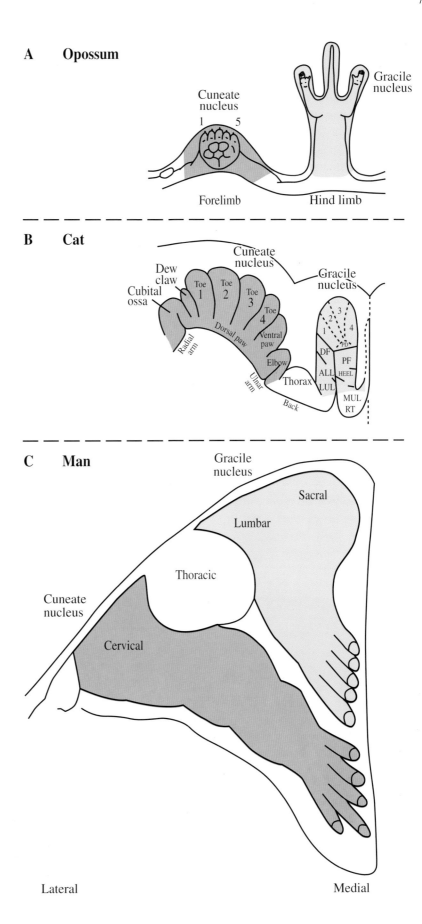

Figure 1-84. **A.** Somatotopic representation of the hind limb and the forelimb in the gracile and cuneate nuclei of the opossum. After Hamilton and Jones (1973). Extensive areas are assigned to the forelimb, hind limb, and their digits (1-5), while trunk representation is meager. **B.** Somatotopic representation in the gracile and cuneate nuclei of the cat. After Millar and Basbaum (1975). **C.** Somatotopic representation in the human gracile and cuneate nuclei. After Humphrey (1955). Figures are not to scale. Abbreviations: ALL, anterior lower leg; DF, dorsal foot; LUL, lateral upper leg; MUL, medial upper leg; PD, foot pad; PF, plantar foot; RT, root of tail.

The Lateral Corticospinal Tract. The lateral corticospinal tract of higher primates and man is the crossed component of the classical pyramidal tract (Tower, 1949). In man, roughly 60% of the pyramidal tract fibers are myelinated, the rest are unmyelinated (Lassek, 1954). The majority of the myelinated corticospinal fibers are of small diameter. The degeneration of the corticospinal fibers following massive bilateral cortical insult in a man is illustrated in Figure 1-85. (Note the sparing of the spinocerebellar fibers in the marginal fasciculus far-laterally.) A high proportion of the lateral corticospinal tract fibers originate in the precentral motor and premotor areas (Lassek, 1954; Nyberg-Hansen, 1969). However, a fair proportion of corticospinal fibers originate in postcentral "nonmotor" areas (e.g., Levin and Bradford, 1938; Peele, 1942; Minckler et al., 1944; Russell and DeMyer, 1961; Murray and Coulter, 1981). In the monkey, according to Russell and DeMyer (1961), 29% of the pyramidal tract fibers originate in the motor cortex (area 4), 29% in premotor cortex (area 6), and 40% in the parietal cortex (sensory association areas). Similar proportions were obtained in the lumbar spinal cord of monkey and cat by Coulter et al. (1976).

The source of corticospinal tract fibers are layer V neurons (Hicks and D'Amato, 1977; Wise and

Jones, 1977; Biber et al. 1978;Brosamle and Schwab, 1997), not only the giant Betz cells but also smaller pyramidal cells (Groos et al., 1978; Murray and Coulter, 1981). In man, the lateral corticospinal tract contains about 1 million fibers on each side of the cord, two-thirds of which are myelinated (Lassek, 1954; DeMyer, 1959). Approximately, 55% of all corticospinal fibers terminate in the cervical cord, 20% in the thoracic cord, and 25% at lumbosacral levels (Weil and Lassek, 1929). The cortical areas representing the forelimb and hind limb preferentially project to corresponding cervical and lumbar levels in the spinal cord (Coulter and Jones, 1977; Groos et al., 1978; Tigges et al., 1979; Wise et al., 1979; Murray and Coulter, 1981). However, there is evidence for considerable segmental overlap in this projection (Armand et al., 1974; Hayes and Rustioni, 1981) due to the extensive longitudinal (rostrocaudal) collateralization of corticospinal fibers (Shinoda et al., 1986).

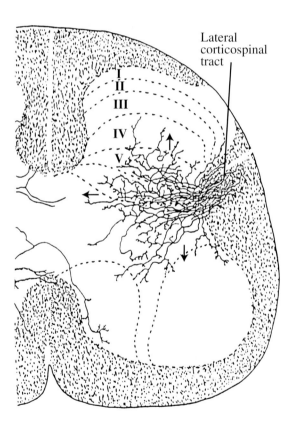

Lateral corticospinal tract

I
II
III
IV
V

Figure 1-86. Collaterals of the lateral corticospinal tract axons that enter the spinal cord in the cat follow three different routes. The dorsal collaterals terminate at the base of the dorsal horn, the central collaterals arborize in the intermediate gray, and the ventral collaterals reach the vicinity of the ventral horn. After Scheibel and Scheibel (1966). Golgi technique.

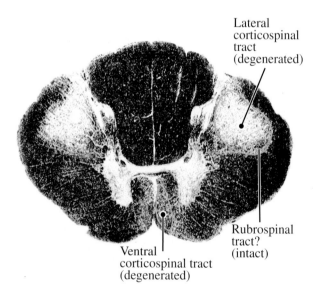

Lateral corticospinal tract (degenerated)

Rubrospinal tract? (intact)

Ventral corticospinal tract (degenerated)

Figure 1-85. Thoracic spinal cord in a man with bilateral degeneration of the lateral corticospinal tract following severe cortical damage. Note that the overlying marginal funiculus is spared. The smaller ventral corticospinal tract is less affected. The possible site of the intact rubrospinal tract is indicated. After Crosby et al. (1962). Weigert technique.

A

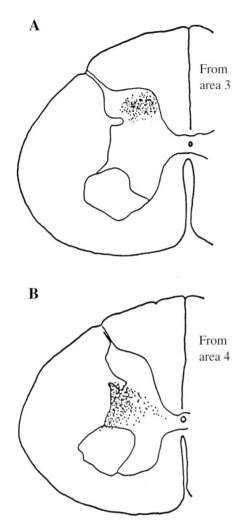

From area 3

B

From area 4

Figure 1-87. Termination of labeled corticospinal fibers in the dorsal horn of a monkey following injection of radioactive amino acids into the somesthetic area of the cerebral cortex (**A**), and in the intermediate gray following injection into the motor area (**B**). After Coulter and Jones (1977). Autoradiographic technique.

In addition to their longitudinal collateralization, corticospinal axons also branch transversely before terminating in different regions of the extended intermediate gray (Scheibel and Scheibel, 1966; Nyberg-Hansen 1966a; Shinoda et al., 1976; Shinoda et al., 1986; Figure 1-86). Some collaterals follow a dorsal trajectory and terminate at the base of the dorsal horn. These may synapse with sensory interneurons. Other collaterals terminate in the core of the intermediate gray, while still others turn ventrally and terminate in the vicinity of the ventral horn motor columns. Liu and Chambers (1964) reported that corticospinal axons from the sensory cortex (the postcentral gyrus) terminate preferentially in the lower laminae of the dorsal horn, whereas corticospinal fibers from the motor cortex terminate chiefly in the intermediate gray and the ventral horn. This differential pattern of collateral distribution has been confirmed by others (Kuypers and Brinkman, 1970; Coulter and Jones, 1977; Tigges et al., 1979; Murray and Coulter, 1981; Cheema et al., 1984; Ralston and Ralston, 1985; Figure 1-87).

Species differences have been noted in the termination of the ventrally coursing corticospinal fibers (Kuypers, 1964; Figure 1-88). In the cat, the corticospinal fibers terminate dorsal to the motoneuron columns, suggesting that they make synaptic contacts with interneurons (the presumed central pattern generators). In the rhesus monkey, many corticospinal axon terminals reach the vicinity of motoneurons, and even more do so in the chimpanzee. The latter pattern characterizes the termination of corticospinal fibers in man (Schoen, 1964). This finding has been interpreted to indicate an evolutionary shift from the

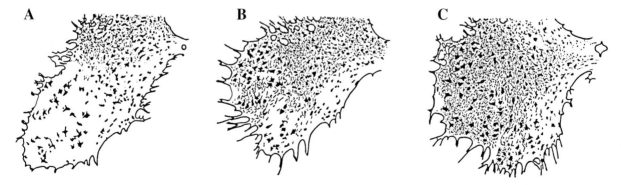

Figure 1-88. Distribution of degenerating corticospinal terminals in the cervical spinal cord in cat (**A**), monkey (**B**), and chimpanzee (**C**), following cortical lesions. In the cat, degenerating terminals are limited to the intermediate gray; in the monkey, the terminals extend to some of the lateral motor columns in the ventral horn; in the chimpanzee, corticospinal terminals surround all the lateral motor columns. After Kuypers (1964). Nauta technique.

indirect cortical control of spinal motoneurons (by way of interneurons) to a direct one.

In contrast to the large lateral corticospinal tract, which is composed mainly of fibers originating in the contralateral cerebral cortex, the smaller ventral corticospinal tract is composed mostly of ipsilateral fibers that descend in the ventromedial funiculus. Fibers of the ventral corticospinal tract are said to arise from the precentral but not the postcentral gyrus (Liu and Chambers, 1964).

The Rubrospinal Tract. The rubrospinal tract is situated ventral to (and may be overlapping with) the lateral corticospinal tract (Hinman and Carpenter, 1959; Kuypers et al., 1962; Nyberg-Hansen and Brodal, 1964; Schoen, 1964; Nyberg-Hansen, 1966b; Poirier and Bouvier, 1966; Edwards, 1972; Miller and Strominger, 1973; Murray and Haines, 1975; see Figure 1-80; right). Collaterals of rubrospinal fibers are distributed in the intermediate gray in a pattern similar to the distribution of corticospinal tract collaterals from the motor cortex (Edwards, 1972; Murray and Haines, 1975). Physiological studies indicate that, in the cat, the rubrospinal terminals synapse with interneurons rather than directly with motoneurons (Hongo et al., 1969, 1972). In contrast, in the monkey, rubrospinal tract fibers make monosynaptic connections with motoneurons (Shapovalov et al., 1971). A possible explanation of the shared course and distribution of corticospinal and rubrospinal fibers is that both function as descending transcerebellar feedback loops. According to this view, the corticospinal tract forms the upper transcerebellar loop, and the rubrospinal tract forms the lower transcerebellar loop (Figure 5-8 in Altman and Bayer, 1997). In man the rubrospinal tract has become vestigial (Massion, 1967; Nathan and Smith, 1982) but its few fibers may occupy the same sites as they do in other mammals (Stern, 1938).

The Hypothalamospinal Tract. Not much information is currently available about hypothalamic projection to the spinal cord. Fibers from the paraventricular nucleus of the hypothalamus have been traced in the dorsolateral funiculus to caudal segments of the spinal cord (Saper et al., 1976; Luiten et al., 1985; Cechetto and Saper, 1988). In the lumbar cord, collaterals of this system leave the main bundle and terminate in the region of the intermediolateral column and in the central autonomic area.

1.8.3   The Intraspinal (Propriospinal) Tracts of the Inferior Circumferential Fasciculus.
The inferior circumferential fasciculus forms a crescent-shaped band around the ventral horn (Figure 1-80; left side). This fasciculus contains, according to the best curently available evidence (Anderson, 1963; Sterling and Kuypers, 1968; Barilari and Kuypers, 1969; Matsushita and Ikeda, 1973; Scheibel, 1984), the bulk of the locally terminating intaspinal (propriospinal) axons of the interneurons of the intermediate gray and ventral horn. The location of this band is suggested by the extensive degeneration in midthoracic cord of a cat following the chronic isolation of the spinal cord by its transection at both the cervical and low thoracic levels (Figure 1-89).

The intraspinal interneurons and their fibers have for some time been assumed to play a major role in the intersegmental organization of spinal reflexes (Sherrington and Laslett, 1903; Lloyd, 1942). Two types of intraspinal axons have been distinguished: (i) short ascending and descending fibers that give off many collaterals (Figure 1-90), and (ii) long ascending fibers that give off fewer collaterals (Matsushita and Ikeda, 1973). Some of the intraspinal fibers are distributed ipsilaterally, others have a predominantly contralateral distribution (Molenaar and Kuypers, 1978). As we shall see later, the inferior circumferential fasciculus is among the earliest myelinating fiber tracts in the human spinal cord.

1.8.4 The Ascending Spinocephalic Tracts of the Inferior Lateral Fasciculus.
In addition to ascending fibers of the gracile and cuneate fasciculi, which are predominantly presynaptic dorsal root fibers, the white matter also contains a large contingent of postsynaptic fibers, traditionally known as the spinothalamic tract. Unlike the fibers of the dorsal funiculus, the fibers of the spinothalamic tract cross to the contralateral side within a few segments of their origin. However, recent studies have established that a large proportion of the fibers of the "spinothalamic" tract, or their collaterals, terminate in the medulla, pons, and midbrain reticular formation. Other fibers of this system proceed to the hypothalamus, and a few even reach some limbic structures of the telencephalon. Accordingly we shall refer to this tract collectively as the spinocephalic tract.

The Spinothalamic Tract. The small caliber, mostly myelinated fibers of the spinothalamic tract

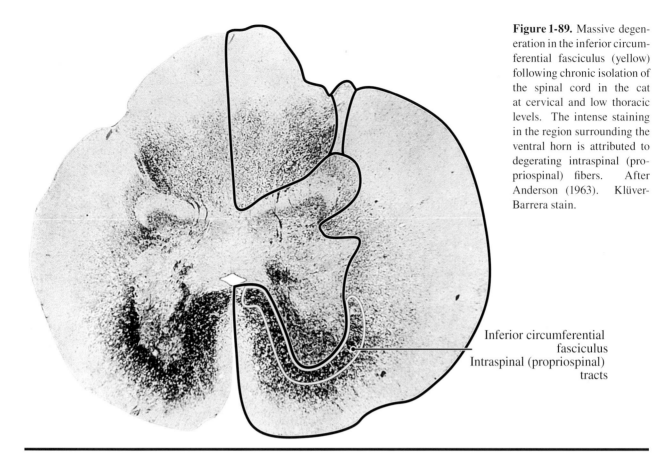

Figure 1-89. Massive degeneration in the inferior circumferential fasciculus (yellow) following chronic isolation of the spinal cord in the cat at cervical and low thoracic levels. The intense staining in the region surrounding the ventral horn is attributed to degerating intraspinal (propriospinal) fibers. After Anderson (1963). Klüver-Barrera stain.

Inferior circumferential fasciculus
Intraspinal (propriospinal) tracts

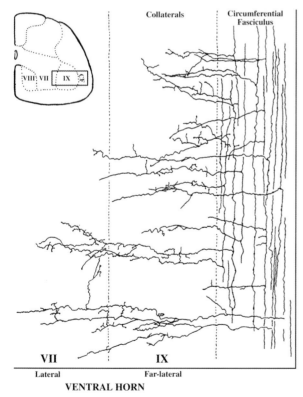

Figure 1-90. Intraspinal (propriospinal) axons in the inferior circumferential fasciculus (CF) and their collaterals that terminate in the ventral horn of a kitten. Location of the horizontal section shown in the inset. After Matsushita and Ikeda (1973). Golgi technique.

located in the inferior lateral fasciculus (Figure 1-80) terminate in the contralateral thalamus (Mott, 1895; Le Gros Clark, 1936; Walker, 1940; Boivie, 1971). Fibers within the spinothalamic tract are topographically organized (Figure 1-91); those originating in caudal spinal segments (the sacral cord) are located dorsolaterally, and those from progressively more rostral levels accumulate ventrolaterally in an orderly sequence (Foerster and Gagel, 1932; Hyndman and Van Epps, 1939; Weaver and Walker, 1941; Gardner and Cuneo, 1945; Morin et al., 1951; Poirier and Bertrand, 1955; Applebaum et al., 1975). However, a recent study indicates that spinothalamic tract fibers shift their position as they ascend from caudal to rostral levels of the cord (Dado et al., 1994b). At C5-C6, the majority (88%) of the physiologically identified spinothalamic axons were located ventrally but further rostraly, at C2, many of them (74%) have shifted their position dorsolaterally.

There is both clinical and experimental evidence that the lateral spinothalamic tract is a principal pathway for the transmission of nociceptive messages to higher levels of the central nervous system. Early clinical observations indicated that lesions or transection of the ventrolateral funiculus in man results in

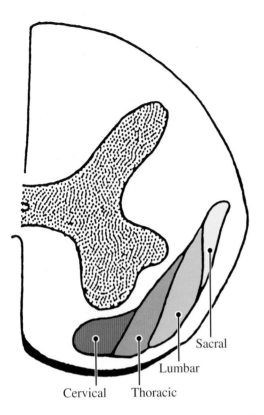

Figure 1-91. Topographic arrangement of ascending spinothalamic fibers in the inferior lateral fasciculus of the human spinal cord. Based on degeneration patterns following clinical chordotomies. After Crosby et al. (1962).

loss of pain and temperature sensation (Petrén, 1910; Spiller and Martin, 1912; Foerster and Gagel, 1932). Indeed, this operation has become a standard surgical procedure for the treatment of intractable pain (White and Sweet, 1969). Supporting this are the clinical reports that electric stimulation of the spinothalamic tract elicits painful sensations in patients (Mayer et al., 1975) while transection of the spinothalamic tract in animals produces analgesia (e.g., Kennard, 1954; Vierck and Luck, 1979). Finally, physiological studies have established that most spinothalamic tract neurons (according to some studies, virtually all) discharge either exclusively or at an increased rate in response to noxious cutaneous stimulation (Beall et al., 1977; Chung et al., 1979a; Kenshalo et al., 1979; Price, 1984; Dado et al., 1994a; Katter et al., 1996b). Spinothalamic cells also respond to noxious stimulation of muscle (Levante et al., 1975) and viscera (Milne, 1981; Katter et al., 1996b).

The spinothalamic interneurons are located principally in the dorsal horn in the cervical cord (Morin et al., 1951; Kerr, 1975), but in the lumbar

cord they are also present in the intermediate gray (Trevino and Carstens, 1975; Willis et al., 1979; Katter et al., 1996a). In the dorsal horn, the spinothalamic neurons are concentrated in laminae I and IV; there are few such cells in the substantia gelatinosa (Willis et al., 1979; Burstein et al., 1990; Dado, 1994a; Figure 1-92). In the intermediate gray, the spinothalamic tract neurons are concentrated in the lateral reticulated area but there are also some in the central autonomic area. As noted before, the axons of spinothalamic interneurons cross to the opposite side within 1-2 segments of their origin and ascend contralaterally in the lateral fasciculus. Many spinothalamic fibers terminate in the ventrobasal complex of the thalamus

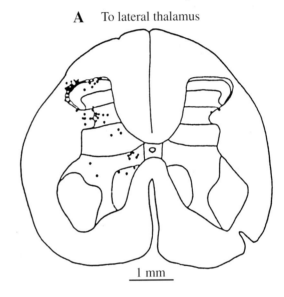

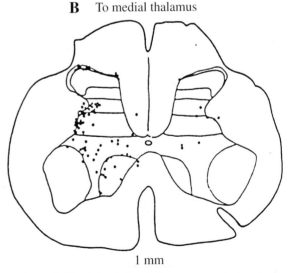

Figure 1-92. Spinothalamic interneurons that project to the lateral thalamus (**A**) and the medial thalamus (**B**) in the monkey. The interneurons are concentrated in lamina I and IV, and the intermediate gray. Spinothalamic neurons in the substantia gelatinosa are rare. From Willis et al. (1979). HRP technique.

(Getz, 1952; Anderson and Berry, 1959; Mehler, 1962, 1974; Lund and Webster, 1967; Boivie, 1971; Jones and Burton, 1974; Giesler et al., 1981; Ma et al., 1987; Ralston and Ralston, 1994). However, it is not resolved whether or not the spinothalamic fibers terminate there at the same locations as do the fibers of the dorsal column nuclei. Most spinothalamic fibers terminate in the medial or intralaminar nuclei of the thalamus, in particular the central lateral nucleus and the ventromedial nucleus.

The Spinoreticular Tract. There are old reports (Mott, 1895; Le Gros Clark, 1936; Bowsher, 1957; Rossi and Brodal, 1957; Anderson and Berry, 1959), and new evidence (Mehler et al., 1960; Lund and Webster, 1967; Casey, 1969; Fields, et al., 1975; Bowsher, 1976; RoBards et al., 1976; Maunz et al., 1978; Kevetter et al., 1982; Haber et al., 1982; Menétrey et al., 1982; Chaouch et al., 1983; Wiberg and Blomquist, 1984; Björkeland and Boivie, 1984) that the fibers of the so-called spinothalamic tract terminate extensively at several other sites than the thalamus, in particular in the medullary, pontine, and mesencephalic reticular formation (Figure 1-93). There are probably several spinoreticular pathways. Spinoreticular fibers have been traced to the dorsal reticular nuclei of the medulla (Lima, 1990; Villanueva et al., 1991); these fibers convey nociceptive messages (Bing et al., 1990). Other spinoreticular fibers project to the medial and/or lateral pontomed-

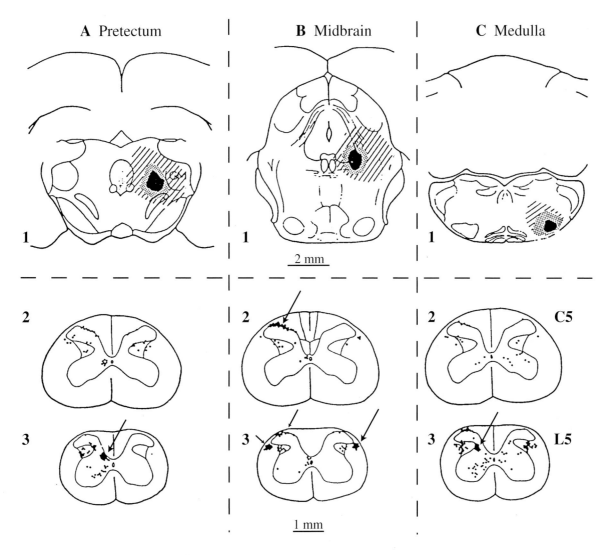

Figure 1-93. Localization of retrogradely labeled spinoreticular neurons at C5 (**2**) and L5 (**3**) of the rat spinal cord following injection of HRP into the reticular formation (**1**) of the the pretectum (**A**), the midbrain (**B**), or the medulla (**C**). In all cases, spinoreticular cells are distributed in the marginal layer of the dorsal horn, the reticulated area, the central autonomic area, and the intermediate gray, though in varying concentrations. Arrows point to sites of high concentration. After Chaouch et al. (1983).

ullary nuclei of the reticular formation (Chaouch et al., 1983; Menétrey et al, 1983, 1984; Nahin and Micevych, 1986). The available evidence indicates that most spinoreticular fibers ascend in the inferior lateral fasciculus and that at least some of them are collaterals of either spinothalamic tract fibers (Haber et al., 1982; Kevetter and Willis, 1982) or spinohypo-thalamic tract fibers (Kostarczyk et al., 1997).

The Spinomesencephalic Tract. The early reports that focused on the thalamic distribution of spinothalamic tract fibers also made reference to termination of the same fiber system in the mesencephalon (Mott, 1895; Le Gros Clark, 1936). A major target of these fibers is the mesencephalic reticular formation but there are also other mesencephalic targets, including the periaqueductal gray, the nucleus cuneiformis, and the intercollicular region (Bowsher, 1957; Rossi and Brodal, 1957; Mehler et al., 1960; Kerr, 1975; RoBards et al., 1976). According to a recent study (Mouton and Holstege, 1998), three times as many lamina I neurons project to the periaqueductal gray as they do to the thalamus. The spinomesencephalic interneurons have the same distribution in the spinal cord as the spinothalamic interneurons do (Mantyh, 1982; Wiberg and Blomquist, 1984) and have similar physiological properties (Hylden et al., 1986; Yezierski and Schwartz, 1986; Yezierski et al., 1987; Djouhri et al., 1997). This poses the question whether the spinomesencephalic fibers constitute a discrete tract or are collaterals of the lateral spinothalamic axons.

The Spinohypothalamic Tract. Retrograde tracers injected into the lateral or medial hypothalamus label interneurons in the superficial layers and the depth of the dorsal horn, and in the central gray surrounding the spinal canal (Burstein et al., 1987). All these regions, as we saw earlier, are implicated in nociceptive functions. Few, if any, neurons are labeled in the substantia gelatinosa. The intraspinal distribution of spinohypothalamic neurons resembles that of the spinothalamic neurons but is less extensive (Burstein et al., 1990). The spinohypothalamic fibers reach the preoptic area, the lateral hypothalamus, the dorsal and posterior hypothalamic area, the paraventricular nucleus, the dorsomedial nucleus, and the suprachiasmatic nucleus (Cliffer et al., 1991). Correlated physiological studies indicate that the majority (Burstein et al., 1991), or virtually all (Kostarczyk et al., 1997) of the spinohypothalamic neurons

respond to noxious stimulation. The ascending fibers of the spinohypothalamic tract were located at C1 in the dorsolateral funiculus (Kostarczyk et al. 1997). Some of the spinohypothalamic fibers may be collaterals of spinothalamic axons (Burstein et al., 1991; Katter et al., 1996b).

A Spinotelencephalic Pathway. In addition to the spinocephalic fiber tracts, some spinal cord fibers also reach limbic structures of the telencephalon (Figure 1-94). These include the amygdala, the septal nuclei, the nucleus accumbens, the bed nucleus of the stria terminalis, the substantia innominata, the infralimbic cortex, and the orbital cortex (Burstein et al., 1987; Burstein and Giesler, 1989; Cliffer et al., 1991; Burstein and Potrebic, 1993). Many of the spinotelencephalic neurons are concentrated in the reticulated area and in the central gray surrounding the spinal canal.

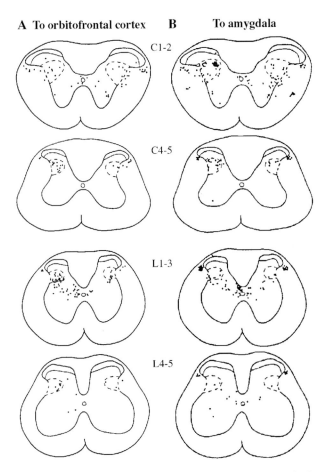

Figure 1-94. Interneurons in the cervical and lumbar spinal cord that project to the orbitofrontal cortex (**A**) and the amygdala (**B**) in the rat. The reticulated area and the intermediate gray appear to be the principal loci of spinotelencephalic interneurons. After Burstein and Potrebic (1993). HRP technique.

In summary, the currently available evidence supports the proposition that the fibers of the so-called spinothalamic tract constitute a more extensive afferent system, aptly called the spinocephalic tract. Unlike the spinolemnsical tract of the dorsal funiculus, which conveys mostly exteroceptive input directly to the neocortex, the spinocephalic tract of the lateral funiculus is a more diffuse pathway that transmits nociceptive input primarily to paleocephalic structures, including the limbic cortex.

1.8.5 The Ascending Proprioceptive Tracts of the Marginal Fasciculus.

The marginal fasciculus (Figure 1-80, left) is composed of three ascending proprioceptive tracts that relay information, directly or indirectly, to the cerebellum. These are the dorsal spinocerebellar tract (Flechsig's tract), the ventral spinocerebellar tract (Gower's tract), and the spino-olivary tract. We have discussed earlier the dorsal spinocerebellar tract in relation to Clarke's column, which is the main source of its fibers in the thoracic cord. Another source of the dorsal spinocerebellar tract is the central cervical nucleus at cervical levels (Matsushita and Ikeda, 1975). The ventral spinocerebellar tract originates in neurons scattered at the base of the dorsal horn and more ventrally in the intermediate gray of the lower thoracic and upper lumbar spinal cord (Hubbard and Oscarsson, 1962), sometimes referred to as the spinal border cells. The fibers of the ventral spinocerebellar tract cross to the opposite side at segmental levels, ascend in the ventral portion of the marginal fasciculus, and reach the cerebellum by way of the superior cerebellar peduncle (Xu and Grant, 1994). This is in contrast to the dorsal spinocerebellar tract that projects mainly to the ipsilateral cerebellum by way of the inferior cerebellar peduncle (Figure 1-95). Brodal (1981) suggested that the dorsal spinocerebellar tract provides fine-grained proprioceptive information to the cerebellum, while the ventral spinocerebellar tract conveys integrated messages about the position of different body parts, particularly the hind limbs. Both the dorsal spinocerebellar tract and the ventral spinocerebellar tract have a segmentally arranged topographic organization (Figure 1-96). The site of origin of spino-olivary fibers has not been established with certainty. It has been suggested that they originate mainly in the ventral horn (Brodal et al., 1950; Mizuno, 1966). Some of the spino-olivary fibers may be collaterals of the spinoreticular fibers (Mizumo, 1966).

1.8.6. Descending Cephalospinal Tracts of the Ventral and Ventromedial Funiculi.

Several descending supraspinal tracts of subcortical origin course in the ventral and ventromedial funiculi. Most commonly mentioned of these are the olivospinal, the vestibulospinal, the tectospinal, and the reticulospinal tracts. Least understood is the presumed olivospinal tract illustrated in Figure 1-97. While the importance of this proprioceptive tract has been advocated by some anatomists (e.g., Crosby et al., 1962), others (e.g., Brodal, 1981) have altogether denied its existence.

The Vestibulospinal Tract. In an anatomical tracer study, Nyberg-Hansen (1966a) distinguished two vestibulospinal tracts, the lateral and the medial. The more extensive lateral vestibulospinal tract originates in the lateral vestibular (or Deiters') nucleus (Pompeiano and Brodal, 1957). The descending fibers of this tract are situated ventrolaterally at cervical levels but shift to the ventral funiculus at lumbar and sacral levels and synapse with dendrites of interneurons in the vicinity of the motor columns (Nyberg-Hansen and Mascitti, 1964). The smaller medial vestibulospinal tract, the so-called sulcomarginal fasciculus, is located in the ventromedial funiculus. It originates in the medial vestibular nucleus and is associated rostrally with the medial longitudinal fasciculus (Nyberg-Hansen, 1964b). These fibers descend no farther than midthoracic levels and apparently contact interneurons in the ventral horn.

Physiological studies have shown that lateral vestibulospinal efferents have monosynaptic connections with extensor motoneurons of the neck (Wilson and Yoshida, 1969) and trunk (Wilson et al. 1970), and polysynaptic connections with flexor motoneurons of the forelimb (Wilson and Yoshida, 1969) and hindlimb (Grillner et al., 1970). Lateral vestibulospinal efferents must play a role in the maintenance of the upright (antigravity) body posture. Shinoda et al. (1986, 1992) used intracellular staining to study the trajectory, collateral branching, and final termination of physiologically identified vestibulospinal axons in the ventral funiculus (Figure 1-98). The axons were traced over a distance of 2.5 to 15.5 mm rostrocaudally. Over these distances, the stem axons give off up to 9 collaterals at a right angle to their trajectory. In the gray matter the axon collaterals ramify extensively and terminate either in the intermediate gray

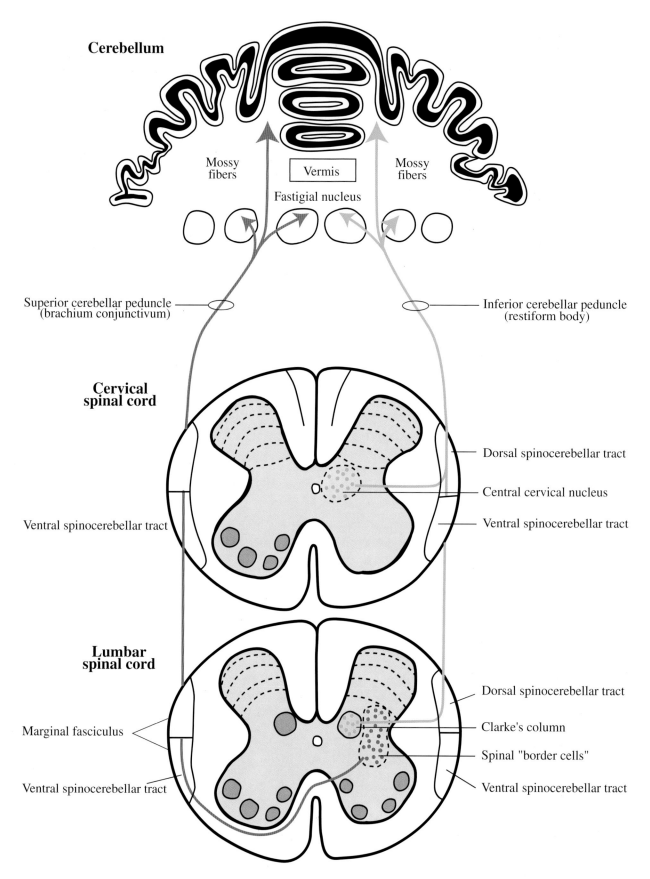

Figure 1-95. The spinal cord origins of the ipsilateral dorsal spinocerebellar tract (**right**) and of the contralateral ventral spinocerebellar tract (**left**), and their course towards the deep nuclei and the cortex of the cerebellum.

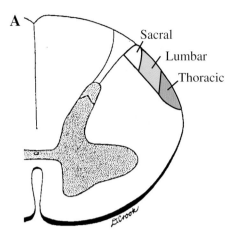

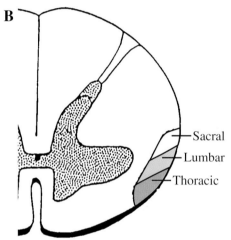

Figure 1-96. Topographic distribution in the human spinal cord of the ascending fibers of the dorsal (**A**) and ventral (**B**) spinocerebellar tracts within the marginal fasciculus. After Crosby et al. (1962).

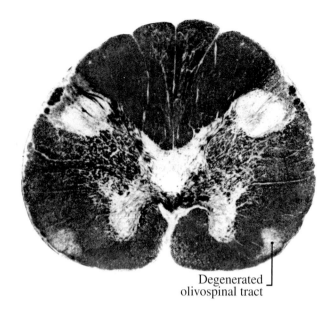

Figure 1-97. Bilateral degeneration of the presumed olivospinal tract in the ventral funiculus of the human spinal cord. After Crosby et al. (1962). Weigert technique.

or the ventral horn (Figure 1-99). Shinoda and associates called the former the medial collaterals and the latter, the lateral collaterals. The lateral collaterals form axodendritic and axosomatic synapses with large neurons. An alternative interpretation of their data is that, in addition to the collaterals terminating in the intermediate zone, there is a medial and a lateral collateral system. The medial collaterals (perhaps components of the medial vestibulospinal tract) synapse with medial panel (axial) motoneurons, while the lateral collaterals (perhaps components of the ventral vestibulospinal tract) synapse with lateral panel (appendicular) motoneurons.

The Tectospinal Tract. Fibers of the tectospinal tract originate in the deep layers of the superior colliculus, cross in the dorsal tegmental decussation, and terminate in the cervical spinal cord (Papez

and Freeman, 1930; Rasmussen, 1936; Tasiro, 1940; Pearce and Glees, 1956; Altman and Carpenter, 1961; Nyberg-Hansen, 1964a). The tectospinal fibers course in the medial aspect of the ventral funiculus (Figure 1-100) and appear to make axosomatic and axodendritic contacts with small and large neurons of the ventral horn (Nyberg-Hansen, 1964a). Considering that most tectospinal fibers terminate in the upper cervical segments, few reach the lower cervical segments, and none reach the thoracic cord (Nyberg-Hansen, 1964a), the old idea that tectospinal efferents are involved in visually guided head turning seems well justified.

The Reticulospinal Tract. An important source of descending cephalospinal efferents to the spinal cord is the extensive medullary and pontine reticular formation. The principal origin of medullary reticulospinal fibers is the nucleus reticularis gigantocellularis and the nucleus reticularis magnocellularis (Nyberg-Hansen, 1965; Basbaum et al., 1978). The principal origin of pontine reticulospinal fibers are large neurons in the nucleus reticularis pontis caudalis and oralis. The pontine reticulospinal tract descends in the ventral funiculus and its fibers contact interneurons, and possibly motoneurons, in the ventral horn (Nyberg-Hansen, 1965). This may be the ventral reticulospinal tract of earlier anatomists (Crosby et al., 1962). The medullary reticulospinal tract is situated laterally (Nyberg-Hansen, 1965); it is probably identical with the medial reticulospinal tract of earlier

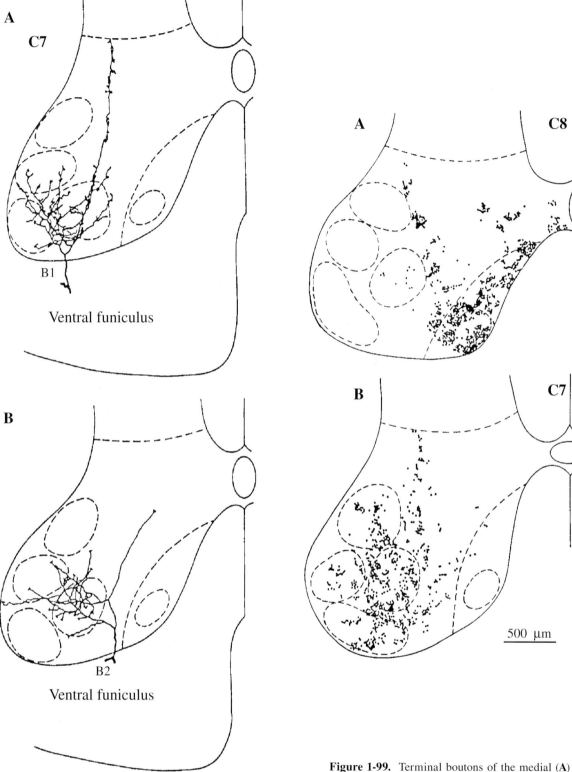

Figure 1-98. Terminal arbors in the far-lateral (**A**) and lateral (**B**) motor columns of the cervical (C7) spinal cord of two collaterals of a single vestibulo-spinal axon in the ventral funiculus of a cat. From Shinoda et al. (1992). Intracellular staining.

Figure 1-99. Terminal boutons of the medial (**A**) and ventral (**B**) vestibulospinal tracts in the cervi-cal spinal cord (C8, C7) of the cat. The medial ter-minals are concentrated in the medial panel of ven-tral horn motor columns. The ventral terminals are concentrated in the lateral and far-lateral panels of the ventral horn motor columns. From Shinoda et al. (1992). Intracellular staining.

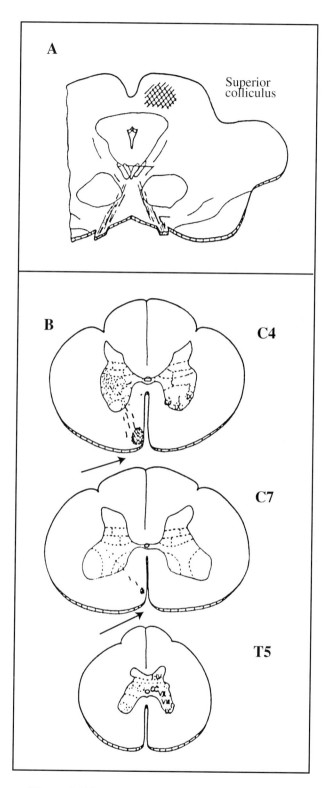

Figure 1-100. Following superior colliculus (tectal) lesions (**A**) in the cat, the degenerating tectospinal tract (**B**) is conspicuous in the ventromedial funiculus at C4 but tapers off at C7, and is not detectable at T5. There is a high concentration of degenerating axon terminals in the intermediate gray and ventral horn at upper cervical levels but only scattered remnants are seen more caudally. After Nyberg-Hansen (1964a). Nauta technique.

anatomists (Crosby et al., 1962). The mesencephalic reticular formation is apparently not a source of reticulospinal efferents (Nyberg-Hansen, 1965; Edwards, 1975).

Early physiological studies indicated that, depending on the exact site of electrical stimulation, neurons of the medullary reticular formation exert either a facilitatory or an inhibitory influence on monosynaptic spinal cord reflexes (Magoun and Rhines, 1946). Lesions of the ventral funiculus abolish this inhibitory influence (Jankowska et al., 1968). It is now known that the pontine and medullary reticular formation is a heterogeneous system and that the different reticular nuclei are involved in different functions. Basbaum et al. (1978) distinguished three components of the medullary reticulospinal system. The nucleus reticularis gigantocellularis, located dorsally in the medullary reticular formation, projects to the spinal cord via the ventral funiculus and its fibers terminate mainly in the ventral horn near the motoneuron columns. This pathway appears to be involved in motor functions. In contrast, fibers originating in the nucleus raphe magnus and in the nucleus reticularis magnocellularis descend in the dorsolateral funiculus, and project to the dorsal horn. These efferents have been implicated (as other fiber tracts in this location) in nociceptive functions (Basbaum et al., 1978). These observations suggest that reticular efferents intermingle with other descending tracts in accordance with their specific functions. Relatively little is known about the reticulospinal tract in man (Nathan et al., 1996).

2 AN EVOLUTIONARY INTERPRETATION OF SPINAL CORD ORGANIZATION

2.1 Phylogeny of the Spinal Cord

2.1.1 The Spinal Cord in Chordates.

The spinal cord is phylogenetically the oldest part of the vertebrate central nervous system since a spinal cord is present in primitive chordates devoid of a true brain (Ariens-Kappers et al., 1936; Bone, 1960; Nieuwenhuys, 1964). Thus, Amphioxus (lancelet), a filter-feeding chordate lacking a head with specialized sense organs, has a spinal cord, albeit a primitve one (Figure 2-1). The spinal cord of Amphioxus is located dorsal to the notochord, the phylogenetic and ontogenetic precursor of the vertebrate spine. Alternating (rather than bilaterally symmetrical) dorsal roots and ventral roots link the spinal cord of Amphioxus with its body. The Amphioxus spinal cord does not have peripherally situated spinal ganglia with specialized sensory neurons. Instead, Rohde cells and Rohon-Beard cells, large neurons distributed inside the spinal cord, convey sensory input from the periphery. Some of these neurons have massive dendrites (Figure 2-1) and a "giant" axon that traverses the length of the body. These primitive neurons probably operate differently than the dedicated sensory ganglion cells of vertebrates. Interestingly, neurons resembling Rohde cells and Rohon-Beard cells are present in the spinal cord of some fish (like the stingray). In some amphibians (like the salamander) these neurons are present during their larval stage of development, then disappear during metamorphosis to be replaced by peripheral sensory ganglion cells. Discrete gray and white matter is not discernible in the spinal cord of Amphioxus. Rather, most neurons either straddle the spinal canal or are located in its vicinity (Figure 2-1). These scattered periventricular neurons may be the precursors of the evolving gray matter in vertebrates.

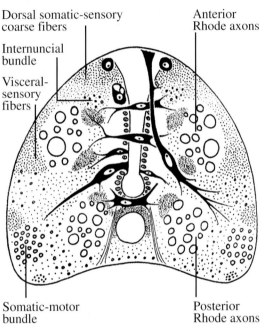

Figure **2-1.** Coronal section of the midportion of the spinal cord of Amphioxus. After Bone (1960).

2.1.2 The Spinal Cord in Cyclostomes.

Cyclostomes, such as the lamprey or hagfish, are the most primitive extant vertebrates. Although fish-like in appearance, Cyclostomes lack jaws and fins. However, they possess a head and specialized sense organs, including eyes and nostrils, and a primitive brain. While there are distinct dorsal root ganglia with sensory ganglion cells in the lamprey (Figure 2-2B), large spherical cells are also present dorsally in the spinal cord with features of sensory neurons (Figure 2-A). As in Amphioxus, dorsal roots and ventral roots alternate in adjacent segments in the spinal cord of the lamprey (Figure 2-2B) but in some cyclostomes the two roots fuse distally into a single spinal nerve. Many of the spinal axons are myelin-

A

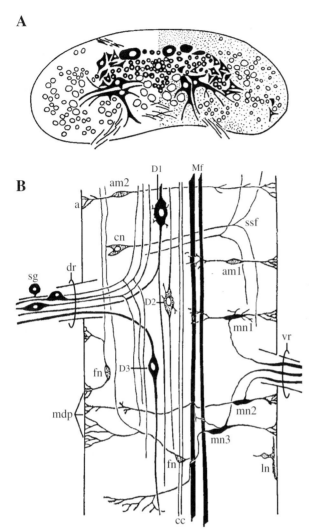

B

Figure 2-2. A. The spinal cord of the lamprey in coronal section. **B.** Survey, in the horizontal plane, of different types of spinal cord neurons and their processes in Cyclostomes. After Nieuwenhuys (1964). *Abbreviations* (some with numbers): a, axon; am, amacrine cell; cc, central canal; cn, commissural neuron; D, dorsal cell; dr, dorsal root; fn, funicular neuron; ln, lateral Retzius neuron; mdp, marginal dendritic plexus; Mf, Müller fiber, mn, motor neurons; sg, spinal ganglion; ssf, somatosensory fibers: vr, ventral root.

ated. The sensory fibers that enter the spinal cord bifurcate into ascending and descending branches but run only for a short distance within the spinal cord (Ariens-Kappers et al., 1936). An incipient gray matter surrounds the central canal, but tracts composed of descending fibers from the medulla and brain stem, including the large Müller fibers, traverse it (Figure 2-2B). Finally, while a discrete dorsal horn and ventral horn is not discernible in the gray matter, the multipolar motoneurons do tend to aggregate ventrally in the the spinal cord (Figure 2-1A). Apparently, rudiments of some features of the spinal cord of higher vertebrates are present in Cyclostomes.

Among many other functions, the spinal cord coordinates swimming in Cyclostomes. In the lamprey, swimming is based on two processes: (i) undulatory movements that are propagated towards the tail and move the animal forward, and (ii) bending of the body from one side to the other at segmental levels that produces turning (Wallén and Williams, 1984). The role played by spinal cord pattern generators in swimming has been investigated in the lamprey with the technique of fictive locomotion (Cohen and Harris-Warrick, 1984; Hagevik and McClellan, 1999). The results suggest that oscillator circuits are distributed on the right and left side along the length of the spinal cord, and the alternation of ventral root bursts (i.e., discharge of motoneurons) is the result of strong reciprocal inhibition across the midline. Buchanan (1996) identified three types of neurons in the lamprey spinal cord: (i) ipsilateral excitatory, (ii) ipsilateral inhibitory, and (iii) contralateral (commissural) inhibitory interneurons. The importance of commissural interneurons in the generation of undulatory movements is indicated by the finding that a midline cut through the spinal cord abolishes the rhythmicity of fictive locomotion (Buchanan, 1999).

2.1.3 The Spinal Cord in Fishes. In the spinal cord of cartilaginous fishes, such as sharks and rays, the gray matter and white matter are partially segregated but, as in Cyclostomes, the gray matter is traversed by prominent fiber bundles (Figures 2-3A, 2-4A). The dorsal horn, the lateral horn, and the ventral horn are distinguishable in this fractionated gray matter. However, the dorsal horn is less well developed in sharks and rays than in teleosts (Figure 2-4B) or higher vertebrates, possibly because it is composed of fewer laminae. Several observations support this assumption. First, the ray's dorsal horn is the target of only small caliber axons, what Lenhossék (1895) called the "dorsal bundle of thin fibers" (Figure 2-3D). The large caliber sensory fibers (the recurving exteroceptive collaterals of mammals) seem to be missing. The large caliber axons, Lenhossék's "ventral bundle of thick fibers," turn ventrally and course toward the intermediate gray. They must be proprioceptive fibers. Second, the dorsal horn of the ray and shark, according to recent immunohistochemical evidence (Ritchie and Leonard, 1983; Rodriguez-Moldes et al., 1993), is the target of sensory fibers containing substance P (Figure 2-3B, left). As we noted earlier, substance P is associated in mammals with small caliber fibers that convey nociceptive messages and terminate in the superficial sub-

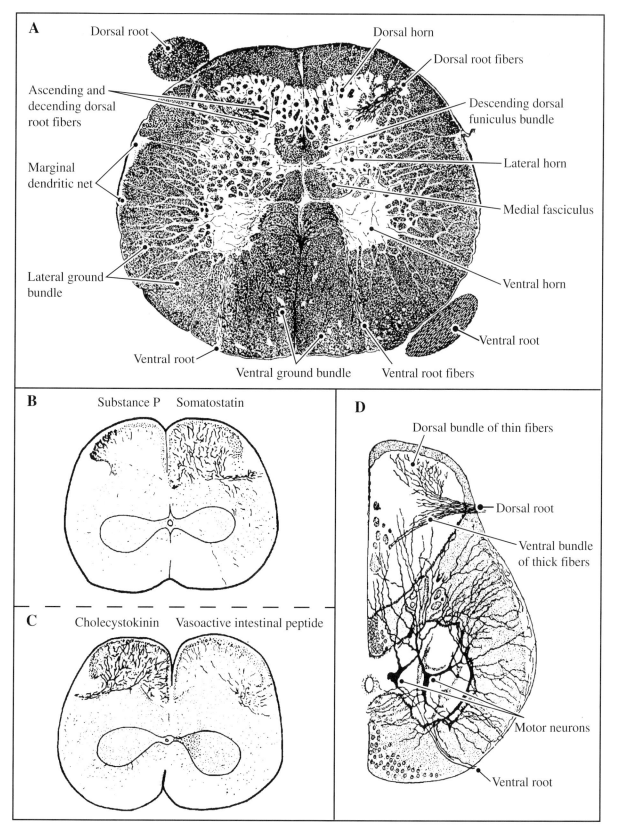

Figure 2-3. A. Coronal section of the spinal cord of the stingray. The gray matter (light) and white matter (opaque) are segregated. A dorsal, a lateral, and a ventral horn is discernable. From Ariens-Kappers et al. (1936). **B** and **C.** Distribution of four immunohistochemically visualized putative neurotransmitters in the spinal cord of the stingray. After Ritchie and Leonard (1983). **D.** Distribution of dorsal root fibers and the dendritic organization of motoneurons in the stingray spinal cord. After von Lenhossék, from Ariens-Kappers et al (1936).

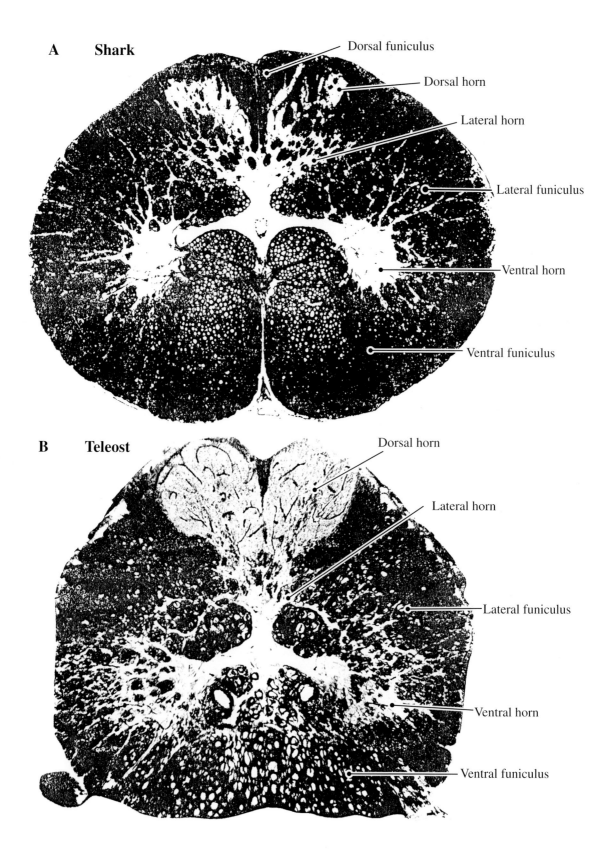

Figure 2-4. Coronal section of the spinal cord in a shark (**A**) and a bony fish (**B**). The dorsal horn is far better developed in the bony fish than in the shark. The ventral and lateral funiculi are prominent in both species while the dorsal funiculus is rudimentary. Weigert-Pal myelin stain. After Nieuwenhuys (1964).

stantia gelatinosa. Third, the entire substance of the stingray dorsal horn reacts positively with putative peptidergic transmitters that have been implicated in nociceptive functions, i.e., somatostatin, cholecystokinin, and vasoactive intestinal peptide (Figures 2-3B, 2-3C).

As noted before, the dorsal funiculus is poorly developed in sharks and rays (Figures 2-3A, 2-4A). The small dorsal funiculus of Cyclostomes, according to Ariens-Kappers et al. (1936), contains the short ascending and descending branches of the bifurcating dorsal root axons; none of them are said to reach the medulla as do the spinolemniscal fibers in mammals. Moreover, dorsal column nuclei, the principal targets of the dorsal funicular fibers, are absent in fishes. Ascending spinobulbar and spinomesencephalic fibers are present but these are postsynaptic axons that originate in second-order dorsal horn neurons and decussate in the ventral commissure (Ariens-Kappers et al., 1936). These afferents may correspond to the spinocephalic fiber system of mammals. Finally, the spinal cord of rays (Figure 2-3A) and sharks (Figure 2-4A) has a prominent lateral horn and a ventral horn. The ventral horn motoneurons have dendrites that arborize extensively in the ventral and lateral funiculi, suggesting that they receive input not only from local proprioceptive afferents but also from intraspinal and supraspinal efferents (Figure 2-3D).

The spinal cord of bony fish resembles that of sharks and rays (Figure 2-4B). Probably all the primary sensory fibers arise from ganglion cell situated in the dorsal root ganglia (Ariens-Kappers et al., 1936). The dorsal horn is more massive in teleosts than in cartilaginous fish but the dorsal funiculus is small. The lateral horn contains preganglionic motoneurons that, in the thoracic cord, send fibers to the sympathetic chain of ganglia. The ventral horn motoneurons closely resemble motoneurons in higher vertebrates. However, there is no indication of a cervical or a lumbar enlargement in the spinal cord of any species of fish.

2.1.4 The Spinal Cord in Amphibians.

A cervical and a lumbar enlargement is evident in the spinal cord of amphibians with limbs (Nieuwenhuys, 1964). In the frog, the lumbar enlargement is particularly prominent, and the spinal nerves are bulkier here than in the thoracic cord (Figure 2-5). Upon

entering the spinal cord, the dorsal root fibers segregate into a dorsomedial and a ventrolateral bundle (Figure 2-6A, left). Fibers of the dorsomedial bundle proceed medially, approach the dorsal horn from the top, and give off local collaterals. The terminal arbors of these dorsal collaterals (Figure 2-6B, right; Figure 2-7) are like the cap terminals that, in mammals, convey nociceptive messages to the dorsal horn (compare with Figure 1-28), and the site where they terminate (Figures 2-6A, B; left side) is similar to the vertical gelatinosal slabs of the human spinal cord (compare with Figure 1-20). It is noteworhty that the amphibian spinal cord lacks recurving collaterals (Stensaas and Stensaas, 1971; Székely and Czéh, 1976). The latter are the terminals of exteroceptive afferents that enter the dorsal horn in mammals from the bottom and end with the distinctive flame terminals (compare with Figures 1-26, 1-27). These considerations suggest that the principal cutaneous input to the amphibian spinal cord (as in fishes) is from nociceptive afferents; exteroceptive input may be scarce or absent altogether.

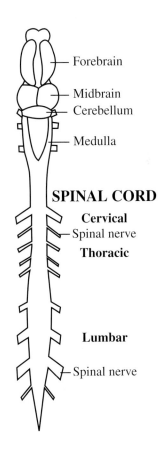

Figure 2-5. Outline of the spinal cord of the frog. Note lumbar enlargement with bulky spinal nerves. After Joseph and Whitlock (1968).

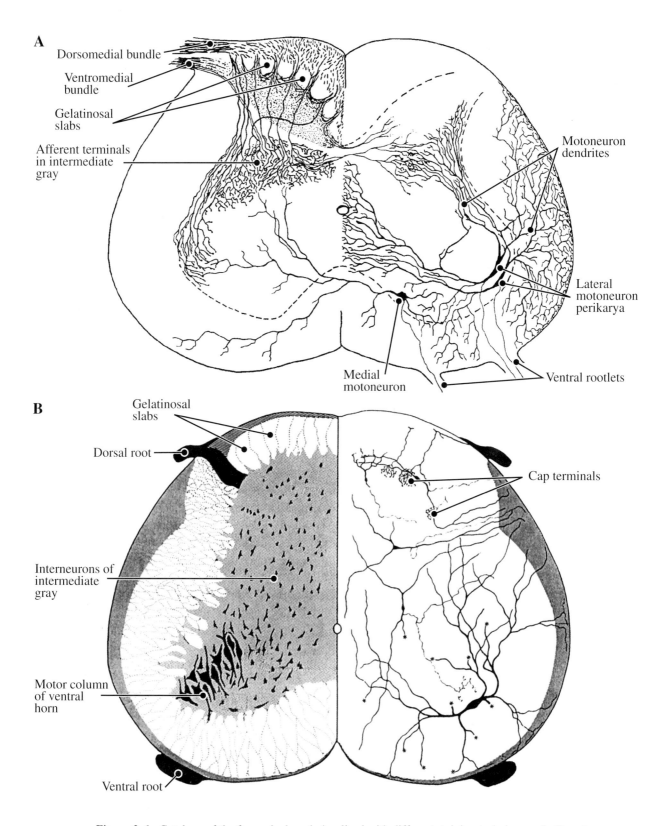

Figure 2-6. Cytology of the frog spinal cord visualized with different staining techniques. **A.** Complementary pattern of dorsal root afferent terminals (**left**) and the dendrites of motoneurons (**right**) in the intermediate gray. After Székely and Czéh (1976). **B.** Motoneuron and interneuron perikarya (**left**), and cap terminals in the dorsal horn (**right**). After Stensaas and Stensaas (1971).

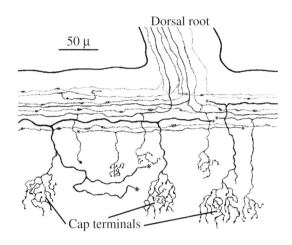

Figure 2-7. Bifurcating dorsal root axons with short collaterals that end as cap terminals in the dorsal horn. Oblique horizontal section of the toad spinal cord. After Stensaas and Stensaas (1971).

Fibers of the ventromedial bundle of the dorsal root turn ventrally, and most of them arborize profusely in the intermediate gray (Figure 2-6A; left side) at a site filled with small interneurons (Figure 2-6B, left) and the dendritic arbors of motoneurons (Figure 2-6A, right). These are proprioceptive collaterals. Other proprioceptive collaterals proceed to the ventral horn (Figure 2-6A, left) and terminate in the vicinity of motoneurons situated in the same location (Figure 2-6B, left). A few collaterals leaving the dorsomedial bundle also seem to terminate in the intermediate gray and the ventral horn (Figure 2-6A, left).

Ventral horn motoneurons of the toad spinal cord have perikarya that are similar to those in higher vertebrates (Figures 2-8A,B). However, the multipolar toad motoneurons have no more that 2-4 main dendrites (Székely and Czéh, 1976), fewer than mammalian motoneurons. Dendritic branches are distributed dorsally and medially within the gray matter, and laterally and ventrally in the white matter (Figure 2-6A, right side). The latter are in the path of fibers of the lateral and ventral funiculi. Incipient rostrocaudally oriented dendritic bundling is indicated in sagittally cut sections (Figure 2-8C). The rostrocaudal length of a motoneuron dendrite may reach 1 mm (Székely and Czéh, 1976) or 2 mm (Stensaas and Stensaas, 1971). The number of boutons on a single frog motoneuron seldom exceeds 20 (Silver, 1942); this contrasts with mammalian motoneurons that may have hundreds of boutons in a single section (Section 1.5.2). The motoneurons of the frog

ventral horn form two discrete columns: a smaller medial column and a larger lateral column (Figure 2-8A). The lateral column of motoneurons is particularly prominent in the cervical and lumbar enlargements (Silver, 1942). Electrophysiological studies indicate that medial column motoneurons innervate trunk muscles, while lateral column motoneurons innervate limb muscles of the extremities (Silver, 1942).

Nemec (1951) distinguished two columns of medial neurons and two columns of lateral neurons in the frog ventral horn (Figure 2-9). In a retrograde degeneration study based on the crushing of nerves that innervate different hind limb muscles in the bullfrog, Cruce (1974) identified twelve motoneuron clusters within the lateral column. He assigned these clusters to three groups, the ventral, the rostrodorsal, and the caudodorsal (Figure 2-10). Although the homologies of amphibian and mammalian muscles are uncertain, the results suggest similarities in the functional organization of motoneuron columns. As in mammals, motoneurons that innervate muscles acting on the hip joint tend to be located more ventrally and rostrally (rostral segments 8 and 9). Motoneurons that innervate muscles that act on the knee joint are located somewhat more dorsally and caudally (segments 8, 9 and 10). Finally, motoneurons acting on ankle and toe joints are located most dorsally and farthest caudally (caudal segments 10 and 11). In a recent study, Ryan et al. (1998) applied HRP to seven homologous muscles in a reptile (iguana) and a mammal (mouse). The results showed that the relative position the motoneuron groups was similar in the two species. This suggests that motoneuron organization is of ancient heritage and has been well preserved in vertebrate evolution. However, there is a difference in the degree of separation of motoneurons between frogs and mammals. In the frog, the motor columns are quite indistinct whereas in mammals many of them are well seperated from one another.

The spinal cord of the frog has extensive ascending and descending connections with the medulla and the brain stem (Joseph and Whitlock, 1968; Ebbeson, 1976). Prominent among the ascending pathways are the spinoreticular, spinovestibular, spinocerebellar, and spinomesencephalic tracts. The mesencephalic reticular formation is a major target of ascending fibers but the details of this projection remain to be determined. A projection from the frog spinal cord to the medullary vestibular complex

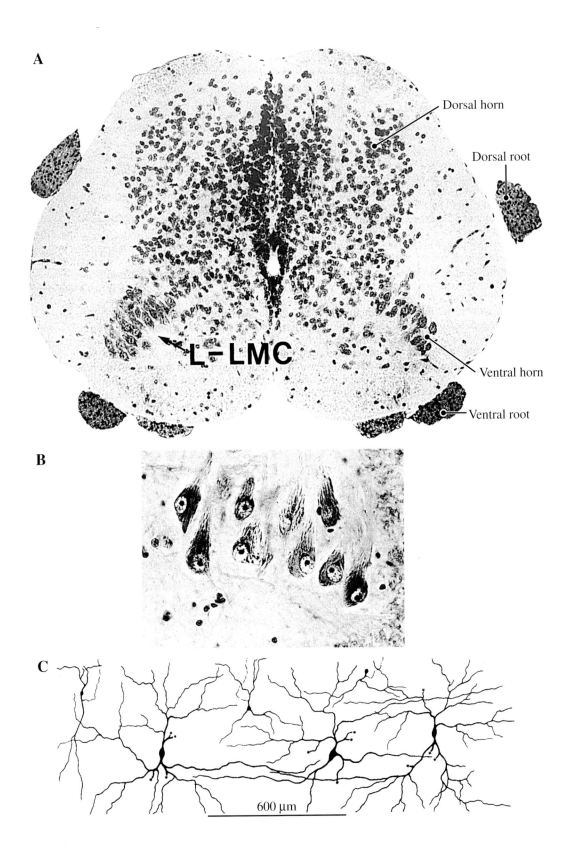

Figure 2-8. A. Gray and white matter in the lumbar enlargement of the toad spinal cord in coronal section with large motoneurons laterally in the ventral horn (L-LMC). **B.** The motoneurons of the lateral motor column at higher magnification. From Sperry and Grobstein (1983). **C.** Incipient motoneuron dendritic bundling in a sagittal section of the toad spinal cord. From Stensaas and Stensaas (1971).

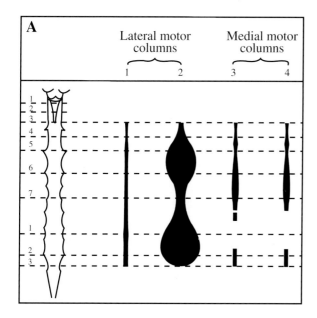

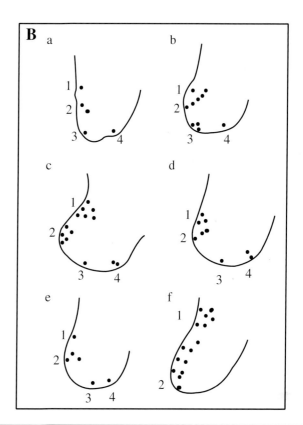

Figure 2-9. A. Reconstruction of the two lateral (1,2) and two medial (3,4) motor columns in the frog spinal cord. **B.** Motoneurons assigned to the different columns at six selected levels of the spinal cord. After Nemec (1951).

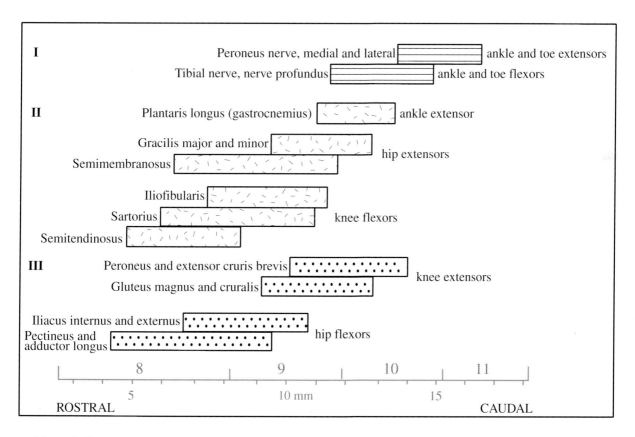

Figure 2-10. Location and spread of 12 motoneuron groups in the lumbar spinal cord of the frog, from rostral to caudal in segments 8-11, in relation to the hind limb muscles they innervate (**left**) and their mode of action (**right**). The motoneurons that innervate proximal knee and hip muscles (I, II) are located rostrally and ventrally, whereas the motoneurons that innervate distal ankle and toe muscles are located more caudally and dorsally (III). After Cruce (1974a).

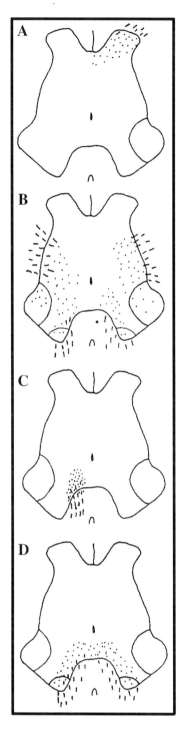

Figure 2-11. Distribution of fibers of the dorsal root (**A**), the reticulospinal tract (**B**), the tectospinal tract (**C**), and the vestibulospinal tract (**D**) in the frog spinal cord. Based on degeneration studies. After Ebbeson (1976).

has been demonstrated physiologically (Precht et al., 1974), and traced anatomically in the frog (Ebbeson, 1976) and the lizard (Ebbeson, 1967). The fibers apparently course in the dorsal funiculus. Some of these fibers may be collaterals of the spinocerebellar tract which, likewise, course in the dorsal funiculus

(Ebbeson, 1976). The spinocerebellar fibers are said to be first order dorsal root axons in the frog (Joseph and Whitlock, 1968b) rather than higher-order (post-synaptic) fibers, as in mammals. The fiber composition of the frog dorsal funiculus is apparently quite different from that of the mammalian dorsal funiculus. Indeed, there is no evidence for the existence of dorsal column nuclei, comparable to the gracile and cuneate nuclei in mammals, or for a medial lemniscal pathway. Finally, the spinothalamic projection is very sparse in the frog (Ebbeson, 1976).

Several descending pathways have been identified in the frog spinal cord, including the tectospinal, vestibulospinal, and reticulospinal tracts (Figure 2-11). The most extensive of all supraspinal descending pathways is the reticulospinal tract (Ebbeson, 1976; Figure 2-11B). Reticulospinal fibers course in the lateral and ventral funiculi and terminate in the intermediate gray and the ventral horn. Reticulospinal tract axons have monosynaptic connections with motoneurons (Cruce, 1974b). The terminals of the vestibulospinal tract are also quite extensive (Figure 2-11D). Vestibulospinal fibers course in the ventral funiculus and penetrate the ventral horn from its basal aspect (Fuller, 1974). That pattern is very similar to the distribution of the lateral vestibulospinal tract fibers in mammals (Figure 1-98). The smaller tectospinal tract courses in the ventral funiculus and penetrates the ventral horn from its base (Figure 2-11C), a pattern that persists in mammals (Figure 1-100). There is no evidence for a telencephalic projection to the spinal cord (Ebbeson, 1976).

2.2 Old and New Components of the Mammalian Spinal Cord

Figure 2-12 illustrates the morphology of the spinal cord in three quadrupeds – frog, turtle and man – at cervical (left) and lumbar (right) levels. Similarities and differences in the structure of the amphibian and human spinal cord are obvious, with the reptilian spinal cord being intermediate between the two. As an evolutionary interpretation of the similarities and differences, we hypothesize that the mammalian spinal cord contains both phylogenetically old and phylogenetically new components. We designate parts of the spinal cord shared by amphibians and mammals as the old, or paleospinal cord, and those parts of the mammalian spinal cord that

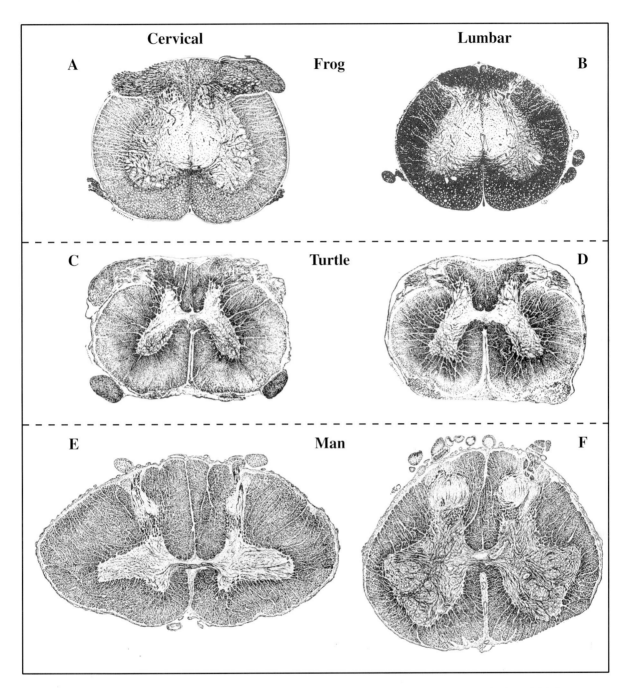

Figure 2-12. Coronal sections of cervical spinal cord (**left column**) and the lumbar spinal cord (**right column**) in frog (**A, B**), turtle (**C, D**), and man (**E, F**). Most notable among the differences is the progressive expansion of the white matter relative to the gray matter, particularly in the cervical cord, from amphibians, to reptiles, to man. Within the white matter, much of this expansion is attributable to the growth of the dorsal and dorsolateral funiculi. Illustrations, not to scale, after Ariens-Kappers et al. (1936).

are absent in primitive vertebrates as the new, or neo-spinal cord. We analyze these two components of the spinal cord in lower and higher vertebrates (specifically, in frog and man) with reference to presumed evolutionary differences in the afferent pathways that relay sensory messages from the spinal cord to old and new brain structures, and differences in the efferent pathways that descend from old and new brain structures and bring motor commands to the spinal cord or modulate its functions.

2.2.1 Paleospinal and Neospinal Sensory Systems. We discussed earlier the functional significance of the small caliber dorsal root afferents. These are the sensory fibers that penetrate the mammalian dorsal horn from the top and end as cap terminals, preferentially in the marginal layer (lamina I) and the upper portion of the substantia gelatinosa (lamina II). Physiological studies established that these fine fibers respond selectively to damaging stimuli, and behavioral and clinical studies implicated this sensory system in pain. Histochemical investigations showed that these fine afferents contain substance P, the puta-

tive nociceptive transmitter, and that the gelatinosal interneurons with which they synapse are rich in peptide neurotransmitters, and their receptors, implicated in the processing of nociceptive messages. In contrast, the large caliber dorsal root afferents have different morphological, physiological, and behavioral properties, and a more complex projection pattern in the dorsal horn. Some of these coarse fibers penetrate the spinal cord from its dorsomedial or medial aspect and proceed ventrally or ventromedially to terminate in the intermediate gray and/or the ventral horn. These are slow adapting, low threshold proprio-

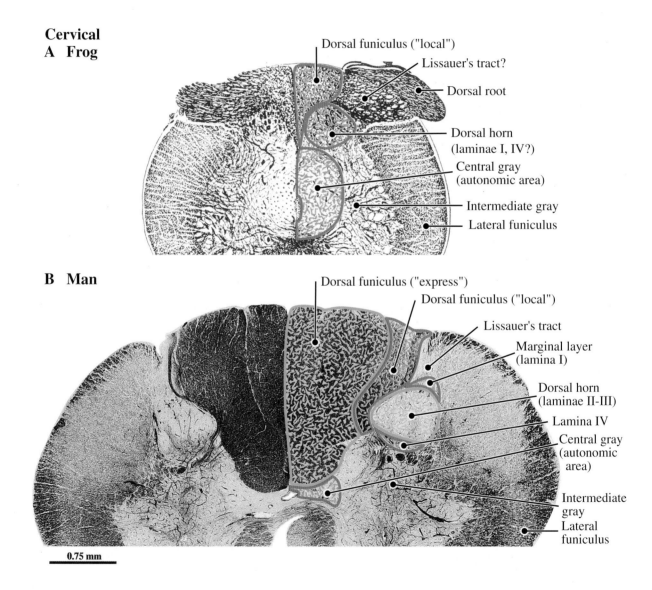

Figure 2-13. A phylogenetic interpretation of old (purple) and new (green) sensory systems in the cervical spinal cord in frog (**A**) and man (**B**). The smaller frog dorsal horn is composed of the phylogenetically older laminae I and IV (purple) while the larger human dorsal horn also contains the phylogenetically younger laminae II-III (green). The small frog dorsal funiculus is composed of short "local" fibers (purple), while the large human dorsal funiculus contains both short "local" (purple) and long "express" (green) fibers. Conversely, the phylogenetically old central autonomic area is relatively large in the frog but small in man. Reproductions not to scale. **A**, from Ariens-Kappers et al. (1936); silver stain. **B**, specimen #Y23-60; newborn; myelin stain.

ceptive fibers that trigger segmental reflexes. Other coarse fibers join the dorsal funiculus and bifurcate into ascending and descending branches that, in turn, give off local collaterals. Most of these fibers are fast adapting, low threshold exteroceptive afferents. The long ascending branch of these axons typically proceeds rostrally to terminate in the dorsal column nuclei and, through relays, convey somesthetic information to higher brain structures. while their local collaterals penetrate the dorsal horn from its medial aspect, recurve beneath the dorsal horn, and pene-

trate it from its bottom. These exteroceptive collaterals terminate with flame endings in the lower portion of the substantia gelatinosa. (We shall return below to the possible functional significance of this dual sensory input to the dorsal horn with cap and flame terminals.)

Some of the morphological differences in the organization of the dorsal spinal cord in frog and man are illustrated in Figures 2-13 and 2-14 at the cervical and lumbar levels, respectively. The first obvious dif-

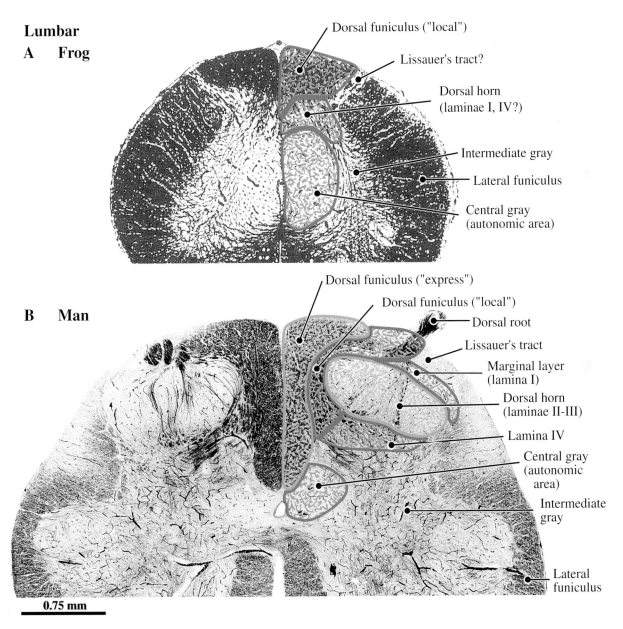

Figure 2-14. A phylogenetic interpretation of old (purple) and new (green) sensory systems in the cervical spinal cord of frog (**A**) and man (**B**) . The differences between the two species seen in the cervical cord (Figure 2-13) are also evident in the lumbar spinal cord. However, the ascending "express" pathway component of the human dorsal funiculus (green) is much smaller at this caudal level than in the cervical cord rostrally. Reproductions not to scale. **A**, from Ariens-Kappers et al. (1936); silver stain. **B**, specimen #Y23-60; newborn; myelin stain.

ference is the relative size of the dorsal horn in the two species: it is small and inconspicuous in the frog, large and bulbous in man. What appears to be absent in the frog dorsal horn is the core of the mammalian dorsal horn. Further studies are needed to substantiate this hypothesis, but it appears that the frog dorsal horn contains only laminae I (the marginal layer) and IV. If so, laminae II and III (the substantia gelatinosa with its multitude of central cells) would be a phylogenetically more recent acquisition in higher vertebrates. Another striking difference is the relative size of the dorsal funiculus and the superior lateral funiculus in the two species: both are small in the frog but very large in man, particularly so in the cervical cord. (We return to this subject below.) The next difference is in the opposite direction: this is the relatively large area occupied by the central gray (central autonomic area) in the frog and its relatively small area in man.

We noted earlier that the dorsal funiculus contains few, if any, long ascending afferents in the frog, and it may also lack dorsal column nuclei. In contrast, the principal fiber constituents of the mammalian dorsal funiculus, which also contains locally distributed fibers, are the long ascending branches of dorsal root fibers that relay exteroceptive messages to higher brain structures via the dorsal column nuclei. This suggests that the dorsal funiculus in frog and man have a different fiber composition. This difference is shown in Figures 2-13 and 2-14. Note that in the frog there is little difference in the size of the dorsal funiculus at lumbar and cervical levels (Figures 2-13A, 2-13B). The lack of incremental growth from caudal to rostral indicates that most (if not all) dorsal funiculus fibers in the frog are short ones that do not ascend to the medulla. In contrast in man the bulk of the dorsal funiculus (the collateralization zone excepted; see below) increases greatly and incrementally from caudal to rostral levels (Figures 2-13B, 2-14B; see also Figure 1-6). Indeed, the fibers originating at lumbosacral levels form a separate structure, the gracile fasciculus, at cervical levels of the cord. Obviously, a significant proportion of the mammalian dorsal funiculus is composed of fibers that proceed uninterruptedly to the dorsal column nuclei. If we may call this large component of the mammalian dorsal funiculus "express" lanes, the inference is warranted that the dorsal funiculus of the frog (and by implication that of lower vertebrates) is composed mainly of "local" lanes.

In Figure 2-15, we illustrate a neglected feature of the organization of the dorsal funiculus in the human spinal cord. What these photomicrographs of myelin-stained, coronal sections reveal is that the fasciculus cuneatus at a cervical level (Figure 2-15A) and the fasciculus gracilis at a lumbar level (Figure 2-15B) contain myelinated fibers that are transected in two different planes. The core of each fasciculus is composed of punctate profiles; these are obviously longitudinally (sagittally) coursing axons transected at a right angle to their trajectory. But also visible is a darker band of semicircular fibers near the dorsal funiculus, both at cervical and lumbar levels, that are sectioned more or less parallel to their trajectory. These transversely oriented fibers are continuous with the dorsal root, enter the dorsal funiculus laterally, course along the medial wall of the dorsal horn, then penetrate the gray matter as individual fascicles underneath the dorsal horn. This circumferential band of fibers is composed of locally terminating branches of the ascending and descending dorsal root axons, to be called the dorsal root collateralization zone. With reference to our current discussion of the different composition of the dorsal funiculus in frog and man, we propose that the frog dorsal funiculus contains only the locally distributed dorsal root fibers, its local lanes, whereas the dorsal funiculus in man also contains a larger complement of supraspinal fibers, the express lanes of the spinolemniscal tract.

2.2.2 Protopathic, Epipathic, and Epicritic Spinal Circuits. There are two classes of large caliber dorsal root afferents, those that convey proprioceptive messages from muscle and joint sensors, and those that convey exteroceptive messages from skin sensors. The latter, the exteroceptors, include Pacinian corpuscles, Merkel discs, and hair follicle endings that respond to delicate mechanical stimuli as one grasps, palpates or handles objects of different shapes, textures, and other physical properties. The exteroceptors and their large caliber afferents have a low stimulus threshold, a small receptive field, and they adapt rapidly to stimuli (i.e., give a transient discharge at the onset and/or cessation of a stimulus, and can track faithfully the amplitude and frequency changes of stimuli). As such, they are well suited to furnish precise "objective" (cognitively useful) information about the static and dynamic properties of external stimuli. In contrast, the small caliber nociceptive afferents with free endings in the skin,

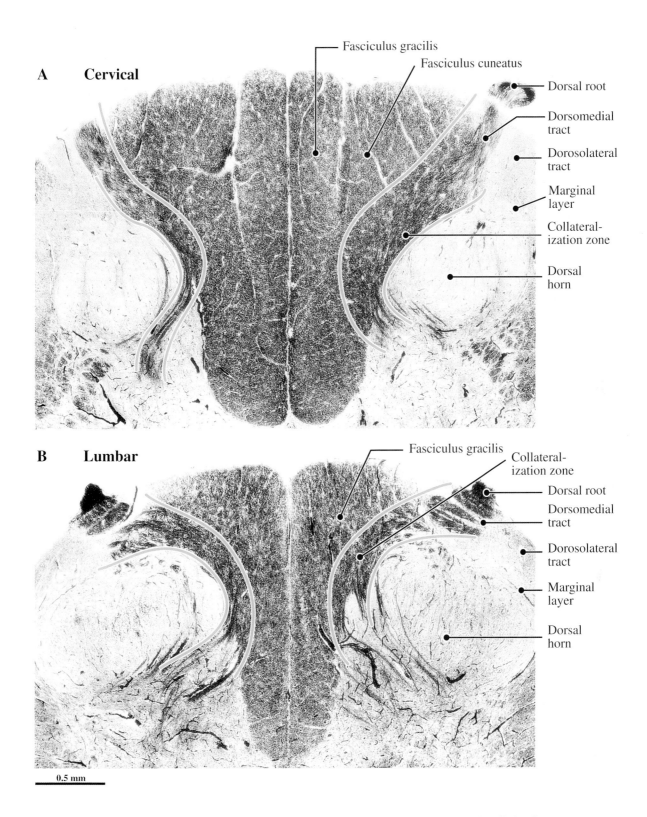

A   Cervical

Fasciculus gracilis
Fasciculus cuneatus
Dorsal root
Dorsomedial tract
Dorosolateral tract
Marginal layer
Collateral-ization zone
Dorsal horn

B   Lumbar

Fasciculus gracilis
Collateral-ization zone
Dorsal root
Dorsomedial tract
Dorosolateral tract
Marginal layer
Dorsal horn

0.5 mm

Figure 2-15. The collateralization zone (blue) of the dorsal funiculus at cervical (**A**) and lumbar (**B**) levels of the human spinal cord. The punctate profiles in the core of the dorsal funiculus are the transversely cut, long branches of dorsal root axons that ascend to the dorsal column nuclei. The circumferential fibers in the lateral portion of the dorsal funiculus are the local collaterals of dorsal root axons that enter the gray matter beneath the dorsal horn. Specimen # Y299-62; 4-day-old infant; myelin stain.

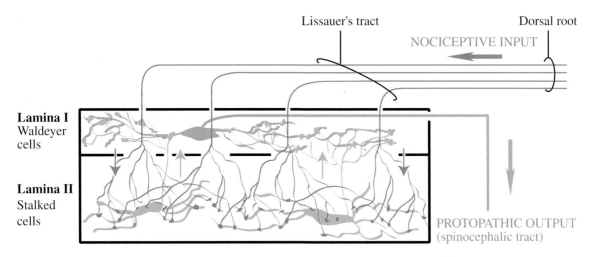

Figure 2-16. The hypothetical synaptic relationship between peripheral *nociceptive* afferents with cap terminals (red) and the dendrites of stalked cells (green) in lamina II. The axon terminals of stalked cells (green) synapse in lamina I with Waldeyer cell dendrites (purple). The ascending axons of the large lamina I neurons (purple) form the central *protopathic* pathway involved in visceral/autonomic regulation.

respond to such stimuli as heat, cold, burns, cuts, bruises, inflammation, and other kinds of threats or damage to body tissues. The nociceptive afferents have a high stimulus threshold, a large receptive field, and adapt slowly to stimuli (i.e., give a sustained discharge throughout stimulation). Instead of providing point-by-point, and moment-by-moment accounts about events that transpire in the external world, they alert the individual to harmful or beneficial effects on the body tissues, that is, they provide "subjective" (emotionally relevant) messages about conditions that affect the individual's well-being and health.

Further consideration of the role that nociceptive messages could play in the control of behavior suggests two different functions: (i) what might be called a visceral housekeeping function, and (ii) a perceptual informative function. For instance, in order to control the constancy of body temperature in warm-blooded animals, it is necessary to monitor continuously any changes in the temperature gradient across the skin, i.e., signal heat loss or heat gain under different ambient conditions. The responses to these signals – heat production or heat dissipation – are to a large extent dependent on visceral reactions that are controlled by the autonomic nervous system (e.g., shivering, sweating, panting). However, temperature is also an important sensory attribute of the palpated or manipulated object, much like its shape or texture. That is, thermal signals can also serve perceptual functions that are controlled by higher levels of the central nervous system. The same applies to

messages about tissue damage. On the one hand, tissue damage requires the initiation and maintenance of appropriate protective and regenerative reactions; this is the visceral function of nociception. On the other hand, the noxious quality of the touched or handled object (for instance, its hardness, sharpness, abrasiveness) is also an important perceptual feature that calls for cognitive assessment. We propose that these two functions, the visceral/autonomic and the perceptual/cognitive, are elaborated by two different neural circuits in the dorsal horn, and are conveyed to different supraspinal brain structures through different afferent channels.

Figure 2-16 provides a diagram of our hypothesis how nociceptive fibers terminate in the superficial laminae of the dorsal horn with cap endings and provide input to one of the dorsal horn circuits. As we noted earlier (Section 1.3.3), the cap endings of small caliber axons are distributed in the upper part of lamina II, where the perikarya and the dendritic arbor of stalked cells are located. The axons of stalked cells terminate dorsally in lamina I. The target of these axons, we propose, are the dendrites of large nociceptive Waldeyer cells in lamina I whose long axons join the spinocephalic tract in the dorsolateral funiculus and reach various supraspinal structures, in particular the periaqueductal gray (Section 1.3.2). (The other large cells of lamina II, like the islet cells, whose axons terminate within lamina II, are not shown in the diagram.) Since nociceptive afferents have large receptive fields and many cap

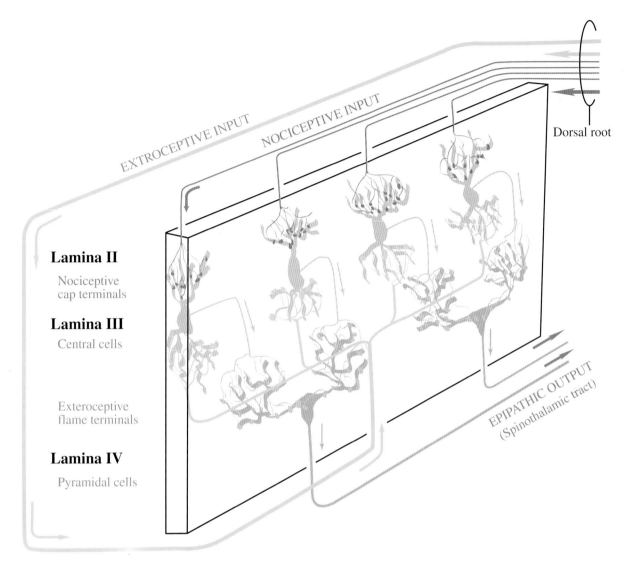

Figure 2-17. The hypothetical synaptic relationship of *nociceptive* (red) and *exteroceptive* (light blue) dorsal root fibers with the dendrites of the double-tufted central cells (purple) in the dorsal horn. The nociceptive fibers end with cap terminals on the dorsal dendrites, whereas the recurring exteroceptive fibers end with flame terminals on the ventral dendrites. The locally arborizing axons of central cells synapse with lamina IV pyramidal cells (violet) whose axons form the ascending *epipathic* pathway.

terminals may converge on a single stalked cell, this pathway is not suited for the conveyance of fine-grained information about the properties of a stimulus. However, the coarse grained messages conveyed by them would be suitable for visceral regulation. Following Head (1920), we refer to this circuit and its afferents as the protopathic pathway. Protopathic sensations are, by definition, highly arousing affective or emotional experiences but, like referred pain, lack such perceptual attributes as topographic or somatotopic localization ("local sign") and iconic representation of the overt features of a stimulus ("object discrimination").

Figure 2-17 provides a diagram of second hypothetical circuit in the dorsal horn with nociceptive input. In this circuit, the central cells of the substantia gelatinosa (Section 1.3.3) are the targets of two afferent inputs, the nociceptive cap terminals and the exteroceptive flame terminals. We may recall that the central cells are the principal interneurons of the substantia gelatinosa that are distinguished by dorsally and ventrally directed (or apical and basal) dendritic tufts. The central cells with this double bouquet of dendrites are well-placed to receive synaptic input from the nociceptive cap terminals dorsally and the exteroceptive flame terminals ventrally. Relevant in this context are the following observa-

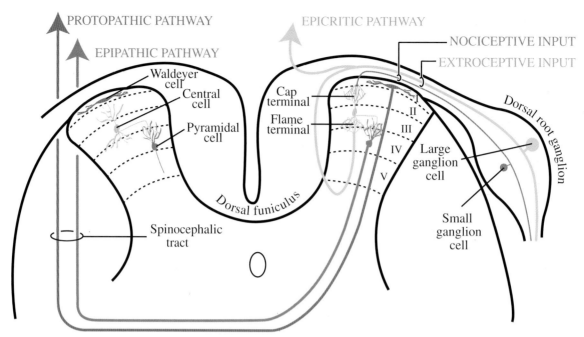

Figure 2-18. Summary diagram of the basic circuitry of two peripheral input channels, the *nociceptive* (red) and *exterocep-tive* (light blue), in relation to two central ascending pathways, the *protopathic* (purple) and the *epipathic* (violet). The relay neurons of the protopathic pathway are principally located in lamina I, those of the epipathic pathway in lamina IV. The axons of both cross to the opposite side within the spinal cord and ascend to the brain. In contrast, the *epicritic* pathway (light blue; shown in detail in Figure 2-20) ascends ipsilaterally and uninterruptedly within the spinal cord to the medulla.

tions (Sections 1.3.3, 1.3.4): First, laminae II and III contain the gelatinosal glomeruli where afferents make synaptic contacts with interneurons with both electron-lucent and electron-dense boutons. Second, the axons of central cells terminate within the sub-stantia gelatinosa. Third, the target of central cell output could be the large pyramidal cells of lamina IV whose dendritic plexus penetrates the substantia gelatinosa. Fourth, lamina IV pyramidal cells are relay neurons that contribute fibers to two ascending tracts, the spinocervical and the spinothalamic tracts.

If the central cells, as suggested, receive both nociceptive and exteroceptive input, they are in a posi-tion to integrate the two to provide supraspinal brain centers with subjective messages that are enriched with objective information, such as the location and physical features of an affect-laden stimulus. We will refer to this integrated circuit and its afferent channel as the epipathic pathway. Figure 2-18 sum-marizes the principal cellular elements of the spinal cord involved in the integration of peripheral nocicep-tive and exteroceptive messages and their transmis-sion to supraspinal levels of the central nervous system by way of two hypothetical pathways, the protopathic and the epipathic. The relationship between these two central pathways and a third afferent system, the neospinal epicritic pathway, is discussed below.

2.2.3   Some Features of the Neospinal Dorsal Funiculus. In addition to the protopathic and epipathic afferent pathways, there is a third ascending channel in the mammalian spinal cord. This chan-nel is composed principally (though not exclusively, as we shall see below) of the main ascending branch of exteroceptive dorsal root fibers that form the bulk of the greatly expanded mammalian dorsal funicu-lus. Head (1920) hypothesized that the dorsal funicu-lus is the epicritic afferent channel that provides the cerebral cortex with objective information about the physical features of things touched and manipulated. However, subsequent clinical observations and exper-imental findings have shown that the dorsal funicu-lus is a far more complex and heterogeneous sensory pathway than it was envisaged by Head. As we shall see, the dorsal funiculus is an inclusive channel that contains not only epicritic afferents but also epipathic afferents.

According to an early comparative study by Brouwer (reported by Ariens-Kappers et al., 1936, vol. 1, p. 260), the dorsal funiculus constitutes 16.6% of the white matter in the opossum, 22% in the cow, 23.9% in the bear, 26.4% in the cebus monkey, and 39% in man. More recently, Bossy and Ferratier (1968) found that the area occupied by the dorsal funiculus relative to the entire white matter (which they measured separately in 28 spinal segments) varies between 15% and 25% in a primitive primate (the bush baby) and between 25% and 45% in man. Expressed as the ratio of the dorsal funiculus to the gray matter, the proportion was 12% for the bush baby and 27% for man. These findings suggest that the progressive increase in mammals in the bulk of dorsal funiculus afferents is an evolutionary trend that has reached its peak in the human spinal cord. What is the significance of the evolutionary expansion of the dorsal funiculus in higher vertebrates and man, and what might be its unique sensorimotor function?

In limbless aquatic vertebrates, like fishes, exteroceptors scattered over the body provide information about ambient conditions in the environment, such as the temperature and salinity of the water, the magnitude of water pressure, the direction of currents and waves, and the like. The cutaneous senses also furnish "passive" (i.e., unsolicited) information about contact with external objects, such as being irritated by a parasite, grabbed by a predator, or nuzzled by a mate. In bottom feeders, tentacles on the head (which are innervated by cranial nerves) provide some actively gathered information about the location of nutrients but, because fishes lack limbs, the spinal exteroceptors do not serve as "active" sensors. In amphibians and reptiles with extremities, the cutaneous spinal afferents may begin to assume an active role. The stretching or grabbing toes, for instance, are in a position to furnish tactile information about the texture of the ground traversed and the physical features of the rock or tree branch touched or grasped. It is in higher vertebrates, particularly those that use their paws to manipulate objects (as rats, squirrels, raccoons, and monkeys do) that the cutaneous exteroceptors acquire a new function, i.e., to gather information about the tactile attributes of objects. For instance, the ability to pick berries or fruits of various sizes, shapes, and textures from a tree branch requires that the digits of the paw are adjusted to the shape of the object, and the force applied is properly adjusted to the task "at hand." This is made possible by the ability to assess by "feel" the varied features of the explored and handled object, such as its configuration, consistency, pliability, and the like.

The ability to palpate, lift, and effectively manipulate objects requires that the passive skin sensors are transformed into active exploratory organs. This evolutionary trend, the development of the haptic sense (sensory infromation obtained by active palpa-

tion), has reached its peak in biped man. In man, the hind limbs are specialized to support the upright stance at rest and during locomotion, and the specialized task of the mobile hands and dexterous fingers is not only to explore and manipulate an endless variety of objects but also to modify, assemble, sculpt, and fabricate them. We shall argue below that this new haptic function of the cutaneous exteroceptors led to the evolutionary transformation of the small paleospinal dorsal funiculus of lower vertebrates into the large neospinal dorsal funiculus of higher mammals and man.

The majority of the long ascending fibers of the dorsal funiculus have a low stimulus threshold, a small receptive field, and they adapt rapidly to the same stimulus. By virtue of these properties, the dorsal funiculus can transmit fine-grained and topographically accurate tactile information to the cerebral cortex by way of dedicated supraspinal relay stations. Indeed, it is the limbs and the digits that have the largest areal representation in the relay stations of this pathway, i.e., in the dorsal column nuclei (Figure 1-84), the ventrobasal complex of the thalamus (Rose and Mountcstle (1959), and the primary somatosensory area of the cerebral cortex (Penfield and Rasmussen (1950). These considerations justify Head's notion that the dorsal funiculus is the epicritic pathway. However, there are some problems with this simple conceptualization. The first comes from clinical and experimental studies of the effects of dorsal funiculus lesions. If the dorsal funiculus is the epicritic afferent system, its destruction ought to produce severe tactile deficits in man, such as the inability to respond to light touch or to localize tactile stimuli applied to different body regions. Neither the older clinical evidence nor current observations support this expectation. Extensive dorsal funiculus lesions in patients do not abolish sensitivity to light touch and do not produce deficits in tactile localization (Dejerine, 1914; Boshes and Padberg, 1953; Cook and Browder, 1965; Gilman and Denny-Brown, 1966; Nathan et al., 1986). Indeed, if the spinothalamic tract is spared, even the prototypical epicritic ability of fine-grained "two-point discrimination" tends to recover. On the other hand, dorsal funiculus lesions do interfere with the ability to identify the shape of an object by palpation (the deficit is called astereognosia), and also with the ability to integrate successive tactile stimulation of the skin into a unitary percept, as when the blindfolded patient is asked to identify numerals traced on his hand (Wartenberg, 1939) or describe the direction of a brush moved over the skin surface (Hankey and Edis, 1989). Moreover, clinical observations indicate that patients with dorsal funiculus lesions tend to be clumsy with their hands, suggesting a deficit in dexterity (Nathan et al., 1986).

Admittedly, few of the dorsal funiculus lesions described in the literature were complete. But the results of better controlled experiments in animals also speak against a simple interpretation of the role of the dorsal funiculus in somesthetic and somatomotor functions. Cats with dorsal funiculus lesions move about quite well on the ground after a period of recovery, and their motor deficiencies do not become evident until they are required to perform difficult tasks, such as turn around on a narrow beam, jump onto a moving platform, or jump over a hurdle on the moving platform (Melzack and Bridges, 1971; Dubrovsky et al., 1971; Melzack and Southmayd, 1974). Such findings support Wall's (1970) hypothesis that the dorsal funiculus afferents play an important role in the coordination of skilled movements.

Impairments of somesthetic functions following dorsal funiculus lesions are also quite specific. Destruction of 90% of the dorsal funicular fibers representing the paw in cats, but not smaller lesions, produce deficits in texture discrimination (Dobry and Casey, 1972). In monkeys, dorsal funiculus lesions produce only transient deficits in two-point tactile discrimination and the detection of stroking of the skin with a brush; however, there is an enduring deficit in the ability to discriminate the direction of the brush stroke (Vierck, 1974, 1977). While the deficits in ballistic reaching movements with the arms is transient, the impairment in the dexterous use of fingers to grasp the object tends to be permanent (Vierck, 1978). Another study showed that monkeys with dorsal funiculus lesions are able to identify simple geometric shapes by touch but cannot distinguish more complex forms that require palpation and successive exploratory movements (Azulay and Schwartz, 1975). Another enduring deficit following dorsal funiculus lesions is the discrimination of vibration frequency (Vierck, et al., 1985). These findings generally confirm the clinical reports in human patients. In a recent study, Vierck and his collaborators (Makous et al., 1996) suggested that dorsal column lesions in monkeys produce enduring deficits only if they have to integrate the successively gathered tactile information over time, which is the case when the animal has

to detect either the direction, the frequency, or the duration of a tactile stimulus.

The finding that dorsal funiculus lesions produce *transient* postoperative deficits in the performance of simple tactile discriminations and routine motor activities indicates that, under normal conditions, the dorsal funiculus is involved in these tasks. The fact that, after some lapse of time the operated animals regain many of their lost abilities, also indicates that the cerebral cortex can use alternate somatosensory afferent channels, if necessary. Finally, the additional finding that dorsal funiculus lesions produce *enduring* deficits in tasks that require palpation and the temporal integration of tactile stimuli, indicate that the dorsal funiculus is essential for certain somesthetic functions. The question is what category these functions might be assigned to. Since the temporal integration of successive tactile stimuli (those actively obtained by serial palpation and manipulation) into a unitary percept presupposes the operation of short-term "working memory" (Baddeley, 1976), and since the acquisition of an extensive repertoire of acquired manipulatory and constructive skills requires long-term memory storage, we propose that the dorsal column pathway of the spinal cord has evolved into a unique afferent channel dedicated to the cognitive processing of tactile information by the cerebral cortex.

What we propose is that the evolutionary transformation of the dorsal funiculus from a locally terminating afferent tract into a supraspinal express pathway, one that selectively conveys tactile information to the cerebral cortex, is linked to the transformation of the grabbing paws with clawed digits of lower vertebrates into the dexterous paws of mammals and the clawless, padded fingers of apes and man (Napier, 1970). The transformation of the locomotor forelimbs into manipulatory arms and hands was not a universal evolutionary trend; it clearly did not take place in herbivores. It is evident in some insectivores, rodents, and carnivores, and in most primates. These species often change their quadruped stance to a squatting or sitting position and thus free their forelimbs and paws for manipulating objects. This somatomotor change, we propose, was coupled with a shift from the *subcortical* control (or automated use) of all limbs for locomotion to a *cortical* control (or voluntary use) of the hindlimbs for standing, squatting or sitting, and the forelimbs for skilled manipulatory tasks.

The ability to use the dexterous hands to palpate, manipulate, and fabricate objects has peaked in man. With a bony structure not unlike that found in lower vertebrates, a man is able to use his hands in an endless variety of ways, sometimes using all fingers in a power grip, and in other applications the tip of the forefinger and the opposed thumb in a precision grip (Napier, 1970). Relying on his dexterous hands, man can spin, weave, and sew to make clothing; split, chip, or polish stone to make tools or weapons; saw planks, hammer nails, and build a house, or a boat; write, draw, or paint; fabricate different components of a machine and assemble them into a working whole; play the guitar, violin, or piano; and so on endlessly. None of these skills comes readymade as an inherited ability; each has to be learned, some quite readily, others through extended practice. The skilled use of the hands would not be possible without the neocortex, which receives a massive sensory input (in particular, visual) by way of a dedicated corticopetal pathway relayed in the thalamus. The tactile component of this dedicated channel is the massive dorsal funiculus.

Although cutaneous afferents with low stimulus threshold and high resolution are the major component of the dorsal funiculus, it also contains other afferent channels. For instance, it has been reported that, in rats, dorsal funiculus lesions reduce the discharge of thalamic neurons to noxious visceral stimuli (Al-Chaer et al., 1996b), and lesions limited to the midline dorsal funiculus alter the behavior of rats suffering from experimentally induced pain (Houghton et al., 1997). With reference to man, a small midline dorsal funiculus lesion was recently reported to abolish visceral pain in a patient (Nauta et al., 1997). The presence of nociceptive afferents in the dorsal funiculus makes good sense if it is true, as we suggested earlier, that the neospinal dorsal funiculus is involved in the learning of tactile discriminations and the mastery of motor skills. According to basic psychological principles, learning is governed by "negative and positive reinforcement," i.e., the punishment effect of pain and the rewarding effect of pleasure. Therefore, the dorsal funiculus may contain nociceptive input to directly convey information to the cortex about negative reinforcement effects (pain, discomfort, injury, malaise, deprivation, exhaustion) and perhaps also positive reinforcement effects (pleasure, relief, comfort, satiation) associated with responses to stimuli. The dorsal funiculus, in this view, is not an *exclusive* epicritic pathway but an *inclusive* afferent channel

dedicated to supply the cortex with all the information that it needs to perform its complex functions. Its largest component is the epicritic pathway but it also contains an epipathic pathway, a proprioceptive pathway (see Figure 1-82), and perhaps others.

Our proposed relationship between two *peripheral* dorsal root input systems (the nociceptive and the exteroceptive) and three *central* cutaneous afferent pathways (the protopathic, epipathic, and epicritic) is summarized in Figures 2-19 and 2-20. The major points are as follows.

(1) One target of the thin and mostly unmyelinated peripheral *nociceptive* dorsal root fibers are the lamina I spinocephalic relay neurons. These relay neurons (such as Waldeyer cells) project to paleocephalic structures: the reticular formation of the medulla and midbrain, the central gray of the medulla, the periaqueductal gray of the midbrain, and the midline nuclei of the thalamus (Figure 2-19). This is the *protopathic* circuit and pathway. This central afferent system receives little or no exteroceptive input. If so, the coarse-grained and affect-laden messages conveyed by this system makes limited contribution to perceptual and cognitive functions. But this pathway could very well be involved in visceral regulation via the autonomic nervous system. We shall consider the coarse sensory signals transmitted by this protopathic pathway as of low "autonomic quality."

(2) The second afferent circuit and channel has a dual input. The double tufted central cells of laminae II-III receive input from both *nociceptive* dorsal root fibers (via the dorsal cap terminals) and *exteroceptive* dorsal root fibers (via the recurving flame terminals). The integrating central cells, in turn, synapse with the pyramidal cells of lamina IV whose ascending axons form the *epipathic* pathway. The principal targets of this channel are the medial and lateral thalamic nuclei (Figure 2-19). This system, in which coarse-grained affective signals of nociceptive origin are enriched with fine-grained exteroceptive signals, could play a role in such hybrid viscero-somatic functions as emotional arousal, behavioral vigilance, and sensory attention. The sensory messages transmitted by this afferent pathway are considered to be of a higher "emotional quality."

(3) The third afferent system, which has progressively evolved from lower mammals to man, receives its principal (though not exclusive) input from

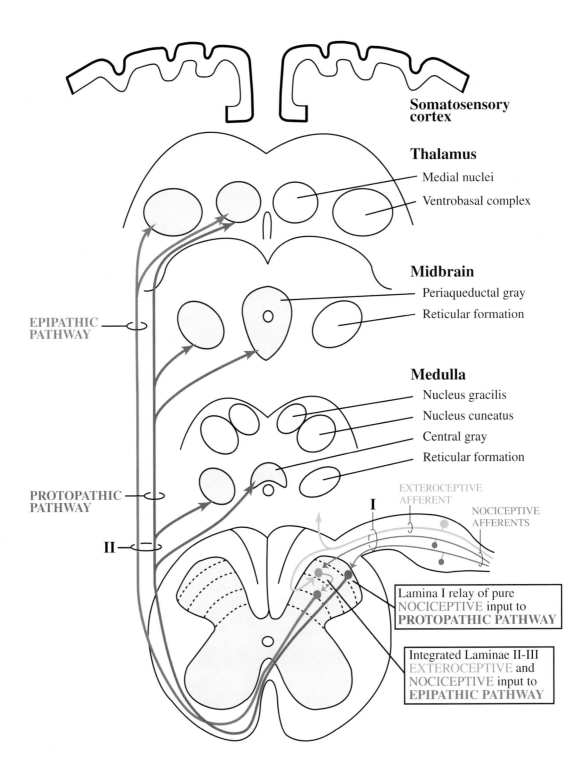

Figure 2-19. Schematic diagram of the spinal circuitry and supraspinal course of the hypothetical *proto-pathic* (purple) and *epipathic* (violet) pathways. Input to the protopathic pathway (I) is from nociceptive dorsal root axons (red) that synapse with relay neurons in lamina I of the dorsal horn. The decussating protopathic afferents (II) terminate in the central gray, periaqueductal gray, the reticular formation, and the medial nuclei of the thalamus. The epipathic pathway receives dual input from nociceptive (red) and extero-ceptive (blue) dorsal root fibers that synapse with central cells in laminae II and III. The preferential targets of the ascending epipathic afferents are the medial and ventrobasal nuclei of the thalamus.

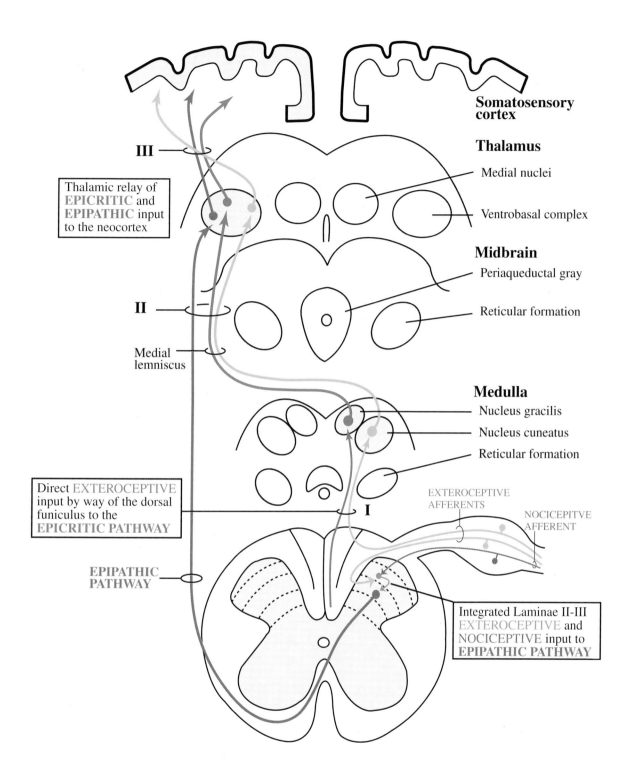

Figure 2-20. Schematic diagram of the supraspinal course of the *epicritic* pathway (dark blue). Input to this pathway is from exteroceptive dorsal root fibers (I) that ascend ipsilaterally to the gracile nucleus (dark blue) and the cuneate nucleus (light blue). The axons of the second order neurons (II) decussate in the medulla and terminate in the ventrobasal complex of the thalamus. The relay neurons of this complex project to the somatosensory cortex and associated cortical areas (III). There is also a smaller *epipathic* (violet) pathway to the cortex by way of the dorsal column nuclei (not shown) and the medial lemniscus; both are relayed in the ventrobasal complex of the thalamus.

exteroceptive dorsal root fibers that proceed directly to the dorsal column nuclei where the messages are relayed, again directly, by way of the ventrobasal nuclei of the thalamus, to the cerebral cortex. This dedicated exteroceptive channel to the cerebral cortex is the *epicritic* pathway (Figure 2-20) and the sensory messages transmitted by this pathway are considered to be of the highest "cognitive quality." The major function of this fine-grained afferent pathway, which maps the extremities and their digits in great detail in the neocortex, is to allow the dexterous use of the hands for palpating, manipulating, and fabricating an infinite variety of objects. This new function is accomplished with the aid of three higher functions. First, the paws or hands are freed for these uses as postural control shifts to the lower body and the hind limbs while squatting, sitting, standing, or walking. Second, the cerebral cortex is provided with detailed information about the properties of the objects touched, grasped, palpated, or otherwise manipulated through a dedicated perceptual channel. Third, through learning and cognitive processing, the cerebral cortex builds and stores an extensive program of manual skills. Importantly, the dorsal funiculus is not a pure epicritic pathway, it also contains epipathic and other afferents. This, we argued, is so because the successful learning of tactile discriminations and manual skills requires negative and positive reinforcement mediated by pain and pleasure.

2.2.4 Paleospinal and Neospinal Efferent Systems.

All vertebrates have a specialized rostral body part, the head. The head contains the special sense organs (those of vision, hearing, smell, taste, and balance) and a brain that processes information gathered by the special senses. Sherrington (1906) called the bilaterally symmetrical olfactory, visual, and auditory sense organs *teleceptors*, and distinguished them from the exteroceptors of the skin as well as the taste buds (which he also called contact receptors). While the skin exteroceptors respond to direct contact made with objects, teleceptors respond to odor, light, or sound emitted and/or reflected by objects located some distance from the body. (Although the vestibular apparatus has affinities with the teleceptors, Sherrington considered it more akin to proprioceptors.) To enable the teleceptors to orient and guide the body toward or away from distant objects, the brain sends motor commands to spinal motoneurons that contract the muscles that turn the head and propel the limbs forwards, sideways, or backwards. This supraspinal control of spinal cord motoneurons is exercised by various "higher-level" (cortical) and "intermediate-level" (subcortical) motor systems, and their motor commands are delivered either to "lower-level" spinal pattern generators or directly to the "final motoneurons" of the ventral horn.

According to a venerable philosophical and psychological tradition, there are two types of motor acts or behavior, the involuntary and the voluntary (for a recent discussion, see Prochazka et al., 2000). A related neurological dichotomy is that between the pyramidal (voluntary) and the extrapyramidal (involuntary) motor systems. The positive terms of "voluntary" and "pyramidal" have definable meanings; the negative terms "involuntary" and "extrapyramidal" are more difficult to define. A voluntary activity is one that a person performs by his own choice or conscious will. When I stand up because I intend to go to the door, or if I consent to stand up when someone asks me to do so, I am acting voluntarily. If I lie unconsciously in bed (as when in a comatose state) I cannot will to stand up; and if I am lying on the sofa semiconsciously (for instance, intoxicated) I may not be able to stand up even if I want to do so. In contrast, involuntary activity is one that I carry out in the absence of my choice or will, and sometimes contrary to my will. There are many kinds of involuntary activities, including muscle twitches, simple reflexes, complex chains of reflexes, autonomic reactions, and emotional expressions and actions over which one has little or no volitional control. It is an old neurological credo, though doubted by many, that voluntary activities are initiated by neocortical mechanisms, and conveyed to the spinal cord by the pyramidal tract (more precisely, the corticospinal fibers of the pyramidal tract), whereas involuntary activities are triggered by subcortical or "extrapyramidal" pathways acting upon the spinal cord.

Below we will seek support for the traditional view that involuntary activities are controlled by subcortical (paleocephalic) motor circuits and efferent pathways of the medulla, pons, midbrain, and diencephalon, whereas voluntary activities are controlled by cortical (neencephalic) mechanisms and conveyed to the spinal cord by way of the corticospinal tract. In our discussion of the paleocephalic motor system, we shall consider only those brain structures that are known to send efferents directly to the spinal cord, i.e., the vestibulospinal, interstitiospinal, reticulospinal, rubrospinal, and tectospinal tracts. We will not deal with the subcortical efferent tracts that exert their influence on the spinal cord indirectly through intermediary brain structures such as the basal telencephalon (striatum, pallidum, amygdala, etc.) or the ventral diencephalon and mesencephalon (hypothalamus, tegmentum) – even though these are often considered major components of the extrapyramidal system.

2.2.5 The Paleospinal Efferent System: The Vestibular, Interstitial, Tectal, and Rubral Tracts.

The vestibulospinal tract is one of the phylogenetically oldest descending tracts of the central nervous system; it has been identified in such a primitive vertebrate as the lamprey (Ariens-Kappers, 1936). In mammals, there are two vestibulospinal tracts. The *lateral vestibulospinal tract* originates in the lateral vestibular (Deiters') nucleus and extends all the way to the lumbosacral cord in animals and man (Brodal, 1981). Stimulation of the lateral vestibular nucleus in cats monosynaptically excites extensor motoneurons and inhibits flexor motoneurons (Lund and Pompeiano, 1965). Lateral vestibulospinal efferents can trigger antigravity reflexes throughout the body and thus play a pivotal role in the maintenance of a rigid posture. The *medial vestibulospinal tract* originates in the medial vestibular nucleus and extends no farther caudally than the midthoracic cord (Nyberg-Hansen, 1964b). As efferents of this tract act upon motoneurons of the neck, shoulder and forelimb muscles, they are likely to play a role in the control of head movement and associated postural adjustments of the upper body. The *interstitiospinal tract* originates in the interstitial nucleus of Cajal located in the midbrain near the oculomotor nucleus (Nyberg-Hansen, 1966b; Kuypers and Maisky, 1975). The interstitial nucleus receives input (directly or indirectly) from vestibular and visual afferents; its efferents extend all the way to sacral spinal cord. The interstitiospinal tract probably controls head position and body posture on the basis of combined messages received from the vestibular and visual systems (Brodal, 1981). Both the vestibulospinal tract and the interstitiospinal tract contribute efferents to the medial longitudinal fasciculus.

The *medial longitudinal fasciculus* is an ancient fiber tract that interconnects the midbrain, the brain stem, and the spinal cord (Ariens-Kappers, et al., 1936; Crosby et al., 1962; Brodal, 1981). (As we shall see later, it is also one of the earliest fiber tracts to myelinate in the developing human brain.) In lower vertebrates, like the lizard, the medial longitudinal fasciculus is not just a "fascicle" but a massive fiber column that extends all the way from the anterior midbrain, through the pons and medulla, to the spinal cord (Figure 2-21). Along the way, it passes by the optic tract, the motor nuclei of the eye muscles, the vestibular nuclei, the acoustic area, and the other medially situated cranial nerve nuclei. Undoubtedly, the medial longitudinal fasciculus is a route for the paleocephalic control of spinal cord activity. In mammals, the medial longitudinal fasciculus is a relatively

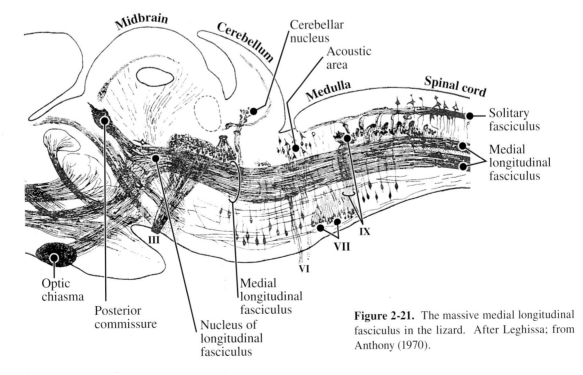

Figure 2-21. The massive medial longitudinal fasciculus in the lizard. After Leghissa; from Anthony (1970).

small fiber tract but it has the same trajectory as in lower vertebrates. At midbrain levels, it is located beneath the aqueduct close to the motor nuclei of the eye muscles. In the pontine region, the medial longitudinal fasciculus turns ventrally, and in the spinal cord it is situated in the ventromedial funiculus where it is known as the sulcomarginal fasciculus (Schoen, 1964). The motor reactions triggered by the vestibular system and the medial longitudinal fasciculus, such as postural adjustments in response to head turning, falling, rotation, acceleration, and deceleration, are typically involuntary reflexes in lower as well as higher vertebrates, including man. These tracts clearly qualify as components of the paleospinal efferent system.

Less well understood is the function of the *reticulospinal tract*. Ariens-Kappers et al. (1936) suggested that the reticular nuclei are the major sensorimotor coordinating centers in the brain stem of lower vertebrates. In lower vertebrates, these nuclei contain large multipolar neurons with extensive dendrites and some interspersed smaller neurons. In Cyclostomes and fishes, the large reticular neurons are scattered in the medulla, pons, and brain stem in the vicinity of the cranial motor nuclei and the medial longitudinal fasciculus. In amphibians and reptiles, reticular cells form identifiable nuclear masses and have received specific names; but their homology with the reticular nuclei of mammals is uncertain. In mammals, three reticular systems have been distinguished: the medullary, the pontine, and the mesencephalic. The principal source of medullary reticulospinal fibers is the nucleus reticularis gigantocellularis and the nucleus reticularis magnocellularis (Nyberg-Hansen, 1965; Basbaum et al., 1978). The principal source of pontine reticulospinal fibers are large neurons in the nucleus reticularis pontis caudalis and the nucleus reticularis pontis oralis. The mesencephalic reticular formation is apparently not a source of reticulospinal efferents (Nyberg-Hansen, 1965; Edwards, 1975). The reticular formation is certainly not the principal sensorimotor coordinating center in mammals, as that role has been taken over by the neocortex. Instead, the reticular formation appears to play a pivotal role in arousal and vigilance (Moruzzi and Magoun, 1949; Hobson and Brazier, 1980), and possibly in emotional reactions. We noted earlier that the reticular nuclei receive a massive protopathic input from the spinal cord by way of the spinocephalic tract. Thus, it is possible that the reticular formation integrates involuntary reactions of a second kind, i.e., those dependent on emotional arousal and behavioral mobilization.

The two other subcortical efferent pathways are the tectospinal and rubrospinal tracts. The *tectospinal tract* originates in neurons located in the deep layers of the superior colliculus. The superior colliculus (optic lobe) is best developed, both in terms of its relative size and laminar complexity, in lower vertebrates. Hence, the tectospinal tract may be the principal pathway from this paleocephalic processing station of the visual system to the spinal cord. In mammals, tectospinal fibers descend in the ventromedial funiculus near the medial longitudinal fasciculus, and most of its fibers terminate in the upper segments of the cervical spinal cord (Nyberg-Hansen, 1964a). It is well known, that unilateral stimulation of the superior colliculus makes the eyes and the head turn contralaterally. The target of tectospinal fibers are probably upper cervical motoneurons that innervate the neck muscles that move the head.

The *rubrospinal tract* originates in the red nucleus of the midbrain. The red nucleus, particularly its magnocellular region, is another phylogenetically old component of the midbrain; it is said to be present in fish and amphibians (Ariens-Kappers, 1936; Pearson and Pearson, 1976). Rubrospinal fibers descend in the superior lateral fasciculus along the entire length of the spinal cord in the goat (Schoen, 1964), cat (Hinman and Carpenter, 1959; Nyberg-Hansen and Brodal, 1964), and the monkey (Kuypers et al., 1962; Poirier and Bouvier, 1966; Miller and Strominger, 1973). Rubrospinal fibers terminate at the base of the dorsal horn, in the intermediate gray, and the interneuronal field surrounding the motor columns (Edwards, 1972; Murray and Haines, 1975) in a pattern that closely resembles the termination of corticospinal tract fibers. While the rubrospinal tract may be phylogenetically younger than the other efferent tracts so far considered (it is well developed in ungulates and carnivores), it is poorly developed in man and is thought to have been "replaced" by the massive corticospinal tract (Schoen, 1964). Stimulation of the red nucleus results in monosynaptic excitation of flexor motoneurons. This effect differs from stimulation of the vestibular nuclei which, as we have seen, causes monosynaptic excitation of extensor motoneurons. The course of the paleospinal efferent system is schematically shown in Figure 2-22.

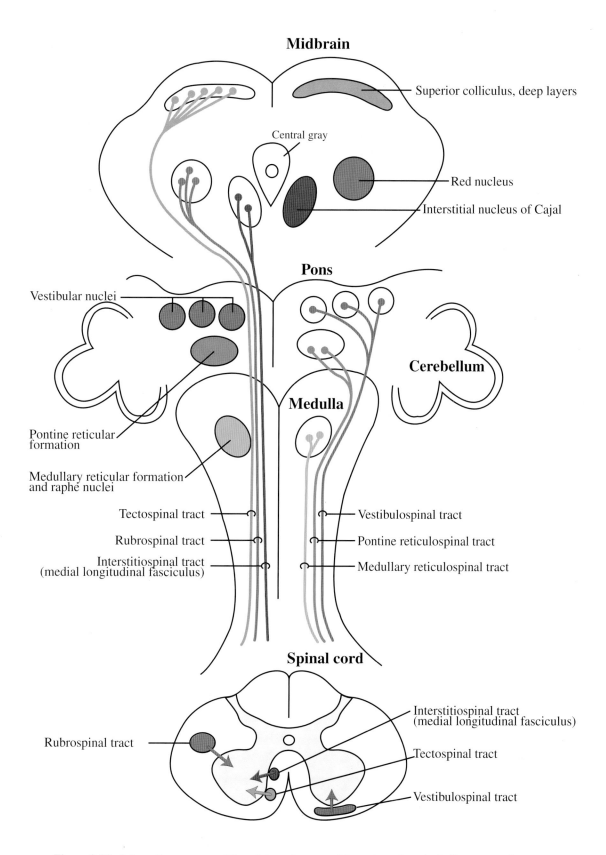

Figure 2-22. Schematic summary of the origin and course of the major paleospinal efferent tracts in mammals. The vestibulospinal and reticulospinal tracts are shown on the right; the tectospinal, rubrospinal, and interstitiospinal tracts on the left. The laterality of these projections is ignored. The site where these tracts penetrate the spinal cord, except the widely distributed reticulospinal tract, is shown at the bottom. Based on Crosby et al. (1962), Brodal (1981), and other sources described in the text.

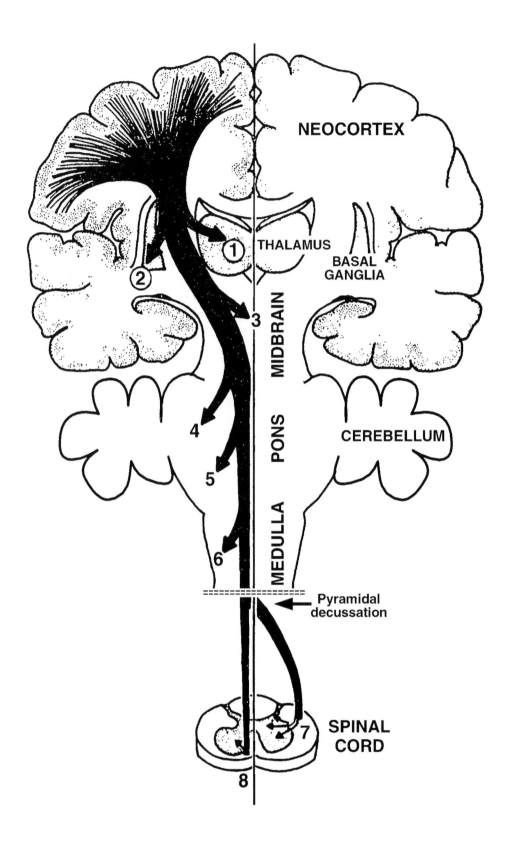

Figure 2-23. The origin and trajectory of fibers of the descending pyramidal tract in the human brain and spinal cord. Numbers indicate the following components of the pyramidal tract: 1, corticothalamic; 2, corticostriatal; 3, corticotectal; 4, corticopontocerebellar; 5, cortico-olivary; 6, corticocuneate and the corticogracile. Beyond the pyramidal decussation: 7, the crossed lateral corticospinal tract, and 8, the uncrossed ventral corticospinal tract. Modified, after Phillips and Porter (1977).

2.2.6 The Neospinal Efferent System: The Corticospinal Tracts. The large lateral corticospinal tract of the human spinal cord is a component of the pyramidal tract (Figure 2-23). The pyramidal tract originates in several areas of the cerebral cortex (Section 1.8.2) and its fibers terminate in several subcortical structures, including the basal ganglia, the thalamus, midbrain, pons, medulla, and the spinal cord. Most of the fibers that descend to the spinal cord, cross to the opposite side in the medulla in a region known as the pyramidal decussation, and form the lateral corticospinal tract. The smaller uncrossed component is the ventral (anterior) corticospinal tract. The corticospinal tract is a phylogenetically recent efferent system that has emerged and evolved in mammals. The relative size and location of the corticospinal tract varies in different mammalian species (Figure 2-24), and there are also species differences in how far the corticospinal tract descends caudally within the spinal cord.

In the hedgehog and the rabbit the crossed corticospinal tract is quite small, it is somewhat larger in ungulates, and in all these species it is situated medially at the base of the dorsal funiculus (rather than in the lateral funiculus) and does not descend beyond the cervical level (Schoen, 1964). In the elephant, the corticospinal tract is likewise situated in the dorsal funiculus but descends as far as the tho-

racic cord (Schoen, 1964). In the tree shrew, an insectivore-like animal with primate affinities, the corticospinal tract of the dorsal funiculus is small and does not seem to descend farther than low thoracic levels (Shriver and Noback, 1967). In contrast, the corticospinal tract in the dorsal funiculus of the rat is quite large (King, 1910; Ranson, 1913b). The location of the crossed corticospinal tract is different in carnivores and primates. In the cat (Chambers and Liu, 1957), in the slow loris, a prosimian (Campbell et al., 1966), and in the macaque monkey (Liu and Chambers, 1964), the crossed corticospinal tract is situated, as in man, in the superior lateral funiculus, and descends through the entire length of the spinal cord. In primates, there is an increase in the relative size of the corticospinal tract from prosimians, through simians, to anthropoids. According to Lassek and Rasmussen (1938), there are about half a million fibers in the corticospinal tract, at the level of the medullary decussation, in the rhesus monkey, and about a million fibers in man. The uncrossed corticospinal tract, if present, is located in all higher mammals in the ventromedial funiculus.

The changing location of the corticospinal tract, and differences in its relative size in different mammalian species, supports the idea that it is a recently evolved efferent system. The observation that the corticospinal tract is relatively large in the rat,

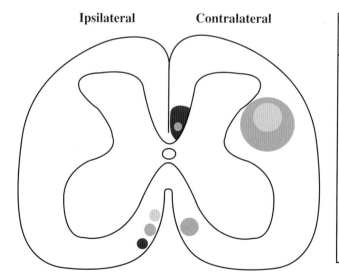

Animal Group	Locations of the Corticospinal Tract
Carnivores	contralateral: lateral funiculus ipsilateral: ventromedial funiculus
Primates	contralateral: lateral funiculus ipsilateral: ventromedial funiculus
Rodents	contralateral: dorsal funiculus; ipsilateral: ventromedial funiculus
Ungulates	contralateral: dorsal and ventro-medial funiculi; ipsilateral: none

Ipsilateral   Contralateral

Figure 2-24. Schematic illustration of the location of the contralateral and ipsilateral corticospinal tracts in different groups of mammals. The crossed corticospinal tract is located in the dorsal funiculus in rodents, in the dorsal and ventromedial funiculi in ungulates, and in the lateral funiculus in carnivores and primates. The smaller uncrossed corticospinal tract (if present) is situated in the ventromdial funiculus. Modified after Schoen (1964), and Phillips and Porter (1977).

while small in ungulates and the elephant, indicates that body size is not a factor in the size of the cortico-spinal tract. The large size of the corticospinal tract in the small rat suggests (as we have argued earlier) that cortical control of spinal motoneurons becomes important in those species that use their extremities and digits not only for locomotion but also for palpating and manipulating objects. Although the elephant has some unusual motor skills, it has a small corticospinal tract presumably because it uses its extremities strictly for locomotion, and employs a special organ, its proboscis, to manipulate objects. (The proboscis, as a modified head structure, is probably under the control of the trigeminal and facial motor nuclei.) The translocation of the corticospinal tract in carnivores and primates from the dorsal funiculus to the lateral funiculus may have been necessitated by two factors. First, the progressive increase in the population of ascending fibers from the lumbar and cervical enlargements in the dorsal funiculus in some orders of mammals may have left less and less room to acco-modate the descending (and, as we shall see, much lateral developing) corticospinal efferents in the same location. Second, the evolutionary increase in the number of descending corticospinal fibers favored a lateral location, since there is more room there for expansion than in the dorsal funiculus, wedged as it is between the dorsal horns. The superior lateral funic-ulus, where the receding rubrospinal tract is located, proved to be a favorable location for the expanding corticospinal tract. The lateral corticospinal tract is uniquely large in the human spinal cord and its fiber terminals are distributed widely in the ventral horn and the intermediate gray (Figure 2-25).

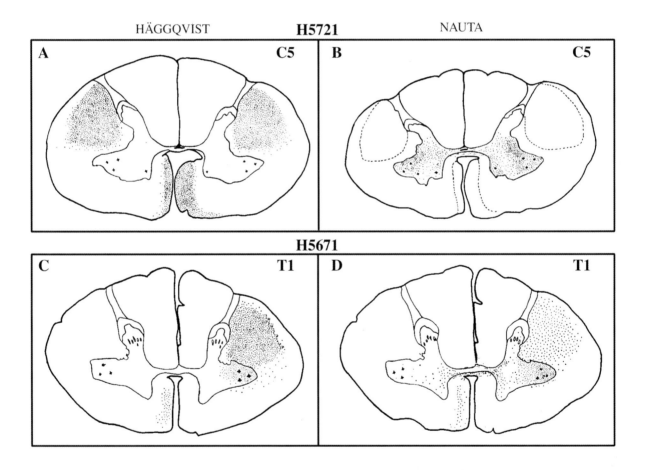

Figure 2-25. Pattern of corticospinal tract degeneration in two clinical cases, each visualized with two techniques at two locations. In case H5721 (**top**), the pyramidal tract was bilaterally damaged in the pons. The Häggquist technique shows extensive bilateral fiber degeneration in the lateral and ventral corticospinal tracts at C5 (**A**) and the Nauta technique reveals preterminal degeneration throughout the ventral horn and the intermediate gray (**B**). In case H5671 (**bottom**), the pyramidal tract was affected only on the left sided at T1. The Häggquist technique shows extensive fiber degeneration in the lateral corticospinal tract contralaterally and modest degeneration in the ventral corticospinal tract ipsilaterally (**C**). The Nauta technique indicates widespread terminal degeneration both in the white and gray matters contralaterally and modest terminal degeneration ipsilaterally in the medial gray matter (**D**). After Schoen (1964).

There is some evidence for species differences in the mode of termination of corticospinal fibers in the ventral horn (Figure 1-88). In the cat, most of the corticospinal fibers synapse with interneurons (Lloyd, 1941), the presumed motor pattern generators (Grillner, 1975; Stein, 1984). This suggests that, in the cat, cortical commands act upon pattern generator circuits rather than individual motoneurons. In primates and man, in contrast, many corticospinal terminals directly contact motoneurons (Bernhard et al. 1953; Kuypers, 1960; Liu and Chambers, 1964; Lawrence and Hopkins, 1976; Schoen, 1964). That monosynaptic cortical-motoneuronal relationship provides a mechanism for the voluntary control of single motor units of the spinal cord for the production of novel skills. There is apparently also a difference between termination patterns of corticospinal fibers with motoneurons that control gross limb movements and those that control fine hand and finger movements (Shinoda et al., 1979; Muir and Lemon, 1983). Thus, corticospinal axons originating in the cortical "hand" area of the monkey establish very few, and possibly only a single synaptic contact with their target motoneuron (Lawrence et al., 1985).

Is the primary function of the corticospinal tract the control of voluntary action or of skilled behavior? The little experimental evidence that we currently have suggests that it is not voluntary movements per se that are interfered with by transection of the pyramidal tract but rather the execution of skilled limb and finger movements. A few examples may suffice. In a marsupial, the bushtail opossum, bilateral transection of the pyramidal tract does not produce abnormalities in posture and locomotion on level ground but does produce deficits in the accurate placement of the limbs on branches of a tree and in grasping food with the digits (Hore et al., 1973). That deficit endured over the observation period of 8 months. Similar observations were made in cats after unilateral or bilateral transection of the pyramidal tract (Liddell and Phillips, 1944). The animals retain, or quickly regain the ability to walk on a flat surface to reach a target but are handicapped in climbing a ladder to do so. The tactile placing reaction, which is tested in blindfolded cats by bringing their paw in contact with a solid surface, is permanently abolished. In rats, near complete section of the pyramidal tract severely interferes with the animals' ability to pick food pellets from a feeder with narrow slots (Castro, 1972). In monkeys, unilateral section of the pyramidal tract produces little deficit in pos-

tural adjustments and in running and climbing but the dexterous use of the fingers becomes impaired (Tower, 1940; Denny-Brown, 1966; Beck and Chambers, 1970). In feeding and grooming, such monkeys prefer to use their normal hand. If forced to use their affected hand, the reaching and grasping movements tend to be stereotyped and the discrete use of fingers is permanently abolished. The deficit in the dexterous use of the fingers is more severe after bilateral transection of the pyramidal tract (Bucy et al., 1966; Lawrence and Kuypers (1968). Normal monkeys can pick morsels through narrow holes with their index finger but the operated animals cannot. Loss of corticospinal control of motoneurons, according to this evidence, does not produce severe and enduring deficits in voluntary (goal-seeking) behavior but seriously interferes with the dexterous use of limb and digits. This, of course, need not imply that the neocortex is not the primary mechanism of voluntary action. Rather, it suggests that the neocortex can make use of alternate efferent pathways to initiate voluntary behavior. It is for this very reason that animals with corticospinal tract lesions in time acquire compensatory action strategies when their dexterity is lost.

Organization of the White Matter: A Summary. In Figure 2-26, we map the three physiologically defined dorsal root afferent systems (exteroceptive, nociceptive, and proprioceptive) in relation to the fiber tracts in which they travel (right) and the fasciculi in which they are located (left) in the white matter of the human cervical spinal cord. *Exteroceptive* input (blue) is conveyed to the brain by the massive gracile and cuneate fasciculi. *Nociceptive* input (red) is conveyed to supraspinal structures in three fasciculi (dorsolateral, inferior lateral, and ventral) by three tracts: Lissauer's tract, the lateral spinocephalic tract, and the ventral spinocephalic tract. The major *proprioceptive* input (brown), is conveyed to the cerebellum by the dorsal and ventral spinocerebellar tracts located in the marginal fasciculus.

In Figure 2-27, we map the three psychologically characterized ascending somatosensory pathways (epicritic, protopathic, and epipathic) and motor pathways (voluntary and involuntary) with reference to the tracts in which they travel (right) and the fasciculi in which they are located (left). The major route of the *epicritic* pathway (blue) with its predominantly exteroceptive input is the gracile fasciculus and cuneate fasciculus. This is the high resolution, "cognitive quality" sensory channel. Lissauer's tract

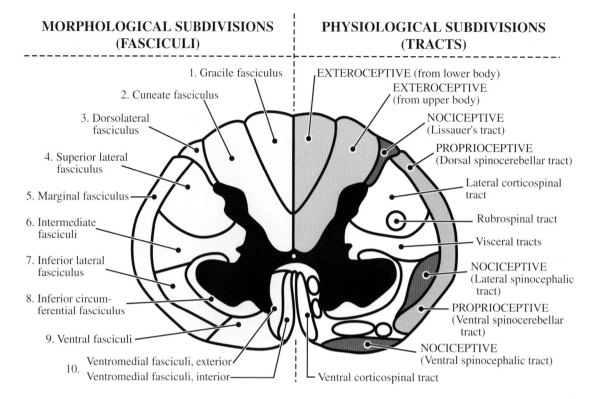

Figure 2-26. Fiber tracts in the white matter of the human cervical cord that transmit principally exteroceptive (blue), nociceptive (red) and proprioceptive (brown) peripheral signals to the brain (**right**) in relation to the fasciculi in which they are located (**left**).

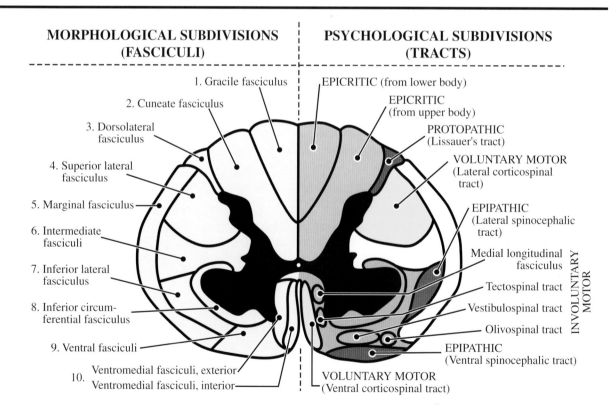

Figure 2-27. Fiber tracts that convey epicritic (blue), protopathic (red), and epipathic (purple) information from the spinal cord to the brain, and descending fiber tracts that bring voluntary (yellow) and involuntary (brown) motor commands from the brain to the spinal cord (**right**) in relation to the fasciculi in which they are located (**left**).

PHYLOGENETIC ORGANIZATION

BEHAVIORAL ORGANIZATION

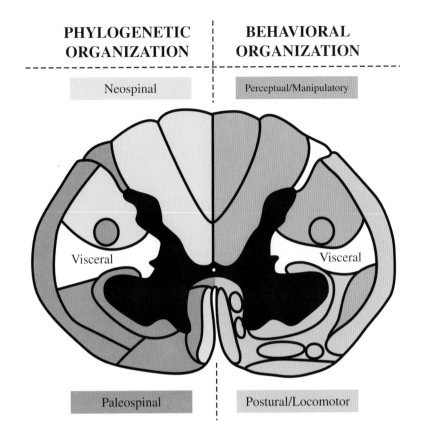

Neospinal

Perceptual/Manipulatory

Visceral

Visceral

Paleospinal

Postural/Locomotor

Figure 2-28. Left. Location in the white matter of the human spinal cord, the *neospinal* sensory and motor tracts (the dorsal funiculus and the lateral corticospinal tract) dorsally and dorsolaterally (green), and of the *paleospinal* sensory (spinocerebellar) and motor (e.g., vestibulospinal, intraspinal) tracts ventrally and ventrolaterally (purple). Obvious exceptions to this generalization are the dorsally situated rubrospinal tract (paleospinal) and the ventrally situated ventral corticospinal tract (neospinal). **Right.** The dorsal and dorsolateral location of the sensory and motor tracts mediating primarily perceptual and manipulatory functions (orange), and the ventral and ventrolateral location of proprioceptive and motor tracts primarily mediating postural and locomotor functions (blue). The identification in this illustration of the rubrospinal tract with perceptual/manipulatory functions, and of the ventral corticospinal tract with postural/locomotor functions is speculative.

with its exclusive nociceptive input and presumed visceral functions is identified as the *protopathic* pathway (red). This is the low resolution, "autonomic quality" sensory channel. The lateral and ventral spinocephalic tracts with their dual nociceptive and exteroceptive input constitute the *epipathic* pathway (purple). This is the intermediate resolution, "emotional quality" sensory channel. The *voluntary* motor command pathways from the cerebral cortex to the spinal cord are the lateral and ventral corticospinal tracts (yellow), while transmission routes for *involuntary* motor commands from subcortical (paleocephalic) structures are located in several ventral and ventromedial fasciculi (brown).

Finally, in Figure 2-28 we distinguish the ascending and the descending fiber tracts of the white matter in terms of their presumed phylogeny (neospinal vs. paleospinal) and global behavioral functions (perceptual/manipulatory vs. postural/locomotor). As shown on the left side, the phylogenetically old sensory and motor systems associated principally with subcortical (paleocephalic) structures are concentrated ventrally and ventrolaterally (purple). The sensory and motor systems linked to the phylogenetically younger (neencephalic) cerebral cortex are located dorsally and dorsolaterally (green). Exceptions are the dorsolaterally located rubrospinal tract (old) and the ventromedially located ventral corticospinal tract (young). This discrepancy is partially resolved by the evidence, illustrated on the right in Figure 2-28, that the ventral domain of the white matter (blue) contains efferents principally involved in the control of posture and locomotion (the tectospinal, vestibulospinal, and interstitiospinal tracts), whereas the dorsal domain (red) contains both sensory and motor tracts involved in the control of perceptual and manipulatory functions (dorsal funiculus and lateral corticospinal tract). If this distinction is a valid one, it may be that the ventral corticospinal tract is located ventrally (perhaps with close connections to medially located axial motoneurons) because it is involved in the voluntary control of biped posture and locomotion, and the rubrospinal tract is located dorsally because it is part of an ancient perceptual/manipulatory motor system. The location of the ventral spinocephalic tract in this presumed postural/locomotor domain is more difficult to explain.

2.3 Organization of the Ventral Horn

2.3.1   The Ventral Horn in Phylogeny.

We have superimposed previously a matrix consisting of 2-4 vertical panels and 2-3 horizontal tiers on the ventral horn motor columns (Figures 1-51, 1-52), and named the motor columns (where present) by a binary method (Figure 1-53) in terms of their location in these panels (medial, central, lateral, and far-lateral) and tiers (ventral, dorsal, and retrodorsal). Some of the panels (i.e., lateral and far-lateral) and some of the tiers (i.e., the retrodorsal) are present only at some levels of the cervical and lumbar enlargement. There are only two panels of motor columns (medial and central) in the upper cervical and thoracic segments, and only two tiers (ventral and dorsal) in the upper cervical and thoracic segments. In the cervical enlargement (the brachial cord) and the lumbosacral enlargement, massive motor columns typically occupy the lateral, far lateral, and retrodorsal sectors of the ventral horn. Recent findings using physiological tracer techniques support the long-held view that the added motor columns in the far-lateral and retrodorsal sectors of the ventral horn innervate distal muscle groups that move the limbs and their digits.

What we know about the evolution of motor columns in vertebrates is in agreement with this interpretation. In aquatic, limbless vertebrates, such as the stingray, the motoneurons occupy a single tier, with a hint of the segregation of smaller motoneurons medially, and larger motoneurons laterally (Figure 2-29A). In tetrapod amphibians, like the frog, the segregation of smaller motoneurons ventromedially and larger motoneurons dorsolaterally is evident at some segmental levels (Figure 2-29B). Finally, in the pigeon, a fair number of large motoneurons are segregated far-laterally, although the presence of a retrodorsal tier of motoneurons is not clearly indicated (Figure 2-29C).

Although there are differences in ventral horn motor column organization in different species of mammals, it is not currently possible to relate these differences to their locomotor specializations and motor capacities. As an illustration of these differences, we compare the organization of motor columns in the lumbar spinal cord of rat and man (Figure 2-30). There are not only much fewer motoneurons in the rat, but there are also fewer motor columns (Figure 2-30A). There is little more than a hint of an incipient segregation of smaller motoneurons in the

medial/central panel, and of larger motoneurons in the lateral/far-lateral panel. In man, as seen in the spinal cord of a newborn (Figure 2-30B), the central panel of small motoneurons is quite inconspicuous but there are many more segregated motor columns-laterally, far-laterally, and retrodorsally. The involve-

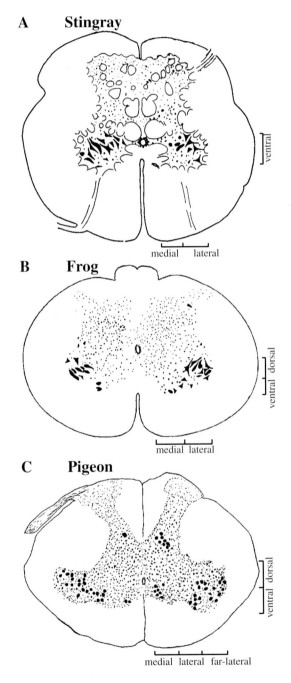

Figure 2-29. Motoneurons in the ventral horn of stingray (**A**), frog (**B**), and pigeon (**C**). There is an increase in the number of segregated motor columns in vertebrate species without and with limbs and in relation to the complexity of their motor apparatus. **A** and **B**, from Nieuwenhuys (1964); **C**, from Ariens-Kappers (1936).

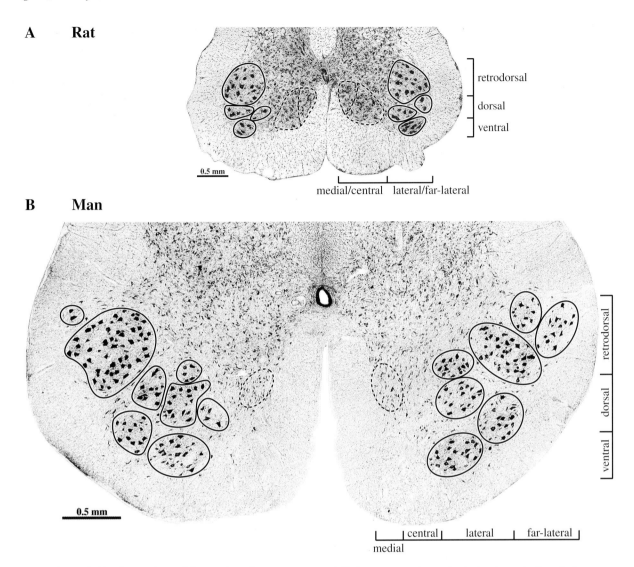

Figure 2-30. Comparison of the number of motoneurons and distinct motor columns in the lumbar spinal cord of an adult rat (**A**) and a newborn child (**B**). There are far more lateral and far-lateral motor columns in the ventral horn in man than in the rat. In contrast, the relative number of motoneurons and size of the medial motor columns is far larger in the rat than in man. **A**, from Paxinos and Watson (1986). **B**, specimen # Y23-60.

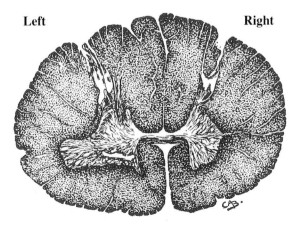

Figure 2-31. The cervical spinal cord of an adult man born without his right arm. The component of the ventral horn containing the lateral and far-lateral motor columns is absent on the affected side. From Elders (1910).

ment in man of the lateral, far-lateral, and retrodorsal motor columns in the control of the muscles of the limbs and digits is dramatically illustrated in Figure 2-31. The lateral enlargement of the right cervical cord is altogether absent in a man who was born without a right arm.

2.3.2   Relationship Between Motor Columns and Motor Subcolumns.

Undoubtedly, the clustering of motoneurons in specific columns, and their segregation from other columns, must be of great structural and functional significance. Motoneurons situated within the same column are liable to be intimately connected with one another by way of recurrent collaterals as well as a shared short-axoned interneurons and overlapping dendritic bundles. While most of these columns can easily be distinguished from one another in normative histological sections (e.g., Figure 1-49), the relationship of the histologically identified discrete columns and the muscle groups innervated by their constituent motoneurons cannot be determined except by using experimental methods (as exemplified by the classical study of Romanes; Figure 1-54). While the recent introduction of retrograde tracer techniques has made this task easier (Figures 1-56 to 1-63), the results obtained have raised difficult problems that are yet to be resolved. First, most of the published tracer studies have not used counterstaining techniques to directly relate the retrogradely labeled motoneurons to the histologically defined motor columns. Second, even where the retrograde labeling has yielded column-like aggregates, these tend to be slimmer and shorter than typical motor columns. Third, aggregates retrogradely labeled from different nerves, muscles or muscle groups – the subcolumns – often overlap with one another in the same location. How are the retrogradely labeled subcolumns that identify the peripheral connections of motoneurons related to the histologically identified motor columns?

In an attempt to provide a provisional correlation between the two sets of data, we took illustrations from several experimental studies and projected them onto maps of histologically delineated motor columns (Figures 2-32 to 2-35). Because cats were used in most of the tracer experiments, we turned for this purpose to Rexed's (1954) cytoarchitectonic atlas of the cat spinal cord. Rexed traced the outlines of the spinal cord and the ventral horn motor columns at every segment from C1 to S2. To fit the present purpose, we made several changes in Rexed's drawings. First, only the outlines of the lower half of the spinal

cord containing the intermediate gray and the ventral horn were retained. Second, Rexed's laminar nomenclature in the ventral horn was abandoned. Rexed labeled all lateral motor columns as lamina IX. Treating the discrete motor columns as a single structural entity is not helpful in the present context. Third, we added the 3x4 grid previously described (Figures 1-51, 1-52) to aid the identification of the motor columns.

The procedure used is illustrated in Figure 2-32. Hörner and Kümmel's (1993) experimental data in cats (Figure 1-57) was projected upon Rexed's outlines of the ventral horn in four segments (C5–C8) of the cervical enlargement. As was described earlier, Hörner and Kümmel applied fluorochrome tracers to 11 separate nerves that supply muscles of the shoulder and arm, and mapped the labeled motoneurons at successive segments from C5 to T1. Granting the limitations of this procedure (combining data from cats raised in different countries and at different times) the illustrations suggest that a single motor column may contain several subcolumns that send their axons to different muscles by way of different peripheral nerves. Thus in C7, the lateral dorsal column (sector l,d) contains motoneurons that send axons to muscles by way of the following local nerves: infraspinatus, supraspinatus, pectoralis major, and pectoralis minor. In the same segment, the far-lateral dorsal column (sector fl,d) contains motoneurons of the spinodeltoid, teres minor, teres major, and acromyodeltoid nerves.

Moreover, since Hörner and Kümmel studied only selected nerves that innervate shoulder and arm muscles, it is possible that a single motor column contains motoneurons of more muscles, including muscles of the forearm, wrist, and possibly digits. This possibility is illustrated in Figures 2-33 and 2-34, where the results of eight other investigations that localized motoneurons innervating selected neck, shoulder, arm, wrist, and paw muscles (see Table for Figure 1-56) were transferred to Rexed's maps from C2 to T12. Thus, in the far-lateral dorsal motor column (coordinates: fl,d) at C8, where Hörner and Kümmel located the motor neurons of teres major, which rotates the arm laterally (Figure 2-32), other investigators located motoneurons of the extensor carpi ulnaris, flexor carpi ulnaris, abductor pollicis longus, and palmaris longus, i.e., muscles that act on joints of the forearm, wrist, and digits (Figure 2-34). These considerations suggests co-localization within

Figure 2-32. Approximate location of retrogradely labeled motoneuron subcolumns of 11 nerves that innervate shoulder and arm muscles in the cat, as found by Hörner and Kümmel (1993) and shown in Figure 1-57, in relation to outlines of brachial motor columns in the cat, as drawn by Rexed (1954). Horizontal and vertical coordinates are schematic. Differences in the size of the color-coded motor subcolumns within a motor column are not indicated, and their location within a column is arbitrary. Abbreviations of ventral horn sectors: c, central, d, dorsal; fl, far-lateral; l, lateral; m, medial; rd, retrodorsal; v, ventral.

LABELED NERVES

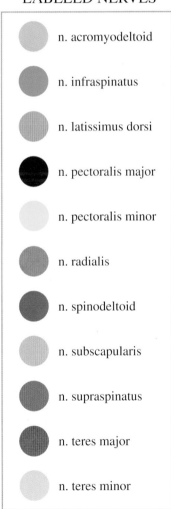

n. acromyodeltoid

n. infraspinatus

n. latissimus dorsi

n. pectoralis major

n. pectoralis minor

n. radialis

n. spinodeltoid

n. subscapularis

n. supraspinatus

n. teres major

n. teres minor

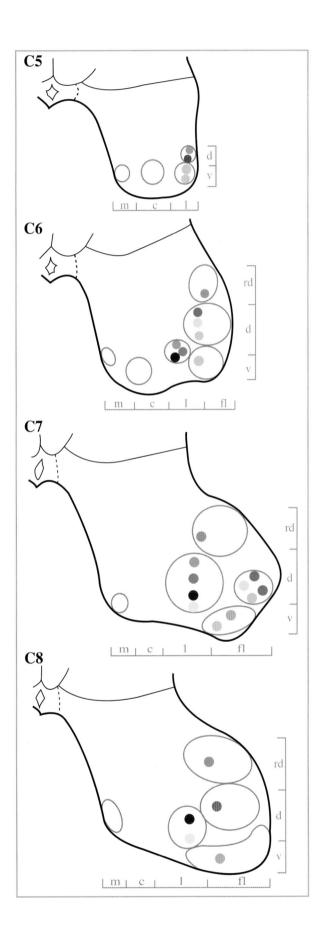

Figures 2-33. Approximate location of retrogradely labeled motor subclolumns in the upper cervical spinal cord of the cat (for source references see, Table for Figure 1-56) that innervate some of the axial muscles of the neck and the muscles of the shoulder girdle, in relation to Rexed's histologically defined motor columns. Horizontal and vertical coordinates are schematic. Differences in the size of the labeled motor subcolumns within a motor column are not indicated, and their location within a column is arbitrary. Abbreviations of the ventral horn sectors: c, central, d, dorsal; fl, far-lateral; l, lateral; m, medial; rd, retrodorsal; v, ventral.

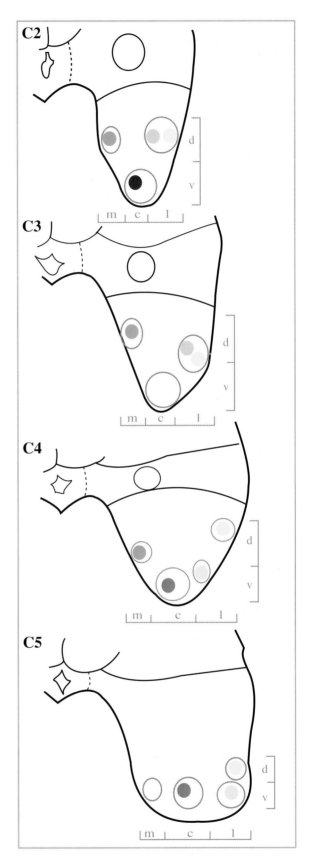

LABELED MUSCLES

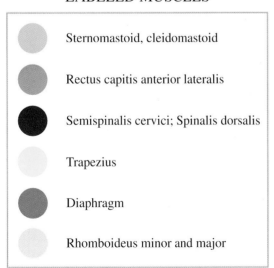

Sternomastoid, cleidomastoid

Rectus capitis anterior lateralis

Semispinalis cervici; Spinalis dorsalis

Trapezius

Diaphragm

Rhomboideus minor and major

Figure 2-34. Approximate location of retrogradely labeled motor subcolumns in the lower cervical (brachial) spinal cord of the cat (for source references, see Table for Figure 1-56) that innervate some of the arm and hand muscles. (An exception is levator scapulae in C6 ventrally, which is a shoulder girdle muscle.) For further details, see Text. Horizontal and vertical coordinates are schematic. Differences in the size of the labeled motor subcolumns within a motor column are not indicated, and their location within a column is arbitrary. Abbreviation of ventral horn sectors: c, central, d, dorsal; fl, far-lateral; l, lateral; m, medial; rd, retrodorsal; v, ventral.

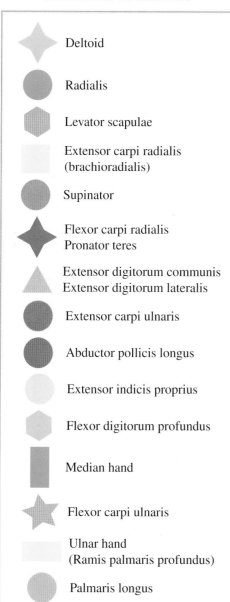

LABELED MUSCLES

Deltoid

Radialis

Levator scapulae

Extensor carpi radialis (brachioradialis)

Supinator

Flexor carpi radialis
Pronator teres

Extensor digitorum communis
Extensor digitorum lateralis

Extensor carpi ulnaris

Abductor pollicis longus

Extensor indicis proprius

Flexor digitorum profundus

Median hand

Flexor carpi ulnaris

Ulnar hand
(Ramis palmaris profundus)

Palmaris longus

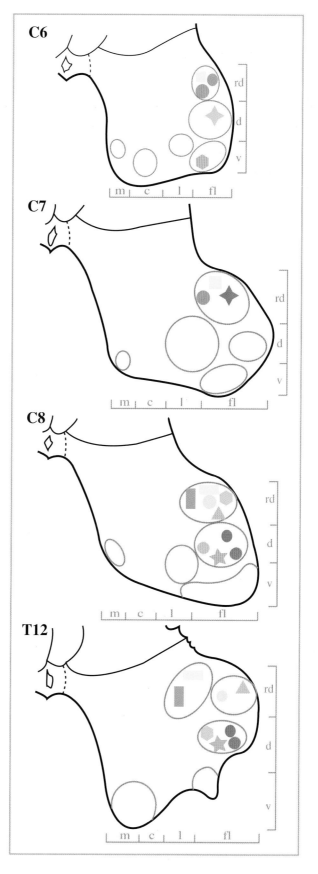

Figure 2-35. Approximate location of retrogradely labeled motor subcolumns in the lumbosacral cord of the cat in relation to Rexed's motor columns. Color-coded circles are based on reports by investigators who studied a select group of muscles (see Figures 1-59 to 1-62). The numbered circles are derived from the comprehensive study of VanderHorst and Holstege (1997). Size and relative location of subcolumns within a motor column are arbitrary. For details, see text. Sector abbreviations as in the previous figures.

LABELED MUSCLES

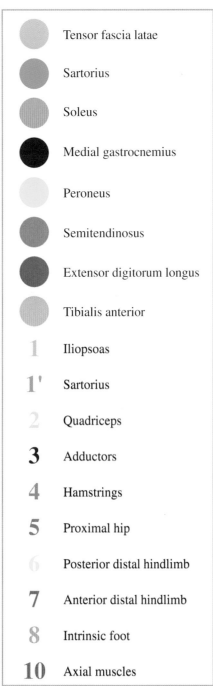

●	Tensor fascia latae
●	Sartorius
●	Soleus
●	Medial gastrocnemius
●	Peroneus
●	Semitendinosus
●	Extensor digitorum longus
●	Tibialis anterior
1	Iliopsoas
1'	Sartorius
2	Quadriceps
3	Adductors
4	Hamstrings
5	Proximal hip
6	Posterior distal hindlimb
7	Anterior distal hindlimb
8	Intrinsic foot
10	Axial muscles

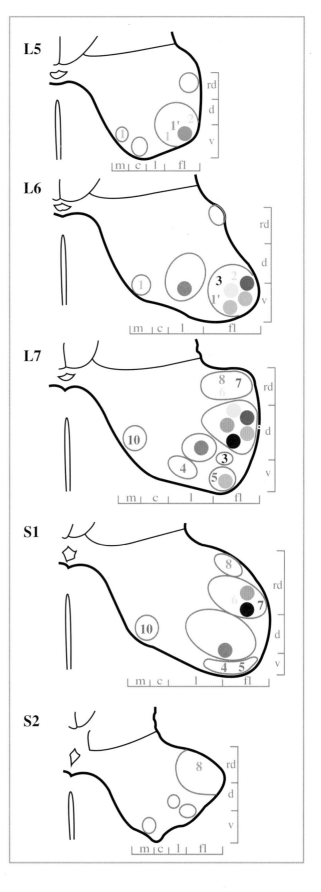

a motor column of subcolumns that act not only on proximal muscles of the arm but also on distal muscles of the paw. Such co-localization may aid the integration of arm, hand, and finger muscles in such an integrated voluntary act as reaching for and grasping an object.

These observations confirm and extend the traditional generalization that motoneurons that innervate the muscles of the neck, shoulder, arm, forearm, and hand in a proximal-to-distal order are located in motor columns that are strung out in the ventral horn in a rostral-to-caudal sequence and extend to the lateral, far-lateral, and retrodorsal sectors in the the cervical and lumbar enlargements. The medial dorsal column (sector m,d) contains the motor subcolumns of a neck muscle, rectus capitis anterior that extends from C1 (not shown here, but seen in Figure 1-56) through C4. Motor subcolumns of two other neck muscles, spinalis dorsalis and semispinalis cervici, are located in the central ventral column (sector c,v) in the upper cervical cord. In the mid-cervical cord (C4-C6), the central ventral column contains the subcolumns of the diaphragm. The lateral dorsal column (sector l,d) contains subcolumns of three shoulder muscles: the sternomastoid, cleidomastoid, and trapezius. Of these, the motoneurons of the trapezius extend as far as C5. The motoneurons of two other shoulder muscles, the rhomboideus minor and major, are located in the lateral ventral column (sector l,v) and extend from C4 to C5. These motoneurons may shift to the far-lateral ventral column (sector fl,v) at C6 where the subcolumns of the levator scapula are located. Subcolumns of the arm muscles extend from C6 to C7 and tend to be located more dorsally and far-laterally. The subcolumns of the deltoid are located in the far-lateral dorsal column (sector fl,d) at C6. The subcolumns of the extensor carpi radialis and brachioradialis are located in the far-lateral retrodorsal column (fl,rd sector) between C6 and C7. In the same motor column are located the motoneurons of the supinator, pronator teres, and flexor carpi radialis. Farthest caudally (C8-T1) and far-laterally are located the subcolumns of the paw and digit muscles. The far-lateral dorsal column (sector fl,d) contains subcolumns of the extensor carpi radialis, flexor carpi ulnaris, palmaris longus, and abductor pollicis longus. The far-lateral retrodorsal column (f,rd sector) contains subcolumns of the ulnar hand, median hand, flexor digitorum profundus, extensor indicus proprius, extensor digitorum communis, and extensor digitorum lateralis.

A similar pattern may hold for the localization of experimentally identified subcolumns in the inferred columns of the lumbosacral enlargement. In Figure 2-35 we have mapped the subcolumns (summarized earlier in Figures 1-59 to 1-63) onto Rexed's drawings of motor columns in the lumbar spinal cord. The color coded circles indicate data from experimenters who localized motoneurons of individual muscles; VanderHorst and Holstege's (1997) report that dealt with motoneurons innervating larger muscle groups are indicated by numbered circles. Although there are some inconsistencies in the data, the results agree that subcolumns of hip and thigh muscles tend to be situated more rostrally and ventrally, whereas those of the leg and foot muscles more caudally and rostrally. Of the subcolumns of proximal thigh muscles, those of the iliopsoas are located in the medial ventral column (sector m,v) at L5 and L6, and those of sartorius in the far-lateral ventral column (sector fl,v), extending as far as L7. The subcolumns of the quadriceps, which act on the thigh and knee, are also located in the same column at L5 and L6, and so are the subcolumns of hip muscles (tensor fascia latae). The subcolumns of the hamstring muscles (biceps femoris, semitendinosus, and semimembranosus) are located more caudally (L7-S1) in the lateral ventral column (sector l,v); although according to one study, the motoneurons of the semitendinosus are located more dorsally in the lateral dorsal column (sector l,d). Surprisingly, the subcolumns of the proximal gluteal muscles are located still more caudally (L7-S1) in the far-lateral ventral column (sector fl,v). The subcolumns of a group of posterior and anterior distal hind limb muscles are located in the far-lateral retrodorsal column (sector fl,rd) at L7-S1. More specifically, subcolumns of the peroneus, soleus, and medial gastrocnemius are located in the far-lateral motor column in L7-S1, and those of the tibialis anterior and extensor digitorum longus either in the far-lateral ventral or far-lateral dorsal motor columns in L6-L7. The subcolumns of the intrinsic foot muscles are located farthest caudally and rostrally in the far-lateral retrodorsal column (sector fl,rd) at L7-S2.

The correlations of this section, of course, are all tentative. A prerequisite for the definitive localization of a set of motor subclolumns within a histologically delineated motor column is that both identifications are made by a single team of investigators and in the same animal. This task remains to to be accomplished.

2.4 Some Structural Features of the Gray Matter

2.4.1   Laminar, Nuclear, and Reticular Components of the Gray Matter. Rexed's (1954, 1964) laminar division of the spinal cord is widely used by investigators in neurobiological research. That scheme is justified and useful for the delineation of components of the dorsal horn. However, the extension of the laminar scheme to the intermediate gray, the central gray, and the ventral horn (as noted earlier) is not justified theoretically and has little practical utility.

In broad terms, and excluding for the moment the spinal cord, there are three types of cell assemblies ("areas" or "structures") in the vertebrate central nervous system: the cortical, the nuclear, and the reticular. (A fourth type, the ganglionic, is limited in vertebrates to the peripheral nervous system.). Each of these cell assemblies can be identified in most cases with little ambiguity. Cortical structures are composed of a superficial sheet of gray matter and a deep core of white matter. The superficial gray matter of cortical structures, sometimes called the pallium, contains cell bodies and their dendrites and axons; the deep white matter is composed of afferent and efferent fibers. Cortical structures are typically laminated because different classes of neurons are assembled in sheets within its gray matter. In some instances, as in the case of the cerebral cortex or the retina, layers rich in cell bodies alternate with cell-free fibrous layers containing dendrites and axon terminals. The cortical organization of neurons is, from a phylogenetic perspective, a progressive neuroarchitectonic feature. This is so because the location of perikarya in superficial sheets permits the enlargement of the neuronal population for increasing processing power through: (i) increase of the width of the cortex, (ii) the addition of new layers to the cortex, and (iii) the folding of the cortical surface through lobulation and fissurization.

Nuclear structures, in contrast, are composed of a central core of neuronal perikarya and an external shell of dendrites and incoming and outgoing axons. Typical brain nuclei are found in the mesencephalon (e.g., cranial nerve nuclei, red nucleus), diencephalon (nuclei of the thalamus and hypothalamus), and the basal telencephalon (nuclei of the amygdala). In instances where the two components, the perikaryal core and the fibrous shell, are clearly dis-

tinguishable from their surrounding, the nuclear complex is sometimes referred to as a "body" (e.g., the medial geniculate body or the lateral geniculate body). From a phylogenetic perspective, nuclear organization is a conservative cytoarchitectonic feature because the expansion of the cell population of a nucleus is constrained by the surrounding gray and white matter. The expansion of the cell population of a brain nucleus is sometimes achieved through its translocation from an internal to a superficial position and through lamination. An example of a superficially displaced and laminated brain nucleus is the lateral geniculate body in carnivores and primates.

In both cortices and nuclei the perikarya of neurons are aligned in an orderly manner, and the dendrites have a distinctive configuration and a regular orientation in relation to the trajectory of the afferents that synapse with them. In contrast, in reticular structures, the perikarya tend to be scattered irregularly among fibers with different trajectories and, correspondingly, the dendrites radiate irregularly and overlap with one another (Leontovich and Zhukova, 1963; Ramón-Moliner and Nauta, 1966). Ramón-Moliner and Nauta called the dendritic pattern of neurons in laminar structures " idiodendritic," and those of reticular structures "isodendritic." A prototypical brain region with a reticular organization is the reticular formation of the pons, medulla, and midbrain. However, there are other reticular regions as well, for instance, the raphe nuclei in the brain stem and the zona incerta in the diencephalon. Whereas cortical and nuclear structures with their regularly arranged perikarya and orderly dendritic fields are well suited for the topographic mapping of sensory input and the somatotopic representation of motor output, reticular structures with their irregularly arranged perikarya and dendritic fields are better suited for more diffuse functions, such as visceral mobilization and behavioral arousal.

Applying this classification to the organization of the spinal cord, we may identify in it, albeit in a greatly modified form, all three types of neuronal assemblies. The fact that the gray matter of the spinal cord is surrounded by the white matter makes it appear as a large nucleus. However, the internal organization of the gray matter reveals the presence of three types of cell assemblies within it. The dorsal horn, even if it does not have the features of a prototypical cortex, is a laminated structure. Rexed's laminae I-V are superficial sheets stacked on top of

Figure 2-36. Laminar and nuclear (columnar) components of the spinal cord gray matter. The dorsal horn is composed of elongated laminae or stacked sheets that contain different types of neurons and have different afferent and efferent connections. The ventral horn has a nuclear organization. Each elongated nucleus (or column) contains an aggregate of tightly packed motoneurons in its core that is surrounded by a singularly organized dendritic field (the dendritic bundles). The heterogeneous intermediate gray, with the exception of a few nuclear structures, has a reticular organization. It is composed of scattered neurons with irregular dendritic fields and is traversed by ascending and descending fibers of diverse origin and presumably diverse functions.

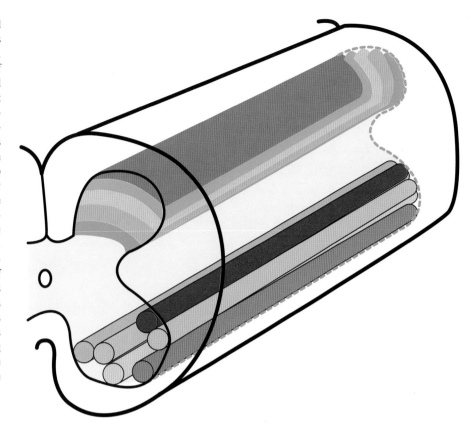

one another (Figure 2-36) that stretch uninterruptedly from the first cervical segment rostrally to the last sacral segment caudally. Each layer of the dorsal horn contains different cell types, each has dendrites oriented in an orderly way in a particular direction, and each is the target of different classes of afferents and the source of efferents with different trajectories. Indeed, the comparative evidence that we have considered earlier suggests that the number of laminae in the dorsal horn has increased in vertebrate phylogeny, and the reviewed physiological evidence has established that the fine circuits of the different laminae have distinct functions.

Although the dorsal horn could be thought of as a laminated nuclear structure, we are inclined to consider its lamination more akin to cortices. The reason is that the dorsal horn is primarily the target of sensory fibers and many sensory receiving areas (such as the olfactory bulb and the retina) have a cortical organization. The argument is not a conclusive one because the targets of the eighth nerve (the cochlear and the vestibular nuclei) are nuclear in organization and lack a visible lamination.

In sharp contrast to the laminated dorsal horn, the ventral horn lacks any laminar features. As seen in coronal sections, the perikarya of motoneurons are

arranged in a compact fashion in the core of discrete nuclei. The motor nuclei, in turn, are surrounded by a fibrous shell (e.g., Figure 1-45) composed of regularly arranged dendrites, much in the same way as are typical brain nuclei. Of course, the spinal cord motor nuclei differ from the spherical brain nuclei by forming long columns within the tubular spinal cord (Figure 2-36). Correspondingly, the dendritic arbor of motoneurons is not radial but stretched rostrocaudally to form longitudinal dendritic bundles, as previously described (e.g., Figure 1-68).

Differing from the laminar dorsal horn and the nuclear ventral horn, the intermediate gray is a heterogeneous field that contains some nuclear structures but many more reticular areas. Clarke's column is a clear instance of a nuclear structure, and so are some of the preganglionic motor columns of the lateral horn. Réthelyi (1984) suggested that the intermediate gray is the "central core" of the spinal cord, to which is attached a sensory appendage dorsally (the dorsal horn), a somatomotor appendage ventrally (the ventral horn), and a visceromotor appendage laterally (the lateral horn). An alternative view is that the intermediate gray is an intercalated reticular region of the spinal cord, composed of a great variety of interneurons with diverse supporting functions.

2.4.2   Micromodules in the Substantia Gelatinosa. To appreciate the significance of the "slabs" of laminae II-III of the dorsal horn that we have alluded to earlier (e.g., Figures 1-25, 2-6), we review briefly our current knowledge of a related cellular complex, or micromodule, the "barrels" of the somesthetic cortex. In lamina IV of the somesthetic cortex, in the region representing the facial vibrissae and sinus hairs, neuronal aggregates have been identified in mice and rats (Woolsey and van der Loos, 1970; Welker and Woolsey, 1974; see Figures 2-37A and 2-39A) and some other small mammalian species (Woolsey et al., 1975). The function of the facial vibrissae is to detect physical features of the envi-

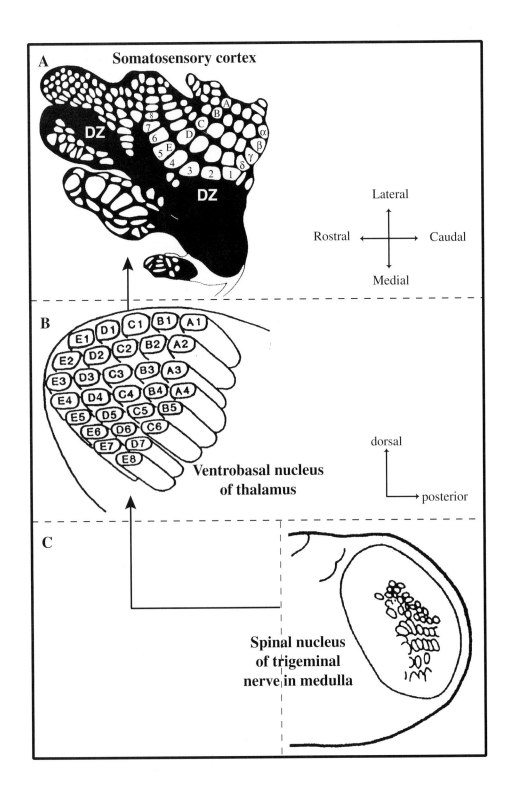

Figure 2-37. **A.** The barrel field in the somatosensory cortex of the rat. Each barrel (identified by letters and numbers) represents a single facial vibrissa. After Tracey and Waite (1995). **B.** Representation of the facial vibrissae in the thalamic ventrobasal complex of the rat. From Sugitani et al. (1990). **C.** Barreloids in the spinal nucleus of the trigeminal nerve of the rat. After Belford and Killackey (1979).

ronment in which the animal moves about through an active palpating process, called "whisking." Each cortical barrel receives somatosensory input from Merkel discs of a single vibrissa. The morphogenetic organization of neurons into barrels is mostly a post-natal phenomenon in rodents, as removal of specific vibrissae interferes with the development of the corresponding barrels (Van der Loos and Woolsey, 1973; Belford and Killackey, 1980). Barrel-like neuronal aggregates (barreloids) have also been identified in the trigeminal nucleus (Figure 2-37C), which is the target of somesthetic afferents from the face area, and in the region of the ventrobasal thalamic complex (Figure 2-37B) where trigeminal afferents synapse with neurons that project to the cortex (Woolsey et al., 1979; Belford and Killackey, 1979).

The cortical barrels have been conceptualized as components of the vertical columns of the somesthetic cortex, earlier identified anatomically by Lorente de Nó (1938) and physiologically by Mountcastle (1957). All neurons within a cortical column represent the same somatotopic location and cutaneous modality, and have similar receptive fields. As such, the vertical columns, including the specialized barrels and barreloids, may be considered *minimodules* of larger cutaneous fields. This raises the question: are there somatosensory minimodules in the dorsal horn comparable to the barrels of the cortex and the barreloids in the thalamus and the trigeminal nucleus? We propose that, indeed, the vertical "slabs" of the substantia gelatinosa illustrated earlier in coronal sections of the substantia gelatinosa of the human spinal cord (Figure 1-25), and the frog spinal cord (Figure 2-6), constitute such minimodules.

The vertical gelatinosal slabs, which are best visualized in preparations with fiber staining techniques, are a ubiquitous feature of the mammalian dorsal horn (Figure 2-38). Components of these slabs may be the dendrites of the double-tufted central cells seen with silver staining in the human dorsal horn (Figures 1-19, 1-20), and the flame terminals of the large caliber tactile afferents visualized with various techniques in animals (Figures 1-26 to 1-28). In a classical study of the morphology of afferent terminals and cell types in the mouse neocortex, Lorente de Nó (1938) illustrated the bushy terminal of "specific" thalamocortical axons in lamina IV, and the complementary bushy dendrites of small granular neurons in the same region (Figure 2-39A). The width of these interlocking sites may correspond to

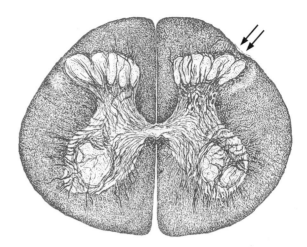

Figure 2-38. Gelatinosal "slabs" in the lumbosacral dorsal horn of the gazelle. After Bianchi, from Ariens-Kappers et al. (1936).

the width of the cortical columns previously alluded to. According to recent studies (Welker and Woolsey, 1974; Jensen and Killackey, 1987; Waite and Tracey, 1995) a similar pattern is discernible in the barrel region of the somesthetic cortex (Figure 2-39B). In line with this evidence, we propose that the somatosensory gelatinosal slabs in the spinal cord are homologous to the cortical columns and barrels of lamina IV but with one structural difference, that the gelatinosal slabs have a different shape than the columns or barrels. This shape, as illustrated in Figure 2-39C, is relatable to the tubular structure of the spinal cord: both the afferent terminals and the dendritic arbor of recipient neurons in the gelatinosal slabs are flattened in the rostrocaudal plane (Figure 2-39C).

In terms of the fine circuitry of the dorsal horn described earlier (see Figure 2-17), the gelatinosal slabs have three principal components: (i) the low threshold, exteroceptive flame terminals in the depth of the substantia gelatinosa; (ii) the high threshold, nociceptive cap terminals superficially; and (iii) the double-tufted central cells with which the flame and cap terminals synapse between them. The evidence obtained by Scheibel and Scheibel (1968), as illustrated in Figure 1-15, indicates that the central cells and the afferent terminals synapsing with them are all elongated in the rostrocaudal plane. It is reasonable to assume, therefore, that the gelatinosal slabs are also elongated in shape, as reconstructed in Figure 2-39C. We noted earlier that the number of gelatinosal slabs do not exceed a dozen in the coronal plane. We do not know exactly how long these slabs are and, therefore,

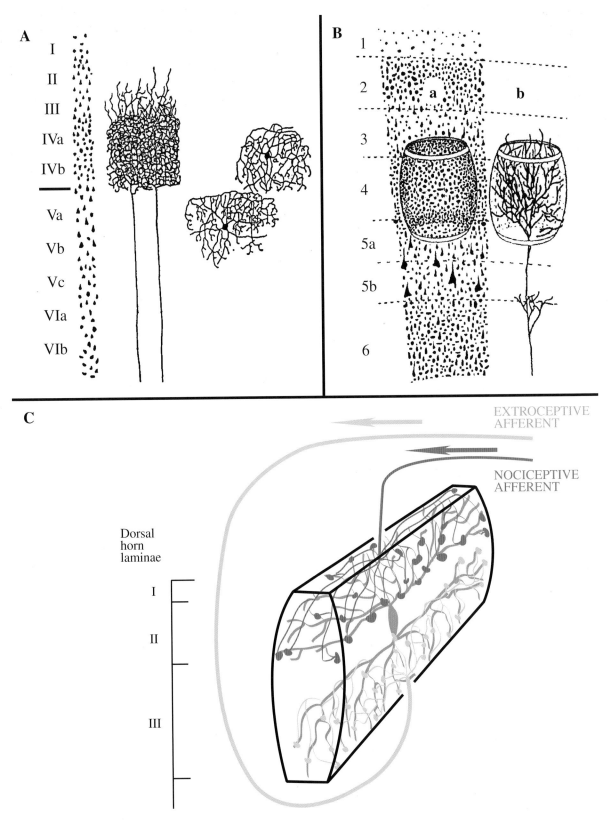

Figure 2-39. A. The bushy terminals of "specific" thalamocortical afferents (**left**) and the complimentary dendritic arbor of the receiving granular neurons (**right**) in lamina IV of the mouse neocortex. After Lorente de Nó (1938). **B.** The hypothetical relationship between the bushy afferent terminals (**right**) and the granular neurons forming a barrel (**left**). After Waite and Tracey (1995). **C.** The hypothetical structure of gelatinosal slabs in the dorsal horn of the spinal cord. Its three pricipal components are the nociceptive afferents with cap terminals (red) the exteroceptive afferents with flame terminals (blue), and the rostrocaudally oriented apical and basal dendritic tufts of central cells (purple). All three components are elongated in the rostrocaudal plane.

how many might fit lengthwise within a segment. But their aligmnment is likely to take the form illustrated in Figure 2-40.

Why would the hypothesized somesthetic micromodules of the substantia gelatinosa become slab-shaped, in contrast to the more spherical somesthetic micromodules found in the brain, like the barrels or barreloids? A possible answer is that this configuration is a space-saving arrangement. While the dorsal root fibers from the periphery enter the dorsal horn in a discontinuous manner through the bottle-

neck of discrete dorsal roots, their collaterals must terminate continuously along the length of the uninterrupted substantia gelatinosa. The utility of the rostrocaudally elongated slabs is therefore obvious. By transforming the more common spherical axonal terminals and dendritic plexuses into elongated complexes, advantage is taken of the ample space available within the spinal cord along the rostrocaudal plane and minimizing the expansion of the dorsal horn in the highly constrained gray matter in the mediolateral plane.

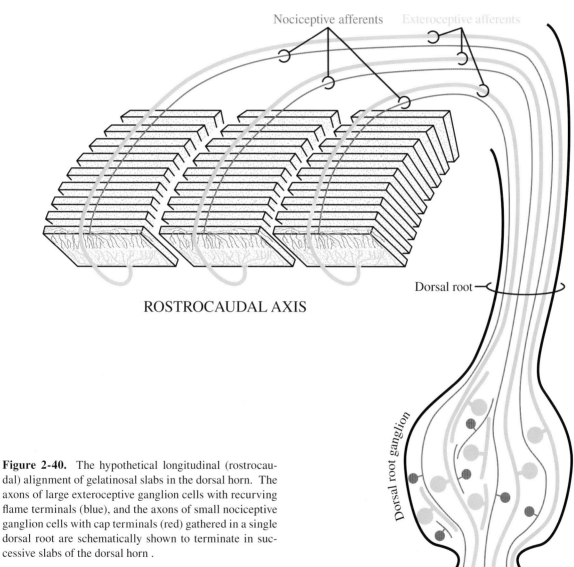

ROSTROCAUDAL AXIS

Figure 2-40. The hypothetical longitudinal (rostrocaudal) alignment of gelatinosal slabs in the dorsal horn. The axons of large exteroceptive ganglion cells with recurving flame terminals (blue), and the axons of small nociceptive ganglion cells with cap terminals (red) gathered in a single dorsal root are schematically shown to terminate in successive slabs of the dorsal horn .

3 EXPERIMENTAL STUDIES OF SPINAL CORD MORPHOGENESIS, NEUROGENESIS, AND NEURONAL MATURATION

3.1 Spinal Cord Morphogenesis: An Overview

3.1.1 Early Histological Observations of Spinal Cord Development. An early study of the development of the spinal cord, using the just introduced technique of staining hardened nerve tissue with chromic acid (Hannover, 1844), was carried out in fetal sheep by Bidder and Kupffer (1857). The investigators reported that the gray matter of the spinal cord develops before the white matter, and inferred from this that the early developing fibers of the spinal cord issue from cells of the gray matter. Bidder and Kupffer also observed that fibers of the spinal ganglia sprout concurrently in both directions, peripherally and centrally. Among well-known subsequent investigations of the embryonic development of the spinal cord were those of His (1886, 1889), von Lenhossék (1889), Retzius (1898), and Ramón y Cajal (1909). Studying the cellular composition of the early spinal cord (commonly referred to as the neural tube), His discovered that its mitotic cells were concentrated near the lumen of the central canal; he named these cells, *Keimzellen* (germ cells, stem cells). His hypothesized that after cell division, one of the daughter cells remains in the vicinity of the lumen and continues to proliferate while the other cell leaves the germinal epithelium and differentiates into a young neuron, or neuroblast. His argued that another cell line, that of the spongioblasts, are the source of neuroglia. His named the germinal neuroepithelium, the inner plate (*Innerplatte*), and distinguished two other layers in the embryonic spinal cord, the mantle layer and the marginal zone. According to His, the mantle layer is composed of differentiating neuroblasts and the marginal zone contains the fibers of the future white matter.

His's conception of the structure of the primitive spinal cord was illustrated by Ramón y Cajal (1909), with added cytological details based on his own studies with the Golgi technique (Figure 3-1A). Writers of textbooks later modified His's scheme by calling the germinal epithelium of the neural tube, or neuroepithelium, the ependymal layer (Figure 3-1B). This was unfortunate because the ependymal layer is composed of highly specialized cells (ependymal cells, tanycytes) that come to line the central canal in the maturing central nervous system, some time after the proliferative neuroepithelium has disappeared. Calling the primordial gray matter the mantle layer, and the primordial white matter the marginal layer is not particularly helpful either because it introduces two unnecessary terms and implies a break in a continuous developmental process. (After all, at what point does the "mantle layer" become the progressively expanding gray matter, and when is the "marginal layer" transformed into the developing white matter?)

With reference to the gross structure of the developing spinal cord, His distinguished four "plates" (Figure 3-1C, left). Flanking the central canal laterally, and divided by the sulcus limitans (*Medianfurche*), is the alar plate (*Flügelplatte*) dorsally and the basal plate (*Grundplatte*) ventrally. Capping the spinal cord is the roof plate (*Deckplatte*), and the floor plate (*Bodenplatte*) forms the base of the spinal cord. The roof plate and floor plate have a different cellular composition than the alar plate and basal plate (or lateral plates). His's distinction between the alar plate and the basal plate is of great significance because it was accepted for a long time that cells generated in the alar plate is the source of neurons of the sensory dorsal horn, while the cells of the basal plate are the

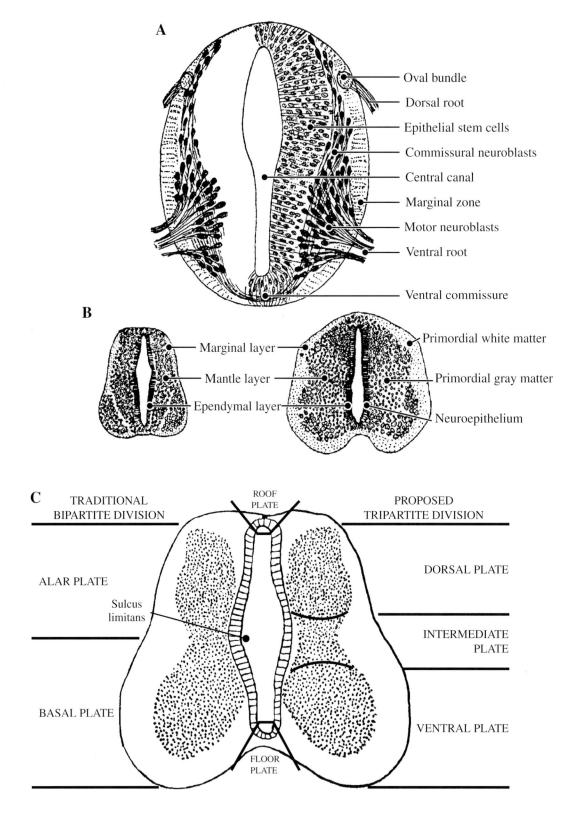

Figure 3-1. A. Schematic drawing by Ramón y Cajal (1909) of His's interpretation of the cytology of the spinal cord in a 4-week-old human embryo. **B.** The "layers" of the spinal cord in a younger (**left**) and an older (**right**) embryo. The traditional names of the layers are in the center, the revised terminology on the right. **C.** His's partitioning of the embryonic spinal cord into the roof plate, the floor plate, and two neuroepithelial plates, the alar plate and the basal plate (**left**). Our proposed division of the embryonic spinal cord into dorsal, intermediate, and ventral plates (**right**) is justified by the observations described and illustrated on the succeeding pages.

source of the motoneurons of the ventral horn (Figure 3-1B). However, we shall provide empirical evidence that the lateral neuroepithelium (the source of all spinal cord neurons) is divisible into three morphogenetic components of equal importance, the dorsal, intermediate, and ventral plates (Figure 3-1C, right). We will show that the dorsal (alar) neuroepithelium is the source of the sensory processing neurons of the dorsal horn, the ventral (basal) neuroepithelium is the source of motoneurons of the ventral horn, and the neglected intermediate neuroepithelium is the source of interneurons of the intermediate gray. We will also show that the sulcus limitans is not an early embryonic landmark but a later developing feature of the maturing spinal cord, the site of the persisting central canal.

3.1.2 Recent Histological Observations of Spinal Cord Development.

In Figures 3-2 to 3-6 we illustrate the morphogenetic development of the cervical spinal cord in the rat at daily intervals from embryonic day 11 (E11) to embryonic day E19 (E19). The specimens were embedded in plastic (methacrylate) for optimal preservation of all tissue components, and stained with a dye (hematoxylin-eosin) that visualizes in this preparation not only the perikarya of primitive cells and differentiating neurons but also, if present, their processes.

On *E11*, about half a day after the closure of the neural tube (E10.5, see Figure 4-31A), the egg-shaped spinal cord surrounds a slit-shaped spinal canal. The spinal canal is surrounded laterally by the pseudostratified neuroepithelium, composed of radially oriented spindle shaped cells (NEP cells). The neuroepithelium is capped dorsally and ventrally by the more tightly packed cells of the roof plate and the floor plate (Figure 3-2). The nuclei of NEP are arranged irregularly about 3-4 deep, and those undergoing mitotic division are situated near the spinal canal. The division of the lateral neuroepithelium into

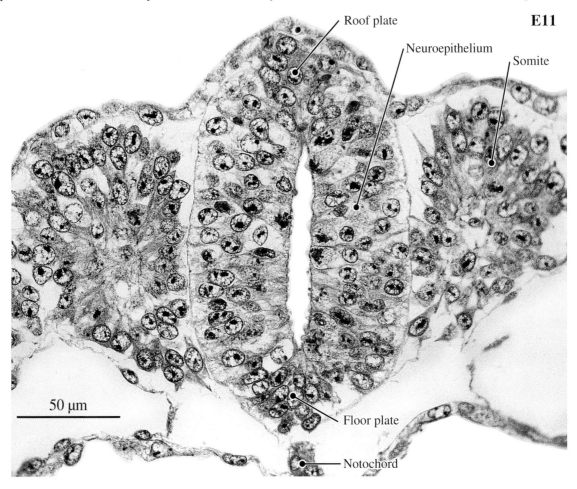

Roof plate   **E11**
Neuroepithelium
Somite
50 μm
Floor plate
Notochord

Figure 3-2. The cervical spinal cord of an E11 rat embryo. The slit-shaped spinal canal is surrounded by the pseudostratified neuroepithelium composed of radially oriented, elongated NEP cells. The nuclei of NEP cells are arranged irregularly 3-4 deep, and those undergoing mitotic division are situated near the lumen. The roof plate and floor plate are composed of smaller, more tightly packed cells. Methacrylate embedding; hematoxylin-eosin stain.

separate compartments is not evident at this stage of development. The spinal cord is flanked by somites, and the notochord is visible a short distance from the floor plate. The dorsal root ganglia have not yet formed and afferent nor efferent fibers are not yet detectable peripherally.

By *E12* (Figure 3-3A), several changes are evident in the cervical spinal cord. First, the slit-shaped spinal canal has changed its shape, due to the swellings forming ventrally, centrally, and dorsally. These divisions of the slit shaped spinal canals are identified as the dorsal, central, and ventral canals. Second, the cell packing density of the neuroepithelium as well as its width and height have greatly increased. Third, there is a hint of the formation of dorsal root ganglia. Fourth, the spinal cord has become broader at its base, looking somewhat like a pear. Fifth, a few differentiating cells with round nuclei have started to accumulate outside the neuroepithelium. (This is more evident at higher magnification; see Figure 3-25.)

By *E13* (Figure 3-3B), most of the features seen in an incipient form on day E12 have become more pronounced. The spinal cord is more obviously pear-shaped, and the three swellings of the spinal canal are more prominent. The size and compactness of the spinal ganglia have increased. Finally, the number of round differentiating cells, particularly in the future ventral horn, has increased.

By *E14* (Figure 3-4A), several new developments are seen in the pumpkin-shaped cervical spinal cord. In spite of the appearance of a few differentiating cells, the spinal cord consists on E13 of a single tissue layer, i.e., the neuroepithelium But by E14, three discrete layers are distinguishable. The first of these is the neuroepithelium itself with its horizontally oriented, spindle shaped cells. The second layer is the primordial gray matter containing a fair population of variably shaped differentiating cells in the incipient ventral horn and in the formative intermediate gray. The third layer is the thin primordial white matter. In the region surrounding the ventral canal, the ventral plate, the areal growth of the incipient ventral horn is associated with a reduction in the width of the neuroepithelium, designated as the ventral neuroepithelium. These changes are less pronounced in the intermediate plate. The formative white matter is most prominent at two points: ventrally, where

the ventral commissure and the ventral funiculus are developing, and dorsally, where dorsal root fibers enter the cord and form His's oval bundle. (We shall show later that this is the region where the dorsal root afferents bifurcate and give rise to ascending and descending branches.) A small bundle of sensory fibers, forming the dorsal root, enter the spinal cord dorsolaterally, and a small contingent of motor fibers, forming the ventral root, leave it ventrolaterally.

By *E15* (Figure 3-4B), the changes seen on the previous day have become more prominent and there are also some new developments. In the ventral plate, the width of the neuroepithelium has shrunken further and, in a reciprocal fashion, the ventral horn has greatly expanded. Among the new develoments that have taken place by E15 are the shrinkage of the intermediate neuroepithelium and the expansion of the intermediate gray. In sharp contrast, the dorsal neuroepithelium has greatly expanded in association with the growth of the dorsal funiculus and thge oval bundle of His.

By *E16* (Figure 3-5A), two significant developments have taken place. The first of these is the evident maturation of motoneurons in the ventral horn and the beginning of their segregation into discrete nuclei (columns). The second is the expansion of the gray matter dorsally. Among some of the other changes are the ongoing shrinkage of the ventral and intermediate neuroepithelia, and the growth of the ventromedial and lateral funiculi.

By *E17* (Figure 3-5B), the expansion of the dorsal horn is quite obvious in the cervical spinal cord and so is the formation of the dorsal funiculus. Other developments include the shrinkage of the spinal canal, the ongoing maturation and segregation of motoneurons in the ventral horn, and the growth of the ventral and lateral funiculi.

By *E18* (Figure 3-6A) and E19 (Figure 3-6B), the spinal cord has begun to assume its mature shape. The changes that contribute to this are the lateral expansion of the gray matter, the growth of the white matter, including the dorsal funiculus, and the shrinkage of the spinal canal in such a way that only the permanent central canal remains. The vestige of the neuroepithelium is the thin band surrounding the shrunken central canal. (This proliferative zone, as we shall see later, is the source of neuroglia.)

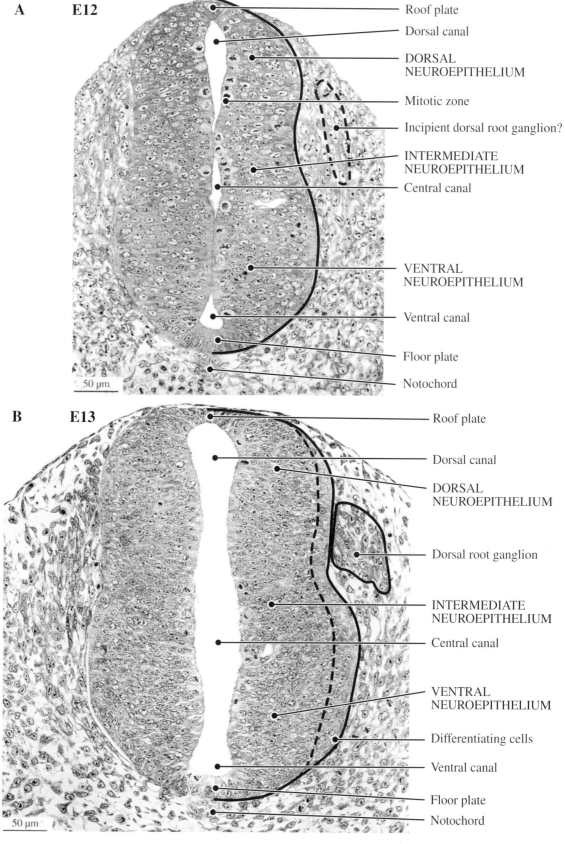

A   E12

Roof plate
Dorsal canal
DORSAL NEUROEPITHELIUM
Mitotic zone
Incipient dorsal root ganglion?
INTERMEDIATE NEUROEPITHELIUM
Central canal
VENTRAL NEUROEPITHELIUM
Ventral canal
Floor plate
Notochord

50 µm

B   E13

Roof plate
Dorsal canal
DORSAL NEUROEPITHELIUM
Dorsal root ganglion
INTERMEDIATE NEUROEPITHELIUM
Central canal
VENTRAL NEUROEPITHELIUM
Differentiating cells
Ventral canal
Floor plate
Notochord

50 µm

Figure 3-3. The cervical spinal cord of an E12 (**A**) and an E13 (**B**) rat. The neuroepithelium is expanding greatly during this period relative to the roof plate and the floor plate. The spinal canal and the neuroepithelium surrounding it are becoming partitioned into dorsal, intermediate (central), and ventral compartments. A thin band of differentiating cells is forming laterally (broken outline).   Methacrylate; hematoxylin-eosin.

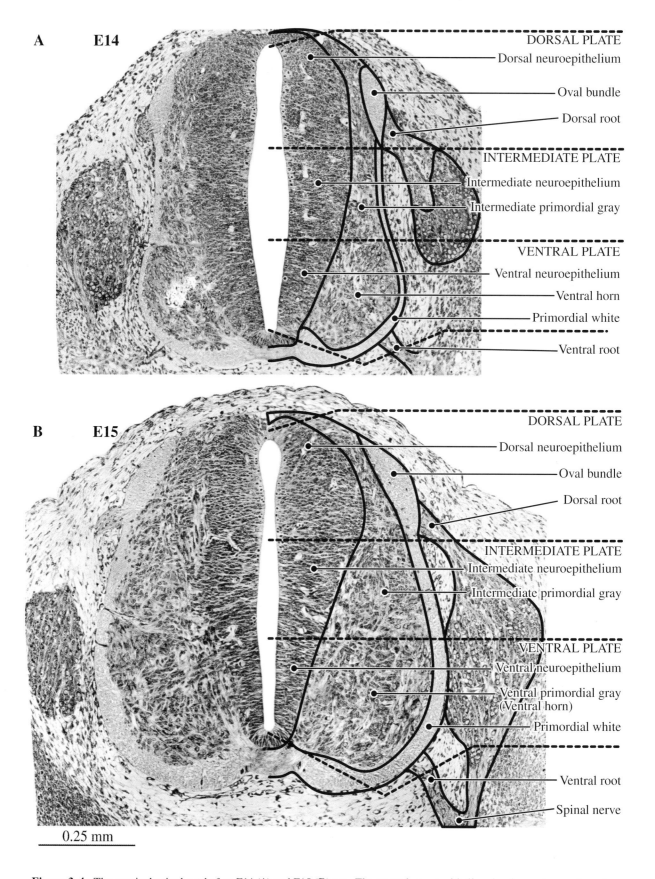

Figure 3-4. The cervical spinal cord of an E14 (**A**) and E15 (**B**) rat. The ventral neuroepithelium has begun to recede and the ventral horn to expand by E14. By E15, the intermediate neuroepithelium has begun to recede, and the intermediate gray to expand; in contrast, the dorsal neuroepithelium is expanding. Another development during this period is the formation and growth of the white matter, including the oval bundle dorsolaterally. Methacrylate; hematoxylin-eosin.

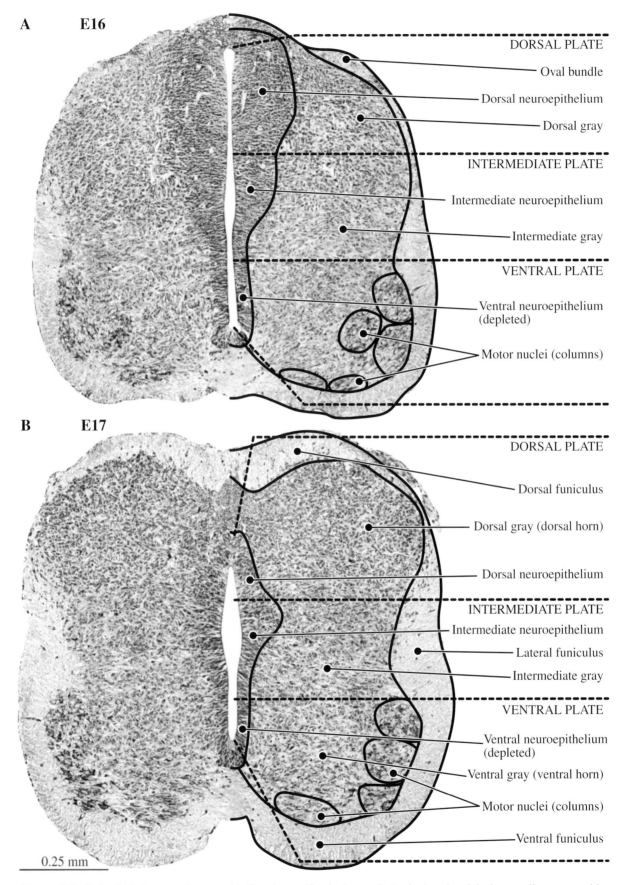

Figure 3-5. A. By E16, the ventral neuroepithelium is receding in the cervical spinal cord and the intermediate neuroepithelium is shrinking; however, the dorsal neuroepithelium remains prominent. **B.** By E17, the dorsal neuroepithelium is receding while the dorsal horn has greatly expanded and the dorsal funiculus is developing. Methacrylate; hematoxylin-eosin.

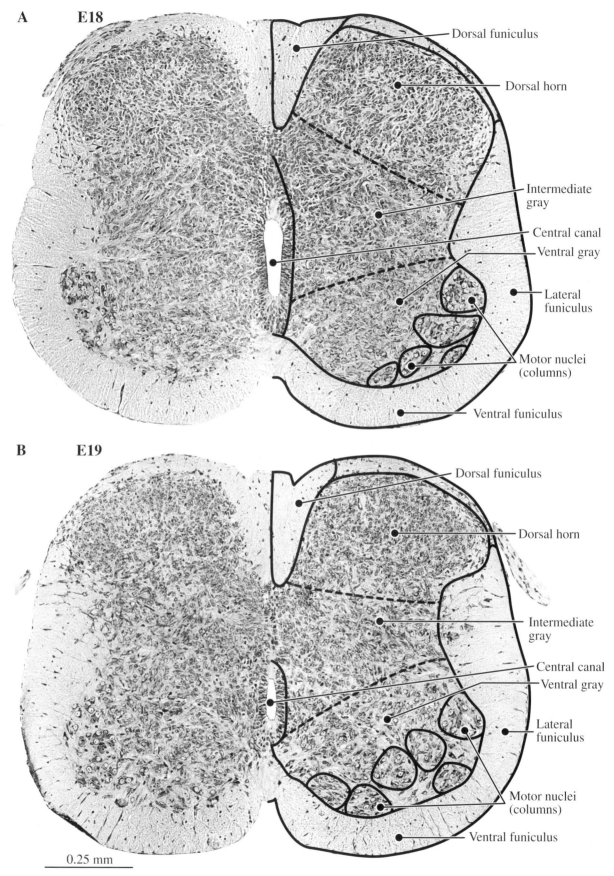

Figure 3-6. The cervical spinal cord is beginning to assume its mature form by E18 (**A**) and E19 (**B**). The dorsal horn is expanding and the dorsal funiculus is deepening. As a result of the shrinkage of the embryonic spinal canal, only the permanent central canal remains. Methacrylate; hematoxylin-eosin.

3.2 Spinal Cord Neurogenesis: A Cytological and Autoradiographic Investigation in the Rat

3.2.1 *The Technique of Thymidine Autoradiography.* Thymidine is a specific precursor of DNA, and if radioactively labeled thymidine (e.g., ³H-thymidine) is administered to an animal, the chromosomes of its proliferating cells will incorporate the radiochemical before mitotic division and their daughter cells will become radioactive. Because the DNA of nondividing cells is metabolically stable, postmitotic cells in the same animal will not be labeled with the radioactive thymidine. In the case of neural tissue, like the spinal cord, the radioactive thymidine will label the proliferating neuroepithelial cells (NEP cells) but the postmitotic neurons (irrespective where they reside) will not be labeled. After their exodus from the neuroepithelium, the tagged NEP cells that differentiate into neurons will retain their radioactive nuclear DNA as long as they survive. However, in the NEP cells that stay in the neuroepithelium and continue to divide after the administration of ³H-thymidine, the concentration of labeled nuclear DNA will be halved with each division. This may lead to a dilution of the radioactive DNA to a level that it is no longer detectable with conventional thymidine autoradiography.

Thymidine autoradiography has been used in developmental neurobiology for three purposes: (1) to locate the site of production of particular classes or groups of neurons; (2) to track the migratory route of these neurons from their production site to their destination, and determine their pattern of settling; and (3) to date the time of origin (or birthdates) of particular classes of neurons. We shall discuss separately the uses of each of these techniques, and some of the results obtained with them regarding spinal cord neurogenesis and morphogenesis.

3.2.2 *Morphology and Cell Dynamics of the Spinal Cord Neuroepithelium.* Short-survival autoradiography is the specific technique used to locate the time and site of neuron production, or neurogenesis. In this procedure, ³H-thymidine is administered to a pregnant animal at a chosen gestational age and her embryos are removed after an interval that is long enough to allow the incorporation of the radiochemical into the DNA of dividing cells but too brief to allow the exodus of the proliferating cells from the neuroepithelium and their differentiation. In our short-survival studies (e.g., Altman and Bayer, 1984), the embryos were consistently killed 2 hours after their mother was injected with ³H-thymidine.

We mentioned earlier His's view that the neuroepithelium is a stratified germinal matrix in which mitotic cells form a discrete cell layer adjacent to the spinal canal and is flanked by another layer of nonmitotic cells. However, Sauer (1935) deduced from his light microscopic observations that the neuroepithelium is, in fact, a pseudostratified germinal matrix. Sauer noted that the cytoplasm of the spindle shaped germinal cells, which are oriented at a right angle to the ventricle, are anchored by polar cytoplasmic processes to the external and internal limiting membrane of the neuroepithelium. He proposed that inside the anchored cytoplasm, the nuclei of the cells move toward the ventricle before dividing and then, after mitosis, the nuclei of the daughter cells move away from the lumen (Figure 3-7A). Sauer called this process "interkinetic nuclear migration." Sauer's hypothesis was later confirmed with short-survival autoradiography by Sidman et al. (1959), and others. The mitotic cycle (Figures 3-7B, 7C) has been calculated to be about 11 hours in the neuroepithelium of young rodent embryos (Atlas and Bond, 1965; Langman et al., 1966). The mitotic cycle may vary at different ages (Kaufman, 1968; Hoshino et al., 1973) and at different neuroepithelial sites (Denham, 1967; Wilson, 1973).

The current interpretation of interkinetic nuclear migration is that the nuclei of NEP cells move to the *synthetic zone* before cell division where they incorporate the thymidine required to duplicate their chromosomes. When the cell is ready to divide, its nucleus translocates to the periventricular *mitotic zone* and produces two daughter cells. This pattern of neuroepithelial cell labeling is illustrated in the spinal cord neuroepithelium of an E15 rat killed 2 hours after the administration of ³H-thymidine (Figure 3-8). The majority of cells are heavily labeled in the synthetic zone. A smaller complement of labeled cells is present in the region between the synthetic zone and the mitotic zone. Only a few lightly labeled cells have reached the mitotic zone near the ventricle. The differentiating zone of the primordial gray matter contains a few heavily labeled cells. These may be precursors of locally multiplying glia.

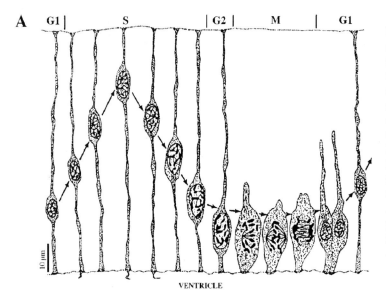

Figure 3-7. **A.** Translocation of the nuclei of NEP cells during the G1 phase of the cell cycle towards the synthetic zone (S) and, during G2, towards the mitotic zone (M) near the lumen of the ventricle. After Sauer (1935), from Jacobson (1978). **B.** Percentage of ³H-thymidine labeled metaphases in the mouse neuroepithelium. From Langman and Welch (1967). **C.** Approximate duration of the phases of the mitotic cycle of proliferating NEP cells. From Altman (1969).

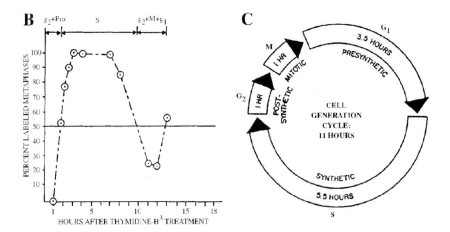

3.2.3 Sojourn, Migration, and Maturation of Spinal Cord Neurons.

In *short survival autoradiograms* of E13 rat (Figure 3-9), the synthetic zone of the neuroepithelium is flanked laterally by a band composed mostly of unlabeled cells. This band is broad in the ventral plate and narrow in the intermediate and dorsal plates. The simplest interpretation is that this band is composed of differentiating (postmitotic) neurons: a large complement of motoneurons ventrally, and a few early-generated interneurons more dorsally. However, short survival autoradiograms of E15 rats (Figure 3-10) indicate that there are, in fact, *two* unlabeled bands: one composed of darkly staining cells that look like neuroepithelial cells, and another band of lightly staining cells that are settling in the incipient gray matter. We will try to show below with sequential survival autoradiography that the postmitotic lateral region of the neuroepi-

thelium is a distinct compartment, its *sojourn zone.* If this conclusion is correct, the current conceptualization of the neuroepithelium as a pseudostratified matrix (i.e., one that consists of a single layer of proliferating cells) will have to be revised.

The technique of *sequential survival autoradiography* is used to trace the movements and settling of young neurons. Groups of pregnant rats of the same gestational age are injected with ³H-thymidine but the embryos of different dams are allowed to survive for different periods thereafter. Figure 3-11 shows the distribution of labeled cells in embryos tagged with ³H-thymidine on E13 and killed 2 hours, 1 day, and 2 days following the injections. After 2 hours survival, the synthetic zone is full of labeled cells but the thin lateral band of cells is unlabeled (Figure 3-11A). After 1 day survival, there are two

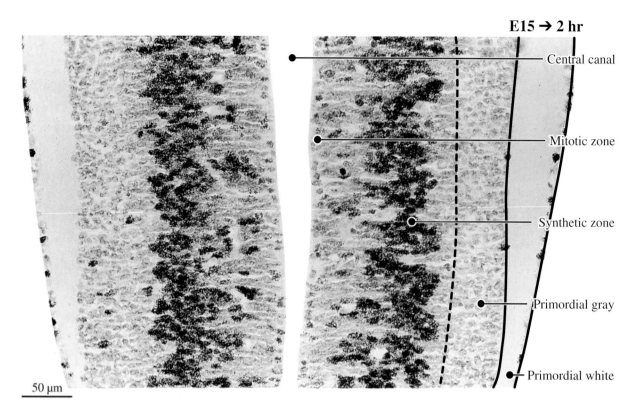

Figure 3-8. Horizontal section through the dorsal spinal cord of an E15 rat embryo killed 2 hours after the administration of ^{3}H-thymidine. The nuclei of NEP cells incorporating the labeled DNA precursor are located in the synthetic zone. Short survival autoradiogram. Paraffin.

bands of less heavily labeled cells in the neuroepithelium, and the expanding gray matter contains both heavily labeled and unlabeled cells (Figure 3-11B). The label dilution in the synthetic zone and the putative sojourn zone is to be expected because the multiplying NEP cells had time to undergo at least two divisions during the 24-hour survival period. The labeling pattern changes after 48 hours survival (Figure 3-11C). In this E15 rat, the heavily labeled cells are widely scattered in the enlarged intermediate gray matter while less heavily labeled cells occupy the inner synthetic zone as well as the greatly expanded outer band of the neuroepithelium. If one considers that the latter region is occupied by unlabeled cells in short survival radiograms in embryos of the same age (Figure 3-10), their labeling in the long survival radiograms establishes that the lateral band of neuroepithelial cells cells are sojourning here prior to their exit and migration into the gray matter.

This sequence of sojourn and migration of differentiating neurons is more obvious in embryos that were tagged with ^{3}H-thymidine on E15 and were killed 2 hours, 1 day and 2 days thereafter (Figure 3-12). In the E15 embryo that survived for 2 hours after tagging, labeled cells abound in the synthetic zone of the intermediate and dorsal neuroepithelia but the cells in the putative sojourn zone of the neuroepithelium are unlabeled (Figure 3-12A). However, after 1 day survival, most of the cells in the putative sojourn zones of the intermediate and dorsal neuroepithelia are labeled (Figure 3-12B). Obviously, labeled cells from the proliferative zone have moved into the lateral band of the neuroepithelium between E15 and E16. Finally, both the synthetic and the sojourn zones of the neuroepithelium are in a process of dissolution 2 days after tagging in the E17 embryos, and by now the labeled cells have penetrated the intermediate gray, and are particularly abundant in the dorsal horn (Figure 3-12C). The conclusion is justified that the postmitotic (differentiating) cells of the intermediate and dorsal neuroepithelia pause for about 1 day in the sojourn zone of the neuroepithelium and then migrate into the expanding gray matter.

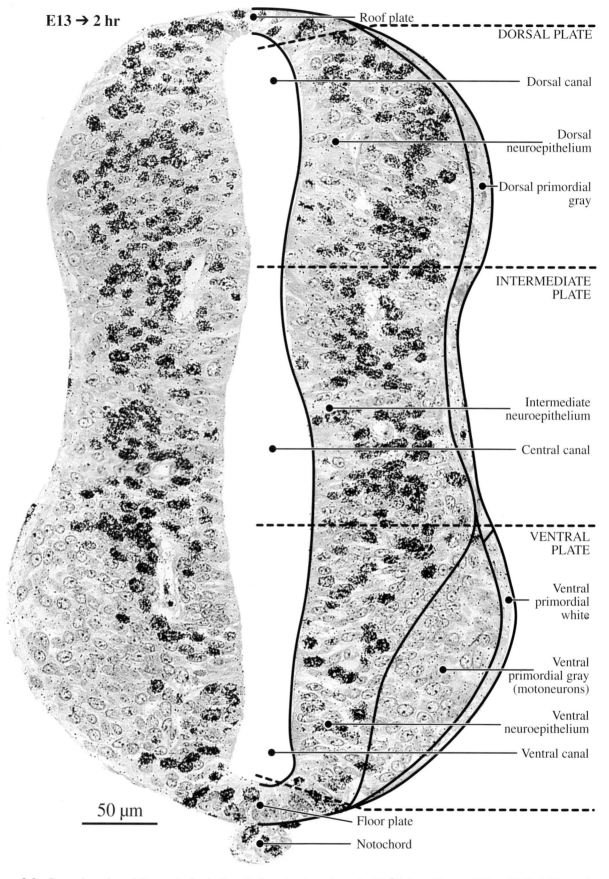

E13 → 2 hr

Roof plate

DORSAL PLATE

Dorsal canal

Dorsal neuroepithelium

Dorsal primordial gray

INTERMEDIATE PLATE

Intermediate neuroepithelium

Central canal

VENTRAL PLATE

Ventral primordial white

Ventral primordial gray (motoneurons)

Ventral neuroepithelium

Ventral canal

50 μm

Floor plate

Notochord

Figure 3-9. Coronal section of the cervical spinal cord of a rat embryo tagged with ³H-thymidine on E13 and killed 2 hours later. Labeled NEP cells abound in the synthetic zone of the dorsal and intermediate neuroepithelia but are less abundant in the ventral neuroepithelium. Except in the incipient ventral horn, there are few unlabeled cells in the incipient gray matter. Methacrylate.

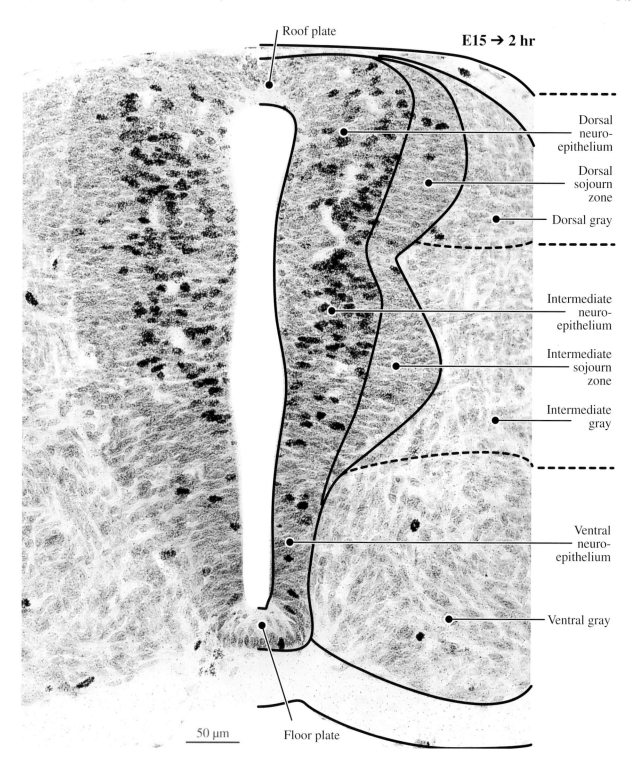

Figure 3-10. Short survival autoradiogram of the cervical spinal cord of a rat that received ³H-thymidine on E15 and was killed 2 hours later. The synthetic zone of the ventral neuroepithelium has the lowest concentration of labeled NEP cells, the intermediate and dorsal neuroepithelia the highest. The intermediate and dorsal neuroepithelia (but not the ventral neuroepithelium) also contain an outer band of darkly staining but unlabeled (young postmitotic cells). These bands are identified as the sojourn zones of the spinal cord neuroepithelium. Only a few scattered labeled cells, presumed neuroglia precursors, are present in the gray matter.

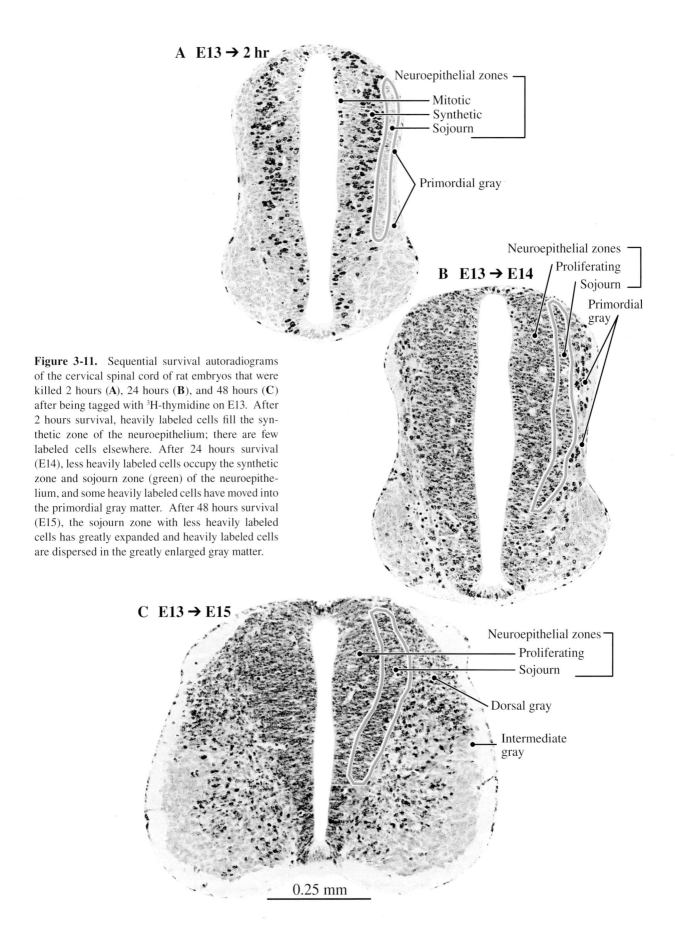

Figure 3-11. Sequential survival autoradiograms of the cervical spinal cord of rat embryos that were killed 2 hours (**A**), 24 hours (**B**), and 48 hours (**C**) after being tagged with ³H-thymidine on E13. After 2 hours survival, heavily labeled cells fill the synthetic zone of the neuroepithelium; there are few labeled cells elsewhere. After 24 hours survival (E14), less heavily labeled cells occupy the synthetic zone and sojourn zone (green) of the neuroepithelium, and some heavily labeled cells have moved into the primordial gray matter. After 48 hours survival (E15), the sojourn zone with less heavily labeled cells has greatly expanded and heavily labeled cells are dispersed in the greatly enlarged gray matter.

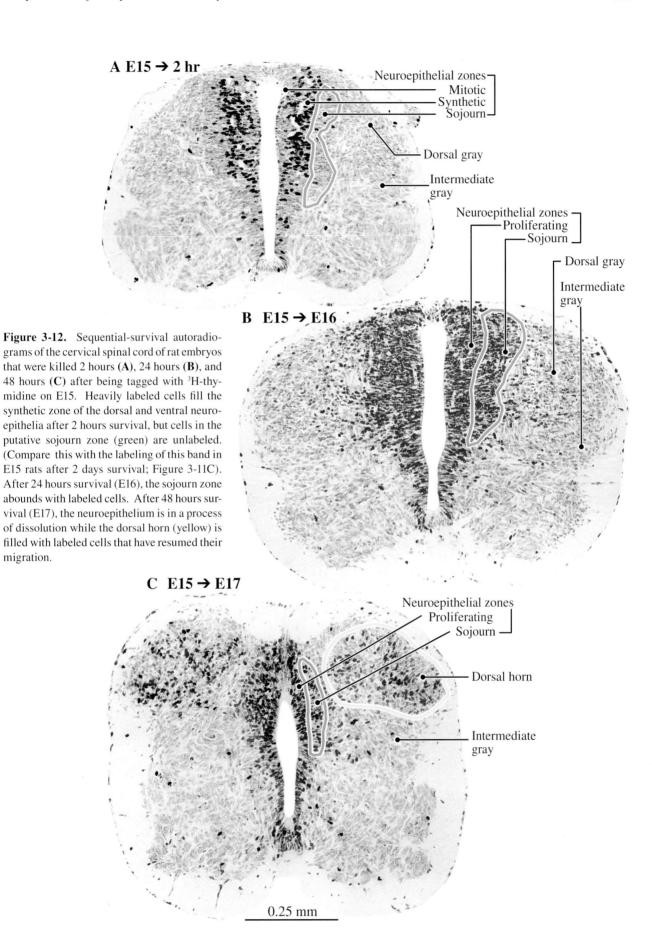

A E15 → 2 hr

Neuroepithelial zones
Mitotic
Synthetic
Sojourn

Dorsal gray

Intermediate gray

Figure 3-12. Sequential-survival autoradiograms of the cervical spinal cord of rat embryos that were killed 2 hours (**A**), 24 hours (**B**), and 48 hours (**C**) after being tagged with ^{3}H-thymidine on E15. Heavily labeled cells fill the synthetic zone of the dorsal and ventral neuroepithelia after 2 hours survival, but cells in the putative sojourn zone (green) are unlabeled. (Compare this with the labeling of this band in E15 rats after 2 days survival; Figure 3-11C). After 24 hours survival (E16), the sojourn zone abounds with labeled cells. After 48 hours survival (E17), the neuroepithelium is in a process of dissolution while the dorsal horn (yellow) is filled with labeled cells that have resumed their migration.

B E15 → E16

Neuroepithelial zones
Proliferating
Sojourn

Dorsal gray

Intermediate gray

C E15 → E17

Neuroepithelial zones
Proliferating
Sojourn

Dorsal horn

Intermediate gray

0.25 mm

3.2.4   Dating the Time of Origin of Spinal Cord Neurons. The time of origin of neurons of the spinal cord has been investigated by several investigators with *long survival autoradiography*. In this procedure animals that are tagged with radioactive thymidine in utero are killed some time between birth and adulthood, at an age when the identity of labeled neurons is easy to specify. Most investigators used the "flash-labeling" technique with a single injection of the radiochemical on a particular day of gestation. Nornes and Das (1974) and Nornes and Carry (1978) reported that, in the mouse spinal cord, neurons originate between E10 and E14 with temporal gradients along the ventrodorsal axis. Ventral motoneurons originate on E10–E11, the neurons of the intermediate gray on E11–E14, and the neurons of the dorsal horn on E12–E14. These investigators suggested that the neurons produced on E10–E11 migrate from the basal plate (ventral neuroepithelium) while those produced on E12–E14 migrate from the alar plate (dorsal neuroepithelium). In contrast, Sims and Vaughn (1979) claimed that motoneurons in the mouse spinal cord are generated mostly between E9 and E10.5, and the earliest interneurons are generated on E9.5. In a study that combined choline acetyltransferase immunocytochemistry with ^{3}H-thymidine autoradiography, Barber et al (1991) found that both somatic and autonomic motoneurons are generated concurrently in the rat spinal cord, with peak production on E11 at thoracic levels, and on E12 and E13 at lumbar and sacral levels. At a given level, cholinergic interneurons ("partition cells" and "cluster cells") are generated 1 or 2 days later than the motoneurons. Nandi et al. (1993) and Beal and Bice (1994), who combined thymidine autoradiography with fluorescence staining, reported that in the rat spinal cord interneurons and relay neurons of the intermediate gray are generated between E13 and E15, and neurons of the upper laminae of the dorsal horn between E13 and E16. Relay neurons with long axons (i.e., those projecting to supraspinal levels) originate before propriospinal (intraspinal) interneurons with short ascending or descending axons (Bice and Beal, 1997). Finally, according to the autoradiographic study in mice by Lawson and Biscoe (1979), peak generation time of dorsal root ganglion neurons is E11.5 at cervical levels and E12.5 at lumbar levels. According to these authors, the large ganglion cells originate before the small ones, and the production of small ganglion cells continues for at least 48 hours after the production of large ganglion cells has ended.

In all these studies, estimates of the birth dates of different classes of neurons was based on counts of "heavily" labeled cells in a population as a function of age at the time of injection. The logic of ignoring "lightly" labeled cells is sound. A class of cells generated for instance on E11, would be labeled not only if ^{3}H-thymidine was administered on E11 but also following earlier administration. However, tagging on E10 or E9 would result in light labeling because the concentration of labeled DNA would decrease as the daughter cells kept dividing before they left the proliferative neuroepithelium. In contrast, administration of ^{3}H-thymidine on E11 would make those cells preparing to differentiate heavily labeled because they would retain all their labeled DNA. (Designating the latter cells as being "born" on E11 requires, of course, that the same class of cells can no longer be labeled with injections made on E12.)

However, the rationale of the "flash labeling" technique is flawed because many factors other than the cessation of cell division can affect the labeling intensity of a cell. Among these factors are: the specific activity of the administered radiochemical (basically the ratio of radioactively tagged and untagged thymidine); the thickness of the histological section (which determines the concentration of cell nuclei within a tissue sample and the absorption of the short range ß particles by the tissue); the size of the cell (cells with large nuclei, in which the chromosomes are more dispersed, are likely to appear less heavily labeled than cells with small nuclei and tightly packed chromosomes); the variable sensitivity of the photographic emulsion (an emulsion with more or larger silver grains will capture more radioactive particles); and, of course, the length of the autoradiographic exposure time (which in different experiments has varied from weeks to months).

To overcome this problem in dating the time of origin of neurons, we introduced some time ago a method called "progressively delayed cumulative labeling" (Bayer and Altman, 1974). In this procedure, groups of pregnant rats are injected with ^{3}H-thymidine on two successive days with an *overlapping schedule* (E11+E12, E12+E13, E13+E14, etc.) and their progeny are allowed to survive either until the perinatal period (E21) or young adulthood (P60). The multiple injections (in practice, two successive daily injections) assure that virtually all (over 95%) multiplying cells are labeled. In coumting the cells, no distinction is made between heavily or lightly labeled cells. Instead, all labeled cells (those that were still proliferating at the time of the injections) and all unlabeled cells (those that have become postmitotic) are counted in a sample and their proportion is calculated as a function of the onset of the injections. Starting the procedure with an injection schedule that labels all cells in a population (typically, E11), the decline in the proportion of labeled cells (#labeled cells / #total cells X 100) in successively delayed injection groups specifies the proportion of neurons generated on succeeding days by using the simple formula: (% labeled cells injection group 1) – (% labeled cells injection group 2) = % neurons "born" between injection groups 1 and 2.

Figures 3-13, 3-14, and 3-15 illustrate the labeling of cervical spinal cord neurons in perinatal rats (E21) that received two successive doses of ^{3}H-thymidine beginning on the morning of day E11, E12, E13, E14, E15, or E16. In the rat that received the radiochemical beginning on E11 (E11+E12→E21) neurons throughout the gray matter are labeled (Figure 3-13A). Most of the labeling is light, but some motoneurons are heavily labeled. In the rat in which the injection was started on E12 (E12+E13→E21), some of the ventral horn motoneurons are no longer labeled (Figure 3-13B). The assumption is justified that the unlabeled motoneurons originated between the morning of E11(when they were heavily labeled) and E12 (when they were no longer labeled). Injection of ^{3}H-thymidine beginning on E13 (E13+E14→E21) greatly reduced the proportion of labeled motoneurons, but most neurons of the intermediate gray are still labeled (Figure 3-14A). In the animal in which injection of the radiochemical was started on E14 (E14+E15→E21), some of the neurons of the intermediate gray are no longer labeled (Figure 3-14B). In the animal in which the initial injection was delayed until E15 (E15+E16→E21), labeled cells are largely limited to the region of the dorsal horn and the central autonomic area (Figure 3-15A). Finally, in the animal that received the radiochemical beginning on day E16 (E16+E17→E21), only a few labeled cells are seen in the latter regions (Figure 3-15B). We concluded from these studies that, indeed, there is a ventral-to-dorsal gradient in spinal cord neurogenesis, and that the process ends on E16 (Altman and Bayer, 1984).

In another investigation, we allowed a group of similarly injected rats to survive until young adulthood (P60). Motoneurons in an adult rat that was labeled with ^{3}H-thymidine on E12 (E12+E13→P60) are shown in Figure 3-16. In the illustrated sample, those motoneurons of the lower cervical cord that have nuclei in the plane of sectioning are filled with reduced silver grains produced by the radioactive particles. However, there are differences in the proportion of labeled motoneurons in the medial motor columns (Figure 3-17A) and the lateral motor columns (Figure 3-17B). There are also differences in the proportion of labeled cells at different rostrocaudal levels of the spinal cord, as illustrated in samples from the upper cervical cord (Figure 3-18A), lower cervical cord (Figure 3-18B), and the lumbar spinal cord (Figure 3-18C).

In Figure 3-19 we summarize our quantitative results with reference to the proportion of motoneurons generated on different days at cervical, thoracic, and lumbar levels of the rat spinal cord. There is evidently a rostral-to-caudal gradient in the time of origin of motoneurons. At cervical levels, 20% of the motoneurons originate on E11 or earlier; peak production (65%) is on E12; and a declining complement of motoneurons is generated between E13 and E14. The production of motoneurons is negligible on E11 at thoracic levels, most of them are produced on E12 and E13. The pattern is similar at lumbar levels, except the peak on E13 is more pronounced. At all levels of the spinal cord, a small fraction of motoneurons is generated on E14. Data regarding differences in the generation of motoneurons in the lateral and medial tiers of the lower cervical cord are summarized in Figure 3-20. There is a pronounced lateral-to-medial gradient in motoneuron production. In the motor columns of the lateral panel, the peak period of motoneuron production is E12, whereas in the medial columns (which represent a small percentage of the total motoneuron population) the peak is on E13 and an appreciable percentage of motoneurons are still generated on E14.

Quantitative data about the time of origin of dorsal root ganglion cells at the three levels of the spinal cord are given in Figure 3-21. The neurons of the dorsal root ganglia are generated over a protracted period between E11 and E16 (Figure 3-21). Here, too, there is a clear rostrocaudal gradient in the production times of neurons. At cervical levels, most ganglion cells (over 80%) are generated between E12 and E14. At thoracic levels, a comparable proportion of ganglion cells is generated between E13 and E15, and at lumbar levels between E14 and E15.

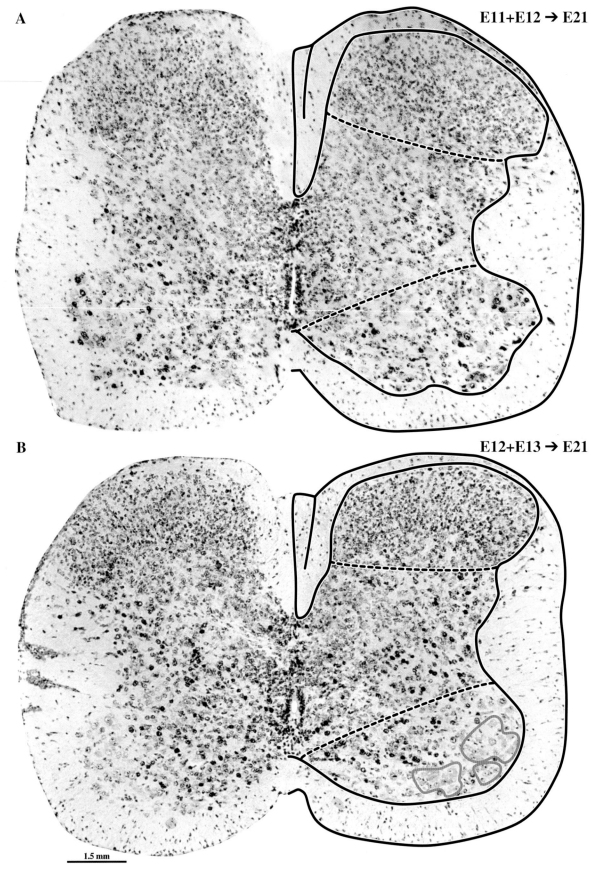

Figure 3-13. A. Long-survival autoradiograms of the cervical spinal cord from an E21 rat that received successive doses of ³H-thymidine on E11 and E12. Virtually all cells are labeled, either lightly or heavily. In the ventral horn, some motoneurons are conspicuous with their heavy labeling and a few are unlabeled. **B.** In the rat in which cumulative labeling was begun on E12, there are many unlabeled motoneurons laterally (outlined area). These motoneurons were generated before E12.

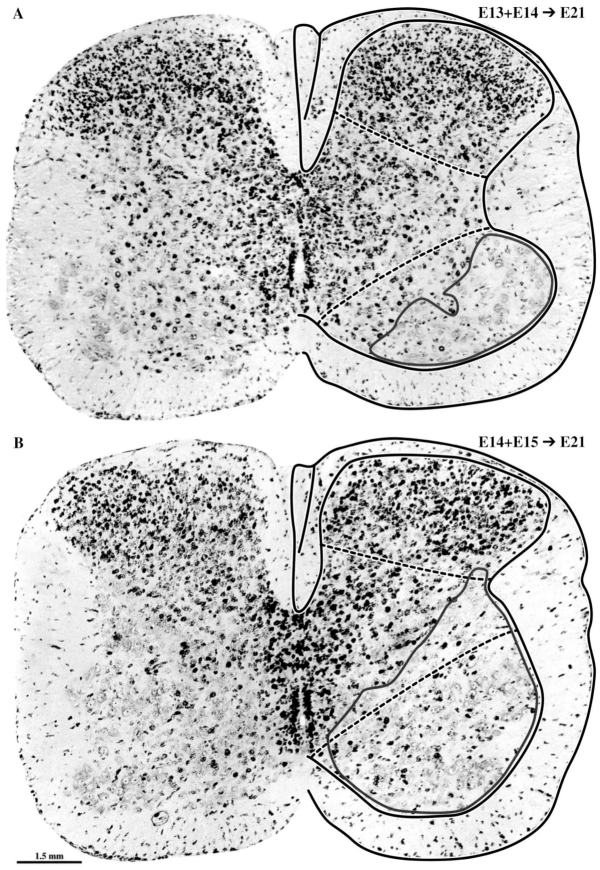

A E13+E14 → E21

B E14+E15 → E21

1.5 mm

Figure 3-14. A. Long survival auroradiogram from an E21 rat tagged with ³H-thymidine beginning on E13. Most lateral motoneurons are no longer labeled (outline). Some medial motoneurons and the cells of the rest of the spinal cord are heavily labeled. **B.** In the rat tagged with ³H-thymidine beginning on E14 , most motoneurons and some of the intermediate gray neurons are no longer labeled while virtually all of the neurons of the dorsal horn and central gray are heavily labeled.

A   **E15+E16 → E21**

B   **E16+E17 → E21**

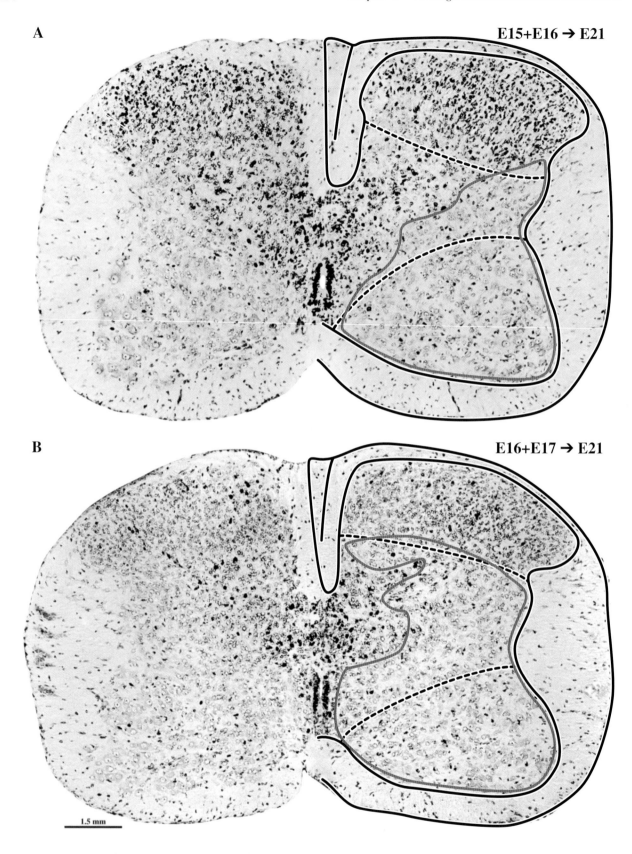

1.5 mm

Figure 3-15. A. Long survival autoradiogram from an E21 rat tagged with ³H-thymidine beginning on E15. Labeled cell are limited to the central autonomic area, the medial portion of the intermediate gray, and the dorsal horn. **B.** In the rat in which ³H-thymidine administration was delayed until E16, many cells are still labeled in the central autonomic area but only scattered cells are labeled in the dorsal horn and the medial intermediate gray.

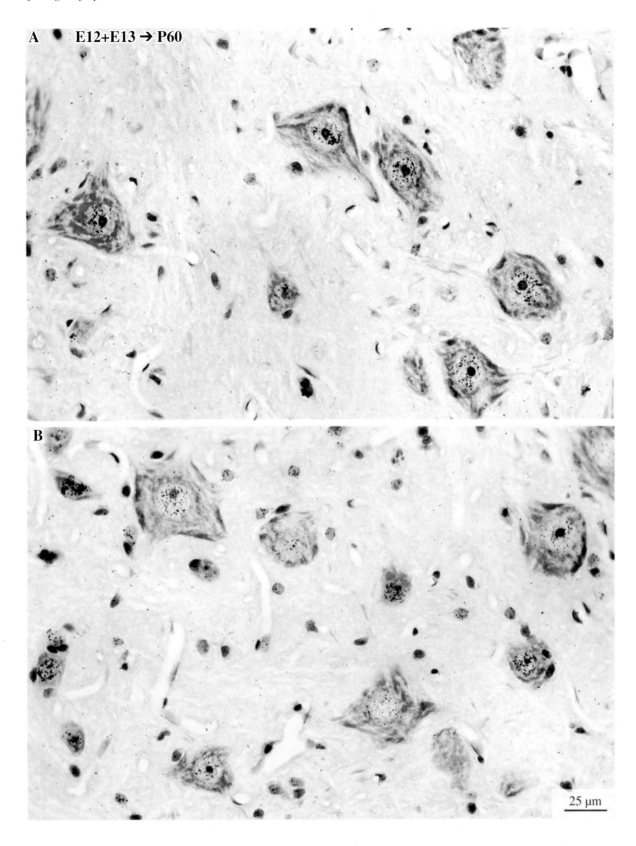

Figure 3-16. A, B. Labeling of lateral panel motoneurons in the upper cervical spinal cord of an adult (P60) rat that received two successive doses of ^{3}H-thymidine on E12 and E13. The opaque silver grains are concentrated over the nuclei of both large (alpha) and small (gamma) motoneurons. Long survival autoradiograms.

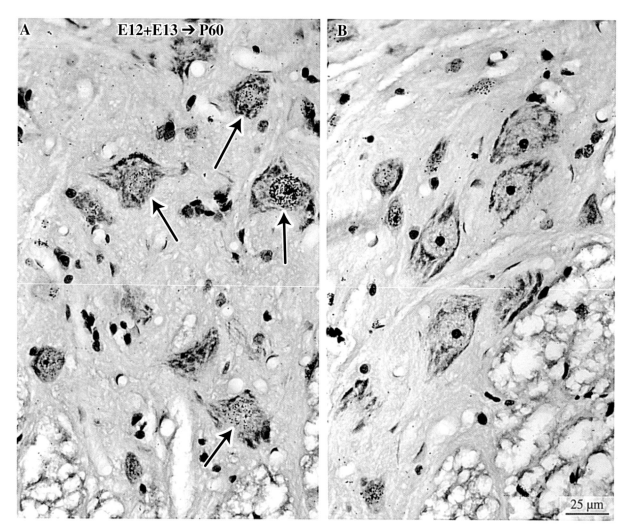

Figure 3-17.   The labeling of cell nuclei of motoneurons in the upper cervical spinal cord of an adult rat that was tagged with ³H-thymidine on E12 and E13. All large motoneurons are labeled (arrows) in a selected medial motor column (**A**) but none in a selected lateral column (**B**). The motoneurons in this lateral column were generated before the morning of E12, whereas the sampled motoneurons in the medial column were generated on or after E12. Long survival autoradiograms.

Figure 3-18. Rostral-to-caudal gradient in the labeling of the cell nuclei of motoneurons in the spinal cord of the same rat shown in Figure 3-17. **A.** Only a single motoneuron (arrow) is labeled in this motor column in the upper cervical cord. The majority of motoneurons were apparently "born" at this rostralmost level before the morning of E12. **B.** In the lower lower cervical cord there is an admixture of labeled and unlabeled motoneurons. **C.** Farther caudally in the lumbar spinal cord, all the motoneurons that have cell nuclei in the plane of sectioning are labeled. These motoneurons were generated on or after E12. Long survival autoradiograms.

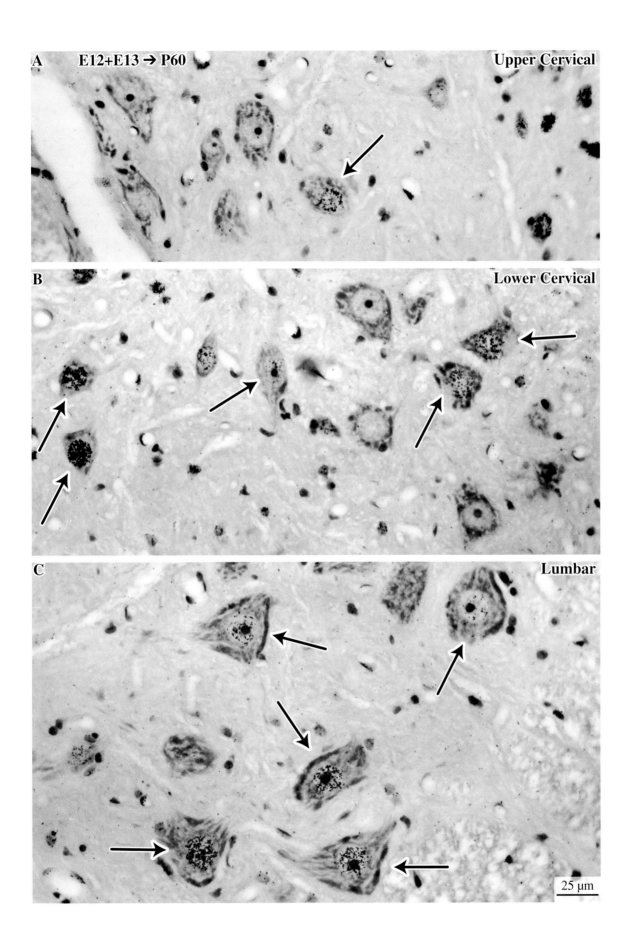

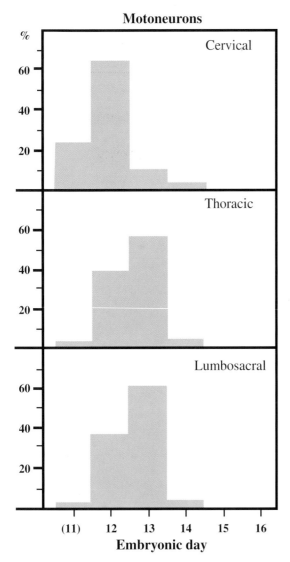

Motoneurons

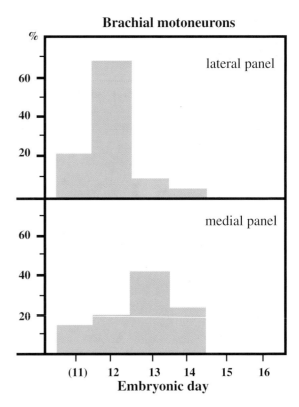

Brachial motoneurons

Figure 3-19. Proportion of ventral horn motoneurons generated between E11 (or earlier) and E14 in the cervical, thoracic, and lumbosacral levels of the rat spinal cord. There is a rostral-to-caudal gradient in the temporal order of neurogenesis. Motoneuron production peaks on E12 in the cervical cord and on E13 in the lumbosacral cord. A small proportion of motoneurons are generated on E14 throughout the spinal cord. After Altman and Bayer (1984).

Figure 3-20. Time of origin of motoneurons in the lateral and medial panels of the lower cervical spinal cord of the rat. There is a pronounced lateral-to-medial gradient in the generation of motoneurons. After Altman and Bayer (1984).

Figure 3-21. Time of origin of dorsal root ganglion cells at cervical, thoracic, and lumbosacral levels of the rat spinal cord. The production of these peripheral sensory neurons is more prolonged than the production of central motoneurons. There is a rostral-to-caudal gradient in the proportion of ganglion cells generated on specific days within the same overall period. After Altman and Bayer (1984).

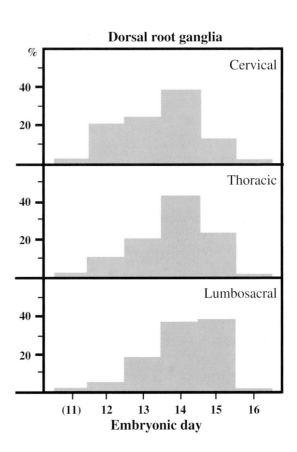

Dorsal root ganglia

3.3 Maturation of Spinal Cord Neurons: A Cytological and Autoradiographic Investigation in the Rat

3.3.1 Maturation of Motoneurons: A Brief Review. The maturation of spinal cord neurons, particularly motoneurons, has been studied by several investigators. Using the Golgi procedure in mice, in which neurogenesis starts about 1-2 days earlier than in the rat, Wenthworth (1984) found that most ventral horn neurons are within or near the neuroepithelium in a less mature E9 embryo (E10, if corrected for dating method) and their neurites are still confined to the spinal cord (Figure 3-22A). However, in a more mature E9 (E10) embryo, a few motoneurons have moved laterally and their axons, led by filopodia are exiting the cord (Figure 3-22B). These are obviously motoneurons. By E10 (E11), the concentration of maturing motoneurons with exiting axons has increased considerably; however, the perikarya of most of these cells are still horizontally oriented (Figure 3-22C). By E11 (E12), the perikarya of many of the differentiating motoneurons have become vertically oriented and some of them show incipient signs of becoming multipolar (Figure 3-22D). This heralds the outgrowth of dendrites.

Chen and Chiu (1992) found in the rat, that monoclonal antibodies of the cell adhesive molecule, NCAM, begin to recognize motoneurons by E11, and that these cells acquire detectable levels of choline acetyltransferase (the marker for cholinergic neurons) by E11.5. By this age, two other markers for developing neurons were also detected in the ventral horn, the growth associated protein GAP-43 and the surface glycoprotein TAG-1. Reactivity with the latter two compounds was transient and disappeared a few days later. The loss of these antigens may coincide with the motoneuron axons reaching and synapsing with their muscle targets. According to another study (Phelps et al., 1990), choline acetyltransferase is first expressed in rat ventral horn motoneurons on E13. The expression of choline acetyltransferase appeared a few days later in the visceral motoneurons of the lateral horn. The authors hypothesized that the cholinergic phenotype is not expressed until the differentiating neurons have settled in their final locations. The expression of neuregulins (NRGs), which are believed to promote the synthesis of postsynaptic acetylcholine receptors and the formation of voltage-gated sodium channels, increases in ventral horn neurons at about the time

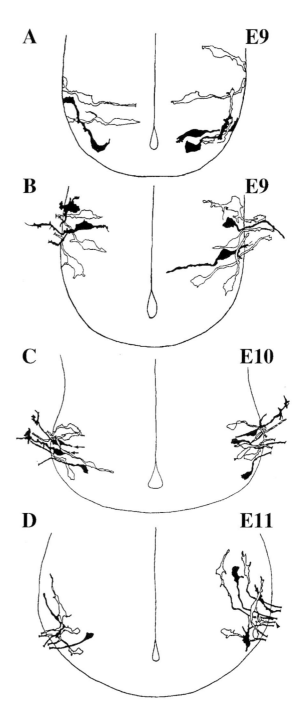

Figure 3-22. Ventral plate motoneurons, with neurites confined to the spinal cord (**A**) and those with exiting axons (**B**) in E9 mice. (Motoneurons are generated 1-2 days earlier in mice than in rats.) Motoneurons with peripheral axons are more common E10 (**C**) and E11 (**D**) mice. By E11, some of the motoneurons have changed their orientation from horizontal to vertical, and their apical poles show signs of the incipient sprouting of dendrites. Modified after Wentworth (1984).

neuromuscular synapses are formed (Loeb and Fisch-bach, 1997),

    The dendritic maturation of motoneurons has been studied mostly after birth. In a pioneering study, Scheibel and Scheibel (1970) showed in kittens that motoneuron dendritic bundles begin to form after birth and continue to develop up to 4 months of age (Figure 3-23). Bellinger and Anderson (1987a, 1987b) obtained similar results in rats, a species in which dendritic bundles are more dense than in the

cat (Figure 3-24). There is some evidence for differences in the rate of dendritic bundle development in different motoneuron columns in the rat spinal cord (Westerga and Gramsberger, 1991; Curfs et al., 1993). Experiments indicate that the development of dendritic bundles is dependent on afferent stimulation (Kalb, 1994) and the preservation of synaptic contact with muscles (O'Hanlon and Lowrie, 1994a, 1994b). Investigations with highly enriched cultures of embryonic motoneurons suggest that glutamate, the excitatory neurotransmitter of spinal cord motoneurons,

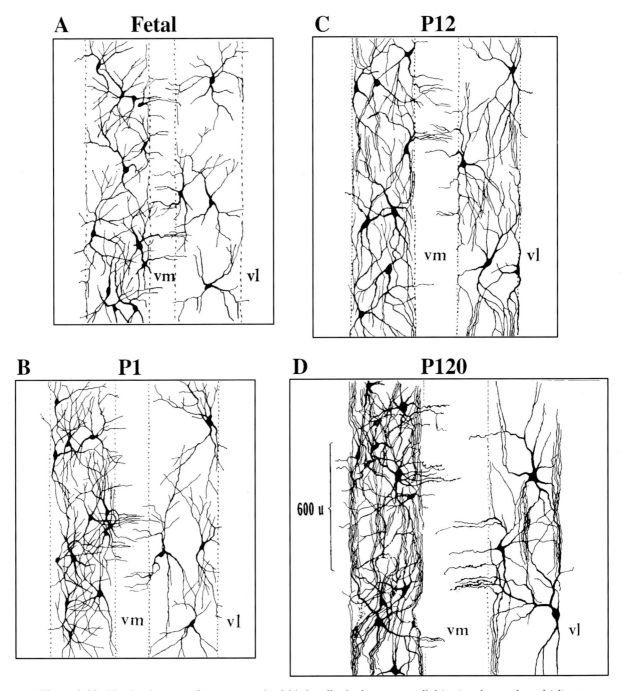

Figure 3-23. The development of motoneuron dendritic bundles in the ventromedial (vm) and ventrolateral (vl) motor columns in fetal (**A**), P1 (**B**), and P12 (**C**) kittens, and a P120 cat (**D**). After Scheibel and Scheibel (1970).

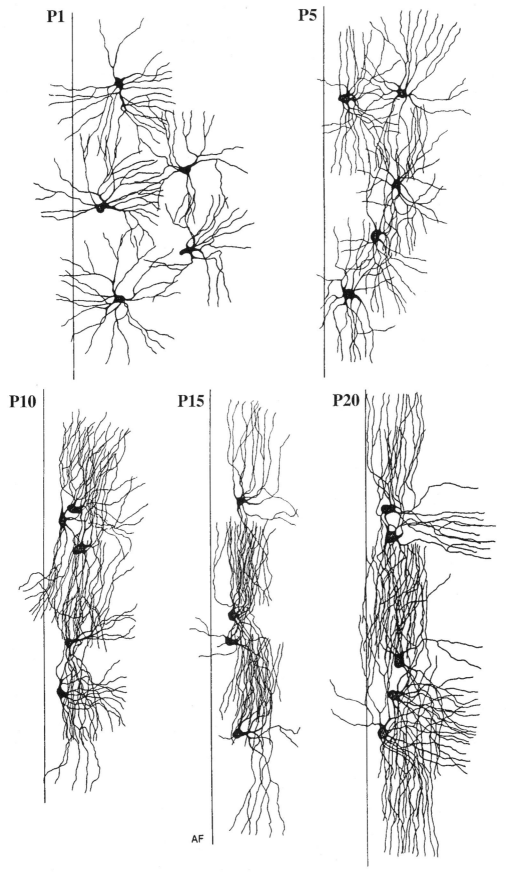

Figure 3-24. Development of motoneurons dendritic bundles in the lateral motor columns of the rat spinal cord between P1 and P20. After Bellinger and Anderson (1987a).

plays a role in the regulation of dendritic development (Metzger et al., 1998). Finally, it has been found that the dendritic growth of sexually dimorphic motoneurons is regulated by testosterone, with differences observed in the androgen sensitivity of neurons of the bulbocavernosus and the dorsolateral nucleus (Goldstein and Sengelaub, 1993).

3.3.2   Phases in the Maturation of Somatic Motoneurons.

We examined the maturation of ventral horn motoneurons in plastic-embedded sections of the rat spinal cord at daily intervals from E12 onwards. We could distinguish five phases in the maturation of motoneurons. On E12, a group of cells appears ventrolaterally in the cervical cord that can be distinguished from the darkly staining and spindle shaped NEP cells by two criteria: the light staining and round shape of their nuclei (Figure 3-25). These ventral plate cells are the earliest differentiating neurons of the spinal cord, and they signal the *first phase* (presumably the postmitotic phase) in the development of motoneurons. By E13, two changes are seen in some cells located in the same position: some acquire a darkly staining cytoplasmic cap directed toward the wall of the spinal cord (Figure 3-26A) while others devoid of a cytoplasmic cap sprout axons that exit the spinal cord (Figure 3-26B). We hypothesize that these two cytological changes represent successive phases, the preparatory accumulation of cytoplasmic material to form axons, the *second phase* (the preaxonal phase), and the subsequent outgrowth of the axon, the *third phase* (the axogenetic phase) of motoneuron maturation.

As seen in coronal (Figure 3-27A) and horizontal (Figure 3-27B) sections, the outgrowth of motoneuron axons on E13 takes place while their peripheral targets are still in the immature myotome phase of differentiation. We do not know whether or not these early axons form synapses with the muscle primordia. It is noteworthy that, by E13, many of the laterally situated motoneurons display a new cytological feature: their perikarya changes from spherical to bipolar as they develop darkly staining apical and basal cytoplasmic caps (Figure 3-28). This is the *fourth phase* in motoneuron maturation (the preparatory stage of incipient dendritic development). By E14, the majority of motoneurons in the enlarged ventral horn are bipolar; however, the orientation of these cells varies in the different segregating clusters of motoneurons (Figure 3-29). This phase in motoneuron maturation is coupled with two events: the onset of maturation of the different muscle masses at increasing distances from the spinal cord (Figure 3-30), and the incipient segregation of bipolar motoneurons into clusters (Figure 3-29). The segregation of the medial/central and lateral/far-lateral clusters is well-advanced in the cervical spinal cord by E15 (Figure 3-31). The orientation of bipolar motoneurons within the partitioning motoneuron clusters are different. The *fifth phase* of motoneuron maturation, with the slow transformation of bipolar cells into multipolar cells, begins on E16 and is more evident by E17 (Figure 3-32). At least two stages may be distinguished during this phase. The first is an increase in the size and staining intensity of the motoneuron cytoplasm. The second, seen by E18 and E19, is a pronounced cytoplasmic hypertrophy and the formation of multiple polar caps (Figure 3-33). These changes in motoneuron maturation are coupled with the progressive partitioning of the clusters of motoneurons into discrete columns.

The sequence of cytoplasmic changes from bipolar hypertrophy to multipolar hypertrophy is illustrated at higher magnification in Figure 3-34. In an ultrastructural investigation of the development of a different neuron, the Purkinje cell of the cerebellar cortex, we found that the hypertrophied dendritic cytoplasmic cap is very rich in such organelles as the endoplasmic reticulum and mitochondria (Altman and Bayer, 1997). We postulate that the bipolar and multipolar hypertrophy represent two phases in the dendritic maturation of ventral horn motoneurons.

Paralleling the rostral-to-caudal gradient in motoneuron production obtained in quantitative studies in adult rats (Figure 3-19A), a similar gradient is seen in motoneuron maturation in embryonic rats. Thus, in the same E14 embryo in which motoneuron development is well advanced in the cervical cord, there is a gradual delay in the cytological maturation of motoneurons at thoracic, lumbar, and sacral levels (Figure 3-35). This gradient also holds for the generation of motoneurons and their migration from the neuroepithelium to the ventral horn, as the autoradiographic evidence indicates (Figure 3-36). In the embryo tagged with radioactive thymidine on E13 and killed on E14 (Figure 3-36A), there are very few labeled cells (late-generated motoneurons) in the ventral horn of the cervical cord, but there are more in the thoracic cord, and still more in the lumbar cord (Figures 3-36B, C).

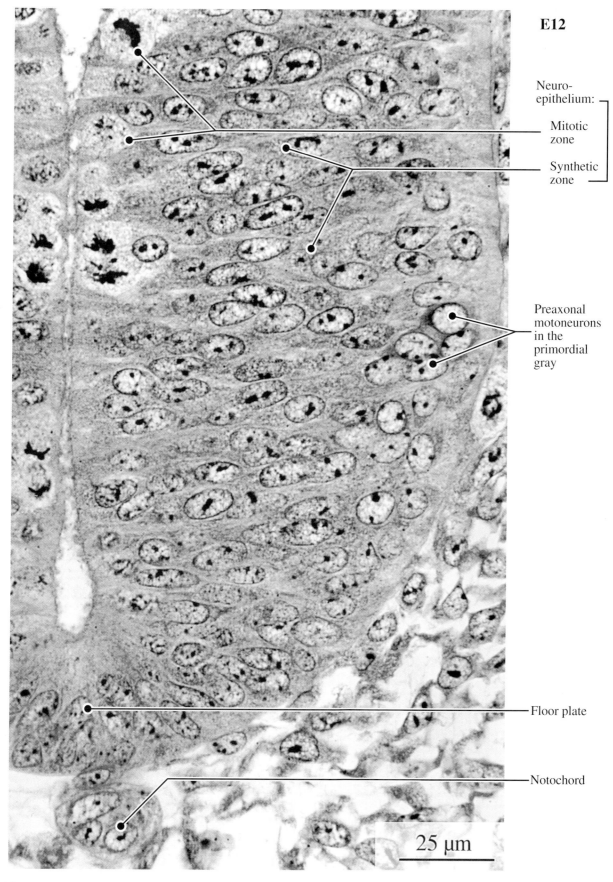

E12

Neuro-
epithelium:

Mitotic
zone

Synthetic
zone

Preaxonal
motoneurons
in the
primordial
gray

Floor plate

Notochord

25 μm

Figure 3-25. First phase in the maturation of motoneurons in the cervical spinal cord of an E12 rat. The darkly staining nuclei of some spindle shaped NEP cells become round and pale as they move laterally. Methacrylate; hematoxylin-eosin.

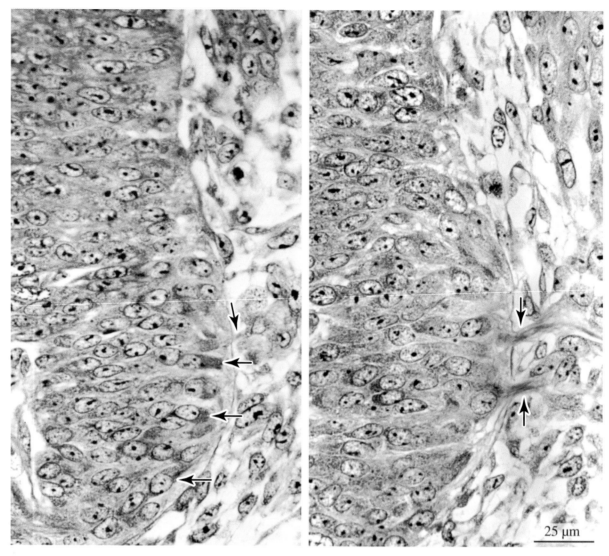

Figure 3-26. A. Motoneurons with darkly staining axonal cytoplasmic caps (horizontal arrows) in the ventral horn of an E13 rat. **B.** Motoneurons without cytoplasmic caps but with an exiting axon (vertical arrows) at another level of the ventral horn in the same embryo. The formation of the cytoplasmic cap and the outgrowth of the axon represent the second and third phases, respectively, in the maturation of motoneurons. Methacrylate; hematoxylin-eosin.

The five phases in the maturation motoneurons are schematically summarized in Figure 3-37. The first three phases (I-III) are associated with axonogenesis, the last two (IV-V) with dendrogenesis. The first phase is the transformation of horizontally oriented, spindle-shaped NEP cells with dark nuclei into postmitotic cells with pale and round nuclei. In the cervical cord of the rat, such cells are first in the incipient ventral horn on E12. The second phase is the growth of a darkly staining, outward pointing cytoplasmic cap. This cap contains the organelles needed for axon growth. The third phase is the sprouting of an axon that exits the ventral horn. As the axon grows toward the differentiating muscles, the motoneuron perikaryon undergoes two changes: it becomes bipolar again and develops darkly staining polar caps. This fourth phase of motoneuron maturation is coupled with the onset of segregation of motoneurons into clusters. The bipolar motoneurons within a cluster tend to have a similar spatial orientation. The development of polar cytoplasmic caps, we presume, signals the initial outgrowth of one or two motoneuron dendrites. The fifth phase is a pronounced hypertrophy of the motoneuron cytoplasm, coupled with the eccentric dislocation of the nucleus and the outgrowth of multipolar cytoplasmic caps. These events are assumed to signal the outgrowth of multiple dendritic branches. Judged by the slow development of dendritic bundles in cats and rats (Figures 3-23, 3-24), the fifth phase of motoneuron maturation must be a lengthy process that does not end until early adulthood.

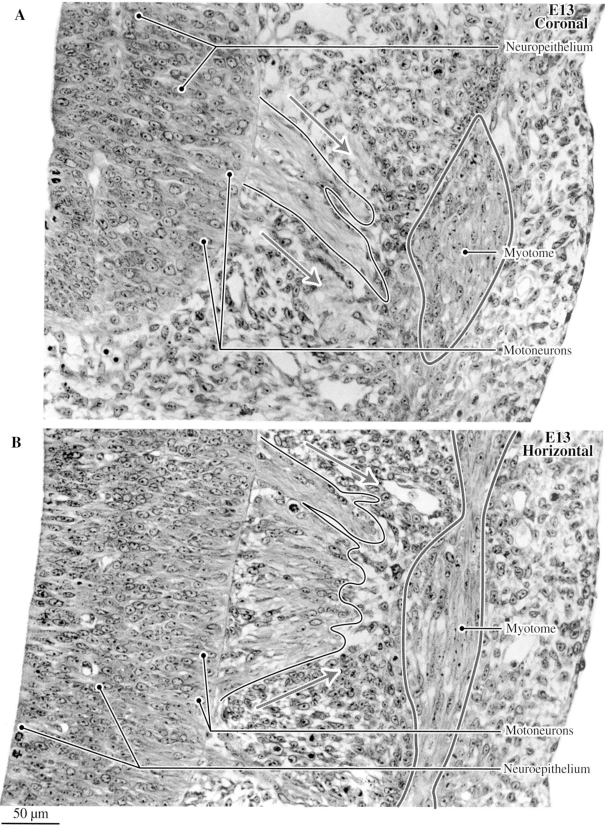

Figure 3-27. Motoneuron axons (between arrows) in the ventral root of the cervical cord growing towards a myotome (outlined) in the coronal (**A**) and the horizontal (**B**) plane in E13 rats. Methacrylate; hematoxylin-eosin.

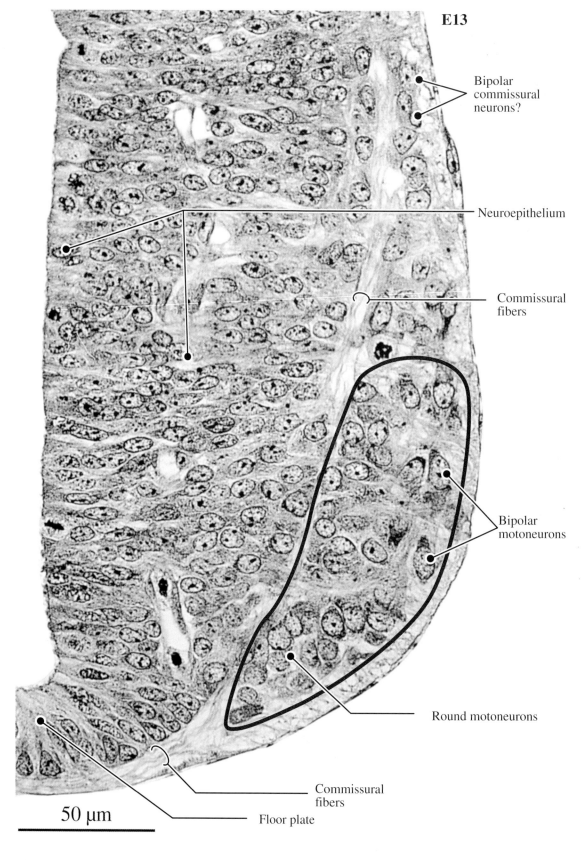

E13

Bipolar commissural neurons?

Neuroepithelium

Commissural fibers

Bipolar motoneurons

Round motoneurons

Commissural fibers

Floor plate

50 μm

Figure 3-28. Development of the incipient ventral horn (outlined) in the cervical cord of an E13 rat. Several of the laterally situated motoneurons have become bipolar and are developing apical or basal darkly staining cytoplasmic caps. This is the onset of the fourth stage in the maturation of motoneurons. Methacrylate; hematoxylin-eosin.

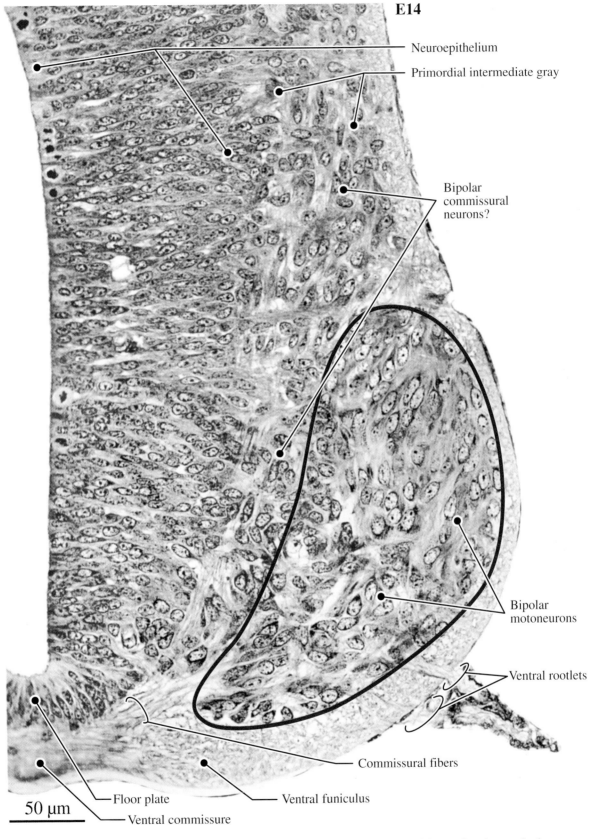

E14

Neuroepithelium

Primordial intermediate gray

Bipolar commissural neurons?

Bipolar motoneurons

Ventral rootlets

Commissural fibers

Ventral funiculus

Floor plate

Ventral commissure

50 μm

Figure 3-29. Considerable increase in the population of bipolar motoneurons with cytoplasmic caps in the expanding ventral horn (outlined) in the cervical spinal cord of an E14 rat. The orientation of bipolar cells varies in the different motoneuron clusters that are beginning to form. Methacrylate; hematoxylin-eosin.

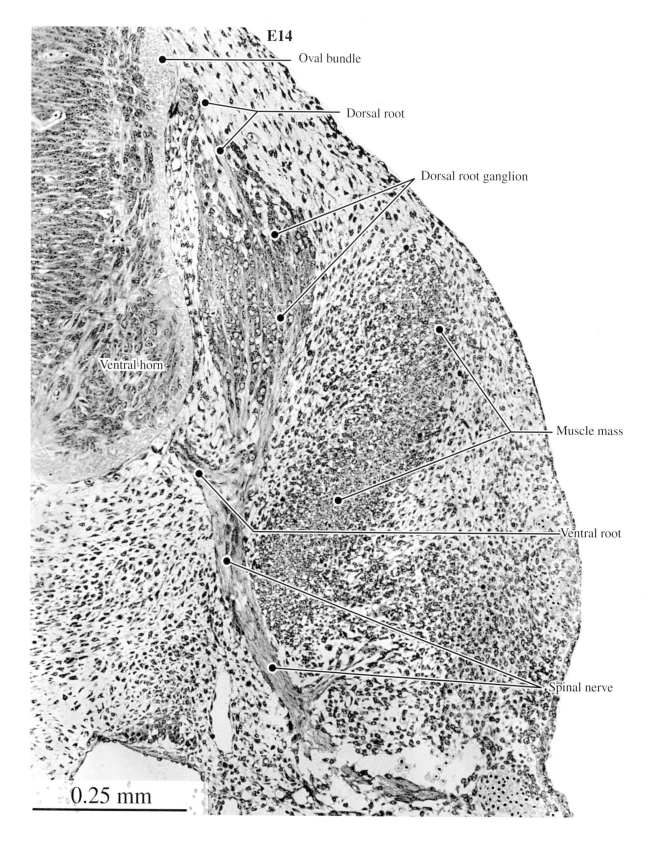

E14

Oval bundle

Dorsal root

Dorsal root ganglion

Ventral horn

Muscle mass

Ventral root

Spinal nerve

0.25 mm

Figure 3-30. The expansion of the ventral horn, and the increase in the population of bipolar moto-neurons in the cervical spinal cord of this E14 rat are associated with the formation of differentiating muscle masses and the lengthening of the spinal nerve. Methacrylate; hematoxylin-eosin.

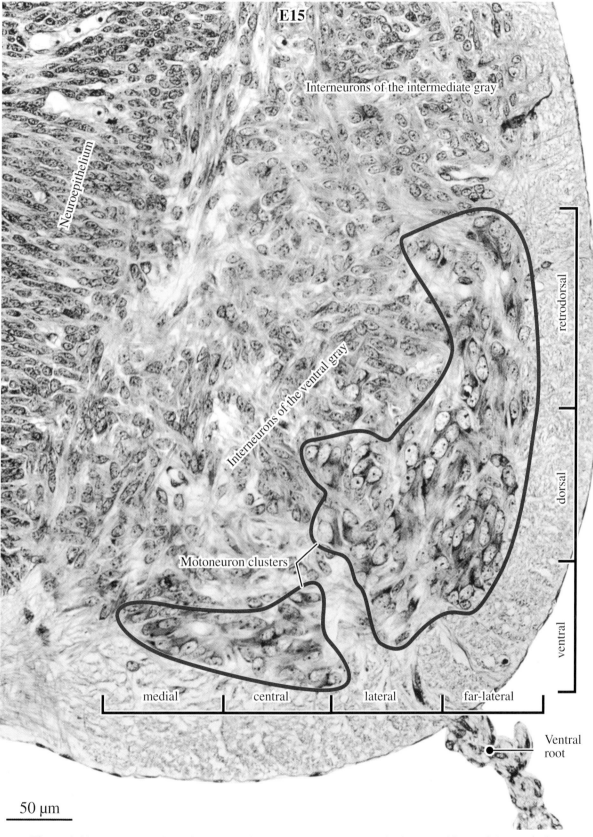

Figure 3-31. The segregation of variably oriented bipolar motoneurons in the ventral horn of the cervical spinal cord of an E15 rat into a medial/central cluster and a lateral/far-lateral cluster (outlined) . There is an increase in the number of interneurons in the expanding intermediate gray. Methacrylate; hematoxylin-eosin.

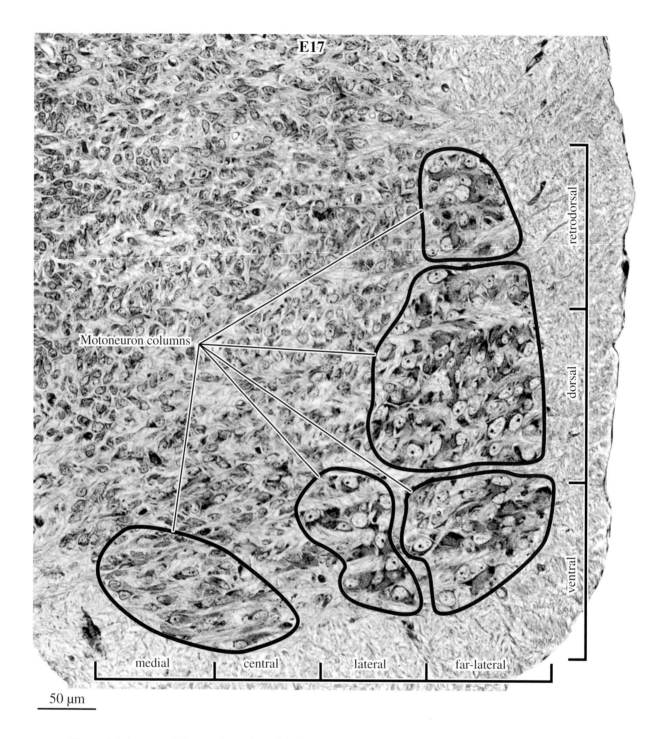

Figure 3-32. Onset of the transformation of bipolar motoneurons into multipolar motoneurons in the cervical spinal cord of an E17 rat. This process involves the formation of hypertrophied cytoplasmic caps and the eccentric dislocation of the motoneuron nuclei. This signals the beginning of the fifth stage of motoneuron maturation. Note the formation of motor columns (outlines). Methacrylate; hematoxylin-eosin.

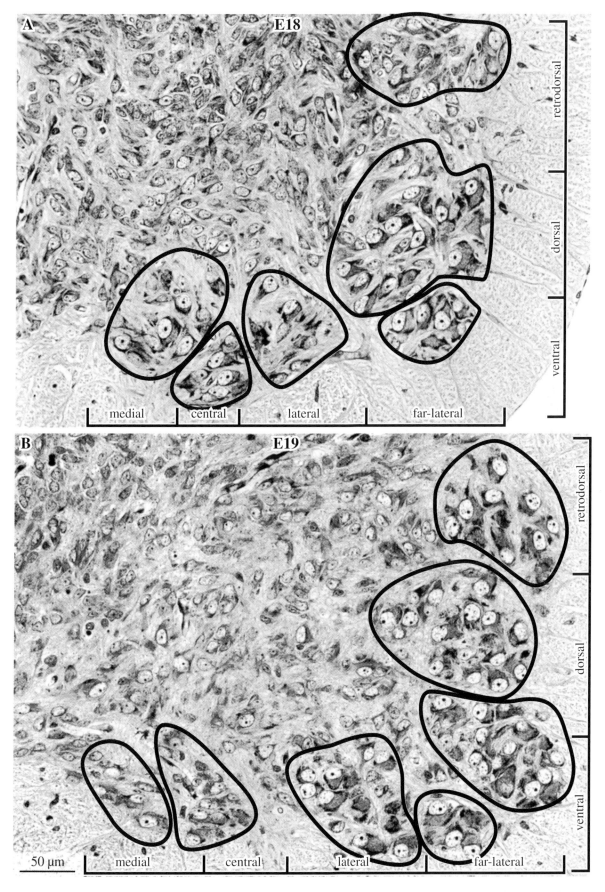

Figure 3-33. Continuing expansion of the ventral horn, segregation of the motor columns, and growth of the eccentric cytoplasmic caps of motoneurons in the cervical cord of an E18 (**A**) and an E19 (**B**) rat. Methacrylate; hematoxylin-eosin.

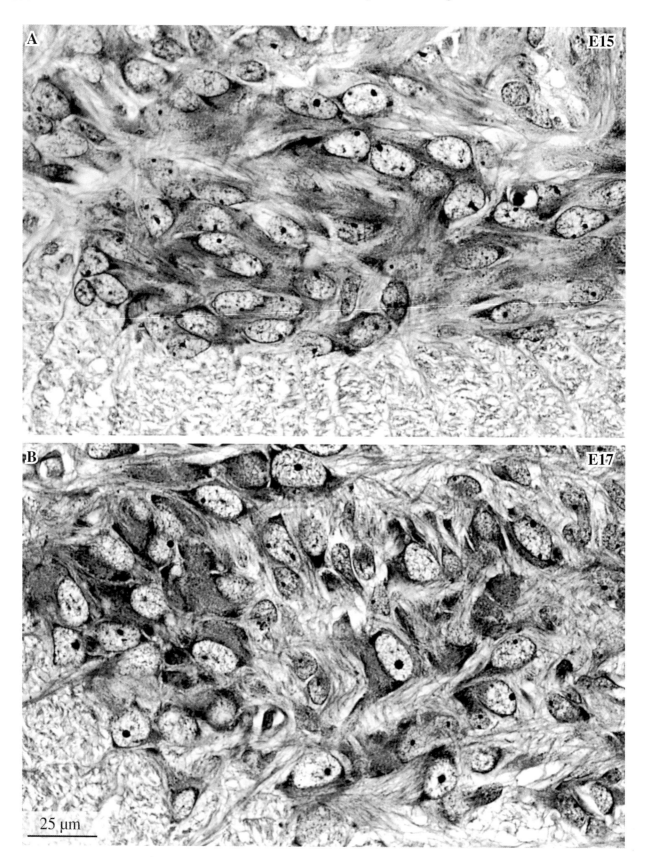

Figure 3-34. Cytoplasmic hypertrophy of motoneurons in the cervical spinal cord of an E15 (**A**) and E17 (**B**) rat. The change of motoneuron perikarya from bipolar on E15 to mutltipolar by E17 reflects the outgrowth of additional motoneurons dendrites from the cell body. Methacrylate; hematoxylin-eosin.   (*Continued on next page*)

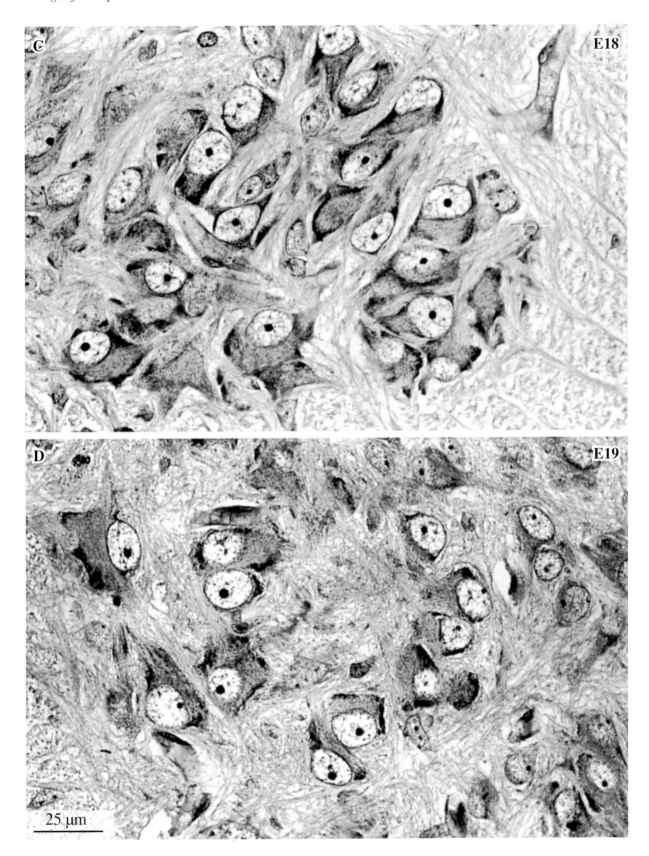

Figure 3-34. Progressive changes in the cytoplasmic hypertrophy of motoneurons in an E18 **(C)** and E19 **(D)** rat. These changes reflect increased perikaryal growth associated with the continuing expansion of the dendrites of multipolar motoneurons. Methacrylate; hematoxylin-eosin.

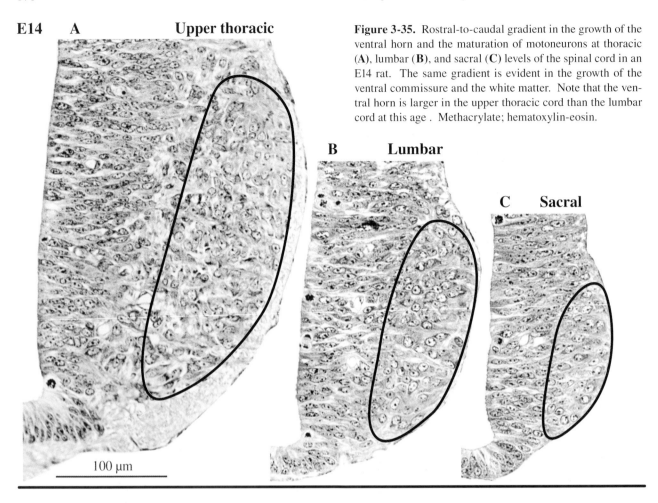

E14   A   Upper thoracic

B   Lumbar

C   Sacral

100 µm

Figure 3-35. Rostral-to-caudal gradient in the growth of the ventral horn and the maturation of motoneurons at thoracic (**A**), lumbar (**B**), and sacral (**C**) levels of the spinal cord in an E14 rat. The same gradient is evident in the growth of the ventral commissure and the white matter. Note that the ventral horn is larger in the upper thoracic cord than the lumbar cord at this age. Methacrylate; hematoxylin-eosin.

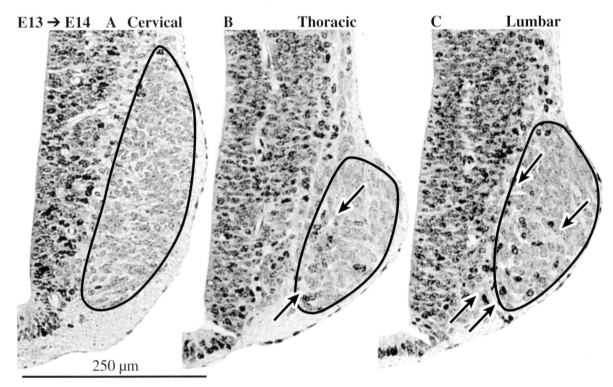

E13 → E14   A   Cervical   **B   Thoracic**   **C   Lumbar**

250 µm

Figure 3-36. Autoradiograms of the ventral horn at cervical (**A**), thoracic (**B**), and lumbar (**C**) levels of the spinal cord of a rat embryo labeled with ^{3}H-thymidine on E13 and killed on E14. Note the increased proportion of labeled motoneurons (those generated on E13) in the ventral horn from rostral to caudal levels of the spinal cord (arrows). Paraffin.

A. Axonogenesis

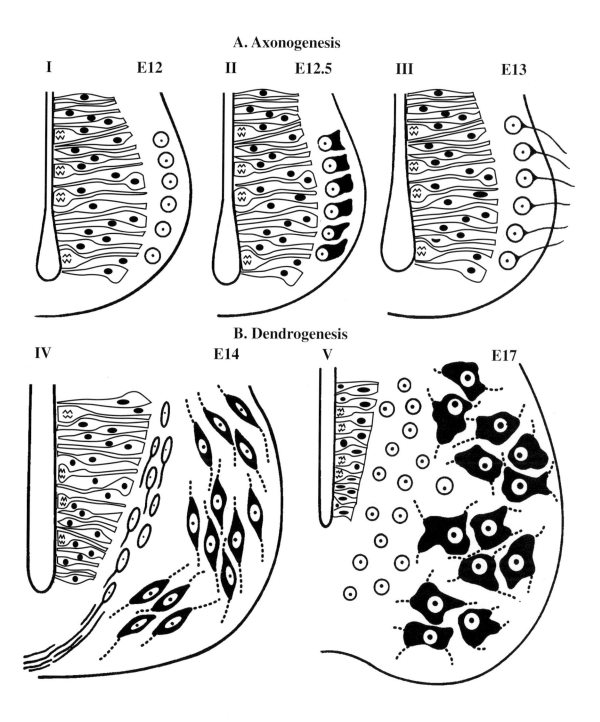

B. Dendrogenesis

Figure 3-37. Five phases in the maturation of motoneurons (with approximate ages) in the early maturing cervical spinal cord of the rat. The cytoplasmic changes from phases I to III are conceptualized as stages of axonogenesis (**A**), whereas the cytoplasmic changes at phases IV and V are conceptualized as stages of dendrogenesis (**B**). **I.** Differentiating (post-mitotic) spherical motoneurons (E12). **II.** Preaxonal motoneurons with peripherally-oriented cytoplasmic caps rich in organelles involved in protein metabolism and membrane production (nominal age, E12.5). **III.** Motoneurons with exiting axons (E13). **IV.** Variably aligned motoneurons with bipolar cytoplasmic caps in segregating motor columns, signaling the onset of dendrogenesis. **V.** Motoneurons with hypertrophied multipolar cytoplasmic caps and more advanced dendrogenesis. The dotted lines shown in IV (E14) and V (E17) are hypothetical dendritic branches not visible in our preparations.

3.3.3 Maturation of Visceral (Preganglionic) Motoneurons.

The autonomic (preganglionic) motoneurons of the lateral horn were originally thought to have a different germinal source than the somatic motoneurons of the ventral horn (Terni, 1924). However, Levi-Montalcini (1950) presented histological evidence that in the embryonic chick spinal cord, the autonomic motoneurons originate in the same ventral location as do the somatic motoneurons, then migrate dorsomedially and settle in the region of the spinal cord, known in birds as the column of Terni. Several decades later, in a combined cytological and thymidine autoradiographic study, evidence was obtained that, in the rat, somatic and visceral motoneurons are generated concurrently in the ventral neuroepithelium, but within a few days the visceral motoneurons migrate dorsally to form the intermediolateral nucleus of the lateral horn (Altman and Bayer, 1984). After their arrival, some of the visceral neurons, the intercalated cells, migrate along a horizontal trajectory from lateral to medial. These findings were later confirmed and extended by Vaughn and his associates (Barber et al., 1991; Markham and Vaughn, 1991; Phelps et al., 1991) who combined thymidine autoradiography with choline acetyltransferase cytochemistry and the HRP tracer technique.

Figure 3-38 shows an autoradiogram of the thoracic spinal cord of a perinatal rat that was tagged with two successive daily doses of ^{3}H-thymidine starting on E13, and was killed on E21. While most cells are labeled in the gray matter, many cells in the ventral horn and some cells in the lateral horn are unlabeled. This indicates that a high proportion of somatic and visceral motoneurons in the thoracic spinal cord are generated before E13. The admixture of labeled and unlabeled cells in the intermediolateral nucleus of the lateral horn in a perinatal rat that

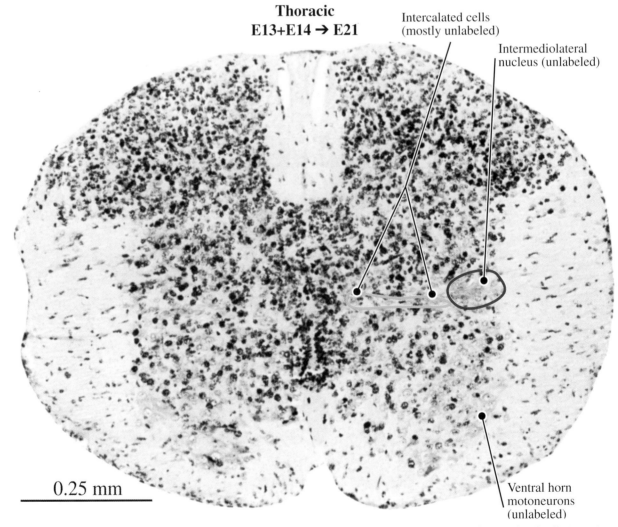

**Thoracic
E13+E14 → E21**

Intercalated cells
(mostly unlabeled)

Intermediolateral
nucleus (unlabeled)

Ventral horn
motoneurons
(unlabeled)

0.25 mm

Figure 3-38. Unlabeled visceral motoneurons in the intermediolateral nucleus (red), and a "rung" of intercalated cells (green), in the thoracic spinal cord in a perinatal rat that was tagged with ^{3}H-thymidine on E13 and E14 (E13+→E21). Many of the somatic motoneurons of the ventral horn are also devoid of radioactive labeling. Paraffin embedding; counterstained autoradiogram.

was tagged with ³H-thymidine starting on E13 is illustrated at higher magnification in Figure 3-39A. The fact that very few of these lateral horn motoneurons are labeled if the administration of the radiochemical is delayed until E14 (Figure 3-39B), indicates that the neurogenesis of visceral motoneurons, like those of somatic motoneurons of the thoracic cord (see Figure 3-19,) comes to a virtual halt during E13.

Few, if any, visceral motoneurons have settled in the future lateral horn by E15 (Figure 3-40A). By E15, they begin to develop apical caps in the formative intermediolateral nucleus (Figure 3-40B). By E16, they form a discrete nucleus with hyeprtrophied perikarya (Figure 3-40C). The migration of inter-

calated cells and the formation of the rung of intercalated neurons on E17, E18, and E19. is traced in Figure 3-41. (For the organization of intercalated cells that form ladder-like rungs in the thoracic spinal cord, see Figure 1-72.)   As seen at higher magnification (Figure 3-42), the spindle shaped putative intercalated cells are migrating dorsomedially E16, and the cytoplasmic hypertrophy of the intercalated bipolar cells that form a discrete rung is evident by E19 (Figure 3-43). The intercalated cells may be the source of a fiber band that joins the lateral funiculus. This pattern of migration of the visceral motoneurons is in good agreement with the results obtained by Phelps et al. (1990) with choline acetyltransferase histochemistry (Figure 3-44).

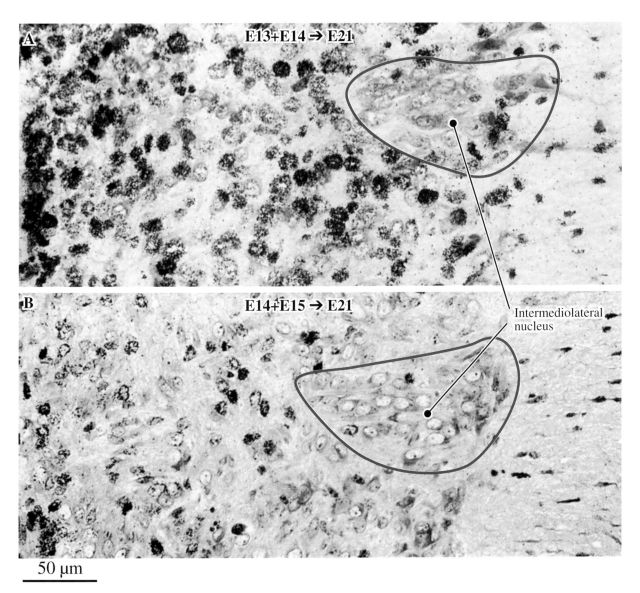

50 μm

Figure 3-39. A. Labeled and unlabeled visceral motoneurons in the intermediolateral nucleus of the thoracic spinal cord of a perinatal rat (E21) that was tagged with ³H-thymidine on E13 and E14. **B.** Most visceral motoneurons are unlabeled in the same location in the perinatal rat that was tagged on E14 and E15. Paraffin; autoradiogram.

Figure 3-40. **A.** Apparent absence of the intermediolateral nucleus in the thoracic spinal cord of an E14 rat. **B.** Presumed migratory route of visceral motoneurons from ventral to dorsal (red arrow), and the formation of the intermediolateral nucleus (red outline) in an E15 rat. **C.** Growth of the intermediolateral nucleus (red) and migratory route of putative intercalated cells (green arrow) in an E16 rat. (Outlined area in C is shown at higher magnification in Figure 3-42.) Methacrylate; hematoxylin-eosin.

Figure 3-41. Migration of the putative intercalated cells from lateral to medial, and the formation of a rung of intercalated neurons (green) in the thoracic cord of E17 **(A)**, E18 **(B)**, and E19 **(C)** rat embryos, in association with the enlargement of the intermediolateral nucleus (red). (Outlined area in C is shown at higher magnification in Figure 3-43.) Methacrylate; hematoxylin-eosin.

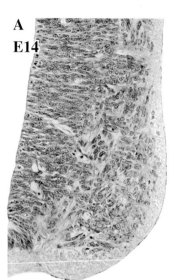
A
E14

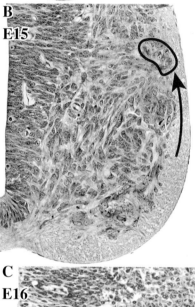
B
E15

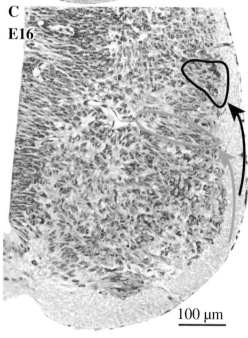
C
E16

100 µm

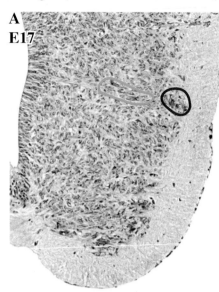
A
E17

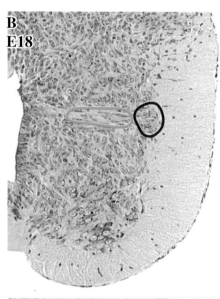
B
E18

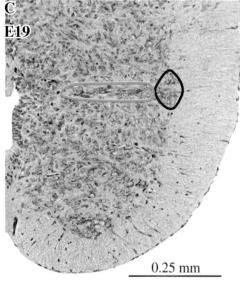
C
E19

0.25 mm

E16

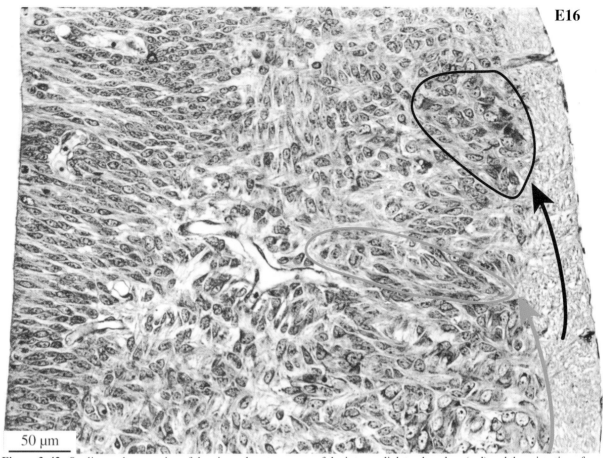

50 µm

Figure 3-42. Settling and maturation of the visceral motoneurons of the intermediolateral nucleus (red) and the migration of bipolar, putative intercalated cells (green) in the thoracic spinal cord of an E16 rat. Methacrylate; hematoxylin-eosin.

E19

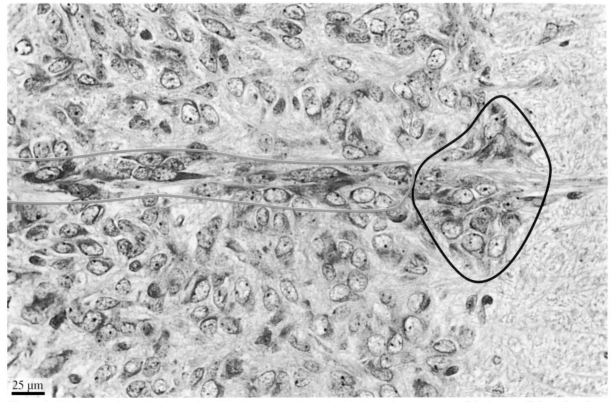

25 µm

Figure 3-43. A rung of maturing intercalated bipolar neurons (green) with visceral motoneurons of the intermediolateral nucleus (red) in an E19 rat. Methacrylate; hematoxylin-eosin.

Figure 3-44. Migration of cholinergic neurons from the ventral horn to the lateral horn in the rat spinal cord between E13 and E21. The organization of the rung of intercalated cells is completed between E17 and E21. From Phelps et al. (1991). Choline acetyltransferase histochemistry.

E13

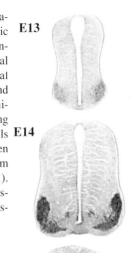

E14

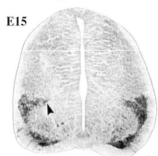

E15

E16

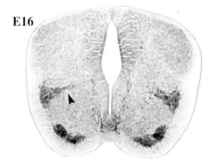

E17

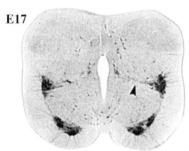

E21

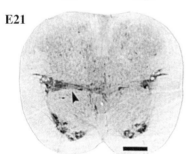

3.3.4   Maturation of the Interneurons of the Intermediate Gray.

The peak in mitotic activity in the ventral neuroepithelium is followed by a surge of mitotic activity in the intermediate neuroepithelium, and by a correlated expansion of the intermediate gray interneuronal field (Figures 3-11 and 3-12). We now examine in greater detail some aspects of the maturation of these intermediate gray neurons in methacrylate sections and autoradiograms at higher magnification.

A narrow band containing lightly staining, vertically oriented spindle-shaped cells begins to form lateral to the intermediate neuroepithelium on E13, while differentiating motoneurons accumulate in increasing numbers in the incipient ventral horn (Figure 3-45). The formation of this band of cells is associated with the appearance of a few strands of fibers that cross to the opposite side underneath the floor plate. The short-survival thymidine radiogram from a rat tagged with ³H-thymidine on the same day shows that these lateral band cells, in contrast to the heavy labeling of cells in the synthetic zone of the intermediate neuroepithelium, are unlabeled (Figure 3-46A). These observations indicate that the postmitotic cells that have moved into this band were generated before the morning of E13. These early generated cells in the primordial intermediate gray are commissural interneurons.

As seen in the autoradiogram of a rat embryo tagged with ³H-thymidine on E13 and killed on E14 (Figure 3-46B), the expanding intermediate gray contains both labeled and unlabeled cells. Evidently, some cells produced after the morning of E13 (Figure 3-46A) have migrated to this site in the elapsed 24 hours. In addition, this autoradiogram also shows that by E14 most of the unlabeled (earlier generated) cells and most of the labeled (later generated) cells have assumed a vertically oriented bipolar shape (Figure 3-46B). These bipolar cells, as seen in a methacrylate section from an E14 rat (Figure 3-47), are the source of the contralaterally projecting commissural axons. Finally, the vertically oriented young commissural interneurons are no longer labeled in short-survival autoradiograms of rat embryoss tagged with ³H-thymidine on E14 (Figure 3-48). We conclude that the commissural interneurons are generated on E12 and E13 in the cervical cord of the rat, and that, by E14, many of them have sprouted axons that cross to the opposite side in the ventral commissure.

E13

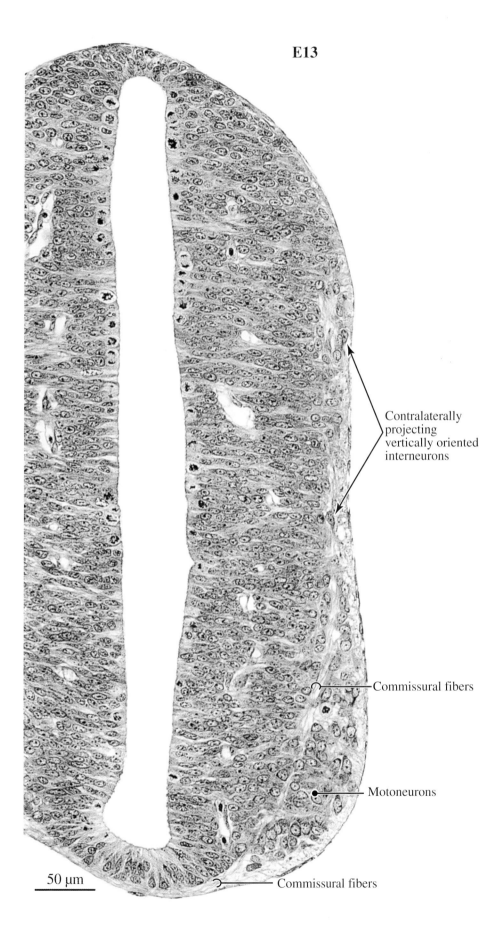

Contralaterally projecting vertically oriented interneurons

Commissural fibers

Motoneurons

Commissural fibers

Figure 3-45. The accumulation in the cervical spinal cord of an E13 rat of a few round cells and vertically oriented bipolar cells in a band lateral to the intermediate neuroepithelium. This is the primordial intermediate gtray. The formation of the primordial intermediate gray is associated with the emergence of a few commissural fibers that cross to the opposite side beneath the floor plate. Methacrylate; hematoxylin-eosin.

50 μm

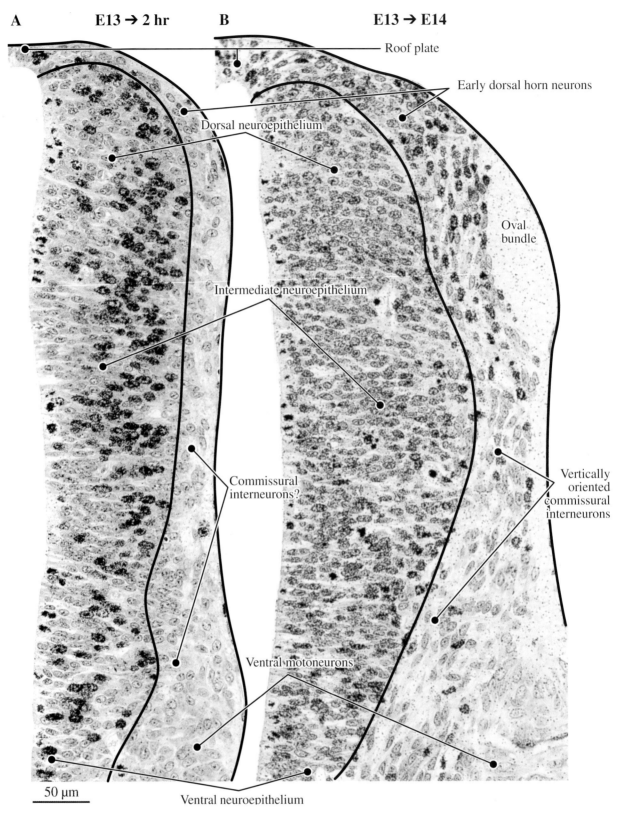

A E13 → 2 hr   **B** E13 → E14

Roof plate

Early dorsal horn neurons

Dorsal neuroepithelium

Oval bundle

Intermediate neuroepithelium

Commissural interneurons?

Vertically oriented commissural interneurons

Ventral motoneurons

50 μm

Ventral neuroepithelium

Figure 3-46. A. Autoradiogram of the cervical spinal cord from a rat embryo tagged with ³H-thymidine on E13 and killed 2 hours later. The horizontally oriented labeled NEP cells are flanked laterally by a narrow band of unlabeled round or bipolar cells. These differentiating cells were generated before the morning of E13. **B.** Autoradiogram from a rat that was tagged with ³H-thymidine on E13 but survived for 24 hours). In this E14 rat, the expanding lateral band contains both unlabeled and labeled cells, and most of them have become bipolar. Paraffin.

E14

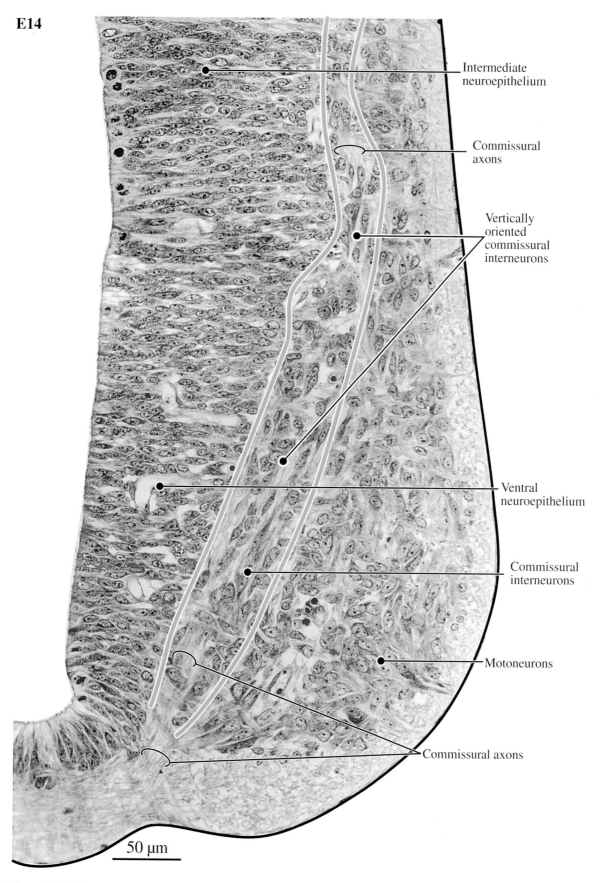

Intermediate
neuroepithelium

Commissural
axons

Vertically
oriented
commissural
interneurons

Ventral
neuroepithelium

Commissural
interneurons

Motoneurons

Commissural axons

50 μm

Figure 3-47. The band of vertically oriented bipolar cells in the cervical spinal cord of an E14 rat in a methacrylate-embedded section. The bipolar cells appear to be the source of commissural axons that cross to the opposite side underneath the floor plate. These cells, some of which may be migrating ventrally, are sandwiched between the neuroepithelium and the expanding gray matter.

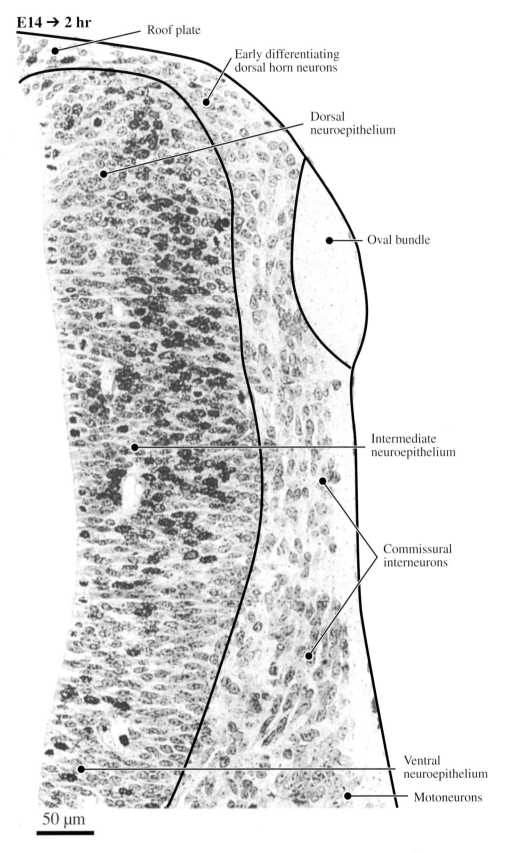

E14 → 2 hr
Roof plate
Early differentiating
dorsal horn neurons
Dorsal
neuroepithelium
Oval bundle
Intermediate
neuroepithelium
Commissural
interneurons
Ventral
neuroepithelium
Motoneurons
50 μm

Figure 3-48. Autoradiogram of the cervical spinal cord of a rat that was tagged with ³H-thymidine on E14 and killed 2 hours later. The vertically oriented bipolar cells flanking the neuroepithelium are not labeled in this short survival radiogram, indicating that the commissural interneurons are generated before E14.

By E15, the band of bipolar commissural interneurons extends all the way from the incipient dorsal horn to the growing ventral horn (Figure 3-49). It is unclear what proportion of them originates in the intermediate neuroepithelium. It is possible that the vertical bipolar shape of commissural interneurons on E13 and E14 signals not only that they are extruding vertically growing axons but that, at least some of them, are migrating from the intermediate plate ventrally. What is clear is that by this age the band of vertically oriented, commissural interneurons is flanked laterally by a new and much larger field of cells, some spherical in shape, others bipolar and horizontally oriented. The radiogram from a rat labeled on E14 and killed on E15 (Figure 3-50) suggests that some horizontal bipolar cells were generated on E14 and are migrating laterally by E15. These horizontally oriented cells may be ipsilaterally projecting interneurons whose axons join the lateral funiculus. The settling of this second wave of cells in the intermediate gray continues on E16 (Figure 3-51). By this age, only fragments of the band of vertically oriented bipolar cells are evident in the intermediate gray, in spite of the persistence of the contralaterally projecting commissural fibers. We presume that after they have completed the extrusion of their axons, the commissural interneurons lose their distinctive vertically oriented bipolar shape.

The hypothesis that the second wave of intermediate gray cells are ipsilaterally projecting interneurons is supported by the progressive expansion of the lateral funiculus (the major conduit of ipsilaterally projecting interneurons, in particular of intraspinal neurons) between E16 and E19 (Figure 3-52). As the interneurons of the intermediate gray continue to develop, most of them lose their bipolar shape (Figure 3-53). This may signal the end of their axonogenesis. The next stage in their maturation is hinted at by the cytology of the radiogram from a perinatal rat labeled with ^{3}H-thymidine on E14 and killed on E21 (Figure 3-54). Many of the interneurons (some labeled, others unlabeled) display variably oriented cytoplasmic caps and multiple poles. This may signal the beginning of dendrogenesis in the interneuronal field of the intermediate gray.

The hypothesis that the transformation of interneurons from bipolar to multipolar reflects the advance from the stage of axonogenesis to the stage of dendrogenesis is supported by the experimental results of Silos-Santiago and Snider (1992) and illustrated in Figure 3-55. These investigators placed crystals of the tracer DiI in various locations on one side of the thoracic spinal cord of fixed rat embryos at E13.5, E15, E17, and E19 to visualize the dendritic development of interneurons. On E13.5, the majority of commissural neurons had a bipolar shape, were vertically oriented, and had rudimentary dendrites (Figure 3-55A). By E15, only a few vertically oriented commissural cells remained; most of them became multipolar with dendrites extending transversely in various directions (Figure 3-55B). The dendritic arbors of interneurons expanded considerably by E19 (Figure 3-55C).

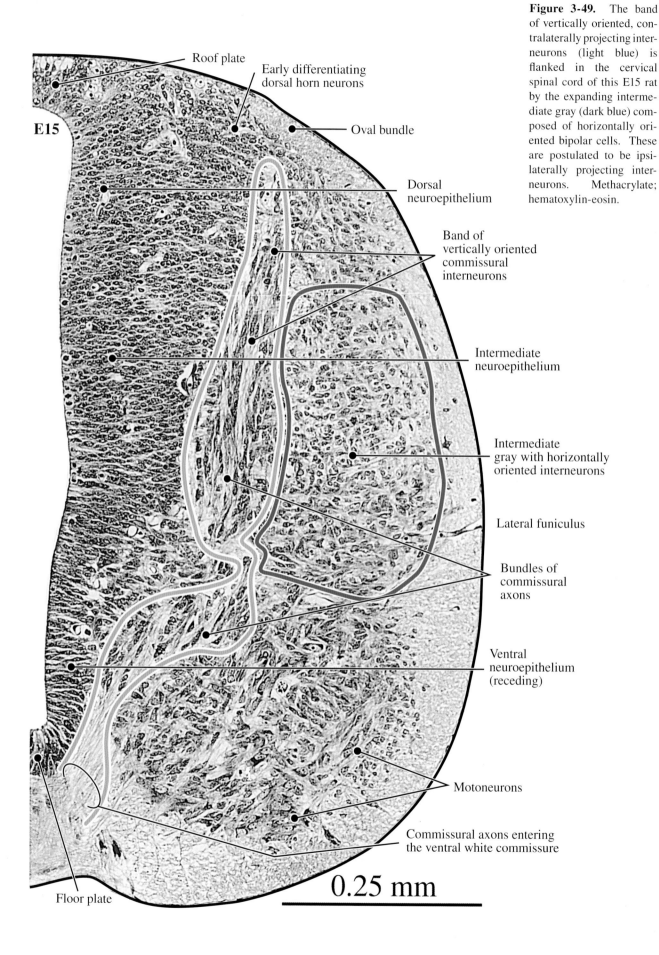

Roof plate

Early differentiating
dorsal horn neurons

E15

Oval bundle

Dorsal
neuroepithelium

Band of
vertically oriented
commissural
interneurons

Intermediate
neuroepithelium

Intermediate
gray with horizontally
oriented interneurons

Lateral funiculus

Bundles of
commissural
axons

Ventral
neuroepithelium
(receding)

Motoneurons

Commissural axons entering
the ventral white commissure

Floor plate

0.25 mm

Figure 3-49. The band of vertically oriented, contralaterally projecting interneurons (light blue) is flanked in the cervical spinal cord of this E15 rat by the expanding intermediate gray (dark blue) composed of horizontally oriented bipolar cells. These are postulated to be ipsilaterally projecting interneurons. Methacrylate; hematoxylin-eosin.

E14 → E15

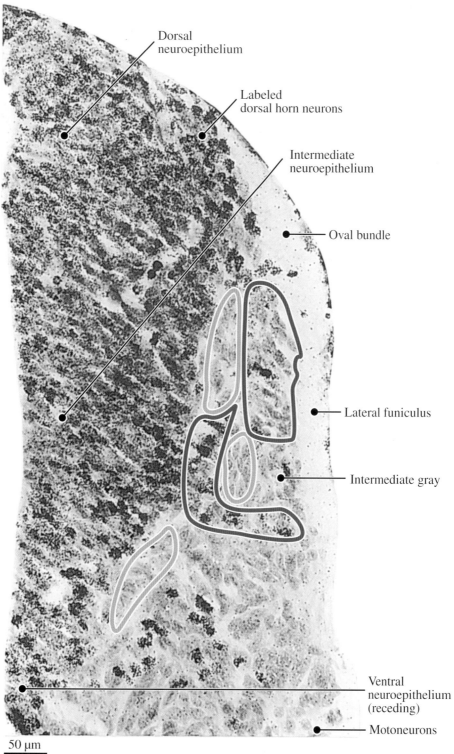

Dorsal
neuroepithelium

Labeled
dorsal horn neurons

Intermediate
neuroepithelium

Oval bundle

Lateral funiculus

Intermediate gray

Ventral
neuroepithelium
(receding)

Motoneurons

50 μm

Figure 3-50. The cervical spinal cord of a rat that was tagged with ³H-thymidine on E14 and was killed 24 hours later (E14→E15). Some horizontally oriented labeled cells (dark blue) traverse the band of vertically oriented unlabeled cells (light blue) in the expanding intermediate gray. Paraffin embedded autoradiogram.

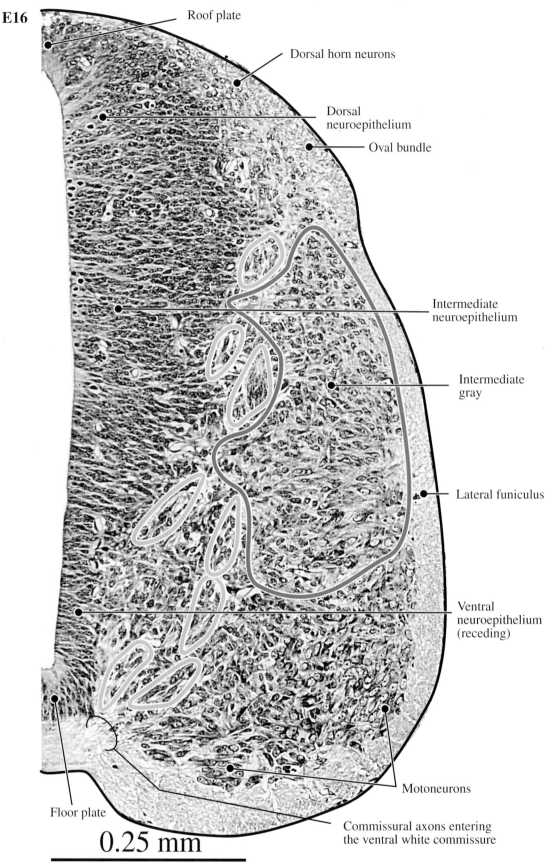

E16

Roof plate

Dorsal horn neurons

Dorsal
neuroepithelium

Oval bundle

Intermediate
neuroepithelium

Intermediate
gray

Lateral funiculus

Ventral
neuroepithelium
(receding)

Motoneurons

Floor plate

Commissural axons entering
the ventral white commissure

0.25 mm

Figure 3-51. Fragments of vertically oriented bipolar cells (light blue) and the expanding intermediate field with horizontally oriented bipolar cells (dark blue) in an E16 rat. The horizontally oriented interneurons are presumed to be ipsilaterally projecting interneurons. Methacrylate; hematoxylin-eosin.

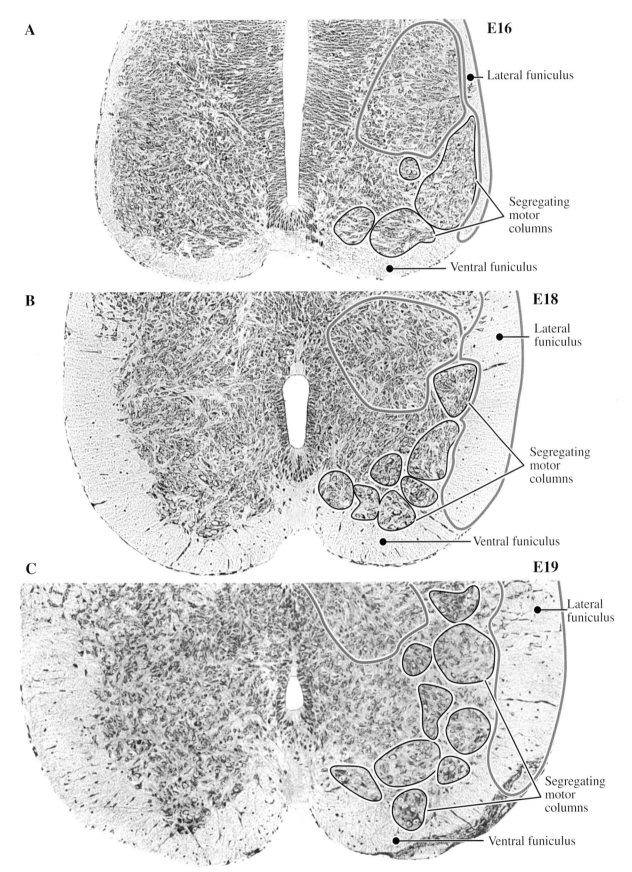

Figure 3-52. Growth of the lateral funiculus (purple) in relation to the maturation of intermediate gray interneurons (blue) and the segregation of motor columns (black) in the spinal cord of E16 (**A**), E18 (**B**), and E19 (**C**) rats. Methacrylate; hematoxylin-eosin.

E19

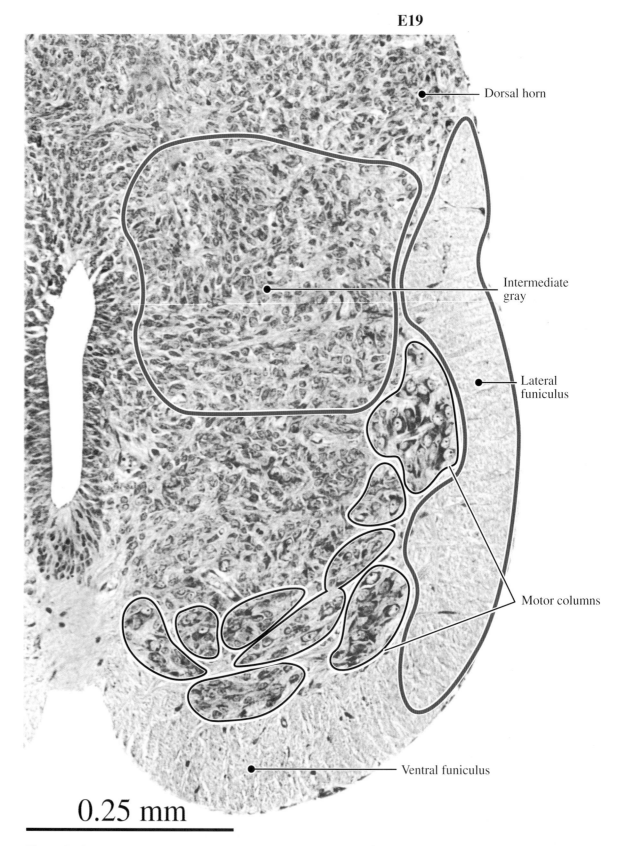

0.25 mm

Figure 3-53. Maturation of the the intermediate gray interneurons (blue) in relation to the growth of the lateral funiculus (purple) and the maturation of motoneurons (black) in an E19 rat. Methacrylate; hematoxylin-eosin.

Intermediate gray **E14+E15 → E21**

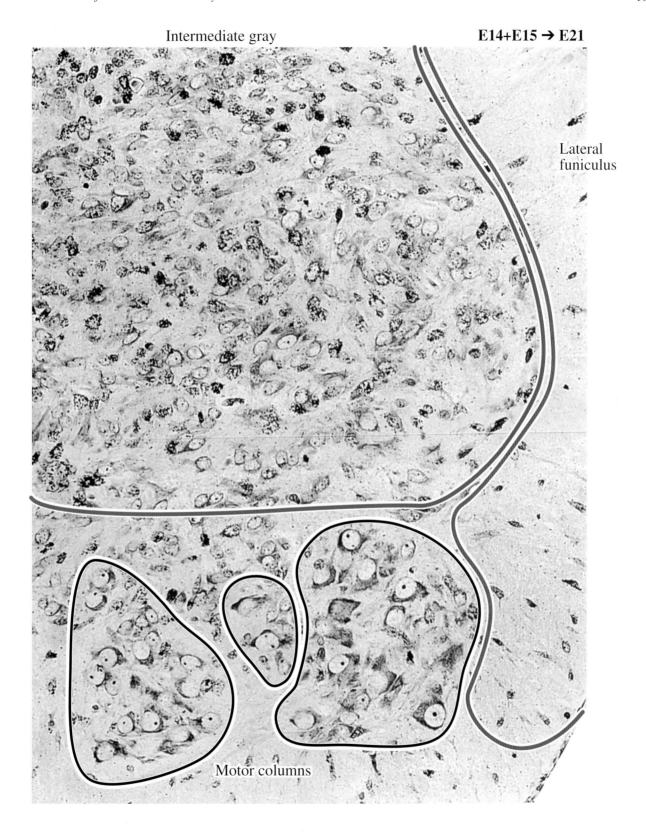

Lateral funiculus

Motor columns

Figure 3-54. Maturation and intermingling of the larger, unlabeled interneurons (those generated before E14) and the smaller, labeled interneurons (those generated on or after E14) in the intermediate gray (blue) of a perinatal rat tagged with ³H-thymidine on E14 (E14+E15→E21). Methacrylate autoradiogram.

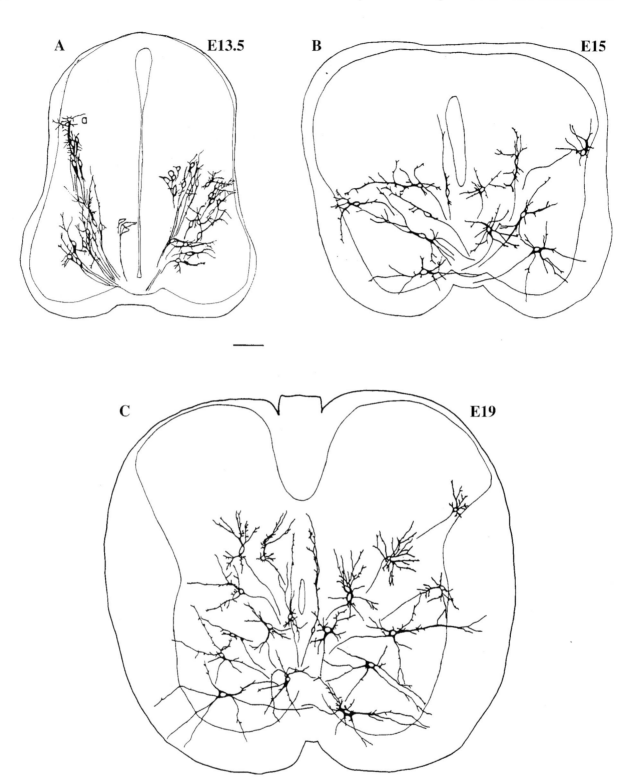

Figure 3-55. Composite drawings of neurons in the thoracic spinal cord of E13.5 **(A)**, E15 **(B)**, E19 **(C)** rats. Note the predominance of bipolar commissural interneurons in the intermediate gray at E13.5. By E15, multipolar interneurons with ramifying dendrites predominate in the intermediate gray. Dendritic development is more pronounced by E19. After Silos-Santiago and Snider (1992). DiI fluorescent technique in fixed tissue.

3.3.5 Maturation of the Large Neurons of the Intermediate Gray.

In addition to the large number of scattered small- and medium-sized interneurons, the intermediate gray also contains larger neurons organized into nuclei or columns. Best known of these are the central cervical nucleus and the lateral cervical nucleus in the cervical cord, and Clarke's column in the thoracic cord. We have sought to determine the time of origin of some of these neurons in the rat spinal cord with autoradiography and the examine the rate of their maturation in methacrylate-embedded sections.

The neurons of the *central cervical nucleus* are labeled in adults rats that were tagged with two doses of ^{3}H-thymidine beginning on E12 (Figure 3-56). They are no longer labeled if the tagging was delayed until E13 (Figure 3-57). This indicates that the production of central cervical nucleus neurons ceases before the morning of E13. Many of the large *lateral cervical nucleus* neurons are labeled in perinatal rats tagged with ^{3}H-thymidine beginning on E13 (Figure 3-58). They are no longer labeled if the

administration of the radiochemical is delayed until E14 (Figure 3-59). This establishes that the production of the lateral cervical nucleus neurons comes to an end on E14. The same applies to the large neurons of Clarke's column in the thoracic spinal cord that are not labeled in rats that were tagged with ^{3}H-thymidine on E14 (Figure 3-60).

The earliest age at which a few multipolar lateral cervical nucleus neurons could be identified in methacrylate sections was E17 (Figure 3-61), suggesting a long delay in settling and maturation. Some bipolar cells with trailing fibers seen in the same region may be neurons still migrating to this site. Putative migrating lateral cervical nucleus neurons were identified in much larger numbers on E18 (Figure 3-62). Both the settled and migrating neurons are either embedded in the gray matter or are scattered in the lateral funiculus. The trajectory of the migrating neurons suggests that lateral cervical neurons originate dorsal to the retracting spinal canal in a region distinguished by a matrix of fibrous material. By E19, a distinctive fiber bundle marks the migratory route

E12+E13 ➔ P60

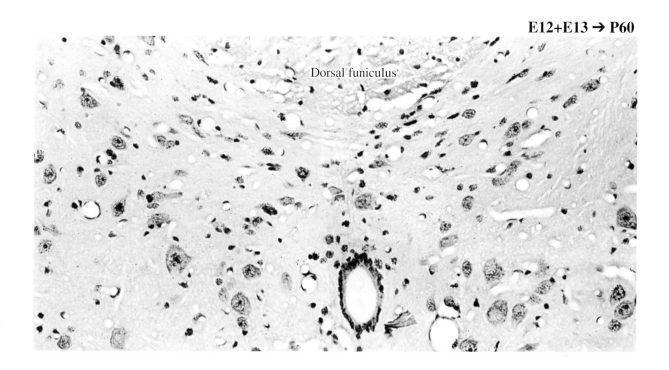

Dorsal funiculus

Figure 3-56. Large and small labeled neurons in the central cervical nucleus of an adult rat that was tagged with ^{3}H-thymidine on E12 and E13 (E12+E13➔P60). Autoradiogram; paraffin.

of these cells (Figure 3-63). Since the axons of the lateral cervical nucleus reach the contralateral thalamus (Morin, 1955; Ha and Liu, 1966; Boivie, 1970), it is possible that these are fibers that decussate in the dorsal commissure of the cervical spinal cord. An occasional differentiating neuron of the central cervical nucleus was first seen on E17, lateral to the spinal canal (Figure 3-64). Their number increased by E18 (Figure 3-65). By this age the spinal canal has receded and the central cervical neurons moved medially with the fusing parenchyma. By E19, the central cervical nucleus neurons appeared quite mature (Figure 3-66). We have not examined the maturation of neurons of Clarke's column in the rat spinal cord. (We present a detailed description of the development of Clarke's column in the human spinal cord in Section 6.4.1.)

E13+E14 → P60

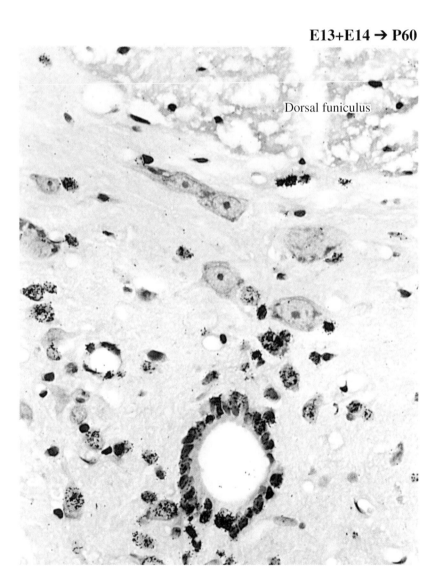

Dorsal funiculus

Figure 3-57. The large neurons of the central cervical nucleus are no longer labeled in an adult rat that was tagged with ³H-thymidine on E13 and E14 (E13+E14→P60). Autoradiogram; paraffin.

E13+E14 ➔ E21

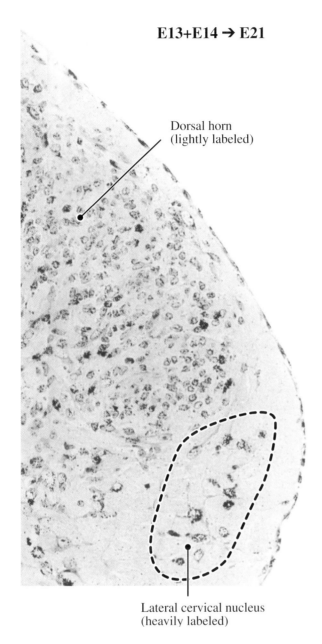

Dorsal horn
(lightly labeled)

Lateral cervical nucleus
(heavily labeled)

Figure 3-58. Admixture of labeled and unlabeled large neurons in the lateral cervical nucleus (outlined area) of a perinatal (E21) rat that was tagged with ³H-thymidine on E13+E14. The late-generated neurons of the dorsal horn are lightly labeled with this early schedule of radiochemical administration. Autoradiogram; paraffin.

E14+E15 ➔ E21

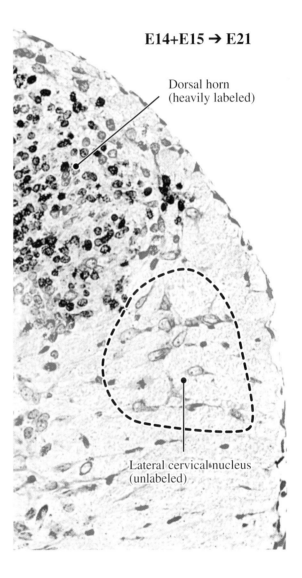

Dorsal horn
(heavily labeled)

Lateral cervical nucleus
(unlabeled)

Figure 3-59. The large neurons in the lateral cervical nucleus are no longer labeled in a perinatal (E21) rat that was tagged with ³H-thymidine on E14 and E15. The small neurons of the dorsal horn are heavily labeled with this late schedule of radiochemical administration. Autoradiogram; paraffin.

E14+E15 → E21

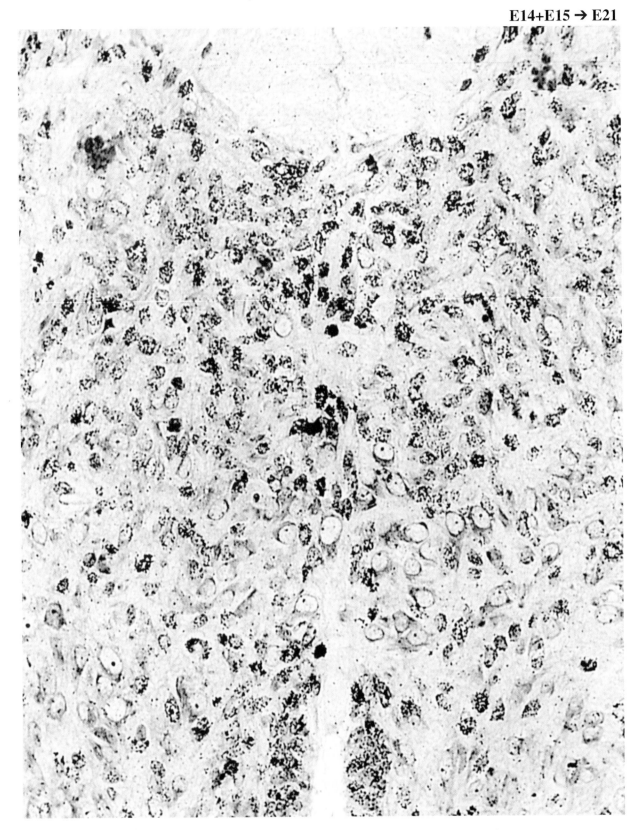

Figure 3-60. The neurons of Clarke's column are not labeled in a perinatal rat (E21) that was exposed to ^{3}H-thymidine on E14 and E15. Autoradiogram; paraffin.

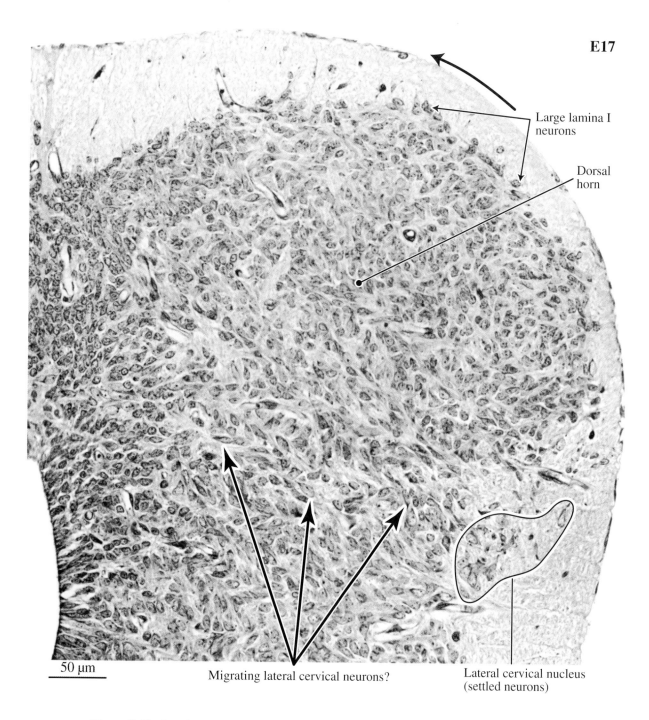

E17

Large lamina I neurons

Dorsal horn

50 µm

Migrating lateral cervical neurons?

Lateral cervical nucleus (settled neurons)

Figure 3-61. Putative migrating neurons (lower arrows) and settled neurons (outlined area) of the lateral cervical nucleus in an E17 rat. Note also the scattered horizontal neurons dispersing over the surface of the dorsal horn (upper arrow). Methacrylate; hematoxylin-eosin.

E18

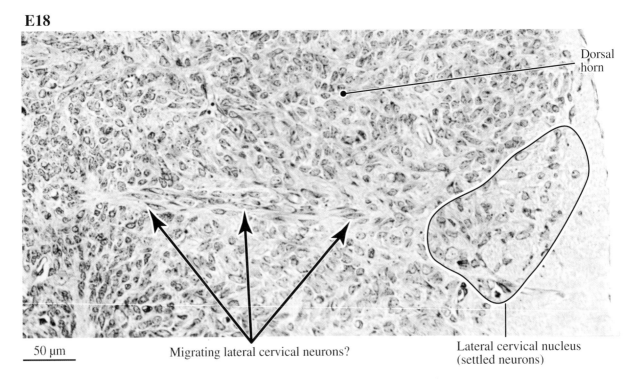

Dorsal
horn

50 µm

Migrating lateral cervical neurons?

Lateral cervical nucleus
(settled neurons)

Figure 3-62. Putative migrating neurons (arrows) and the settled neurons (enclosure) of the
lateral cervical nucleus in an E18 rat. Methacrylate; hematoxylin-eosin.

E19

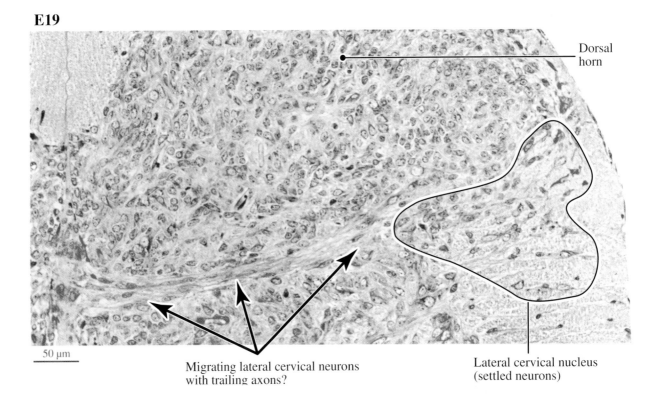

Dorsal
horn

50 µm

Migrating lateral cervical neurons
with trailing axons?

Lateral cervical nucleus
(settled neurons)

Figure 3-63. Putative migrating neurons (arrows) and the settled neurons (enclosure) of the
lateral cervical nucleus in an E19 rat. Note fibers in the possible migratory path of lateral
cervical neurons. Methacrylate; hematoxylin-eosin.

E17

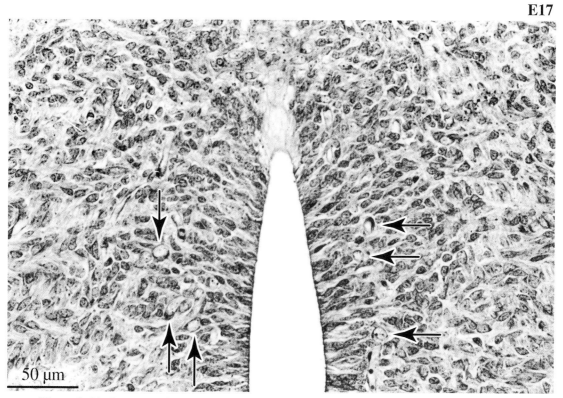

Figure 3-64. Rare maturing central cervical nucleus neurons (arrows) in an E17 rat. Methacrylate; hematoxylin-eosin.

E18

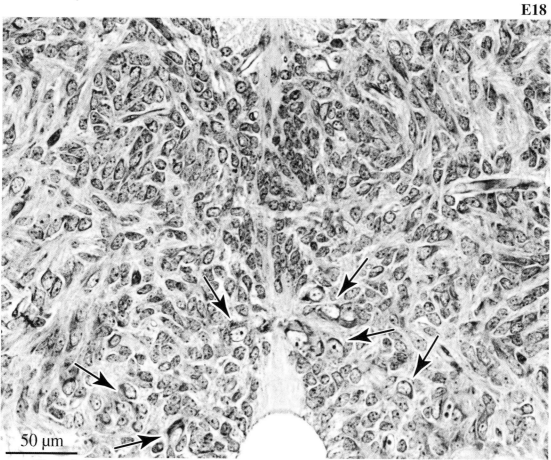

Figure 3-65. Central cervical neurons (arrows), some with prominent cytoplasmic hypertrophy, in an E18 rat. Methacrylate; hematoxylin-eosin.

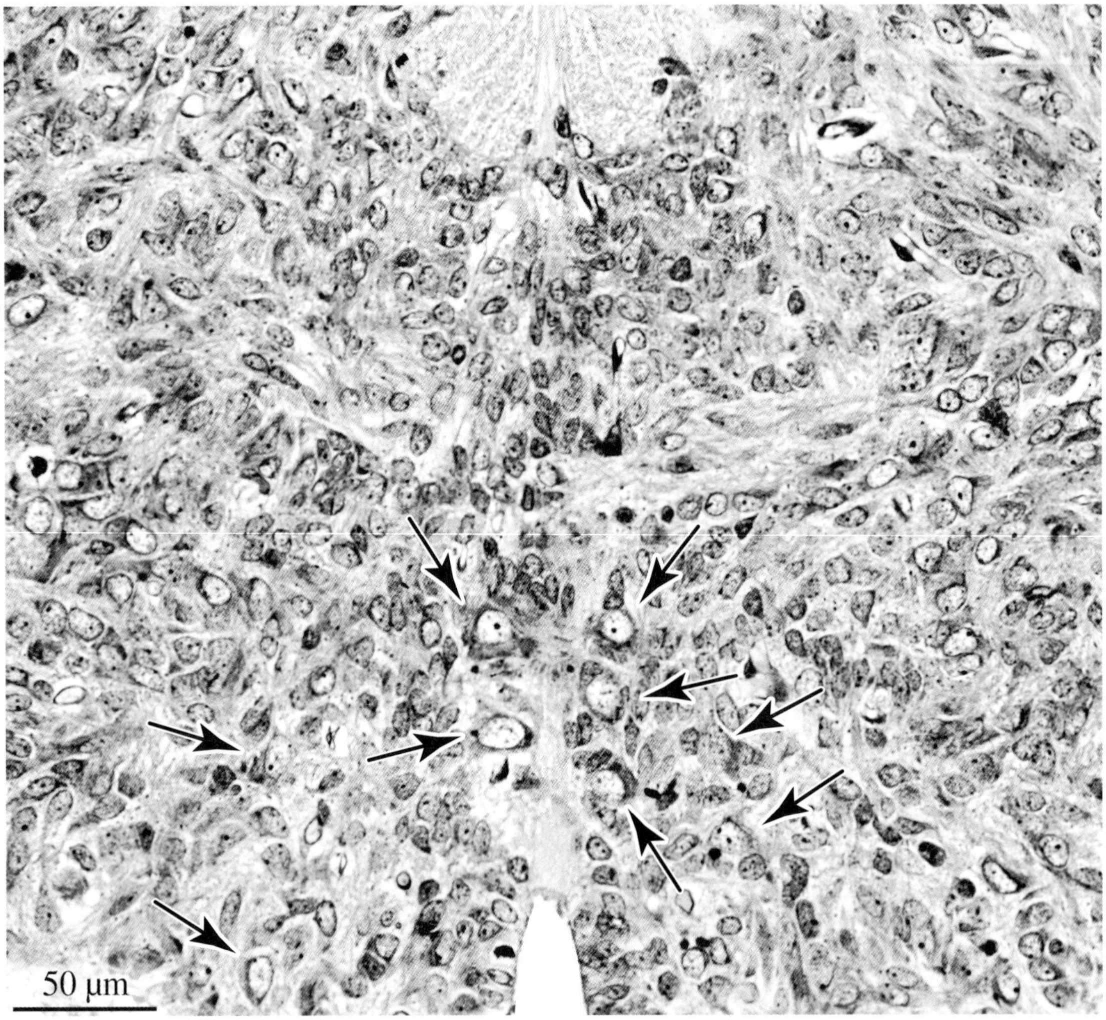

Figure 3-66. Maturing neurons (arrows) of the central cervical nucleus in an E19 rat. Methacrylate; hematoxylin-eosin.

3.3.6 Maturation of the Small Neurons of the Dorsal Horn. The most active proliferative site on E15 is the upper portion of the intermediate neuroepithelium and the dorsal neuroepithelium. As seen in a short-survival radiogram from a rat tagged with ³H-thymidine on the morning of E15 and killed 2 hours later (Figure 3-67), few of the NEP cells are labeled in the thinning ventral neuroepithelium and in the lower portion of the intermediate neuroepithelium. In contrast, the synthetic zone of the upper half of the neuroepithelium is filled with labeled cells. We present evidence here that the dorsal neuroepithelium is the source of the late-generated neurons of

the dorsal horn, and will try to show later (Section 3.3.8) that the upper intermediate neuroepithelium is the source of the last-generated neurons of a different system, i.e., the central autonomic area.

The short-survival autoradiogram of the cervical spinal cord of an E15 rat shows two distinct regions in the dorsal neuroepithelium (Figure 3-67). There is an internal compartment filled with labeled cells and an external compartment containing mostly unlabeled cells. The former region, the synthetic zone, is obviously composed of NEP cells that are still proliferating on E15; whereas the latter region, identified previously as the sojourn zone (Figure 3-10), is composed of postmitotic cells (cells that ceased to divide before the morning of E15). Here we draw attention to the different proliferation dynamics and movements of cells in the sojourn zone of the dorsal neuroepithelium and in the sojourn zone of the upper intermediate neuroepithelium.

In the rat tagged with ^{3}H-thymidine on E15 and killed on E16 (Figure 3-68), both the synthetic and the sojourn zones of the dorsal neuroepithelium are filled with labeled cells and the first contingent of labeled cells has begun to migrate into the adjacent dorsal horn. The dorsal neuroepithelium is evidently the source of the late-generated neurons of the dorsal horn. However, few labeled cells have penetrated the sojourn zone of the upper intermediate neuroepithelium during the same period and even fewer seem to to be migrating into the adjacent intermediate gray. This difference in the cell dynamics of the two neuroepithelial sites is even more obvious in the rat embryo that was tagged with ^{3}H-thymidine on E15 and killed on E17 (Figure 3-69). While the population of labeled cells has increased greatly in the expanded dorsal horn, the labeled cells in the sojourn zone of the upper intermediate gray remain close to the neuroepithelium, suggesting that they constitute a different population of cells with a short migratory route.

The massive migration of young neurons to the dorsal horn on E17 is associated with the dissolution of the dorsal neuroepithelium and the retraction of the spinal canal (Figure 3-69), signaling the end of the production of dorsal horn neurons. Since a sizable sojourn zone persists dorsally, the migration of dorsal horn neurons may continue for a few days. By E21, the labeled dorsal horn neurons (those born on E15) are intermingled with the unlabeled ones (those born before E15) throughout much of the dorsal horn (Figure 3-70). There is only a slight hint that the concentration of labeled (late-generated) neurons may be higher in the substantia gelatinosa (laminae II and III) than in the depth of the dorsal horn. Importantly, the labeled cells of the upper intermediate gray remain close to the neuroepithelium above and around the shrunken central canal.

Higher magnification views of methacrylate autoradiograms in the cervical spinal cord of rats

labeled on E15 and killed on E21 (Figure 3-71) suggest that a fair proportion of the vertically oriented, oval shaped neurons (possibly central cells) are labeled in lamina II and III but few of the larger cell types are labeled. Neurons with larger nuclei in laminae III-IV, possibly stalked cells, are typically unlabeled. It is possible, therefore, that cell type rather than laminar boundary is the determining factor in the temporal order of dorsal horn neuron production (see also Figures 3-73 and 3-74). There is a rostral-to-caudal gradient in the generation of dorsal horn neurons, as seen in the spinal cord from a single perinatal rat that was tagged with ^{3}H-thymidine on E15 (Figure 3-72). The proportion of labeled (later generated) neurons increases in the dorsal horn as one proceeds to the thoracic, lumbar and sacral levels of the spinal cord.

Whereas many small neurons are labeled in laminae II-V of the dorsal horn with ^{3}H-thymidine administered on E15, the large neurons of lamina I, presumably Waldeyer cells, are not labeled (Figure 3-71). In Figures 3-73 and 3-74 we compare the concentration of labeled cells in lamina I in perinatal rats that were tagged with ^{3}H-thymidine beginning on E13 and E15. Most cells, whether small or large, are labeled in lamina I in the rat tagged with the radiochemical on E13 but most of the larger cells of lamina I are unlabeled in the rat in which the administration of the radiochemical was delayed until E15. The majority of large neurons of lamina I must be generated some time between E13 and E14. The possible source of the early-generated large lamina I neurons, and perhaps some other early-generated dorsal horn neurons, was illustrated in Section 3.3.4. There is an aggregate of labeled cells lateral to the roof plate and above the oval bundle in E14 rats that were tagged with ^{3}H-thymidine on E13 (Figure 3-46B) but the same aggregate of differentiating cells is devoid of label in short survival radiograms from E14 rats (Figure 3-48). However, although generated relatively early, the maturation of these neurons appears to take a long time. Not until E17 do the horizontally oriented cells start to disperse from lateral to medial in lamina I of the dorsal horn (Figure 3-61). Initially, these cells are barely larger than the late-generated neurons of the dorsal horn. The large Waldeyer cells do not become distinctly different from the smaller neurons of lamina I and the rest of the dorsal horn until E19 (Figure 3-75).

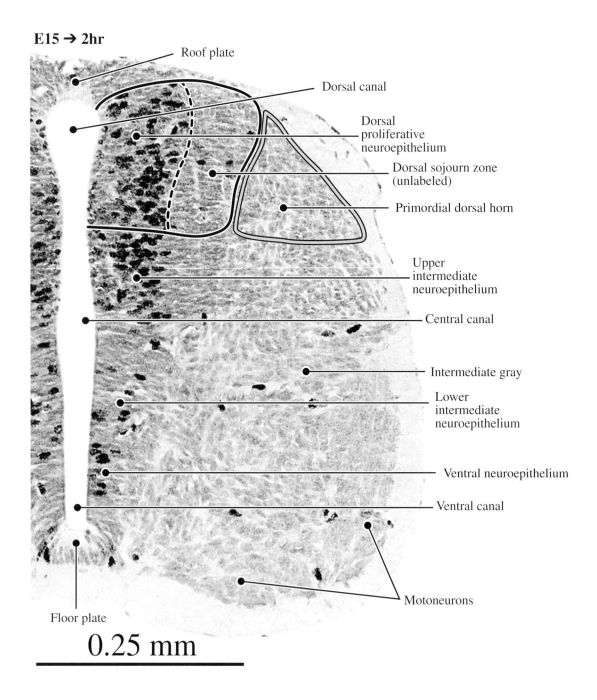

E15 → 2hr

Roof plate

Dorsal canal

Dorsal proliferative neuroepithelium

Dorsal sojourn zone (unlabeled)

Primordial dorsal horn

Upper intermediate neuroepithelium

Central canal

Intermediate gray

Lower intermediate neuroepithelium

Ventral neuroepithelium

Ventral canal

Motoneurons

Floor plate

0.25 mm

Figure 3-67. Short-survival autoradiogram of the cervical spinal cord of an E15 rat that was killed 2 hours after the administration of ³H-thymidine. A high proportion of NEP cells in the proliferative zone of the dorsal neuroepithelium and in the upper intermediate neuroepithelium are labeled. In the same regions, most of the darkly staining cells in the sojourn zone of the neuroepithelium are unlabeled. These are postmitotic cells generated before the morning of E15. The primordial dorsal horn (yellow outline) is also devoid of labeled cells; the cells present were evidently generated before E15. The scattered labeled cells in the gray matter ventrally are locally multiplying glia.

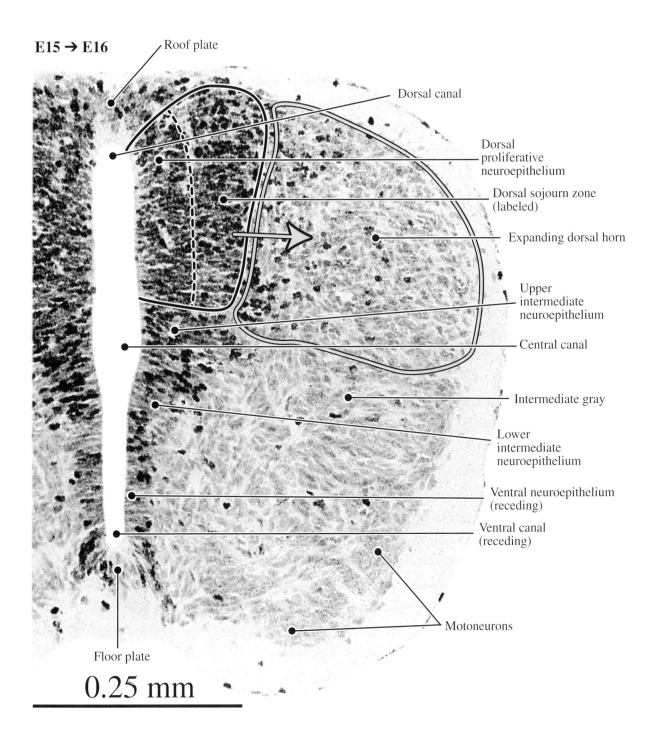

Figure 3-68. Sequential-survival autoradiogram of the cervical spinal cord of a rat that was tagged with
³H-thymidine on E15 and was killed 24 hours later (E15→E16). The unlabeled (earlier generated) cells
seen on the previous day in the dorsal sojourn zone (Figure 3-67) have been replaced by labeled cells
(cells generated on E15). The dorsal horn (yellow outline) is expanding and contains a small contingent
of migrating labeled cells (those generated after E15; yellow arrow). The scattered labeled cells in the
intermediate gray and the ventral horn are presumed to be locally multiplying glia.

E15 → E17

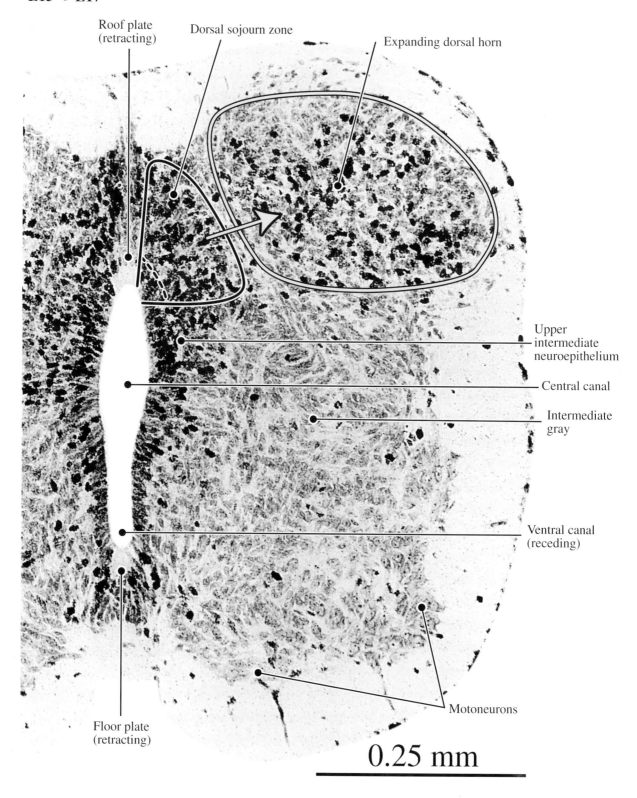

Figure 3-69. Sequential-survival autoradiogram of the cervical spinal cord in a rat that was tagged with ^{3}H-thymidine on E15 and survived 48 hours (E15→E17). The dorsal neuroepithelium is receding while the enlarged dorsal horn (yellow) is filled with labeled cells (those generated on or after E15). The scattered labeled cells in the intermediate gray and the ventral horn are presumed to be locally multiplying glia.

E15+E16 → E21

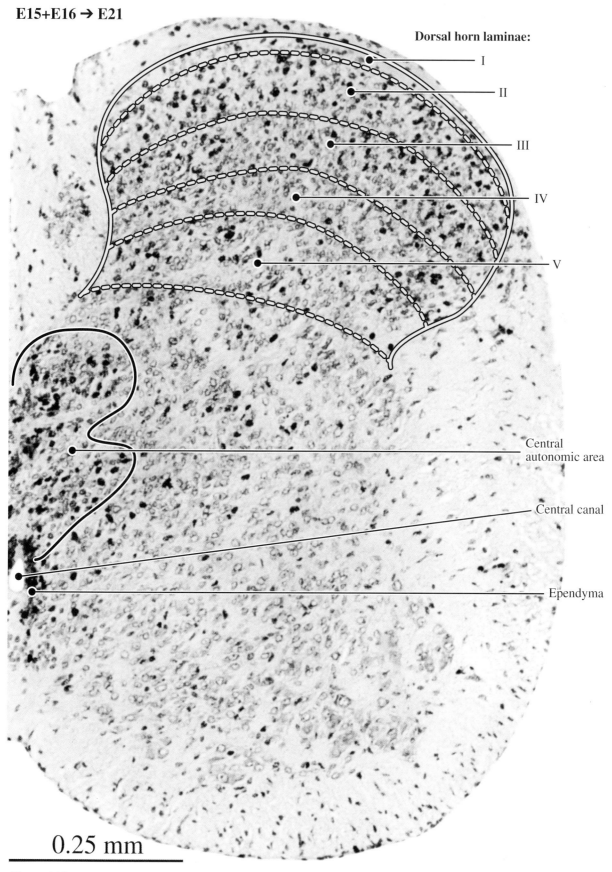

Dorsal horn laminae:
I
II
III
IV
V

Central autonomic area

Central canal

Ependyma

0.25 mm

Figure 3-70. Laminar distribution of labeled cells in the cervical spinal cord of a perinatal rat that was tagged with ³H-thymidine hon E15 and E16. The concentration of labeled cells is somewhat higher in laminae II-III than in laminae IV-V. The labeled cells of the upper intermediate neuroepithelium form the central autonomic area. Autoradiogram; paraffin.

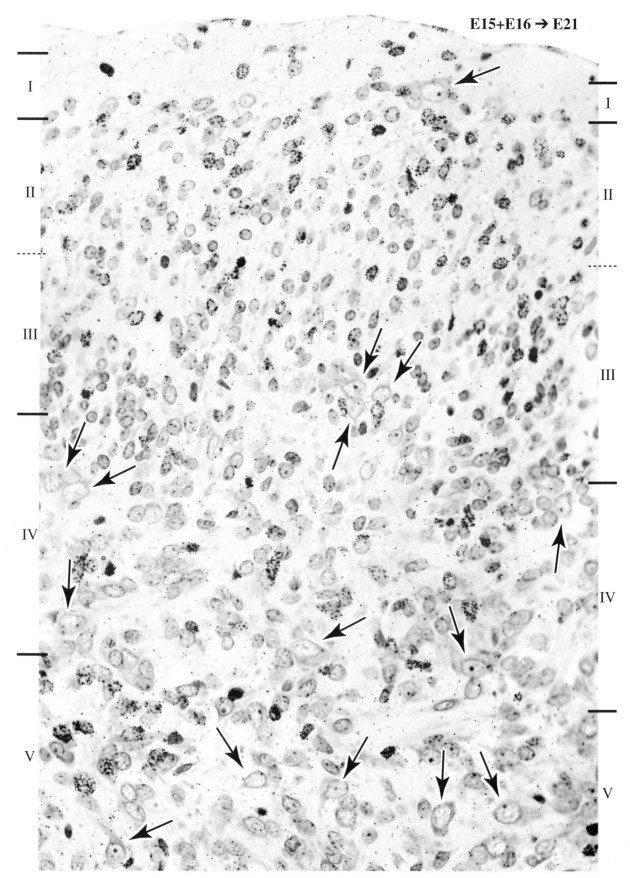

Figure 3-71. Long-survival autoradiogram of the dorsal horn in the cervical spinal cord of a perinatal rat that was tagged with ^{3}H-thymidine beginning on E15. Some small oval cells (perhaps the central cells of the substantia gelatinosa) are labeled. Most of the larger neurons (arrows) are unlabeled. Methacrylate.

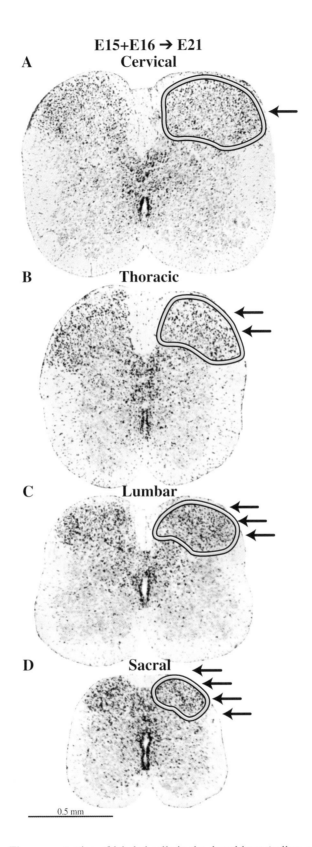

E15+E16 → E21

A   Cervical

B   Thoracic

C   Lumbar

D   Sacral

0.5 mm

Figure 3-72. The concentration of labeled cells in the dorsal horn (yellow outline) of the cervical **(A)**, thoracic **(B)**, lumbar **(C)**, and sacral **(D)** spinal cord of a perinatal (E21) rat that was tagged with ³H-thymidine on E15 and E16. There is an increase in the proportion of labeled cells in the dorsal horn (as well as in the central autonomic area and the intermediate gray) from rostral to caudal levels of the spinal cord. Autoradiograms, paraffin.

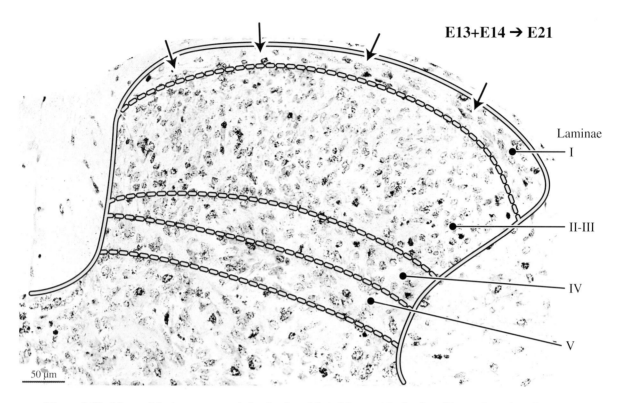

Figure 3-73. Many of the large neurons in lamina I are labeled (arrows) in the dorsal horn of a perinatal rat (E21) that was tagged with ³H-thymidine on E13 and E14. Heavily labeled cells also abound in the lower laminae of the dorsal horn. Autoradiogram; methacrylate.

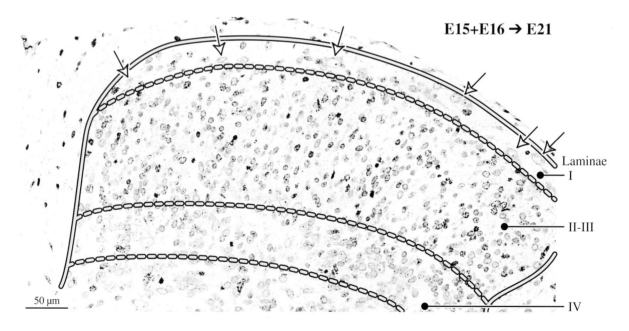

Figure 3-74. In the dorsal horn of the perinatal rat tagged with ³H-thymidine on E15 and E16, most of the large neurons in lamina I are no longer labeled (arrows). Few cells are labeled in lamina IV, but many of the laminae II-III cells are heavily labeled. Autoradiogram; methacrylate.

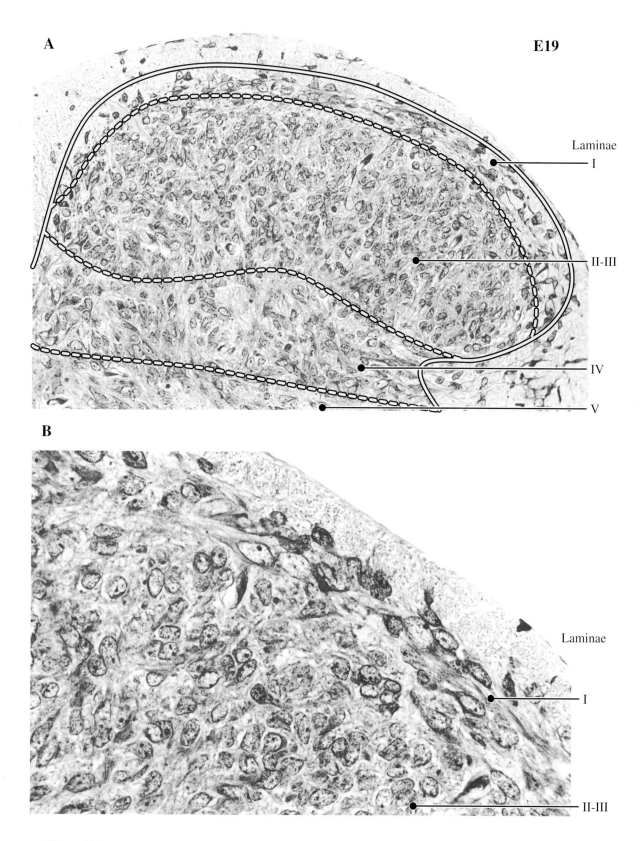

Figure 3-75. Maturation of the large horizontal neurons of lamina I in the cervical spinal cord of an E19 rat at lower (**A**) and higher (**B**) magnification. Methacrylate; hematoxylin-eosin.

3.3.7   Transverse Bands of Migrating and Maturing Intermediate Interneurons.

Figure 3-76 illustrates serial horizontal autoradiograms, from dorsal to ventral, of the cervical spinal cord of a rat that was tagged with ³H-thymidine on E14 and killed on E15. The first two sections are cut through the upper and lower intermediate gray, the third section through the ventral horn. In the autoradiograms that transect the intermediate gray, the proliferative neuroepithelium is composed of a continuous sheet of labeled cells, while the sojourn zone is composed of alternating perpendicular bands (or microsegments) of labeled cells (those generated on or after E14) and unlabeled cells (those generated before E14). The banding pattern of labeled and unlabeled cells is less obvious or is altogether absent far-laterally (Figures 3-76A, B), as if the files of labeled and unlabeled cells rejoin one another near the white matter. There are few labeled cells in the ventral horn and no indication of any microsegmentation (Figure 3-76C).

The banding pattern of labeled and unlabeled cells is illustrated at lower and higher magnification, in a rat embryo that was similarly tagged with ³H-thymidine on E14 and killed on E15, in a parasagittal section that transects the intermediate gray and the ventral horn laterally (Figure 3-77A). The intermediate gray is composed of alternating vertical bands of densely packed labeled or unlabeled cells. As seen at higher magnification (Figure 3-77B), the labeled cells tend to be spherical in shape (their size may be exaggerated by the halo of opaque autoradiographic grains) whereas the unlabeled cells tend to be bipolar and vertically oriented. A comparison with the fine cytology of the spinal cord on E15 in a coronal section (Figure 3-49) indicates that the unlabeled (early generated) bands of vertical bipolar cells are composed of contralaterally projecting commissural interneurons. The labeled (late generated) cells, as suggested by combined histological and autoradiographic evidence (Figures 3-49, 3-50), are probably ipsilaterally projecting interneurons migrating laterally.

We have investigated the microsegmentation of the early- and late-generated interneurons of the intermediate gray in E15 rats with different histological and experimental techniques (Altman and Bayer, 1984). Figures 3-78 and 3-79 illustrate the histology of the normal E15 rat spinal cord in thick (100 μm) celloidin-embedded sections cut in the horizontal and sagittal planes. The horizontal section (Figure 3-78) shows that the synthetic zone of the neuroepithelium is composed of a continous sheet of darkly staining (primitive or younger) cells. In contrast, the sojourn zone displays a sawtooth pattern with alternating bands of darkly staining and lightly staining (more mature or older) cells. Thick parasagittal sections through the lateral spinal cord (Figure 3-79) show that the broader strips composed of darkly staining (younger and presumably migrating) cells correspond to the broader strips containing labeled cells in autoradiograms (Figure 3-77).

Since young neurons, particularly those that migrate (Altman et al., 1968), are extremely radiosensitive, we exposed E15 rats to 150R of whole-body X-irradiation. The animals were killed 6 hours after exposure to locate the radiosensitive (dead) cells and the radioresistant (surviving) cells in the spinal cord. Figure 3-80 shows in the spinal cord of an E15 irradiated rat, alternating bands of radioresistant (intact) and radiosensitive (pyknotic) cells. The radioresistant cells have a predominantly bipolar shape and are aligned in vertical bands that alternate with bands in which all that if left is round pyknotic cells or their debris. Our hypothesis is that the vertically aligned radioresistant cells are the earlier generated (older) contralaterally projecting interneurons, while the radiosensitive cells in the alternating bands are the later generated (younger) ipsilaterally projecting interneurons. An examination of the fine cytology of the spinal cord in horizontally cut, thin methacrylate sections confirms that the two microsegments are associated with fiber bundles that are oriented perpendicularly to one another (Figure 3-81). The bands of horizontally oriented bipolar cells are associated with similarly aligned fibers that proceed toward the lateral funiculus; these are the ipsilaterally projecting interneurons. The bands of small round cells are composed of vertically oriented commissural interneurons transected perpendicularly (compare with the coronal section in Figure 3-49) and the fine dots in their vicinity are the similarly transected contralaterally projecting axons.

In an autoradiographic double-labeling experiment, Nandi et al. (1991, 1993) tested our hypothesis that the contralaterally projecting commissural interneurons are generated earlier than the ipsilaterally projecting relay neurons. Their results showed that in laminae I, VII and VIII, which are the source of ascending supraspinal axons of different lengths, the interneurons with long axons are generated earlier than the interneurons with short axons, irrespective

E14 → E15/HORIZONTAL

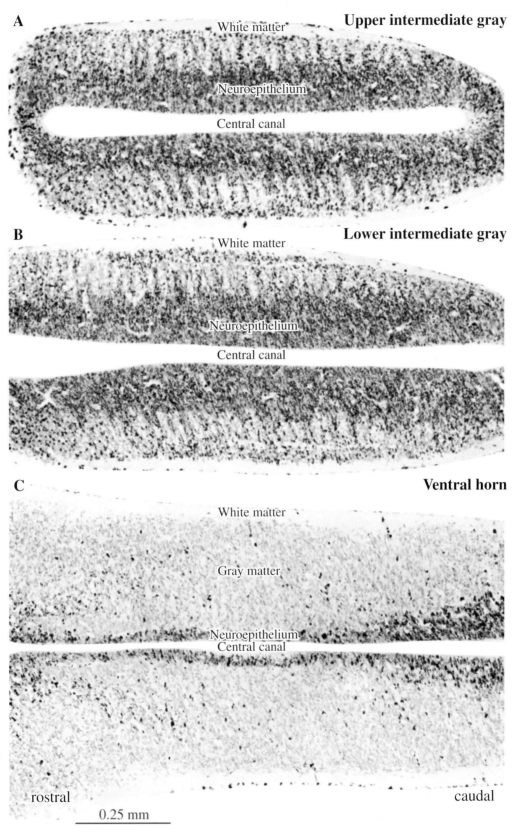

A Upper intermediate gray

White matter

Neuroepithelium

Central canal

B Lower intermediate gray

White matter

Neuroepithelium

Central canal

C Ventral horn

White matter

Gray matter

Neuroepithelium
Central canal

rostral   caudal

0.25 mm

Figure 3-76. Serial horizontal autoradiograms, from dorsal to ventral, of the cervical spinal cord of an E15 rat that was tagged with ³H-thymidine on E14. **A, B.** Alternating bands, or microsegments, composed of labeled cells (those generated after E14) and unlabeled cells (those generated before E14) in the sojourn zone and adjacent intermediate gray. **C.** There are few labeled cells in the ventral horn and no indication of any microsegmentation.

E14 → E15/SAGITTAL

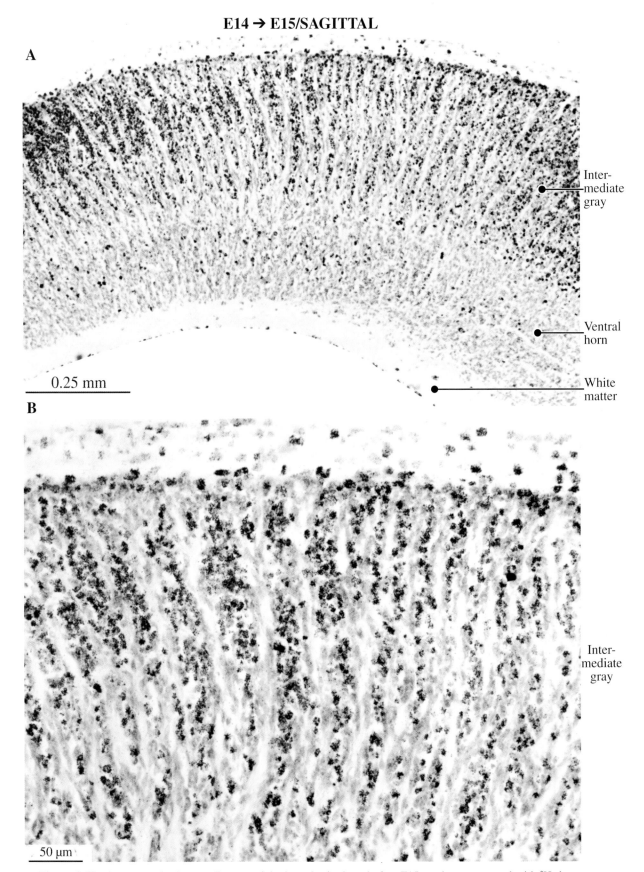

Figure 3-77. A. Parasagittal autoradiogram of the lateral spinal cord of an E15 rat that was tagged with ³H-thymidine 24 hours earlier. Labeled and unlabeled cells form alternating bands in the intermediate gray. There are few labeled cells and no hint of banding in the ventral horn. **B.** The alternating bands of round labeled cells and elongated unlabeled cells in the intermediate gray at higher magnification.

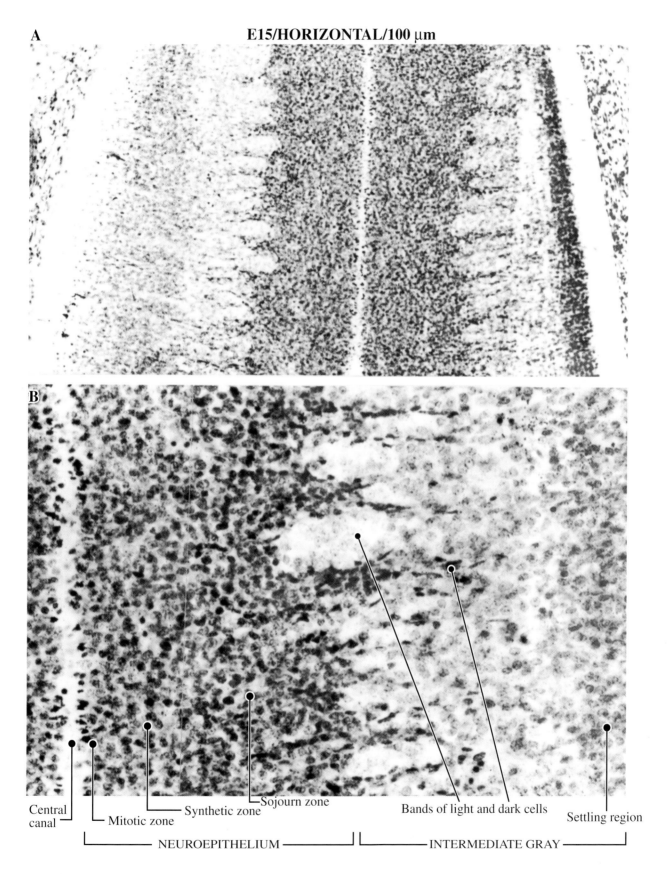

E15/HORIZONTAL/100 μm

Central canal
Mitotic zone
Synthetic zone
Sojourn zone
Bands of light and dark cells
Settling region

NEUROEPITHELIUM — INTERMEDIATE GRAY

Figure 3-78. Thick (100μm), oblique horizontal section through at the level of the intermediate gray in an E15 rat, with alternating bands of darkly staining (presumably more primitive or younger) and lightly staining (older) cells in the sojourn zone and adjacent intermediate gray, at lower **(A)** and higher **(B)** magnification. Celloidin; hematoxylin-eosin.

E15/SAGITTAL/100 μm

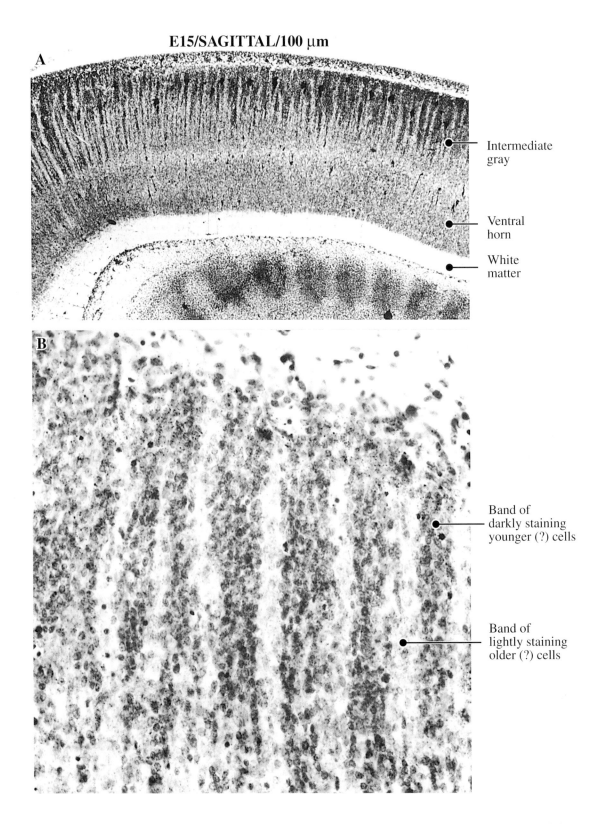

Intermediate
gray

Ventral
horn

White
matter

Band of
darkly staining
younger (?) cells

Band of
lightly staining
older (?) cells

Figure 3-79. A. Thick (100μm) parasagittal section through the lateral spinal cord of an E15 rat. Darkly staining (presumably more primitive or younger) cells and lightly staining (more mature or older) cells form alternating vertical bands (microsegments) at the interface of the sojourn zone and the intermediate gray matter. The banding is not evident in the ventral horn. **B.** Microsegmentation in the intermediate gray at higher magnification. Celloidin; hematoxylin-eosin.

E15/SAGITTAL/X-RAY

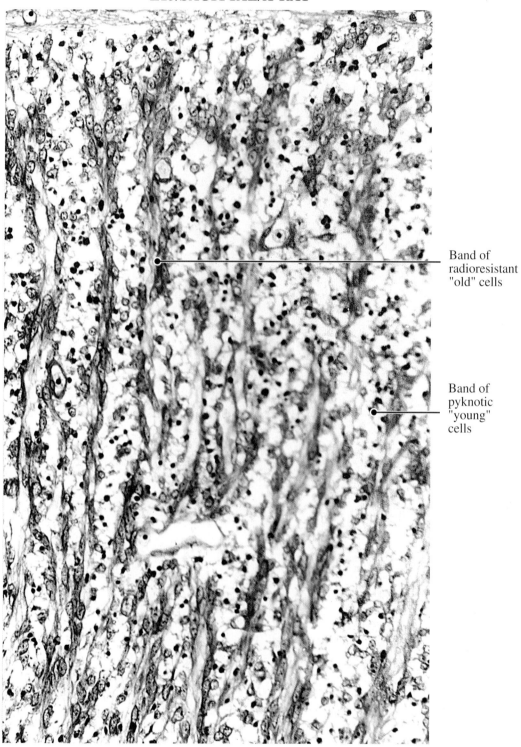

Band of
radioresistant
"old" cells

Band of
pyknotic
"young"
cells

Figure 3-80. Parasagittal section through the lateral spinal cord of an E15 rat, 6 hours after irradiation with 150R X-ray that differentially kills primitive (younger) cells but spares more mature (older) cells. The vertically oriented, spindle shaped cells of the earlier generated contralaterally projecting commissural interneurons survived, while the cells in the alternateng microsegments, presumably the later generated ipsilaterally projecting interneurons, were killed (pyknotic cells and their debris). Methacrylate; hematoxylin-eosin.

E15/HORIZONTAL/3 μm

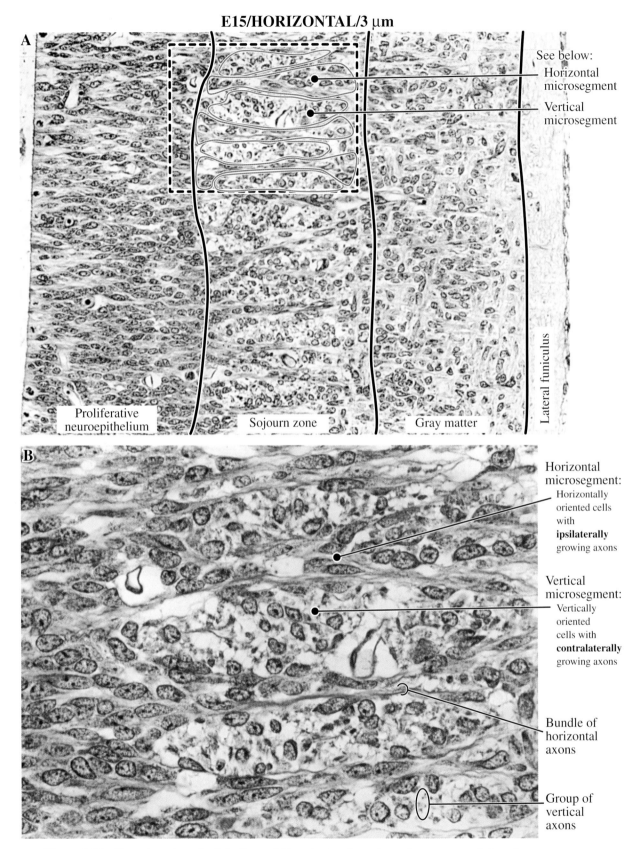

Figure 3-81. The orientation of cell bodies and fibers in the alternating microsegments of the sojourn zone and intermediate gray, in a horizontal section of an E15 rat, at lower **(A)** and higher **(B)** magnification. The microsegments composed of horizontally oriented spindle-shaped cells (red in **A**), are associated with horizontal fibers **(B)**. The microsegments composed of cells with small round profiles (blue in **A**) and fine dots **(B)** are vertically oriented, contralaterally projecting commissural interneurons. Methacrylate; hematoxylin-eosin.

whether they project contralaterally or ipsilaterally. Only in regions containing interneurons with short axons – lamina IV and the nucleus dorsalis – did they find that the contralaterally projecting relay neurons are generated earlier than the ipsilaterally projecting relay neurons. There is evidently a discrepancy between the experimental results of Nandi et al. and our observations. A possible resolution of this discrepancy (which has to be tested experimentally) is that the sequential generation of contralaterally and ipsilaterally projecting neurons (as indicated by thymidine autoradiography) and their sequential maturation (as suggested by cytological observations and the X-ray experiments), applies only to the intraspinal (propriospinal) neurons with locally terminating axons. The generation of contra- and ipsilaterally projecting interneurons with long axons that project to supraspinal targets located at various distances from the spinal cord may obey the principles discovered by Nandi et al. Our interpretation of the microsegmentation of the ipsilaterally and contralaterally projecting (and possibly locally terminating intraspinal) interneurons in the sojourn zone of the neuroepithelium is schematically summarized in Figure 3-82.

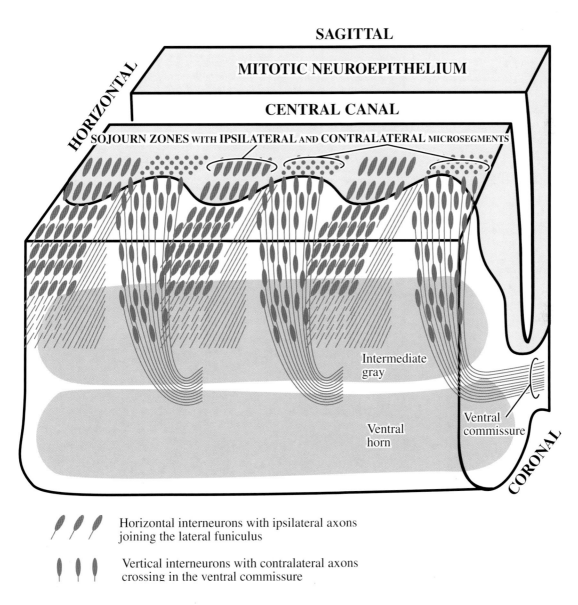

Horizontal interneurons with ipsilateral axons joining the lateral funiculus

Vertical interneurons with contralateral axons crossing in the ventral commissure

Figure 3-82. Schematic illustration of the alternating bands (microsegments) of ipsilaterally projecting (red) and contralaterally projecting (blue) interneurons of the dorsal horn. Microsegmentation is not evident in the mitotic neuroepithelium. In the sojourn zone and adjacent intermediate gray the banding is indicated by the orientation of bipolar cells either horizontally or vertically. The horizontal interneurons extrude axons that course laterally and join the lateral funiculus (not shown). The vertically oriented interneurons extrude axons that course ventrally and cross to the opposite side in the ventral commissure.

3.3.8   Maturation of Neurons of the Central Autonomic Area.

In the rat fetus that was tagged with ^{3}H-thymidine on E16 and was killed 2 hours later, labeled NEP cells surround the receding dorsal canal and the upper part of the central canal (Figure 3-83A). The population of labeled cells is higher in these locations in the fetus that survived for 24 hours after the treatment (Figure 3-83B). Finally, in the rat that survived for 48 hours after the administration of the radiochemical (Figure 3-83C), the labeled cells occupy the formative central autonomic area in the fused area above the regressed spinal canal. (There is also a small complement of late-generated dorsal horn neurons in this fetus.) Figure 3-84 illustrates the distribution of labeled cells in the central autonomic area in a perinatal rat that received two successive doses of ^{3}H-thymidine on E16 and E17. The concentration of labeled cells is appreciable in the central autonomic area but there are few labeled cells in the dorsal horn. Evidently, the central autonomic area contains the latest generated neurons of the spinal cord.

We follow the maturation of the late generated neurons of the central autonomic area in methacrylate sections. On E16 (Figure 3-85), two regions may be distinguished above the central canal: the fibrous roof plate medially and a small lateral area with a few scattered cells. By E17 (Figure 3-86), the fibrous roof plate has receded with the regressing spinal canal and the fused midline is now occupied by a mass of densely packed small cells. These are the young neurons of the central autonomic area that migrate dorsomedially as well as dorsolaterally. By E18 (Figure 3-87), there are two distinct regions in the central autonomic area: (i) an arm around the growing dorsal funiculus with circumferentially oriented cells, and (ii) a midline core region composed mostly of vertically oriented cells. This is the maturing central autonomic area. The distribution of the latest generated neurons in the core and arms of the central autonomic area in an adult (P60) rat that was tagged with ^{3}H-thymidine on E15 and E16 is seen in Figure 3-88. The labeled cells occupy an area that we have previously described as the internal trajectory of visceral afferents (Figures 1-32, 1-33, 1-34).

3.3.9   Summary: Neuroepithelial Mosaicism in the Spinal Cord.

After the neural groove has fused, the primordial spinal cord consists of three components, the roof plate, the floor plate, and the neuroepithelium (the lateral plates). The proliferative neuroepithelium, the sole source of all the neural elements of the spinal cord, initially expands uniformly along the slit-shaped spinal canal. However, subsequent changes in the shape of the spinal canal, in the proliferative dynamics of NEP cells, and in the sequential order of neurogenesis indicate that the spinal cord neuroepithelium is a mosaic germinal matrix. The spinal canal first expands ventrally, and the active ventral neuroepithelium that surrounds the enlarged ventral canal generates the motoneurons of the ventral horn. The ventral neuroepithelium then recedes, and heightened proliferative activity shifts to the lower intermediate neuroepithelium, the source of the bulk of the intermediate gray interneurons. Next, proliferative activity shifts to the dorsal neuroepithelium, and that is followed by the generation of the sensory microneurons of the expanding dorsal horn. Finally, a persisting active neuroepithelial site that surrounds the receding dorsal canal is the source of the latest generated neurons of the central autonomic area.

According to this interpretation, the sequential production of different classes of spinal cord neurons is due to shifts in maximal proliferative activity from one neuroepithelial mosaic to another as development proceeds. Whether or not, or to what extent, these shifts in proliferative dynamics are due to intrinsic genetic mechanism or to extrinsic epigenetic influences, is a question that has to be determined experimentally. Nor do we know whether the differences in the time of production of different subclasses of neurons within the large divisons of the spinal cord – e.g., motoneurons of the lateral and medial columns; small and large neurons of the intermediate gray; and small and large neurons of the dorsal horn – are also due to finer-grained mosaicism within the different neuroepithelial compartments or are due to extrinsic influences.

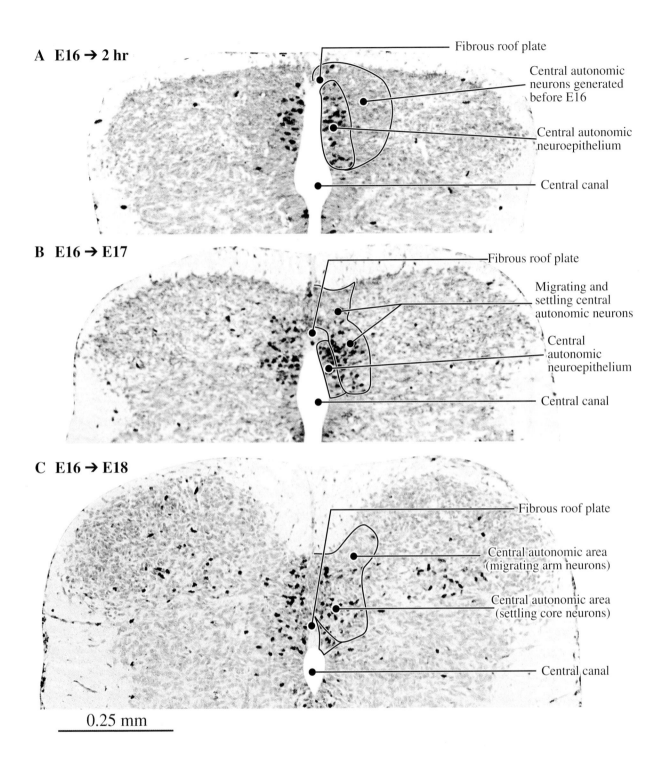

A E16 → 2 hr

Fibrous roof plate

Central autonomic
neurons generated
before E16

Central autonomic
neuroepithelium

Central canal

B E16 → E17

Fibrous roof plate

Migrating and
settling central
autonomic neurons

Central
autonomic
neuroepithelium

Central canal

C E16 → E18

Fibrous roof plate

Central autonomic area
(migrating arm neurons)

Central autonomic area
(settling core neurons)

Central canal

0.25 mm

Figure 3-83. A. In the rat tagged with ³H-thymidine on E16 and killed 2 hours later, labeled cells abound in a portion of
the dorsal neuroepithelium. **B.** In the rat that was tagged on E16 and killed on E17, the labeled cells start to penetrate the
fusing midline area above the receding dorsal canal. **C.** In the rat that was tagged on E16 and killed on E18, the labeled
cells are settling in the central autonomic area above the permanent central canal. Autoradiogram; paraffin.

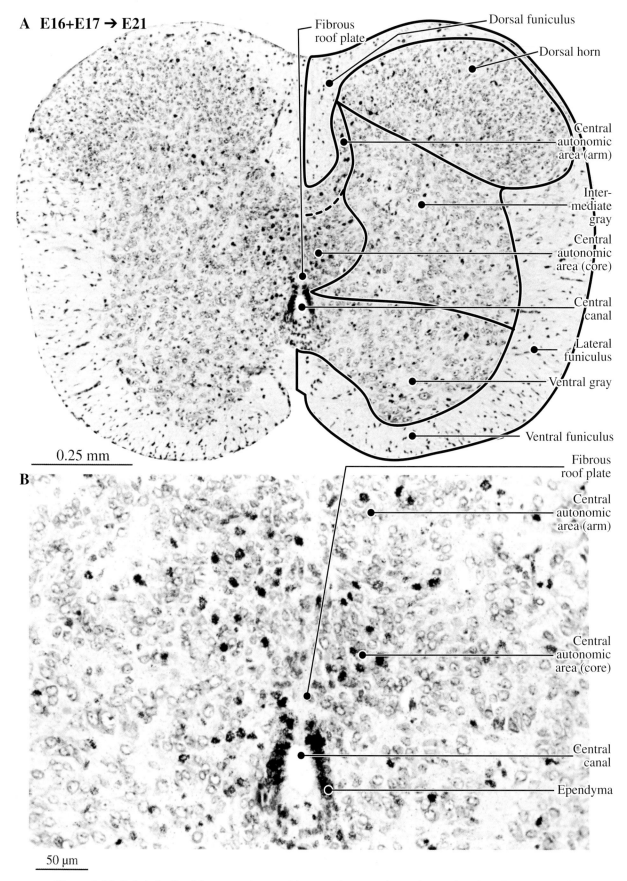

Figure 3-84. Labeled cells of the core and arms of the central autonomic area in a perinatal rat that was tagged with ^{3}H-thymidine on E16 at lower (**A**) and higher (**B**) magnification. The concentration of cells generated on E16 is higher in the central autonomic area than in the dorsal horn. Autoradiogram; paraffin.

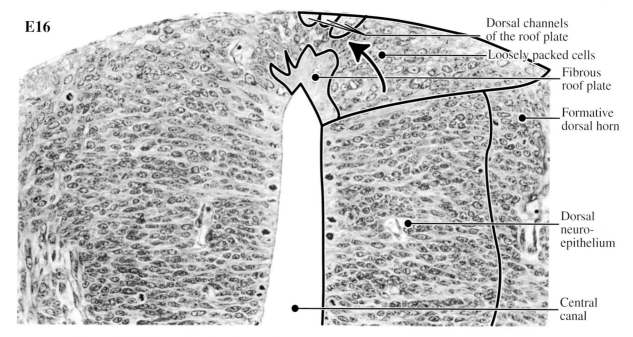

E16

Dorsal channels
of the roof plate

Loosely packed cells

Fibrous
roof plate

Formative
dorsal horn

Dorsal
neuro-
epithelium

Central
canal

Figure 3-85. The region above the dorsal canal is occupied by the roof plate medially and some loosely packed cells laterally in this E16 rat. Methacrylate; hematoxylin-eosin.

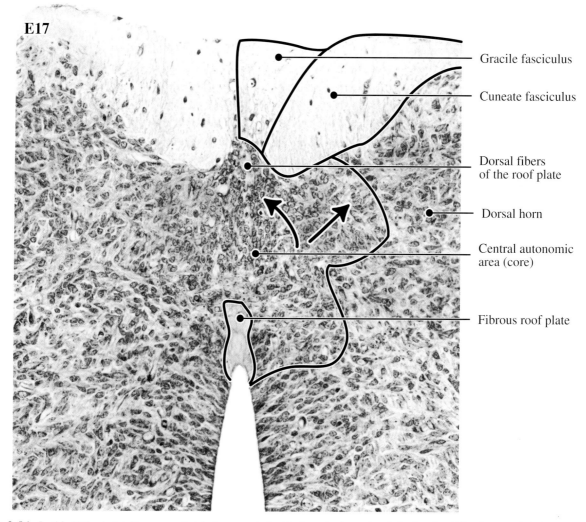

E17

Gracile fasciculus

Cuneate fasciculus

Dorsal fibers
of the roof plate

Dorsal horn

Central autonomic
area (core)

Fibrous roof plate

Figure 3-86. In this E17 rat, the fibrous roof plate has receded with the spinal canal and the fused midline is occupied by the cells of the central autonomic area that migrate dorsomedially and dorsolaterally (arrows). Methacrylate; hematoxylin-eosin.

E18

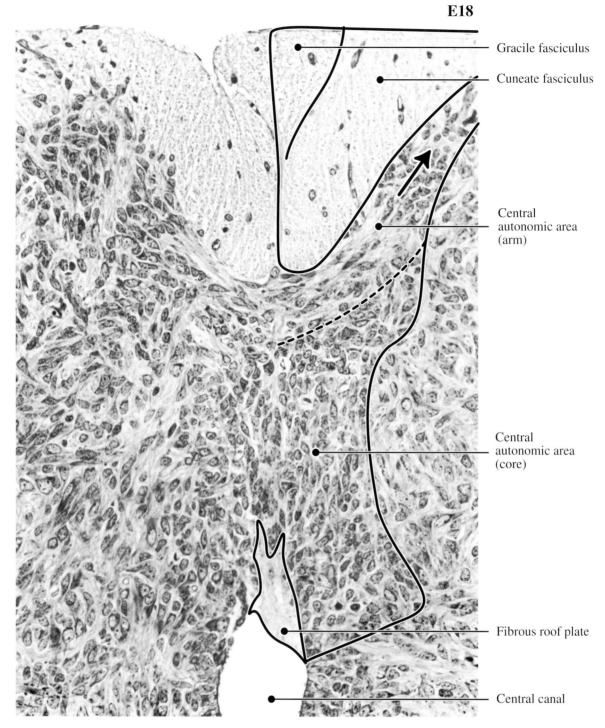

Gracile fasciculus

Cuneate fasciculus

Central
autonomic area
(arm)

Central
autonomic area
(core)

Fibrous roof plate

Central canal

Figure 3-87. In this E18 rat, the core region of the central autonomic area contains vertically oriented cells, and its arms contain circumferentially oriented cells beneath the deepening dorsal funiculus. Methacrylate; hematoxylin-eosin.

Figure 3-88. Autoradiogram from an adult (P60) rat that was tagged with ^{3}H-thymidine on E15 and E16. Note the high concentration of labeled neurons in the core and the arm of the central autonomic area.

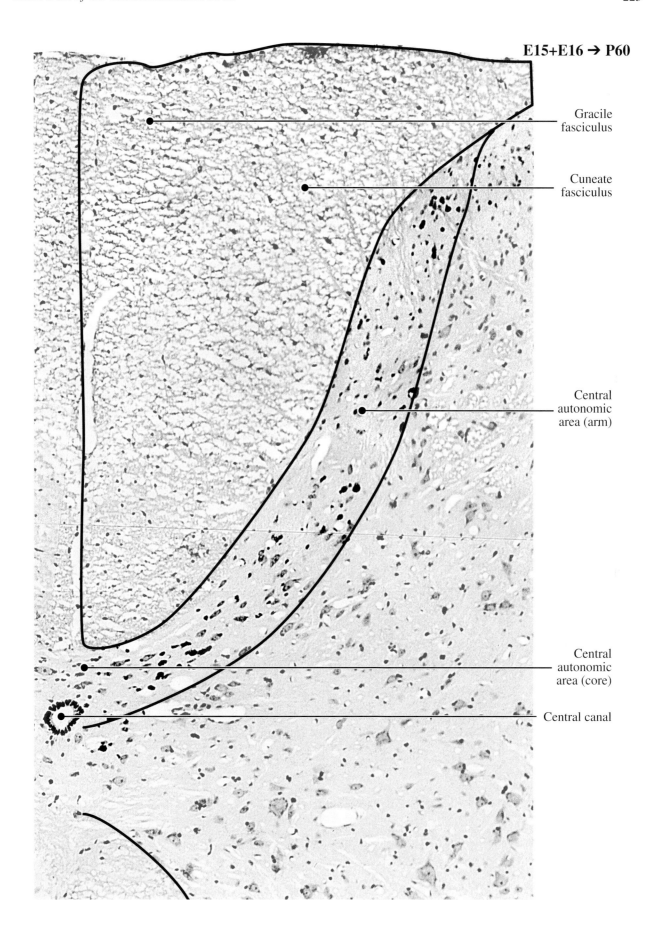

E15+E16 → P60

Gracile
fasciculus

Cuneate
fasciculus

Central
autonomic
area (arm)

Central
autonomic
area (core)

Central canal

4 EXPERIMENTAL STUDIES OF THE GROWTH OF THE ASCENDING AND DESCENDING AXONS AND FIBER TRACTS OF THE SPINAL CORD

4.1 Maturation of Ganglion Cells and the Initial Growth of Dorsal Root Axons

4.1.1 Differentiation and Maturation of Ganglion Cells. According to our quantitative data (Figure 3-21) about 20% of the dorsal root ganglion cells differentiate (become postmitotic) at the cervical level of the rat spinal cord by E12. However, ganglion cell production is a prolonged process and peak production does not occur until E14. In the autoradiogram from a rat labeled with ³H-thymidine on E13 and killed on E14 (Figure 4-1), labeled and unlabeled cells are randomly distributed within the spinal ganglion, indicating that there is no special compartment where the precursors of sensory neurons proliferate. But there is a difference between the production of large and small ganglion cells. In perinatal (E21) rats in which of ³H-thymidine administration was begun on E13 (Figure 4-2A), the majority of both large and small ganglion cells are labeled at cervical levels. In rats in which exposure to the radiochemical was delayed until E14 (Figure 4-2B), most of the small ganglion cells are labeled but only a few of the large ganglion cells. Evidently, the generation of most of

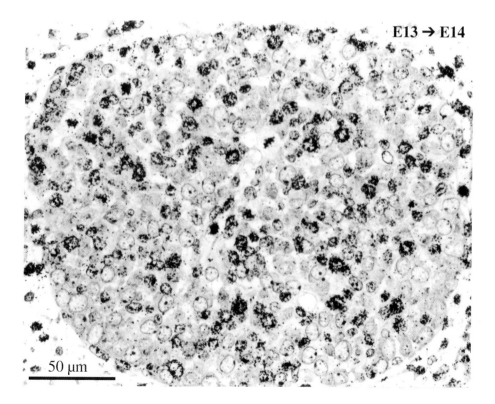

E13 → E14

Figure 4-1. Distribution of labeled dorsal root ganglion cells at the cervical level of the spinal cord in a rat tagged with ³H-thymidine on E13 and killed on E14. The unlabeled cells (those that have become postmitotic before the morning of E13) and the labeled cells (cells still proliferating on E13) are randomly distributed within the ganglion. Autoradiogram; paraffin.

50 μm

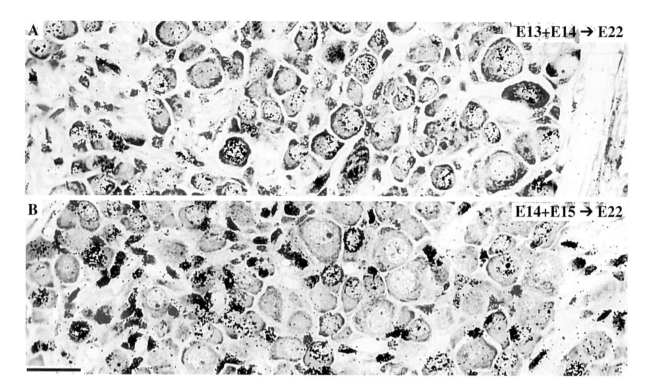

Figure 4-2. A. Most dorsal root ganglion cells are labeled at the cervical level of the spinal cord in the perinatal (E22) rat that was tagged with ³H-thymidine beginning on E13. **B.** Many of the large ganglion cells are no longer labeled in the perinatal rat that was tagged with ³H-thymidine beginning on E14. Autoradiogram. (Scale = 30 μm)

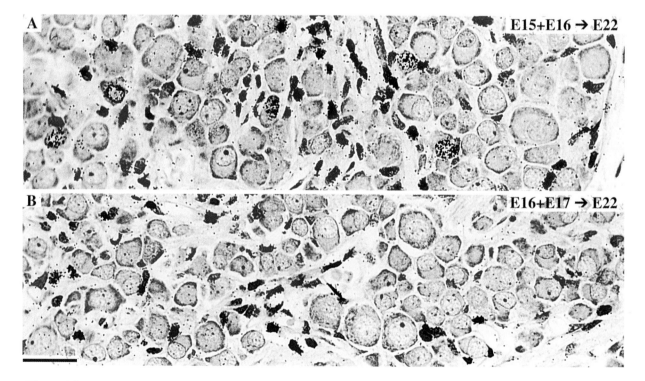

Figure 4-3. A. In the perinatal rat that was tagged with ³H-thymidine beginning on E15, the proportion of labeled small ganglion cells has decreased. **B.** In the perinatal rat in which the administration of ³H-thymidine was delayed until E16, none of the ganglion cells but virtually all the spindle-shaped Schwann (satellite) cells are labeled. Autoradiogram. (Scale = 30 μm)

the large ganglion cells ends before the morning of E14. In rats exposed to ³H-thymidine beginning on E15 (Figure 4-3A), only a few of the small ganglion cells are labeled, and in rats in which the administration of the radiochemical was delayed until on E16 the small ganglion cells are no longer labeled (Figure 4-3B). It is concluded, therefore, that the production of ganglion cells ends on E15. However, since most of the spindle-shaped interfascicular glia cells are labeled, gliogenesis (the production of Schwann cells) must trail neurogenesis in the peripheral spinal ganglia much in the same way as it does in the central nervous system.

The first hint of the formation of dorsal root ganglia at cervical levels of the spinal cord is seen in methacrylate sections on E12 (Figure 4-4); this correlates with the first day of ganglion cell neurogenesis. There is as yet no indication of the sprouting of dorsal root fibers. By E13, the dorsal root ganglia have become appreciably larger and contain tightly packed bipolar cells and an occasional mitotic cell (Figure 4-5). The bipolar ganglion cells are vertically aligned within the dorsal root ganglion (Figure 4-6); these cells must be the source of the proximal axons (neurites) that reach the spinal cord (Figure 4-5) and the distal axons (neurites) that grow peripherally (Figure 4-6). While some of the ganglion cells are still spindle-shaped on E14, others are becoming spherical, and some display an eccentric cytoplasmic swelling (Figure 4-7). There are still many mitotic cells. By E15, the proportion of ganglion cells with a swollen and darkly staining eccentric cytoplasm increases, as seen in coronal (Figure 4-8) and horizontal (Figure 4-9) sections.

The continuing growth and transformation of spinal ganglion cells at cervical levels of the spinal cord between E16 and E19 is seen in horizontal sections in Figures 4-10, 4-11, 4-12. On E16 (Figure 4-10A), the closely spaced dorsal root ganglia are filled with tightly packed ganglion cells with round

E12 Cervical

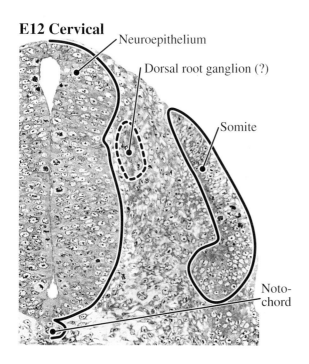

Figure 4-4. The formative dorsal root ganglion at the cervical level of the spinal cord in an E12 rat. The somites are still present at this stage of embryonic development. Methacrylate; hematoxylin-eosin.

E13 Cervical

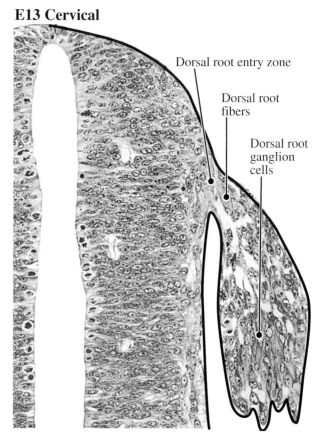

Figure 4-5. Growth of the dorsal root ganglion and the arrival of a few dorsal root fibers at the dorsal root entry zone of the cervical spinal cord in an E13 rat. Methacrylate; hematoxylin-eosin.

A   **Sagittal**   **E13**

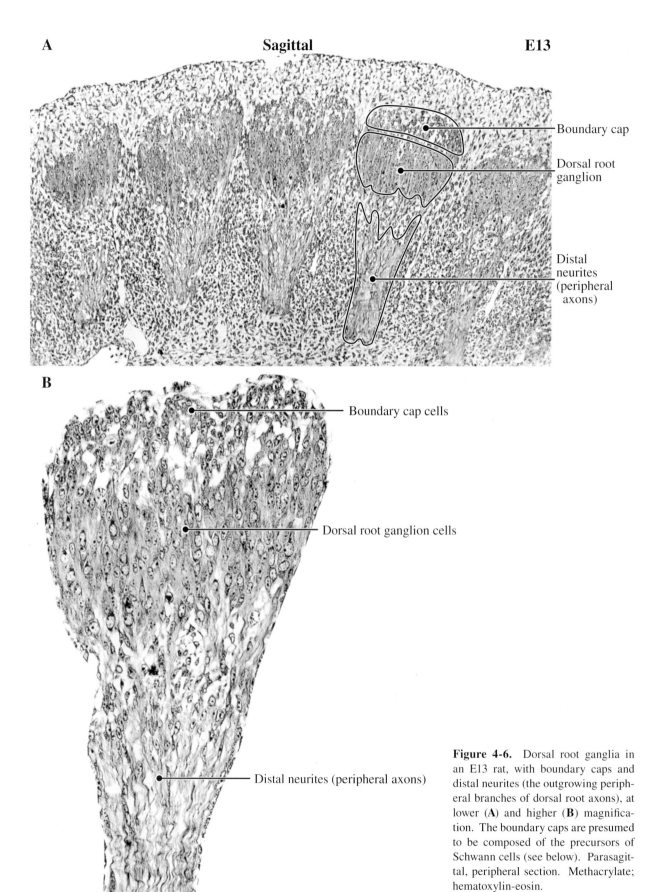

Figure 4-6. Dorsal root ganglia in an E13 rat, with boundary caps and distal neurites (the outgrowing peripheral branches of dorsal root axons), at lower (**A**) and higher (**B**) magnification. The boundary caps are presumed to be composed of the precursors of Schwann cells (see below). Parasagittal, peripheral section. Methacrylate; hematoxylin-eosin.

E14 Coronal

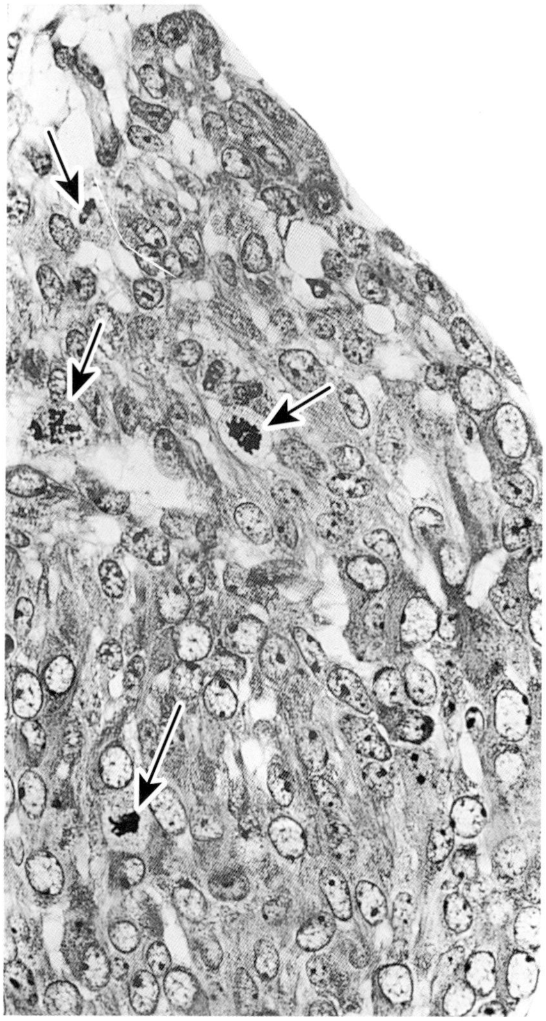

Figure 4-7. Spherical, bipolar, and mitotic (arrows) cells in a coronal section of the dorsal root ganglion in an E14 rat. Methacrylate; hematoxylin-eosin.

E15 Coronal

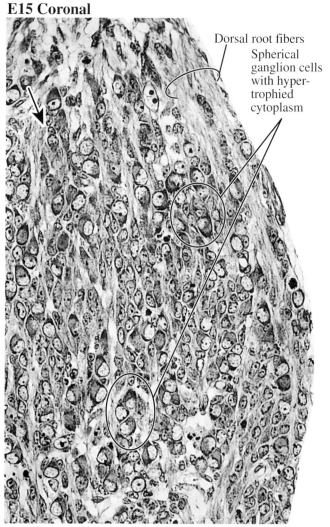

Dorsal root fibers

Spherical ganglion cells with hypertrophied cytoplasm

Figure 4-8. Ganglion cells with spherical nuclei and hypertrophied cytoplasm in a coronal section of the dorsal root ganglion in an E15 rat. Methacrylate; hematoxylin-eosin.

E15 Horizontal

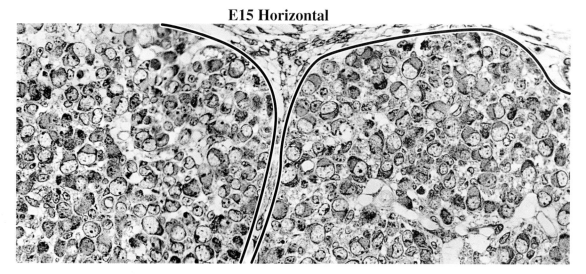

Figure 4-9. Two contiguous dorsal root ganglia in horizontal section in an E15 rat. Many of the ganglion cells have spherical nuclei and darkly staining, hypertrophied cytoplasm. Methacrylate; hematoxylin-eosin.

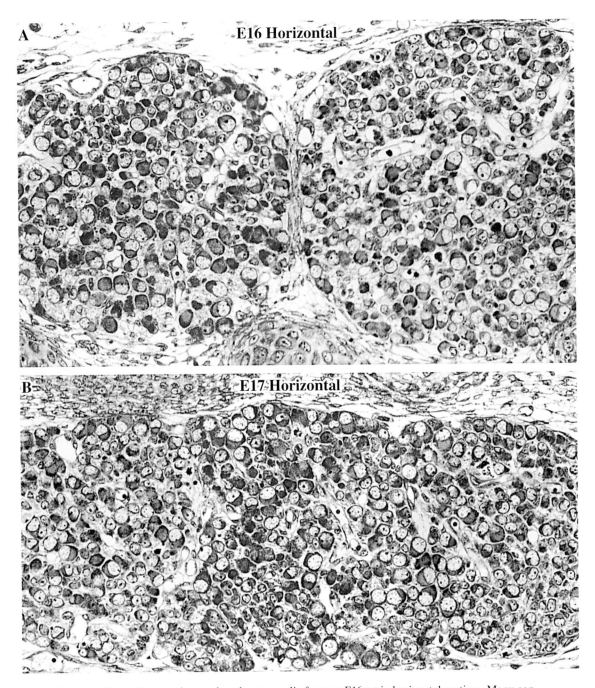

Figure 4-10. A. Two contiguous dorsal root ganglia from an E16 rat in horizontal section. Many ganglion cells have a spherical nucleus and an eccentric hypertrophic cytoplasm. **B.** A larger dorsal root ganglion in with similar cytological features in an E17 rat. Methacrylate; hematoxylin-eosin.

nuclei and an eccentric, hypertrophied darkly staining cytoplasm. By E17 (Figure 4-10B), the dorsal root ganglia elongate in the rostrocaudal plane but the eccentric cytoplasm of ganglion cells remains as prominent as on the previous day. By E18 (Figure 4-11A) and E19 (Figure 4-11B), the packing density of ganglion cells starts to decrease and the cytoplasm of many ganglion cells have become more concen-

tric. By E19, the fibers that traverse the spinal ganglion contain spindle shaped Schwann cells oriented in various planes (Figure 4-12). The progressive segregation of dorsal ganglia in the longituninal plane between E15 and E19 in relation to the growth of the bony vertebrae is seen in Figure 4-13. Finally, the rostrocaudal gradient in the maturation of ganglion cells, in terms of the decreasing size and increasing pack-

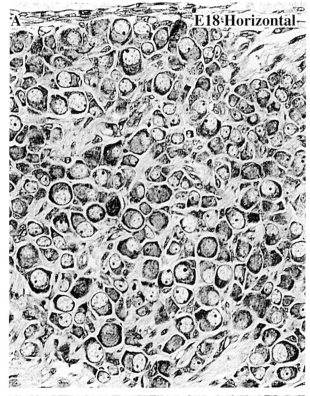

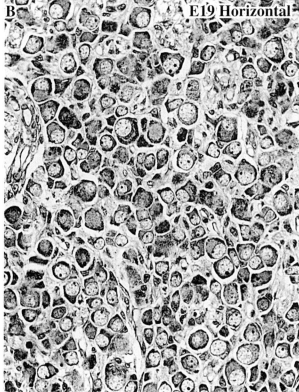

Figure 4-11. Growth of dorsal root ganglion cells in an E18 (**A**) and an E19 (**B**) rat. The proportion of ganglion cells with a spherical nucleus and hypertrophied cytoplasm has increased. Methacrylate; hematoxylin-eosin.

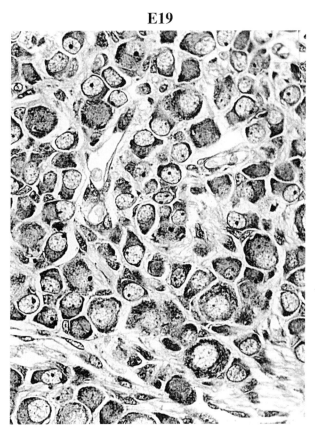

Figure 4-12. Small and large ganglion cells, and some spindle-shaped satellite cells in the dorsal root ganglion of an E19 rat. Methacrylate; hematoxylin-eosin.

ing density of ganglion cells, is illustrated in Figure 4-14 in a single animal at the cervical, the lumbar, and the sacral levels of the spinal cord.

Barber and Vaughn (1986) injected HRP into the developing spinal cord of mouse embryos to retrogradely label spinal ganglion cells (Figure 4-15). They found that on E12 (the mouse spinal cord matures about 2 days earlier than the rat), the spindle-shaped spinal ganglion cells had neurites sprouting at the two poles. By E13, the cytoplasm of ganglion cells became eccentric (they called this the early transitional bipolar stage) and the polar neurites began to slide sideways. That change became more pronounced by E14 (late transitional bipolar stage), and by E15 many ganglion cells became pseudounipolar. Based on the findings of Barber and Vaughn and our own observations, the sequence in the maturation of ganglion cells, with reference to the corresponding embryonic ages in rats, is summarized in Figure 4-16.

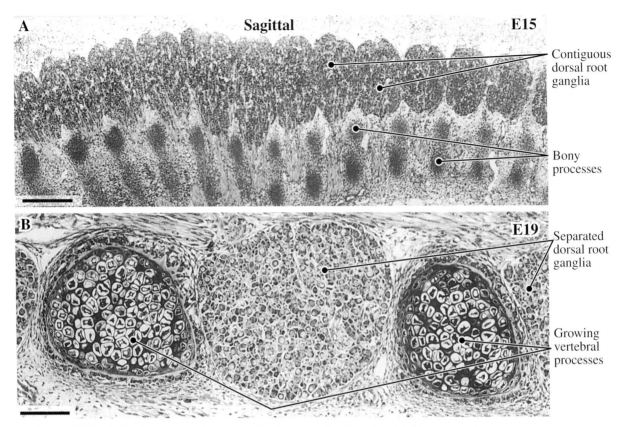

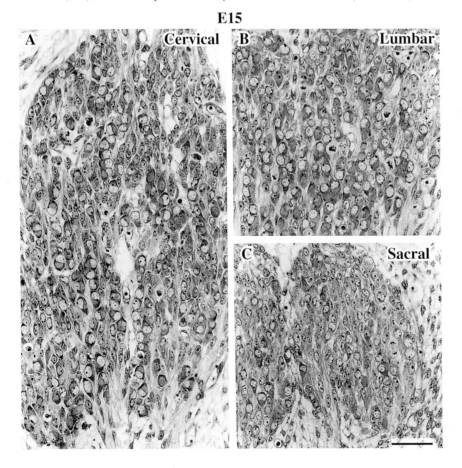

Figure 4-13. **A.** Contiguous dorsal root ganglia with ventrally situated vertebral processes in a sagittal section of an E15 rat. **B.** Separation of the dorsal root ganglia by the expanding vertebral processes in an older (E19) rat. Methacrylate; hematoxylin-eosin. (Scales: **A**, 300 μm; **B**, 100 μm)

Figure 4-14. Rostral-to-caudal gradient in the growth of the dorsal root ganglia, and in the size and maturation of ganglion cells, in an E15 rat at cervical (**A**), lumbar (**B**), and sacral (**C**) levels of the spinal cord. Sagittal sections. Methacrylate; hematoxylin-eosin. (Scale = 50 μm)

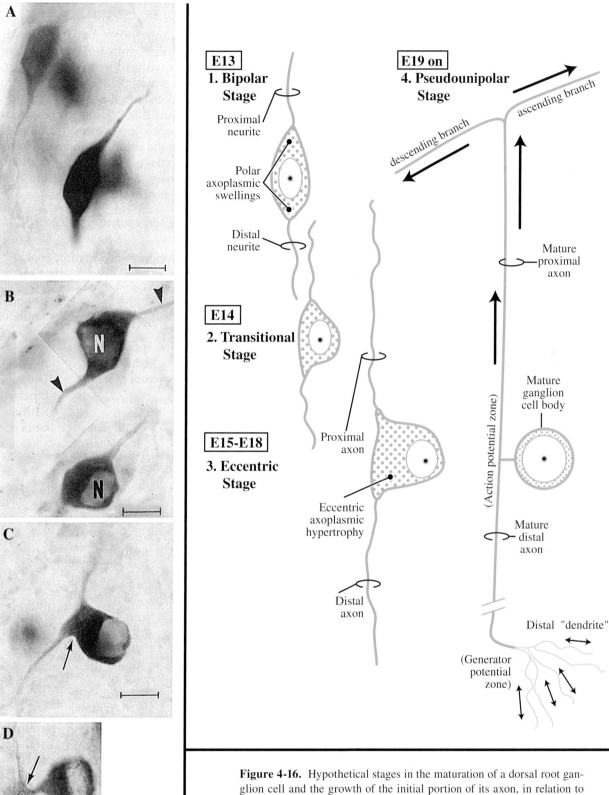

A

B

N

N

C

D

Figure 4-15. Transformation of dorsal root ganglion cells in the mouse from the primitive bipolar stage (**A**) to the mature pseudounipolar stage (**D**). After Barber and Vaughn (1986). HRP technique.

E13
1. Bipolar Stage

Proximal neurite

Polar axoplasmic swellings

Distal neurite

E14
2. Transitional Stage

Proximal axon

E15-E18
3. Eccentric Stage

Eccentric axoplasmic hypertrophy

Distal axon

E19 on
4. Pseudounipolar Stage

descending branch

ascending branch

Mature proximal axon

(Action potential zone)

Mature ganglion cell body

Mature distal axon

Distal "dendrite"

(Generator potential zone)

Figure 4-16. Hypothetical stages in the maturation of a dorsal root ganglion cell and the growth of the initial portion of its axon, in relation to the embryonic ages in the rat. The regional physiological properties of the axon indicated on E19 are based on studies in adults. (For the subsequent central branching of the dorsal root axon, see Figures 4-41 to 4-43.)

4.1.2   Arrival of Dorsal Root Axons at the Spinal Cord. The earliest proximal dorsal root axons reach the dorsolateral wall of the cervical spinal cord by E13 and begin to penetrate the spinal cord at a site called the dorsal root entry zone (Figure 4-17). By E14 (Figure 4-18A), the dorsal root axons that entered the spinal cord form a distinct structure, traditionally known as the oval bundle of His. Oblique sagittal sections (Figure 4-18B) reveal that the oval bundle

of His is the site where the dorsal root axons bifurcate into ascending and descending branches. For this reason we called this site the dorsal root bifurcation zone (Altman and Bayer, 1984). That section also shows that the dorsal root fibers enter the cord as small rootlets distributed rostrocaudally. By E14, the distal branches of dorsal root axons have joined the spinal nerve that proceeds some distance peripherally (Figure 4-19).

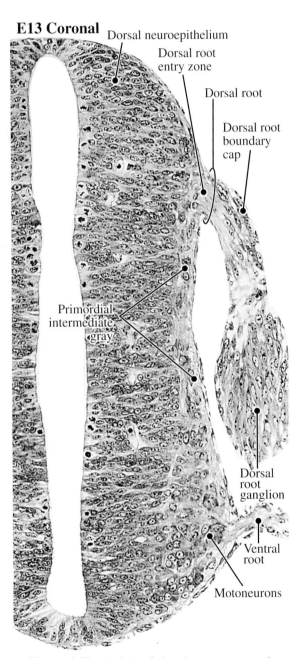

E13 Coronal

Dorsal neuroepithelium
Dorsal root entry zone
Dorsal root
Dorsal root boundary cap
Primordial intermediate gray
Dorsal root ganglion
Ventral root
Motoneurons

Figure 4-17. Arrival of dorsal root axons at the cervical spinal cord in an E13 rat. The primary afferent fibers pass through the boundary cap outside the spinal cord and form inside it the dorsal root entry zone. Methacrylate; hematoxylin-eosin.

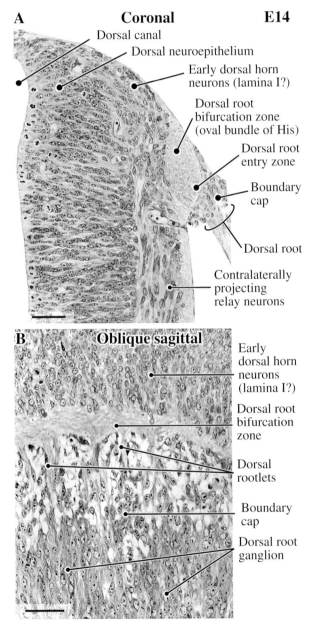

A   Coronal   E14

Dorsal canal
Dorsal neuroepithelium
Early dorsal horn neurons (lamina I?)
Dorsal root bifurcation zone (oval bundle of His)
Dorsal root entry zone
Boundary cap
Dorsal root
Contralaterally projecting relay neurons

B   Oblique sagittal

Early dorsal horn neurons (lamina I?)
Dorsal root bifurcation zone
Dorsal rootlets
Boundary cap
Dorsal root ganglion

Figure 4-18. The dorsal root bifurcation zone (oval bundle of His) in coronal (**A**) and oblique sagittal (**B**) sections in E14 rats. In the sagittal section the bifurcating fibers are cut parallel to their trajectory. Methacrylate; hematoxylin-eosin. (Scales = 50 μm)

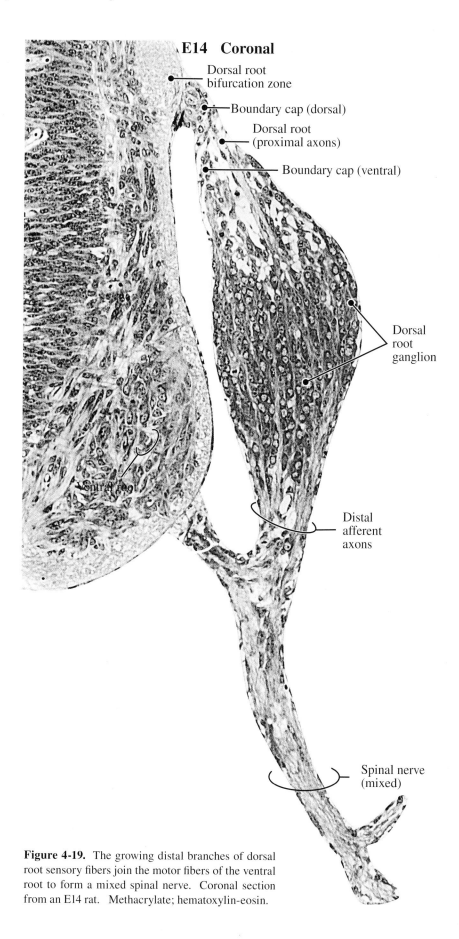

E14 Coronal

Dorsal root
bifurcation zone

Boundary cap (dorsal)

Dorsal root
(proximal axons)

Boundary cap (ventral)

Dorsal
root
ganglion

Ventral root

Distal
afferent
axons

Spinal nerve
(mixed)

Figure 4-19. The growing distal branches of dorsal
root sensory fibers join the motor fibers of the ventral
root to form a mixed spinal nerve. Coronal section
from an E14 rat. Methacrylate; hematoxylin-eosin.

4.1.3   *Components of the Boundary Cap.*

The dorsal root sensory fibers pass through an aggregate of cells adjacent to the external wall of the spinal cord, called the boundary cap (Altman and Bayer, 1984). The boundary cap is identifiable by E13 (Figure 4-20A), before the spinal cord bifurcation zone (the oval bundle of His) forms (see Figure 4-17). On E13, the boundary cap consists of a well developed dorsal component with caplets (Figure 4-20A) and an incipient ventral component (Figure 4-21). By E14, the ventral component starts to expand (Figure 4-20B) in association with the great expansion of the dorsal root ganglion(Figure 4-19). We shall see later that the dorsal boundary cap remains attached to the wall of the spinal cord as long as it persists, whereas the cells of the ventral boundary cap disperse among the lengthening proximal fibers of the dorsal root as the ganglion descends ventrally. The dorsal boundary cap cells form discrete clusters, called caplets (Figures 4-21 and 4-22). Each caplet may be the matrix through which the dorsal rootlets pass as they penetrate the spinal cord (Figure 4-23).

Boundary cap cells and dorsal root ganglion-cells have different cytological features. In particular, boundary cap cells lack the extensive cytoplasm of maturing spinal ganglion cells (compare the two types of cells in Figures 4-22A and 4-22B). While both the boundary cap cells and the ganglion cells are mitotically active, the rate of boundary cap cell proliferation is much higher. This can be seen in autoradiograms of rat embryos that were labeled with ^{3}H-thymidine on E14 and killed 2 hours later (Figures 4-24, 4-25).

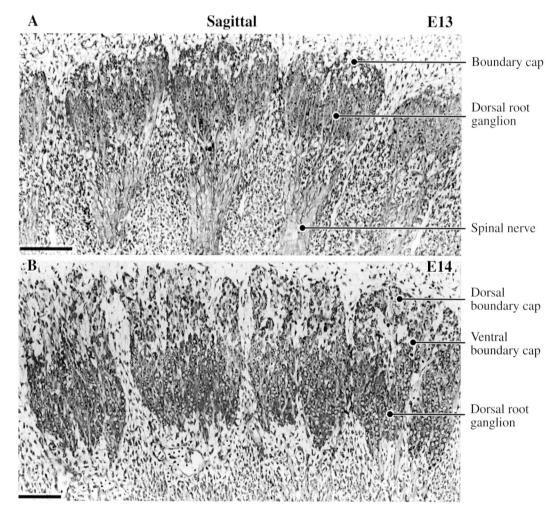

Figure 4-20. A. Boundary caps overlying individual dorsal root ganglia at the cervical level of the spinal cord in an E13 rat. **B.** Separation of the boundary caps into a dorsal and a ventral component in an E14 rat. Methacrylate; hematoxylin-eosin. (Scales = 500 μm)

We postulate that the dorsal and ventral divisions of the boundary cap are composed of two different types of multiplying Schwann cell precursors. The round cells of the dorsal division are stationary satellite cells that never pass through the wall of the spinal cord with the entering and bifurcating fibers of the dorsal root (Figures 4-26, 4-27). They are either immobile elements or are denied entrance into the central nervous system. The cells of the ventral boundary cap, in contrast, become elongated and join the fibers of the lengthening proximal dorsal root (Figure 4-26). These ventral cells multiply at a high rate as they spread peripherally with the growing fascicles of the dorsal root (Figure 4-27). However, as seen in the latter illustration, the satellite cells of both divisions of the boundary cap continue to proliferate briskly after ganglion cell neurogenesis has stopped on E16 (Figure 4-27).

Relevant in this developmental context is the recent experimental finding that Schwann cells exert a trophic influence on the growth of regenerating

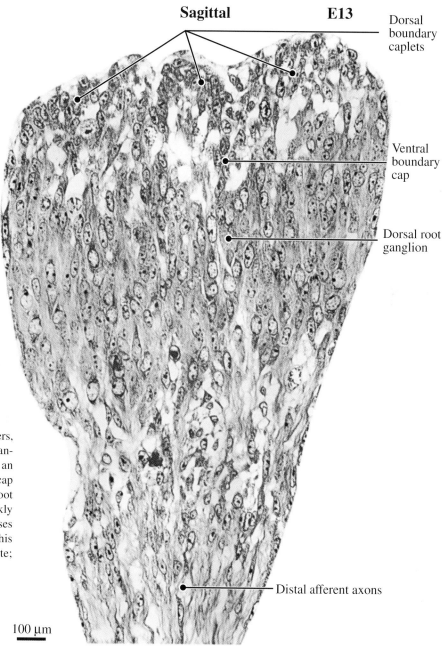

Sagittal   **E13**

Dorsal boundary caplets

Ventral boundary cap

Dorsal root ganglion

Distal afferent axons

100 μm

Figure 4-21. Boundary cap clusters, or caplets, of a single dorsal root ganglion, in a sagittal section from an E13 rat. Note that the boundary cap cells are smaller than the dorsal root ganglion cells and lack the darkly staining bipolar cytoplasmic processes that characterize ganglion cells at this stage of development. Methacrylate; hematoxylin-eosin.

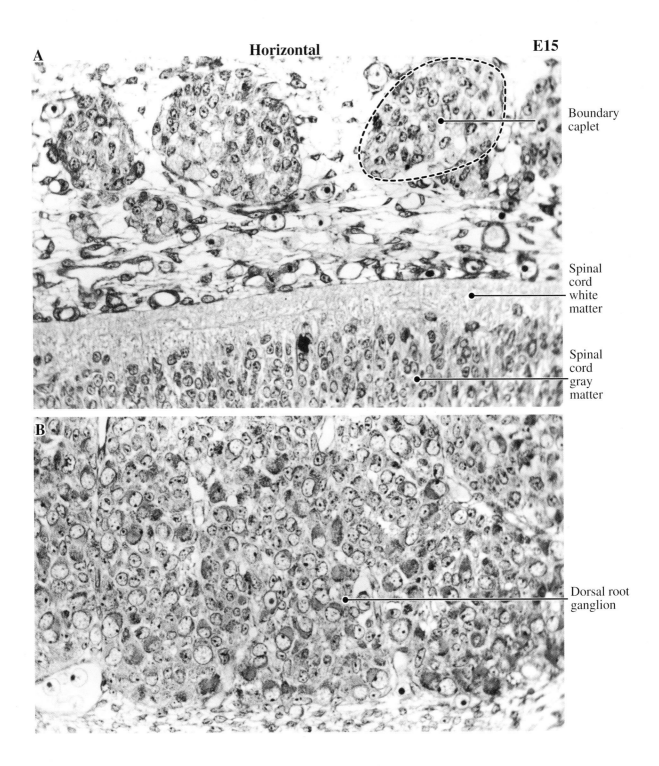

Figure 4-22. Horizontal sections at a dorsal (**A**) and a ventral (**B**) level of the cervical spinal cord in an E15 rat show the topographic relationship between several boundary caplets above a single dorsal root ganglion The small size of the boundary cap cells and the large size of ganglion cells (which now display an eccentric nucleus and a hypertrophic cytoplasm) is more obvious than at earlier ages. Methacrylate; hematoxylin-eosin.

peripheral nerves (Fawcett and Keynes, 1990). Moreover, the addition of Schwann cells to the spinal cord of normal adult rats is reported to induce the sprouting of nearby axons (Li and Raisman, 1994). In a direct test of the role of boundary cap cells in the guidance of peripheral fibers, Golding and Cohen (1997) found that neurites of dorsal root ganglion cells that enter the spinal cord do so preferentially over boundary cap cells. We shall return later to the fate of the dorsal boundary cap cells in the course of spinal cord development.

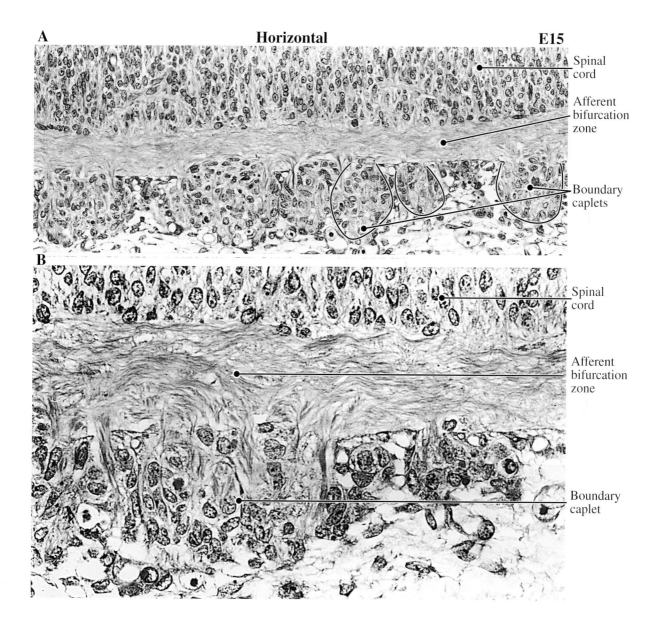

Figure 4-23. A horizontal section through the cervical spinal cord of an E15 rat, at lower (**A**) and higher (**B**) magnification, showing the relationship between individual boundary caplets and the bifurcating fibers of dorsal rootlets. The proximal dorsal root fibers traverse the boundary caplets (where the pial membrane of the spinal cord is seemingly absent) and, upon entering the cord, split into ascending and descending branches. Methacrylate; hematoxylin-eosin.

Coronal   **E14 → 2hr**

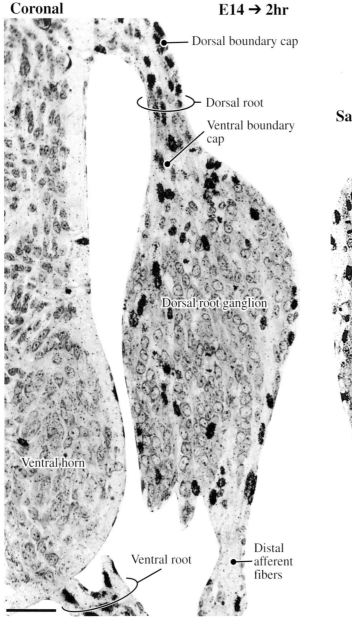

Figure 4-24. Labeled (proliferating) cells of the dorsal and ventral division of the boundary cap in a short-survival coronal autoradiogram from an E14 rat. Methacrylate embedded tissue. (Scale = 50 μm)

Sagittal   **E14 → 2hr**

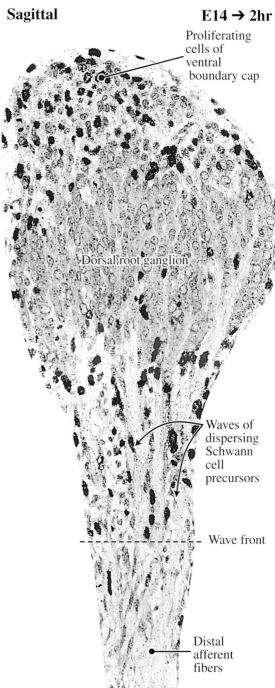

Figure 4-25. Labeled (proliferating) cells in the ventral division of the boundary cap, and the advancing wave of dispersing Schwann cell precursors in the distal portion of the sensory nerve, in a short survival sagittal autoradiogram from another E14 rat. Methacrylate embedded tissue.

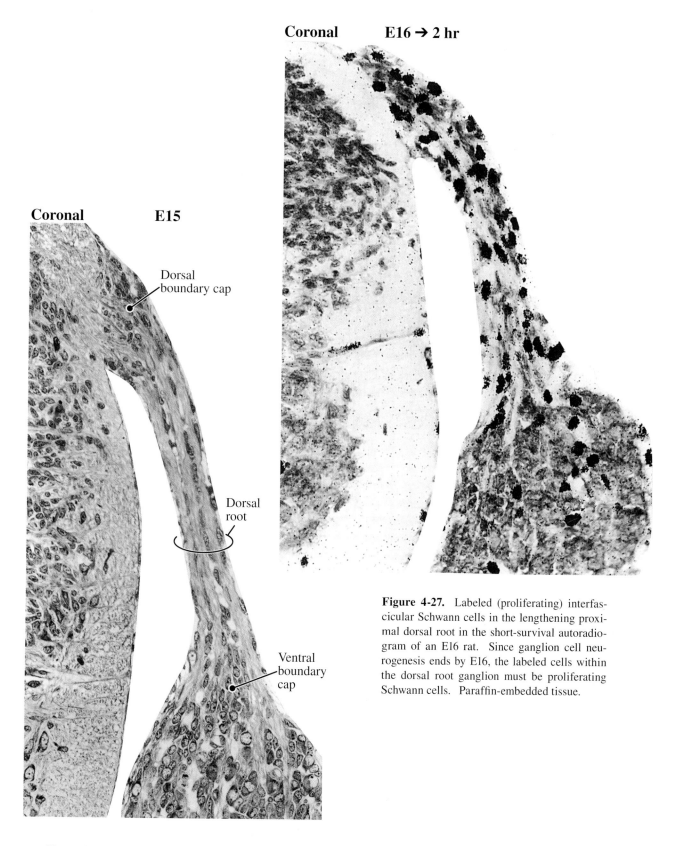

Coronal   **E16 → 2 hr**

Coronal   **E15**

Dorsal
boundary cap

Dorsal
root

Ventral
boundary
cap

Figure 4-27. Labeled (proliferating) interfascicular Schwann cells in the lengthening proximal dorsal root in the short-survival autoradiogram of an E16 rat. Since ganglion cell neurogenesis ends by E16, the labeled cells within the dorsal root ganglion must be proliferating Schwann cells. Paraffin-embedded tissue.

Figure 4-26. The round cells of the dorsal boundary cap and the elongated interfascicular Schwann cells of the ventral boundary cap in the lengthening proximal portion of the dorsal root, in a coronal section from an E15 rat. Methacrylate; hematoxylin-eosin.

4.1.4 *Expansion of the Dorsal Root Bifurcation Zone.*

The dorsal root bifurcation zone is in a dorsolateral position on E14, and its shape (Figure 4-28A) justifies its name as the oval bundle of His. By E15, however, the bifurcation zone expands dorsomedially and assumes a semilunar shape (Figure 4-28B). Late arriving and bifurcating dorsal root fibers (the axons of late-generated ganglion cells) may be pushing the earlier bifurcating fibers dorsomedially. The dorsomedial expansion of the bifurcation zone continues on E16 and the white matter capping the expanding dorsal horn flattens (Figure 4-28C). Since the location of the boundary cap does not change for several days, the distance between it and the leading edge of the bifurcation zone increases in the process.

The white matter capping the dorsal horn changes its configuration between E17 and E20 (Figures 4-29, 4-30). On E17, it develops a club-like extension (Figure 4-29A). We will provide some evidence later that the deep portion of this "club" consist of sprouting collaterals of the ascending and descending dorsal root fibers (Section 4.2.2). Hence this region is designated as the collateralization zone. The medial portion of this "club" may be formed by ascending fibers of the growing cuneate fasciculus. On the subsequent days, the collateralization zone deepens and forms a semicricle around the medial wall of the dorsal horn (Figure 4-29B). At about the same age, the semicircular fibers of the collateralization zone are joined medially by the core portion of the dorsal funiculus (Figure 4-29B). This may contain some of the ascending fibers of the gracile fasciculus. Concurrently, the boundary cap shifts dorsomedially. The latter change may be associated with two ongoing events: (i) the expansion of the dorsal horn (which would "stretch" the overlying dorsal root fibers), and/or the formation of Lissauer's tract lateral to the dorsal root entry zone. Soon after its translocation dorsomedially, as seen in the E20 rat (Figure 4-30), the boundary cap starts to dissolve. This could signal the end of the arrival of the latest forming dorsal root fibers, presumably the axons of the last generated small ganglion cells that contribute branches to Lissauer's tract.

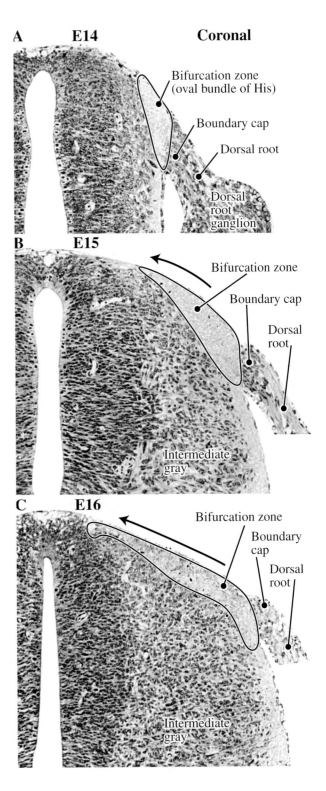

Figure 4-28. Expansion of the dorsal root bifurcation zone (the "oval bundle" of His) in E14 (**A**), E15 (**B**), and E16 (**C**) rat embryos. As the bifurcation zone spreads dorsomedially it becomes semilunar in shape. The location of the boundary cap and the dorsal root entry zone remains unchanged during this period. Methacrylate; hematoxylin-eosin.

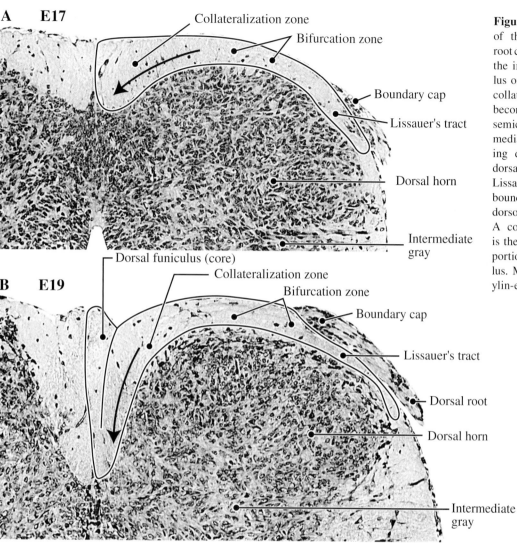

A   E17

Collateralization zone

Bifurcation zone

Boundary cap

Lissauer's tract

Dorsal horn

Intermediate gray

Dorsal funiculus (core)

B   E19

Collateralization zone

Bifurcation zone

Boundary cap

Lissauer's tract

Dorsal root

Dorsal horn

Intermediate gray

Figure 4-29. A. Emergence of the club-shaped dorsal root collateralization zone in the incipient dorsal funiculus on E17. **B.** By E19, the collateralization zone has become deeper and forms a semicircular arc around the medial wall of the expanding dorsal horn. As the dorsal horn expands, and Lissauer's tract develops, the boundary cap shifts from dorsolateral to dorsomedial. A concurrent development is the formation of the core portion of the dorsal funiculus. Methacrylate; hematoxylin-eosin.

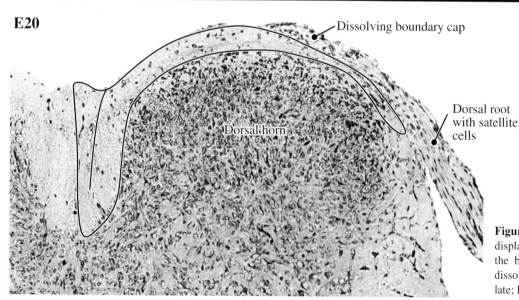

E20

Dissolving boundary cap

Dorsal root with satellite cells

Dorsal horn

Figure 4-30. Following its displacement dorsomedially, the boundary cap begins to dissolve by E20. Methacrylate; hematoxylin-eosin.

4.2   The Roof Plate and the Growth of the Dorsal Funiculus

4.2.1   The Roof Plate and the Dorsal Funiculus. The principal fiber components of the dorsal funiculus in carnivores and primates are the ascending afferents that terminate ipsilaterally in the dorsal column nuclei of the lower medulla. In the rat, as we noted earlier (Section 2.2.6), the dorsal funiculus also contains the descending efferents of the corticospinal tract. Because in the rat the corticospinal tract does not reach the spinal cord until the postnatal period (see below), we will be dealing here only with the development of the ascending afferents of the dorsal funiculus. We saw earlier that the dorsal funiculus emerges in the cervical spinal cord as a relatively shallow, midline structure on E17 (Figure 4-29A), and deepens progressively on the succeeding days (Figures 4,-29B, 4-30). Below we shall show that the fibers of the dorsal funiculus use the extracellular channels of the roof plate as a conduit, and as the axons of the dorsal funiculus fill these channels, the roof plate is pulled downward with the shrinking spinal canal.

The spinal cord neuroepithelium is still open on E10.5 (Figure 4-31A). The roof plate forms as the leading edges of the open neural groove fuse on E11 (Figure 4-31B). The cells of the roof plate are packed more densely than the NEP cells of the lateral plates at this stage of development and mitotic cells are less frequent in the roof plate than in the neuroepithelium. While the neuroepithelium expands greatly on the succeeding days (see Figure 3-3), the thickness of the roof plate changes little, except that its cells are becoming elongated (Figure 4-32). There is also a hint of the development of a fibrous matrix and some cavities above the tip of the dorsal canal by E13 (Figure 4-32). By E14, the fibrous matrix abutting the dorsal canal, and the channels near the surface are more prominent (Figure 4-33). As the autoradiogram from a rat labeled with ³H-thymidine on E14 and killed on E15 indicates (Figure 4-34), the expansion of the roof plate channels is associated with high level of cell proliferation in the roof plate. By E16 (Figure 4-35A), the number of cells in the roof plate has increased appreciably, and it is evident at higher magnification (Figure 4-35B) that the pale matrix near the lumen is composed of fibers whose end feet protrude into the spinal canal. This suggests that the spindle-shaped cells of the roof plate are not

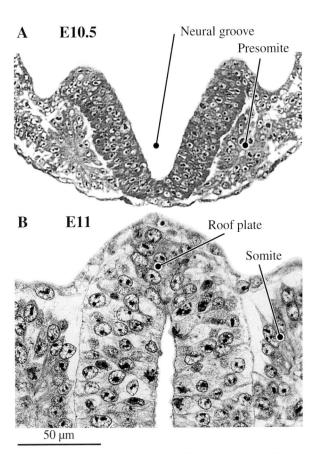

Figure 4-31. A. The unfused spinal cord neuroepithelium (neural groove) in an E10.5 rat. **B.** Formation of the roof plate after closure of the neural tube in an E11 rat. The cells of the roof plate look different than the pseudounipolar NEP cells laterally. Methacrylate; hematoxylin-eosin.

neurons but some type of "skeletal" glia. Whether or not the fibrous processes of the same cells form the walls of the overlying channels is uncertain. As seen in another, perhaps more mature E16 rat (Figure 4-36), the roof plate channels extend laterally and are invaded by the medially spreading branches of the dorsal root afferents (for lower magnification overview, see Figure 4-28C).

The roof plate undergoes several changes by the morning of E17 (Figure 4-37; see also Figure 4-29A). First, the spinal canal recedes and the vacated space is now occupied by a mass of darkly staining cells. These were identified before as the cells of the late-generated neurons of the central autonomic area (see Figure 3-86). Second, most of the roof plate channels disappear as they become filled with the transversely cut axons (seen as fine dots) of the dorsal funiculus. Third, the fibers with end feet in the ventricular lumen move ventrally as the spinal canal

E13

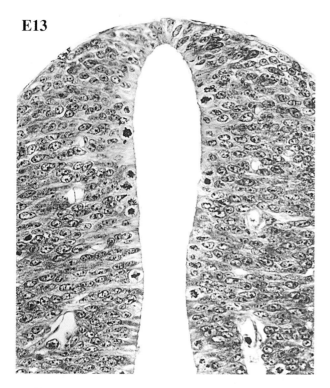

Figure 4-32. Spindle shaped cells of the roof plate in the cervical spinal cord of an E13 rat. There is a hint of the formation of a fibrous matrix and some channels. Methacrylate; hematoxylin-eosin.

E14 ➔ E15

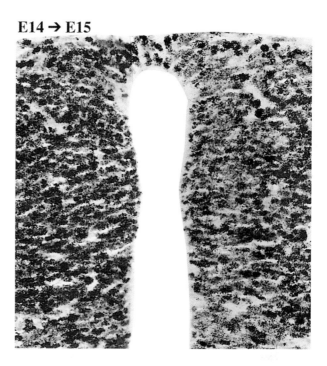

Figure 4-34. Labeled proliferating cells of the roof plate in an E15 rat that was tagged with ^{3}H-thymidine on E14. Autoradiogram; paraffin.

E14

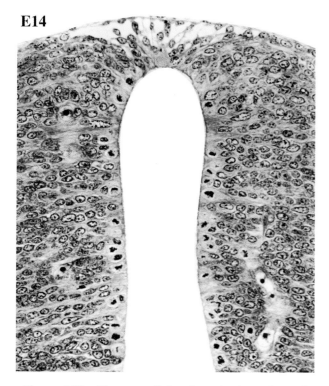

Figure 4-33. The extracellular channels above the roof plate cells and the fibrous matrix near the lumen of the spinal canal in an E14 rat. Methacrylate; hematoxylin-eosin.

recedes. As these changes take place, the fibrous matrix remains anchored at the lining of the spinal canal ventrally , and the pial surface dorsally. Some of the vertically oriented midline cells may be the perikarya of the fibers that elongate at the midline.

Three more noteworthy changes take place on E18 and E19 (Figures 4-38, 4-39). The first is the progressive expansion of the dorsal funiculus. The second is the deepening of the dorsal median septum. The third is the continuing shrinkage of the spinal canal and the ventral displacement of the fibrous matrix tied to it. The result of these changes is that as the spinal canal recedes, the distance between the base of the dorsal funiculus and the apex of the spinal canal – that is, the width of the parenchyma overlying the spinal canal – remains more or less constant. This suggests that the skeletal fibers of the roof plate are not only anchored both dorsally and ventrally but also serve as taut cables that pull the dorsal median septum (and the attached pial and meningeal membranes) downward as the spinal canal recedes.

E16 Coronal

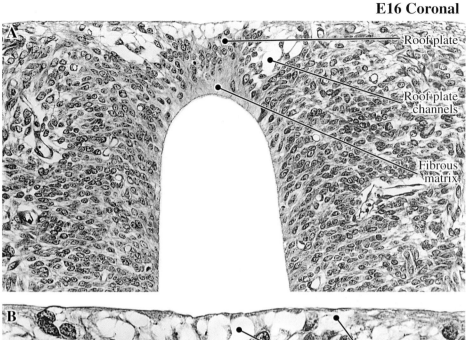

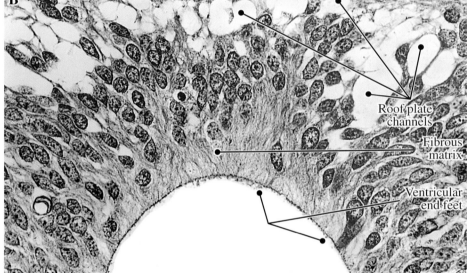

Figure 4-35. The empty extracellular channels and the fibrous matrix of the roof plate in an E16 rat, at lower (**A**) and higher (**B**) magnification. Some of the skeletal fibers of the roof plate have end feet in the lumen of the spinal canal. Methacrylate; hematoxylin-eosin.

E16 Coronal

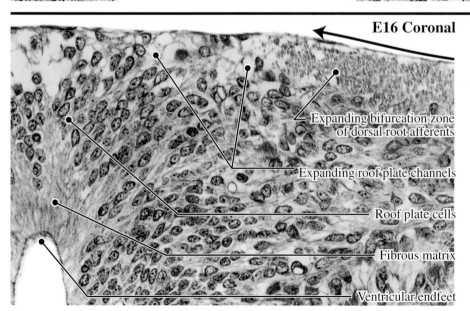

Figure 4-36. The extracellular channels of the roof plate are occupied by the growing fiber branches of the dorsal root bifurcation zone (arrow) in this E16 rat. (For lower magnification of the expanding bifurcation zone, see Figure 4-28C.) The roof plate channels may serve as conduits for the ascending branches of dorsal root axons that will form the dorsal funiculus. Methacrylate; hematoxylin-eosin.

E17 Coronal

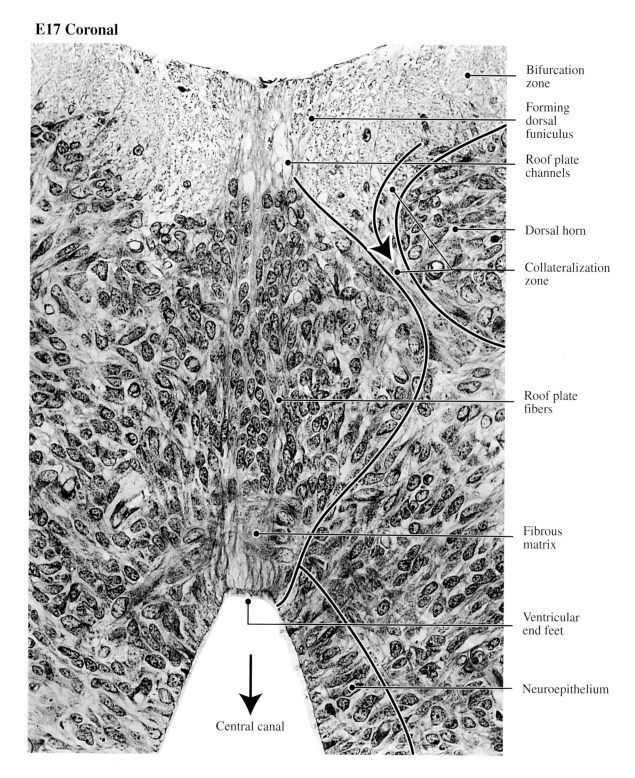

Bifurcation
zone

Forming
dorsal
funiculus

Roof plate
channels

Dorsal horn

Collateralization
zone

Roof plate
fibers

Fibrous
matrix

Ventricular
end feet

Neuroepithelium

Central canal

Figure 4-37. The fibrous matrix of the roof plate recedes with the shrinking spinal canal (bottom arrow) in this E17 rat. The skeletal fibers of the fibrous matrix capping the regressing spinal canal may remain anchored to the midline pial surface. A few empty channels remain near the formative dorsal medial septum but most of them are occupied by transversely cut fibers (small dots) of the growing dorsal funiculus. Some dorsal root collaterals curve around the dorsal horn (curved arrow). Methacrylate; hematoxylin-eosin.

E18 Coronal

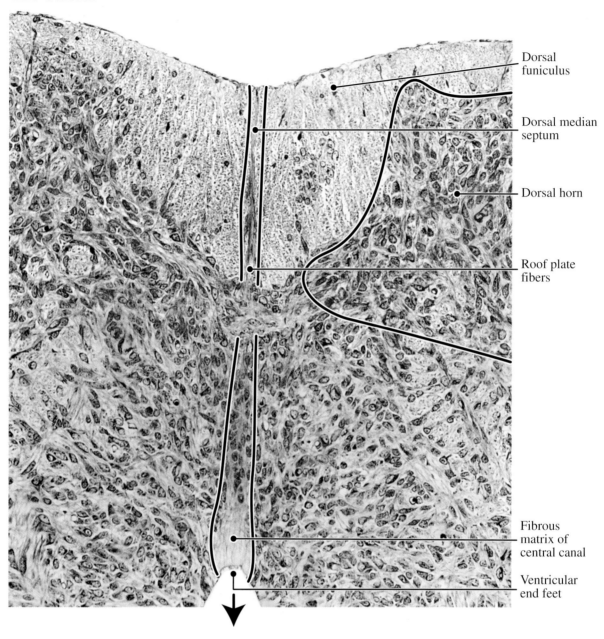

Dorsal funiculus

Dorsal median septum

Dorsal horn

Roof plate fibers

Fibrous matrix of central canal

Ventricular end feet

Figure 4-38. Among the developmental changes evident in this high cervical section of an E18 rat are the deepening of the dorsal funiculus, the shrinking of the spinal canal (bottom arrow), the invagination of the dorsal surface of the spinal cord, and the formation of the dorsal median septum. The possible continuity of the fibrous matrix capping the receding central canal and the fibers associated with the developing dorsal median septum is indicated. The dorsal root collaterals are not evident at this level. Methacrylate; hematoxylin-eosin.

E19 Coronal

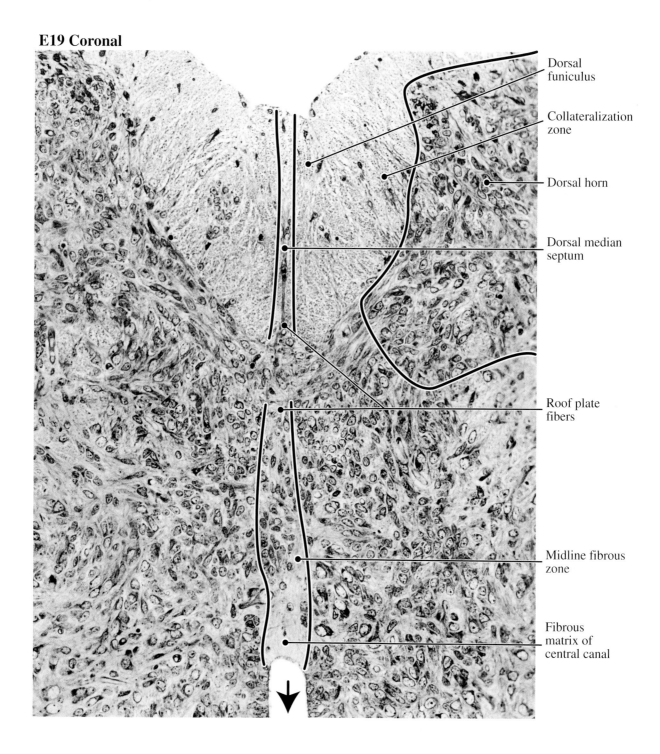

Dorsal funiculus

Collateralization zone

Dorsal horn

Dorsal median septum

Roof plate fibers

Midline fibrous zone

Fibrous matrix of central canal

Figure 4-39. The ongoing withdrawal of the spinal canal (bottom arrow) is associated with the continuing deepening of the dorsal funiculus and the invagination of the dorsal median septum in an E19 rat fetus. The skeletal fibers of the roof plate may be anchored at the pial surface dorsally and at the spinal canal ventrally, and as the spinal canal recedes the pial surface is pulled downward in the midline. Methacrylate; hematoxylin-eosin.

4.2.2   Growth of the Local Collaterals of the Dorsal Funiculus.

Studies of the growth and maturation of spinal cord afferents began early in the twentieth century because of a widespread interest in the embryology of behavior. One issue studied was the earliest time when sensory stimulation elicits reflexes (e.g., Coghill, 1929; Angulo y Gonzalez, 1932; Hooker, 1942; Hamburger, 1963; Humphrey, 1964; Carmichael, 1970). Related anatomical studies dealt with the time when the "reflex arc" closes (e.g., Windle and Orr, 1934; Windle and Baxter, 1936; Windle and Fitzgerald, 1937; Vaughn and Grieshaber, 1973; Smith 1983). Using the silver staining technique, Windle's (1944) findings suggested that the closure of the reflex arc follows a retrograde sequence, starting with the maturation of motoneurons in the ventral horn and ending with the maturation of sensory interneurons in the dorsal horn. Recent experimental studies with tracer techniques (such as HRP and carbocyanine dyes) indicate that the maturation of the dorsal root afferent system is somewhat more complex than it was originally envisaged, since fibers of different sensory modalities and with different spinal cord connections develop at different ages(Kudo and Yamada, 1987; Mirnics and Koerber, 1995a, 1995b; Ozaki and Snider, 1997).

Kudo and Yamada (1987), who labeled the dorsal root in the lumbar spinal cord of rats ranging in age from E15.5 to birth, found that some pioneering fibers penetrate the dorsal horn by E15.5 (our E16; Figure 4-40A). By E16.5, collaterals grow into the dorsal horn in large numbers and displace the bifurcation zone dorsomedially (E17; Figure 4-40B). By E18.5, two collateral bundles can be distinguished: (i) a long medial bundle that reaches the ventral horn, and (ii) a short lateral bundle that penetrates the dorsal horn from below (E19; Figure 4-40C). By E20.5, many long collaterals are arborizing in the ventral horn (E21; Figure 4-40D). These must be proprioceptive fibers (compare with Figures 1-29 to 1-31). Observations by Snider et al. (1992) suggest that the proprioceptive fibers growing toward the medial and lateral motoneuron columns, respectively, sort themselves out before reaching their targets. In contrast, the short collaterals recurve and enter the dorsal horn from beneath. These must be the large caliber exteroceptive fibers with flame endings (compare with Figures 1-26, 1-27).

The synaptic development of proprioceptive fibers follows their arrival in the ventral horn. The number of synaptic boutons in comparable sample areas in the ventral horn increased as follows: 16 synapses on E17.5; 600 on E18.5; 2,000 on E19.5; and 8,000 on E20.5 (Kudo and Yamada, 1987). Ziskind-Conhaim (1990) found that proprioceptive fibers reach the domain of motoneuron dendrites by E16, and boutons were recognized there by E17. Correlated physiological studies showed that stimulation of dorsal root fibers produced excitatory postsynaptic potentials (EPSPs) as early as E16 but with long latencies and slow rise times (Ziskind-Conhaim, 1990). By E17, EPSPs with shorter latencies and faster rise times were obtained. These physiological responses are mediated by NMDA (N-methyl-D-glutamate) receptors. The maturation of inhibitory synapses is more complex (Wu et al., 1992). Miki (1995) studied synaptic maturation in the rat ventral horn with reference to immunocytochemical expression of the alpha, beta- and gamma subspecies of protein kinase C. Synaptic maturation begins on E15 with a few immature synapses and continues through the early postnatal period. According to Knyihar-Csillik et al. (1995), synaptogenesis starts in the ventral horn of the macaque monkey on E27 (gestation period in this species is 165 days) and on E29 more dorsally.

The results of the preceding investigations in the rat suggest that proprioceptive axons reach their targets in the ventral horn and begin to form synapses there as early as E17 (Ziskind-Conhaim, 1990) and no later than E19 (Kudo and Yamada, 1987). The little evidence that is currently available suggests that the large caliber exteroceptive fibers and the small caliber nociceptive fibers reach their targets in the spinal cord several days later. According to Fitzgerald (1987), small diameter fibers do not begin to enter the spinal cord until E19, and do not reach the substantia gelatinosa until E20. Likewise, Mirnics and Koerber (1995b) observed a late wave of entering small caliber fibers. The latter investigators also found that the first wave of these collaterals stays within the segment of entry on the first day and grows to neighboring segments at a rate of one segment per day (Mirnics and Koerber, 1995b). Finally, according to Golden et al. (1997), most synapses in laminae I and II of the dorsal horn (the terminal domain of nociceptive fibers) form after birth.

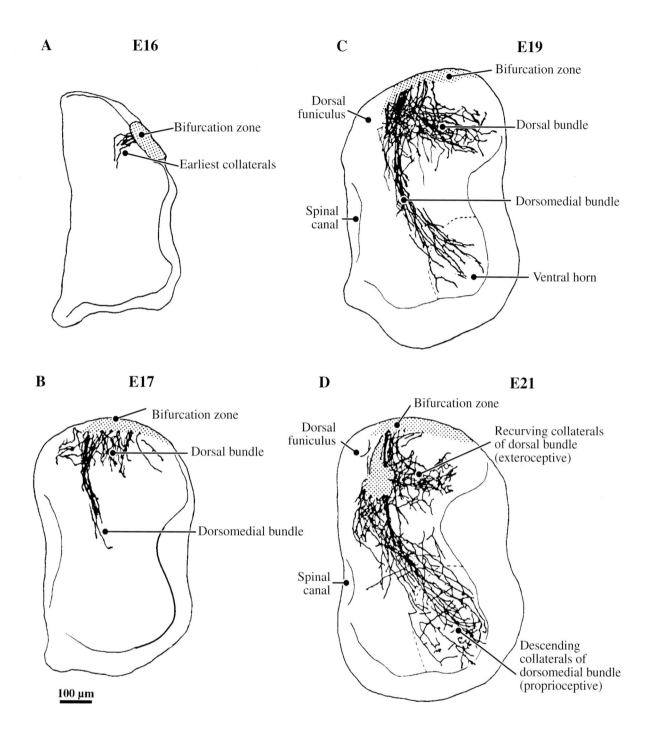

A   E16

Bifurcation zone

Earliest collaterals

B   E17

Bifurcation zone

Dorsal bundle

Dorsomedial bundle

100 μm

C   E19

Bifurcation zone

Dorsal funiculus

Dorsal bundle

Dorsomedial bundle

Spinal canal

Ventral horn

D   E21

Bifurcation zone

Dorsal funiculus

Recurving collaterals of dorsal bundle (exteroceptive)

Spinal canal

Descending collaterals of dorsomedial bundle (proprioceptive)

Figure 4-40. The development of dorsal root collaterals, traced with Di I in vitro, in rat fetuses ranging in age from E16 (E15.5 in the original) to E21 (E20.5). The earliest collaterals appear dorsolaterallly beneath the bifurcation zone on E16 **(A)**. The number of collaterals growing downward from the dorsomedially displaced bifurcation zone has greatly increased by E17 **(B)**. The collaterals forming the dorsomedial bundle (evidently proprioceptive collaterals) begin to penetrate the ventral horn in large numbers by E19 **(C)**, and arborise there profusely by E21**(D)**. The collaterals of the dorsal bundle penetrate the dorsal horn by E19 and start to recurve by E21. These must be exteroceptive collaterals with flame endings. After Kudo and Yamada (1987). Ages corrected, captions modified, and figures rotated from left to right.

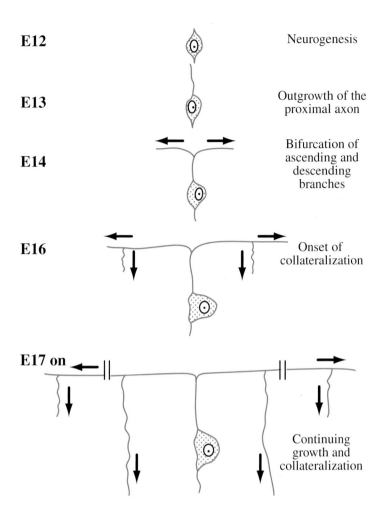

E12   Neurogenesis

E13   Outgrowth of the
                                    proximal axon

E14   Bifurcation of
                                    ascending and
                                    descending
                                    branches

E16   Onset of
                                    collateralization

E17 on

                                    Continuing
                                    growth and
                                    collateralization

Figure 4-41. Hypothetical sequence of events, with approximate dates, in the formation of the local branches of a dorsal root axon from a large ganglion cell in the rat cervical spinal cord. The process begins with the initial outgrowth of the proximal axon on E13. That is followed on E14 by the bifurcation of the axon that enters the spinal cord into ascending and descending branches. The sprouting of locally terminating collaterals begins at about E16 and they start to penetrate the gray matter in appreciable numbers on E17 and thereafter.

These findings, combined with the available evidence about the time of origin of large and small ganglion cells, suggest the following sequence of events (Figure 4-41). According to the autoradiographic evidence, the large dorsal root ganglion cells are generated at cervical levels of the spinal cord between E12 and E13, and the small ganglion cells between E14 and E15 (Figures 4-2, 4-3). Pioneering dorsal root fibers penetrate the spinal cord on E13 (Figures 4-5 and 4-17) and by E14 form the dorsal root bifurcation zone (Figure 4-18). Assuming that the pioneering axons that reach the spinal cord belong to the earliest produced large ganglion cells (those generated on E12), it takes about 1 day for a differentiated ganglion cell to form a proximal axon (E13), and another day to sprout bifurcating ascending and descending branches (E14). Since the bifurcating axons do not begin to sprout local collaterals until E16 (Figure 4-40A) and the collateralization zone is not detectable until E17 (Figure 4-29A), it must take another 2-3 days for this to take place. Finally, since proprioceptive afferents do not reach the ventral horn in sufficient numbers until E19 (Figure 4-40C), and

do not arborize there until E21 (Figure 4-40D), several more days must elapse before the reflex arc is closed.

The time course for maturation of the fine caliber axons of the late-generated small ganglion cells is less certain. But if they follow the same developmental sequence as the large ganglion cells, than the axons of small ganglion cells generated on E15 would begin to bifurcate in Lissauer's tract on E17 (see Figure 4-29A), and their collaterals dip into the substantia gelatinosa on E19. This matches the date given for the ingrowth of these fibers by Fitzgerald (1987). Indeed, it is possible that the translocation of the dorsal division of the boundary cap dorsomedially about E19 and E20 (Figures 4-28, 4-29) is related to the bifurcation of small caliber fibers during this period. If so, the changing shape of the bifurcation zone between E14 and E19 is due to the progressive displacement of proprioceptive and exteroceptive collaterals dorsomedially by the entering nociceptive fibers that form Lissauer's tract. Figure 4-42 illustrates this hypothetical sequence of events.

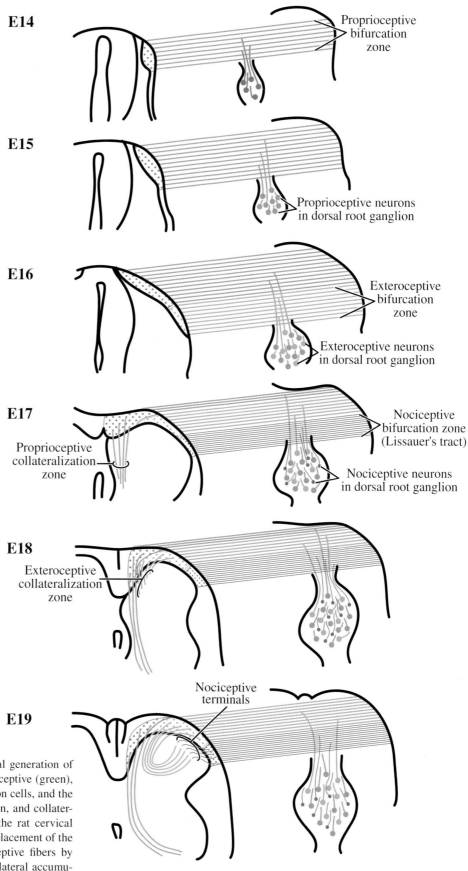

E14

Proprioceptive bifurcation zone

E15

Proprioceptive neurons in dorsal root ganglion

E16

Exteroceptive bifurcation zone

Exteroceptive neurons in dorsal root ganglion

E17

Nociceptive bifurcation zone (Lissauer's tract)

Proprioceptive collateralization zone

Nociceptive neurons in dorsal root ganglion

E18

Exteroceptive collateralization zone

E19

Nociceptive terminals

Figure 4-42. The sequential generation of proprioceptive (blue), exteroceptive (green), and nociceptive (red) ganglion cells, and the successive arrival, bifurcation, and collateralization of their axons in the rat cervical spinal cord. The medial displacement of the earlier bifurcating proprioceptive fibers by exteroceptive fibers and the lateral accumulation of nociceptive fibers is speculative.

4.2.3 Growth of the Ascending Express Lanes of the Dorsal Funiculus. The main constituents of the dorsal funiculus are dorsal root axons that proceed to the dorsal column nuclei of the medulla. But what is the relationship between these long ascending axons and those that are the source of local collaterals? We propose that the ascending dorsal root fibers switch course from the "local lanes" in the lateral aspect of the dorsal funiculus to the "express lanes" in its core after they give off the local collaterals. The basis of this hypothesis is as follows. It is well established that the ascending dorsal root fibers from the sacral and lumbar cord form the gracile fasciculus, and those from thoracic and cervical form the cuneate fasciculus, and the two terminate, respectively, in the ipsilateral gracile nucleus and cuneate nucleus of the medulla. These ascending fibers in the "core" of the dorsal funiculus are an unlikely source of collaterals because this region always appears to be uniformly composed of punctate profiles in coronal sections both in myelin-stained (e.g., Figures 1-12, 1-25, 2-15) and silver-stained (e.g, 1-20) preparations. That is, all these fibers are cut perpendicular to their longitudinal trajectory. In contrast, many fibers in the lateral aspect of the dorsal funiculus, as seen in the same illustrations, are cut obliquely or parallel to their sectioning in the coronal plane. Indeed, these features allowed us to identify this unique region of the dorsal funiculus as its collateralization zone. Another consideration is the fact that the width of this zone remains unchanged as one proceeds from lumbar to cervical levels of the cord, implying that roughly as many fibers leave this region as are added to it at succeeding segments of the cord from caudal to rostral. This is in sharp contrast to the progressive expansion of the gracile and cuneate fasciculi from caudal to rostral, evidently because new ascending fibers are added to it at succeedingly more rostral levels of the spinal cord.

If an ascending dorsal root fiber occupies the collateralization zone only locally, what happens to it at higher segments? It could conceivably terminate locally. But where, then, does the branch that ascends to the dorsal column nuclei come from. It is, therefore, more likely that after it gives off collaterals, the ascending branch shifts its course from lateral to medial and joins the core of the gracile or cuneate fasciculus. If this is correct, there are two lanes in the dorsal funiculus: (i) *local lanes* in the collateralization zone, and *express lanes* in the gracile and cuneate fasciculi (Figure 4-43). The topographic organization of fibers in the local lanes must be segmental. It is possible that the change from segmental to somatotopic organization (as described earlier) occurs as the ascending axons switch from the local to the express lanes.

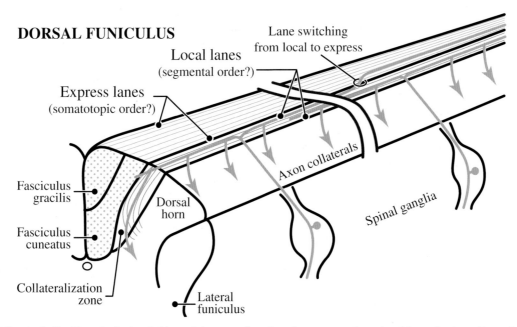

Figure 4-43. Hypothetical switching of the ascending dorsal root axons from local lanes in the collateralization zone of the cervical spinal cord to express lanes in the cuneate fasciculus. The change within the dorsal funiculus from segmental representation of the body surface to somatotopic representation may occur during this switching.

4.3 Growth of Descending Fiber Tracts to the Spinal Cord

4.3.1 Growth of Descending Fiber Tracts from Subcortical Structures.

Studies of fiber growth from the brain stem, mesencephalon, and diencephalon to the spinal cord have been carried out in the chick (Glover, 1993), the opossum (Wang et al., 1992; Cassidy and Cabana, 1993; Martin et al., 1993), and the rat (Lakke and Marani, 1991; Auclair et al. 1993; Kudo et al., 1993; Lakke, 1997). Auclair et al. (1993), using implanted DiI crystals in fixed rat embryos, reported that descending fibers from the medullary reticular formation, the lateral vestibular nucleus, and the interstitial nucleus of Cajal reach the upper cervical cord as early as E13–E14. Kudo et al. (1993), who injected HRP into the thoracic spinal cord of rats ranging in age from E14.5 to E20.5, studied the arrival of supraspinal efferents at thoracic levels. In E14.5 rats, a small number of neurons were retrogradely labeled in the lateral vestibular nucleus, the medullary and pontine reticular formation, and the interstitial nucleus of the medial longitudinal fasciculus. By E15.5, retrogradely labeled neurons were seen in the medullary raphe nuclei, the locus coeruleus, Barrington's nucleus, and the central gray of the midbrain. Red nucleus neurons were labeled following HRP injection on E16.5, and neurons of the nucleus of the solitary tract were labeled on E17.5. Neurons of the gracile nucleus were labeled in rats injected on E19.5, and the neurons of the paraventricular nucleus of the hypothalamus were labeled in rats injected on E20.5. Lakke and Marani (1991) traced the descent of efferents from the red nucleus through the length of the spinal cord (Figure 4-44). Rubrospinal fibers reached the upper cervical segments by E17, thoracic segments by E18, and upper lumbar segments by E19. Fibers from different subdivisions of the red nucleus grew toward their spinal targets at different speeds.

Lakke's (1997) extensive retrograde neuronal tracer study in the rat spinal cord indicates the following order in the arrival of subcortical efferents in the lumbosacral cord. Efferents from the lateral vestibular, raphe magnus, and gigantocellular reticular nuclei arrive on E17. Fibers reach the lumbosacral cord from the following structures by E18: the spinal vestibular and ventral medullary reticular nuclei, the raphe obscurus, the interpolar spinal

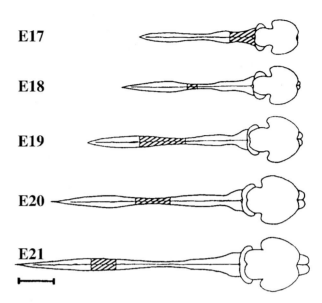

Figure 4-44. Descent of rubrospinal fibers (shaded area) through the length of the rat spinal cord between E17 and E21. From Lakke and Marani (1991).

trigeminal, caudal pontine reticular, mesencephalic reticular and laterodorsal tegmental nuclei, and the interstitial nucleus of Cajal. By E19 fibers arrive from the nucleus ambiguus, and the oral reticular, parvocellular reticular, and ventral gigantocellular nuclei of the pons. By E20 fibers arrive from the nucleus of Darkschewitsch, the locus coeruleus, the dorsal medullary reticular and paramedian reticular nuclei, and the paralemniscal and parabrachial nuclei. Among efferents that reach the lumbosacral cord just prior to birth (E21) are those from the medial vestibular and solitary nuclei, the red nucleus, the nucleus of the posterior commissure, and the Edinger-Westphal nucleus. Descending fibers from the paraventricular hypothalamic nucleus and the lateral hypothalamic area do not reach lumbosacral levels until the first postnatal day. This sequence is similar to that reported in the opossum by Wang et al. (1992). Comparing the time of arrival of descending axons with the time table of neuron production in these subcortical structures, Lakke concluded that the order .of neurogenesis is not a prime determinant of the speed with which their axons grow into the spinal cord. However, axons from the medulla, pons, and midbrain arrive before efferents from the diencephalon and, in particular, from the cerebral cortex.

4.3.2   Growth of Descending Fiber Tracts from the Neocortex.

The development of the corticospinal (or pyramidal) tract has been the subject of many investigations in several mammalian species. These include: the rat (Donatelle, 1977; Schreyer and Jones, 1982; Stanfield et al., 1982; Stanfield and O'Leary, 1985; DeKort et al., 1985; Gribnau et al., 1986; Chung and Coggeshall, 1987; Joosten et al., 1987, 1989, 1992; Gorgels et al., 1989; Gorgels, 1990; Curfs et al., 1994); the hamster (Reh and Kalil, 1981); the opossum (Cabana and Martin, 1985); the cat (Satomi et al., 1989; Alisky et al., 1992); the ferret (Meissirel et al., 1993); and the monkey (Armand et al., 1994, 1997). Of all the descending tracts in the spinal cord, the corticospinal tract is the last to form and takes the longest time to mature.

Most studies of the development of the corticospinal tract were carried out in mammals in which the corticospinal tract is situated in the dorsal funiculus. Donatelle (1977) used amino acid autoradiography and the Fink-Heimer technique in postnatal rats to trace the speed of descent of pyramidal tract fibers into the spinal cord (Figure 4-45). She found that corticospinal axons reach the dorsal funiculus of the contralateral cervical cord by P1, the thoracic cord by P3, the upper lumbar cord by P5, and the coccygeal cord by P9. Axon collaterals do not penetrate the gray matter of the cervical cord until P5, indicating a delay of as much of 4 days between the arrival of axons and their terminal arborization. Reh and Kalil (1981), using amino acid autoradiography and the HRP technique in hamsters, traced the descent of pyramidal

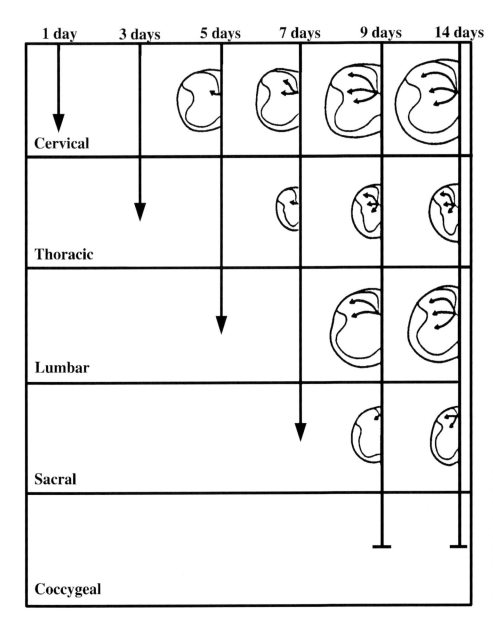

Figure 4-45. Growth (vertical arrows) and collateralization (small curved arrows) of the medial corticospinal tract in the rat spinal cord from cervical to coccygeal levels between P1 and P14. After Donatelle (1997). Autoradiographic tracing.

tract fibers from the somatosensory cortex through various subcortical structures to the spinal cord (Figure 4-46). Corticofugal fibers reach the pons by P1, decussate in the medulla on P3, reach the dorsal funiculus of the cervical cord by P4, the thoracic cord by P6, and the lumbar cord by P8. Reh and Kalil followed the penetration of corticospinal tract fibers into the dorsal horn of the cervical spinal cord (Figure 4-47). The fibers that arrive in the dorsal funiculus of the cervical cord on P4 do not penetrate the dorsal horn until P6. By P8, scattered corticospinal terminals disperse in the dorsal horn and adjacent regions, but it is not until about P14 that a plexus of dense terminals fills the dorsal horn.

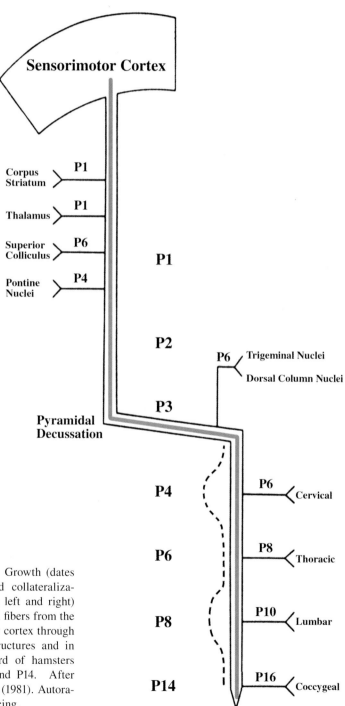

Figure 4-46. Growth (dates in center) and collateralization (dates on left and right) of corticofugal fibers from the somatosensory cortex through subcortical structures and in the spinal cord of hamsters between P1 and P14. After Reh and Kalil (1981). Autoradiographic tracing.

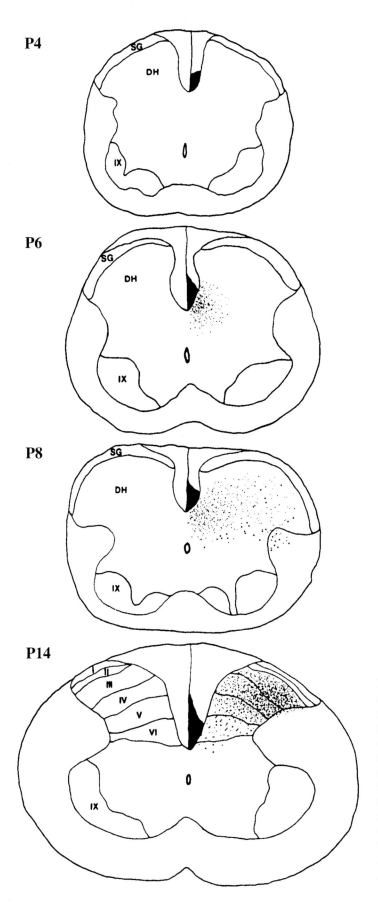

Figure 4-47. The descent and terminal arborization of medial corticospinal tract fibers from the somatosensory cortex in the cervical spinal cord of hamsters between P4 and P14. Blackened region in the dorsal funiculus indicates the location of descending corticospinal axons; fine dots in the gray matter show the distribution of terminals. Autoradiographic tracing. After Reh and Kalil (1981).

Schreyer and Jones (1982) found a similar sequence in the rat, except that they reported an earlier descent. Pyramidal tract fibers reach the pons by E19.5, the medulla by 20.5, and crossed corticospinal fibers appear in the dorsal funiculus of the upper cervical cord by P1. Corticospinal fibers reach the thoracic cord by P3, the lumbar cord by P6, and the sacral cord by P9. It takes 2–3 days for the fibers to penetrate the gray matter at any given segmental level. The formation of terminal arbors may take a few more days (Joosten et al., 1994). Reh and Kalil (1981) suggested that the corticospinal tract fibers descend as a compact bundle rather than as a staggered collection of fibers. Others report the incremental growth of corticospinal fibers at a given locus over a period of several days (e.g., Schreyer and Jones, 1982; Curfs et al., 1994). The late growth of corticospinal axons relative to axons from subcortical structures is reflected in their prolonged staining with immunocytochemical markers of growth cones (Kalil and Skene, 1986; Gorgels et al., 1987; Kalil and Perdew, 1988). There is evidence that many corticospinal terminals are eliminated during development (Reh and Kalil, 1982; Stanfield et al., 1982; Cabana and Martin, 1984; Chung and Coggeshall, 1987; Schreyer and Jones, 1988; Gorgels et al., 1989; Gorgels, 1990; Meissirel et al., 1993; Curfs et al., 1994). The shrinkage of the corticospinal projection may be due to the elimination of efferent terminals from certain areas of the cortex (Figure 4-48).

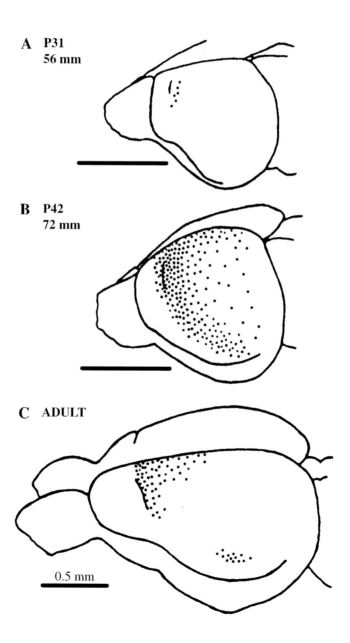

Figure 4-48. Distribution and number of corticospinal projection neurons in the cerebral cortex of the opossum retrogradely labeled from the spinal cord at P31 (**A**), P42 (**B**), and adulthood (**C**). There is an expansion of neurons projecting to the spinal cord between P31 and P42, followed by a retraction by adulthood. After Cabana and Martin (1984).

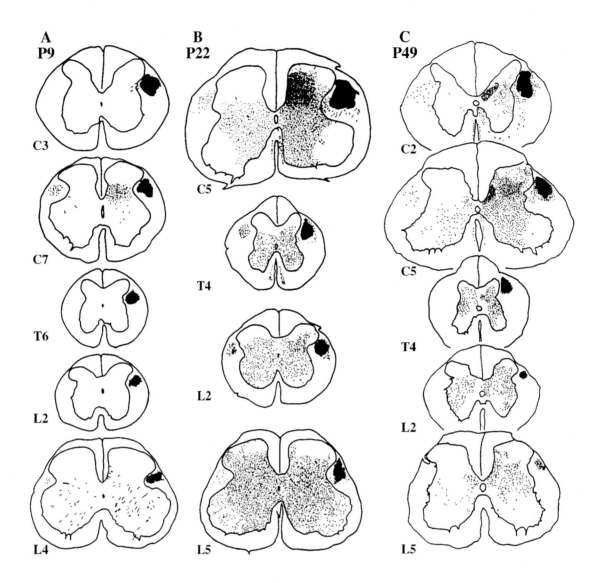

Figure 4-49. Three phases in the growth of fibers of the descending lateral corticospinal tract and their terminal arborization in the spinal cord of the cat. **A.** During the first phase, corticospinal fibers descend in the lateral funiculus (blackened area). **B.** During the second phase, there is an "exuberant" outgrowth of collaterals that penetrate the gray matter (fine dots). **C.** During the third phase, a high proportion of the axon collaterals are "pruned." Anterograde HRP technique. After Alisky et al. (1992).

Only a few studies are available about the growth of the corticospinal tract in species where this efferent system descends in the lateral funiculus rather than the dorsal funiculus. In cats, Alisky et al (1992) identified three phases in the development of the corticofugal projection from the parietal cortex (Figure 4-49). During the first phase (P1–P10), cortical fibers already present in the white matter begin to penetrate the gray matter. In the second phase (P14–P35), the corticospinal axons develop terminal collaterals that are widely distributed throughout much of the gray matter. In the third phase (P42–P49), some of the corticospinal terminals disappear. During the first three weeks, the corticospinal tract is strongly immunoreactive to a molecular marker of axonal growth (MAP 1B). That immunoreactivity declines by the fourth week, and disappears by the fifth week. Kuypers (1964) reported that corticospinal terminals in newborn rhesus monkeys are limited to the intermediate gray (where premotor interneurons are located) and the adult pattern of terminal distribution in the vicinity of ventral horn motoneurons appears in juveniles. Armand et al. (1994, 1997) used the HRP technique in rhesus monkeys to address the question when direct connections between corticospinal terminals and motoneurons may form. These investigators found that corticospinal terminals were distributed in the intermediate zone (at C8/T1 level the spinal cord) in neonates. A modest labeling appeared near the motor columns that control the hand muscles by P5 (Figure 4-50). By 2.5 months, a ring of dense labeling surrounded the dorsal and lateral motor columns but was sparse in the central region. That labeling was still sparse at 11 months when compared with adults. Armand et al. (1994, 1997) found no evidence for an exuberant early corticospinal projection in the monkey, in sharp contrast to the findings by others in several mammalian species. The slow growth of corticospinal collaterals in the monkey spinal cord is associated with a lack of "exuberant" initial growth that is followed by "pruning." It is generally assumed that direct contact of corticospinal axons with motoneurons in primates makes possible the acquisition of voluntary control of individual hand muscles for tasks that require manual dexterity.

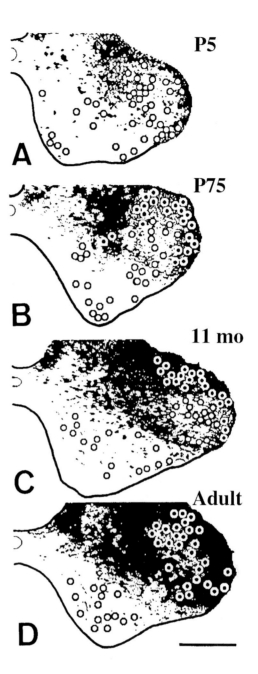

Figure 4-50. Expansion of axon terminals from the hand area of the motor cortex in the cervical ventral horn at 5 days (**A**), 75 days (**B**), 11 months (**C**) and adulthood (**D**) in the monkey. The progressively expanding terminal field of corticospinal fibers is indicated by the opaque area surrounding the lateral motoneurons that innervate the hand muscles. This growth is a protracted process, and there is no indication (as in the cat) of any "pruning" of terminals with age. Anterograde HRP technique. After Armand et al. (1997).

4.4   Spinal Cord Gliogenesis and Myelination

4.4.1 Oligodendroglia and Myelination in the Central Nervous System.

Oligodendroglia (oligodendrocytes) are the myelinating cells of the central nervous system. Mature oligodendroglia have multiple cytoplasmic processes that ensheath axons coursing in their vicinity. In the case of unmyelinated axons, the cytoplasmic processes of oligodendroglia insulate axons gathered in a nerve bundle from one another, and thus reduce interference during impulse propagation. In the case of myelinated axons, the membranes of compacted cytoplasmic processes wrap around the axon in the form of tightly packed spiral lamellae between the nodes of Ranvier. The internodal myelin makes possible the propagation of action potentials at increased velocity with the aid of a saltatory conduction mechanism. Myelin is composed of about 70 percent lipid, and 30 percent protein. The myelin proteins, which are mostly structural constituents, include proteolipid protein, basic myelin protein, glycoproteins, and some other minor constituents (Gilles et al., 1983). Peripheral myelin, but not central nervous myelin, also contains protein zero in abundance (Monuki and Lemke, 1995).

The formation of myelin in the developing nervous system is preceded by the proliferation and differentiation of oligodendroglia called myelination gliosis (Roback and Scherer, 1935; Fleischauer and Hillebrand, 1966). Myelination gliosis, coupled with an increase in the activity of several oxidative enzymes (Friede, 1961; Schonbach et al., 1968; Matthews and Duncan, 1971), precedes the myelination of fiber tracts in the central nervous system. The differentiation of a progenitor cell, called the oligodendrocyte type 2 astrocyte (0-2A), is considered to be the precursor of myelin producing oligodendrocytes (Richardson et al., 1996; Baron et al., 1998). The O-2A cell, depending on environmental conditions and on induction processes, can differentiate either into an astrocyte or an oligodendrocyte (Yu et al., 1994; Trousse et al., 1995; Orentas and Miller, 1996). Once the O-2A cell differentiates into an oligodendrocyte, its shape changes from bipolar to multipolar, and commences to manufacture myelin basic protein, myelin-associated glycoprotein, and proteolipid protein (Pfeiffer et al., 1993).

4.4.2 The Problem of the Origins of Oligodendroglia in the Spinal Cord.

Recent experimental studies have suggested that the oligodendrocyte progenitor cells originate in the ventral region of the spinal cord. Thus when the dorsal and the ventral regions of the spinal cord of E14 rats are grown in different tissue cultures, oligodendrocytes develop in the ventral culture but not in the dorsal culture (Warf et al. 1991). At a later stage of development, the dorsal region also acquires the capacity to produce oligodendrocytes. Using a marker for proliferating cells (BrdU), Noll and Miller (1993) found that the majority of labeled cells in E16.5 rats were located in discrete clusters in the ventral midline region of the spinal cord. The BrdU labeled cells increased in number 12–24 hours after administration of the marker in both the lateral and dorsal regions of the spinal cord. Some of the cells became astrocytes, others differentiated into oligodendrocytes. The ventral neuroepithelial origin of oligodendrocytes is supported by the studies of several investigators (Yu et al. 1994; Ono et al. 1995, Dickinson et al. 1995; Hall et al. 1996; Pringle et al. 1998). However, Cameron-Curry and Le Douarin (1995), using a different experimental procedure, concluded that oligodendrocytes originate from all regions of the spinal cord neuroepithelium. As a possible resolution of this controversy, Warf et al., (1991) suggested that oligodendrocyte progenitor cells are generated in the ventral neuroepithelium during early spinal cord development but disperse later throughout the gray matter and continue to produce oligodendrocytes locally.

The neuroglia of the spinal cord, like its neurons, are derived from the neuroepithelium that surrounds the spinal canal. However, it has not been resolved whether the NEP cells are initially pluripotent and after several cycles of division lose that potency to produce both neurons or glia, or whether different types of NEP cells are committed from the outset to produce either neurons or glia. Some researchers using tissue culture methods have argued that the early NEP cells are pluripotent and extrinsic conditions determine the fate of their progeny. For instance, Kalyani et al (1997) reported that cells from E10.5 rat spinal cord cultured under one set of conditions do not differentiate into neurons or glia. However, the same cells plated on laminin in the absence of chick embryo extract differentiate into neurons, astrocytes, or oligodendrocytes. When these committed cells are cloned, they retain their identity; for instance, some display immunoreactivity for choline acetyltransferase, a marker of differentiating motoneurons and certain other spinal cord neurons. Rao et al. (1998) reported that cells from the spinal cord of older rats (E13.5) will differentiate as oligodendrocytes and two types of astrocytes, but not as neurons, depending on the medium used for their maintenance. The authors referred to these cells as glial-restricted precursors.

As a prelude to our morphological approach to the problem of the origins of oligodendroglia, we will distinguish two types of primary germinal matrices in the central nervous system, the *homogeneous neuroepithelium* and the *heterogeneous neuroepithelium*, and two stages in neuroepithelial development, from manifest pluripotency to a gradual restriction of that potency. A good example of a homogeneous neuroepithelium is the germinal mosaic that produces the hippocampus (Altman and Bayer, 1990). One region of the hippocampal neuroepithelium generates the pyramidal neurons of Ammon's horn, another the granular neurons of the dentate gyrus, still another the neuroglia of the large hippocampal fiber tract, the fimbria. We called the latter the fimbrial *glioepithelium*. In that study we also proposed a distinction between the terms *neuro*epithelium, defined as a pluripotent matrix of NEP cells that generates all types of cells specific to the nervous system (neurons, neuroglia, ependymal cells, tanycytes) and *neurono*epithelium, a germinal matrix dedicated to the exclusive production of *neurons*. In the highly mosaicized germinal matrix of the hippocampus (and there are other such sites in the brain), neuronoepithelia and glioepithelia become spatially segregated from one another early during development and each becomes homogeneous. However, far more common is the heterogeneous (less mosaicized) neuroepithelium that is initially a source of both neurons and glia and which, in the course of time, loses its pluripotency and becomes restricted to the production of glia and other nonneuronal elements.

The autoradiographic evidence to be described below suggests that the spinal cord neuroepithelium (excluding the roof plate and the floor plate, and more particularly the ventral neuroepitheloum) is initially a heterogeneous *neuro*epithelium, one that will generate in the course of time all classes of spinal cord cells – neurons, glia, ependymal cells and tanycytes. As development proceeds,

that potency is reduced in a temporal order. In the first round of cell proliferation, the principal progeny of NEP cells are neurons. After a specified number of divisions, the NEP cells of the ventral neuroepithelium begin to produce glia. Finally, as the cycle winds down, the NEP cells produce ependymal cells and tanycytes that line the central canal. As the production of these highly specialized ventricular cells ends, the proliferative neuroepithelium disappears and cell proliferation shifts to the maturing gray and white matter. However, a distinction must be made in this context between the evident pluripotency of the spinal cord neuroepithelium de toto, and the potency of individual NEP cell lines. The morphological evidence does not resolve the important question whether the sequential loss in neuroepithelial potency is due to a transformation of the same NEP cells over a cycle of divisions or a staggered activation of different classes of NEP cells that are all present from the outset.

4.4.3 The Time and Site of Origin of Spinal Cord Neuroglia.
Neurogenesis ends in the cervical spinal cord of the rat on E16 when the last neurons of the dorsal horn and the central autonomic area are produced (Figure 3-83). By E17, the dorsal canal starts to recede (Figure 3-5B) and the surrounding dorsal neuroepithelium disappears on the succeeding days (Figures 3-6A, B). However, as seen in the short survival autoradiogram from an E17 rat (Figure 4-51A), a portion of the ventral canal neuroepithelium continues to be labeled. Labeled NEP cells are also seen in that location in the short survival radiograms of an E18 rat in which the dorsal canal has begun to recede (Figure 4-51B). By E19, the remnant of the ventral neuroepithelium has disappeared and the labeled cells have shifted to the persisting central canal (Figure 4-52A). A similar labeling pattern, with proliferating cells around the enduring central canal, is seen in the short survival radiograms of rats tagged with ^{3}H-thymidine on E20 (Figure 4-52B) and E21 (Figure 4-53). Thus, up to E17, many days after the cessation of motoneuron production in the ventral neuroepithelium (E14; Figure 3-19) other cell types are still being produced here and, then, for several more days in the neuroepithelium surrounding the permanent central canal. We propose that the ventral neuroepithelium is the original source of the neuroglia of the spinal cord, and the neuroepithelium around the permamnent central canal is the source of ependymal cells.

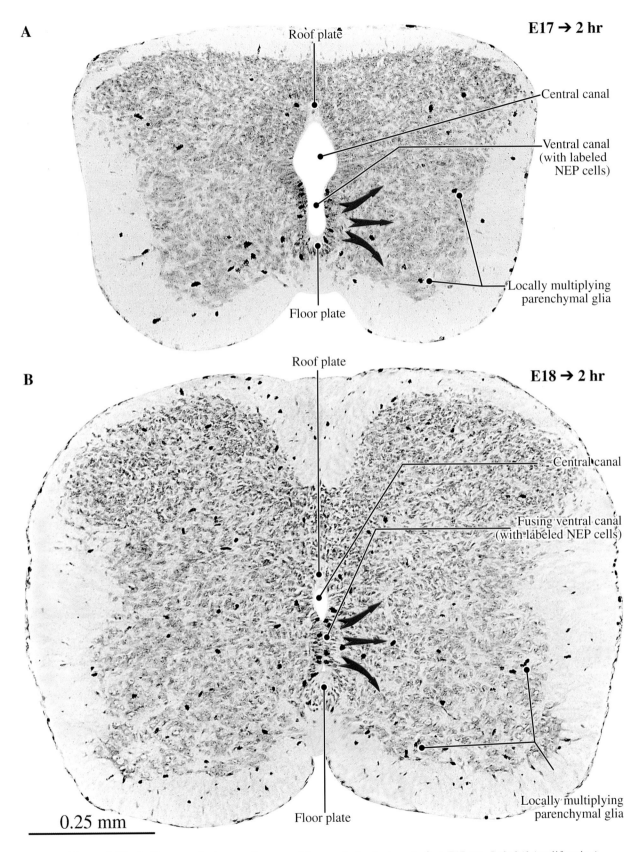

A. E17 → 2 hr

Roof plate

Central canal

Ventral canal (with labeled NEP cells)

Locally multiplying parenchymal glia

Floor plate

B. E18 → 2 hr

Roof plate

Central canal

Fusing ventral canal (with labeled NEP cells)

Locally multiplying parenchymal glia

Floor plate

0.25 mm

Figure 4-51. A. Short survival autoradiogram of the cervical spinal cord of an E17 rat. Labeled (proliferating) cells are concentrated in the ventral neuroepithelium but there are also scattered labeled cells in the surrounding gray matter. **B.** Short survival autoradiogram of the cervical spinal cord of an E18 rat. Labeled cells are still present in the receding ventral neuropeithelium, others are located in the surrounding gray matter. The locally multiplying (parenchymal) glia are postulated to derive from the ventral neuroepithelium (arrows).

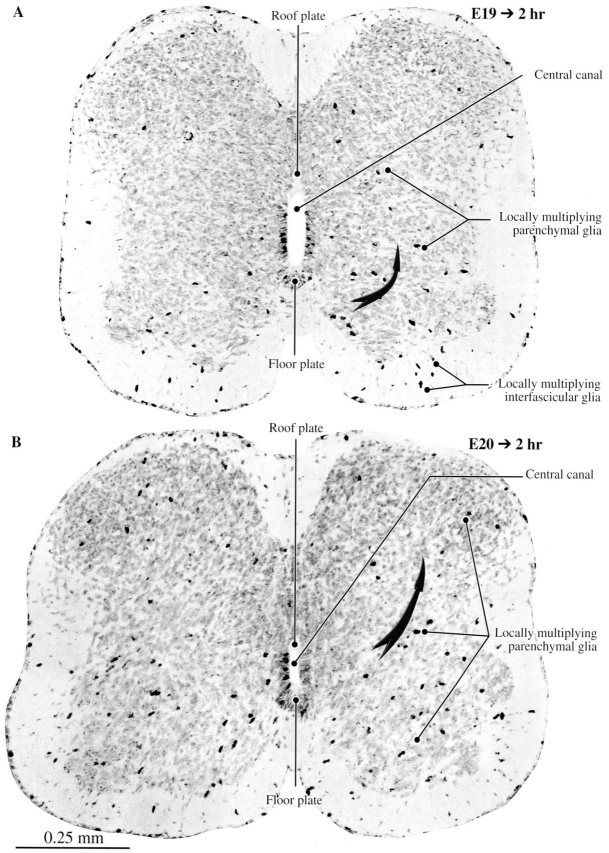

A

Roof plate

E19 → 2 hr

Central canal

Locally multiplying
parenchymal glia

Floor plate

Locally multiplying
interfascicular glia

B

Roof plate

E20 → 2 hr

Central canal

Locally multiplying
parenchymal glia

Floor plate

0.25 mm

Figure 4-52. Short survival autoradiogram of the cervical spinal cord of an E19 **(A)** and E20 **(B)** rat. After regression of the ventral canal and dissolution of the ventral neuroepithelium, labelled (proliferating) cells in the neuroepithelium are limited to the central canal but there are many labneled cells in the gray matter and white matter of the lower half of the spinal cord. Arrows indicate the presumed spread of locally proliferating neuroglia precursors from ventral to dorsal.

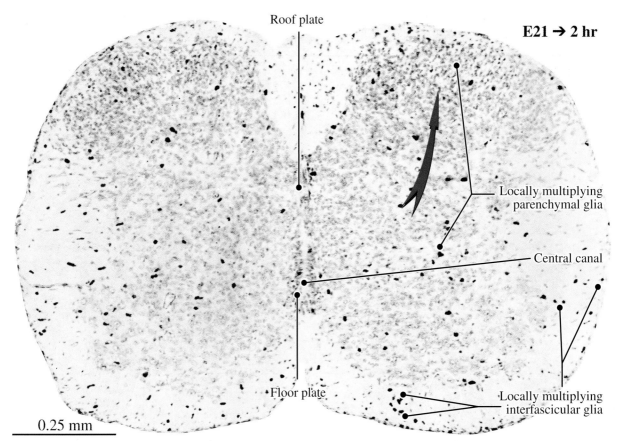

Figure 4-53. Short-survival autoradiogram of the cervical spinal cord of an E21 rat. Note the presence of labeled cells around the central canal and their spread dorsally in the gray and white matter (arrow).

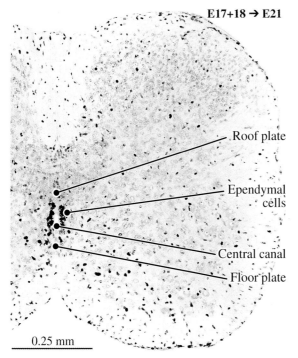

Figure 4-54. Autoradiogram of the cervical spinal cord of a perinatal (E21) rat that was tagged with ³H-thymidine on E17 and E18. Labeled cells are present in the ependymal layer of the central canal, and there is a fair concentration of labeled neuroglia throughout the gray and white matter.

In addition to the labeled cells of the ventral neuroepithelium, labeled cells are present in short-survival radiograms of E17 rats in the adjacent gray matter and a few also more dorsally (Figure 4-51A). These are locally multiplying cells, presumably neuroglia that have originated in the adjacent ventral neuroepithelium. These locally multiplying cells spread in increasing numbers laterally with the expanding ventral horn by E18 (4-51B) and E19 (Figure 4-52A) and begin to penetrate in larger numbers the intermediate gray by E20 (Figure 4-52B) and the dorsal horn by E21 (Figure 4-53). Locally multiplying cells are also present by now in the ventral and lateral funiculi. We identify the former as locally multiplying parenchymal glia, the latter as locally multiplying interfascicular glia.

An interpretation of the foregoing observations is that the production of neuroglia is a two-stage process. After termination of neuron production in the cervical spinal cord on E16, the active ventral neuroepithelium continues to generate precursors of neuroglia. The cells that leave the ventral neuroepithelium disperse larerally and then dorsally in the succeeding days and continue to proliferate at a low rate locally. After dissolution of the ventral neuroepithelium, the generation of glial precursors becomes strictly a local affair. This is the second phase of glial production, that persists in the central nervous system through adulthood (Altman, 1966). However, proliferative cells persist for several days in the thin germinal matrix surrounding the central canal. These, according to our hypothesis, are the precursors of the ependymal cells and tanicytes of the central canal. Indeed, as seen in the autoradiogram of a perinatal rat that was tagged with ³H-thymidine on E17 and E18 (Figure 4-54), the cells labeled in the wall of the central canal are sedentary elements that show little label dilution after several days.

So far we have dealt with the time course of neuroglia production after the cessation of spinal cord neuron production (E17). The question remains when glial production commences in the spinal cord. The radiograms illustrated in Figure 4-55 provide a tentative answer. In the short-survival radiogram of the E13 rat (Figure 4-55A), the ventral horn that flanks the mitotically active ventral neuroepithelium is devoid of labeled cells. A few locally labeled cells appear in the ventral horn in the short survival radiogram of the E14 rat (Figure 4-55B), and many more in the short survival radiogram of the E15 rat (Figure 4-55C). This suggests that glial proliferation starts in the parenchyma of the ventral horn after motoneuron production ends. The hypothesis that the locally mutlipying glia are derived from the ventral neuroepithelium is supported by the following observations. First, although diminishing in size, the ventral neuroepithelium (but not the floor plate) contains many proliferative NEP cells on E15 (Figure 4-55C). Since the production of motoneurons has come to an end on E14 (Figure 3-19), these cells cannot be neuron progenitors. Second, since the ventral canal will disappear within a few days (Figures 4-51B, 5-52A), it is unlikely that ependymal cells are produced at this site. Third, there are few or no labeled cells in the ventral horn on E13 and E14 (Figures 4-55A, B) but a fair number of them appear by E15; this is compatibe with the idea that the locally multiplying precursors originated in the ventral neuroepithelium. Combining all these observations, we propose that the precursors of spinal cord neuroglia proliferate in the ventral neuroepithelium between E15 and E18, and after the ventral neuroepithelium disappears, the production of neuroglia shifts to the gray and the white matter.

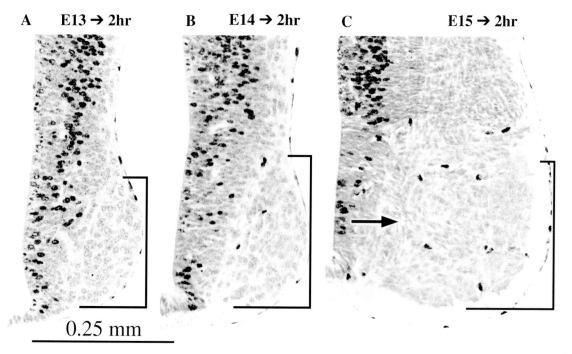

Figure 4-55. A. The incipient ventral horn (bracket) is devoid of labeled (locally multiplying) cells in the short survival autoradiogram of the E13 rat. **B.** A few labeled cells are present in the ventral horn in the short survival autoradiogram of the E14 rat. **C.** The concentration of labeled cells (presumed precursors of glia) has increased in the ventral horn in the short survival autoradiogram of the E15 rat.

4.4.4 *The Floor Plate*. As we have seen earlier (Section 4.2.1), the roof plate is a specialized region of the neural tube. It is much thinner and has a different cell composition than the lateral neuroepithelium that generates neurons. Likewise, the floor plate has a different cellular composition than the neuroepithelium but it also differs from the roof plate. Figure 4-56A shows the cytology of the floor plate in the cervical spinal cord of an E12 rat, 1 day before the commissural fibers start to cross beneath it. On this day the floor plate is composed of a 2-3 cell-deep epithelium of radially oriented, spindle shaped cells. Unlike the adjacent ventral neuroepithelium, the floor plate is typically devoid of mitotic cells. The apex of the floor plate has a fibrous composition, consisting of fibrous processes that extend to the lumen of the ventral canal. The base of the floor plate abuts the notochord, to which it is linked by an intercellular bridge. By E13 (Figure 4-56B), a few commissural fibers have started to cross the midline beneath the floor plate, and the bridge between the floor plate and the notochord has disapeared. On the succeeding days, as the number of decussating fibers in the ventral commissure is growing, two regions can be distinguished in the floor plate: a midline compartment flanked and a pair of lateral compartments (Figure 4-56C). The midline compartment is composed of more densely packed cells that have have short fibrous processes projecting to the lumen. The cells of the lateral compartment are lined up in a single file and have longer processes projecting to the lumen. Mitotic cells are often seen in the lateral compartments but rarely, if ever, in the midline compartment.

Observations in short survival radiograms of E14 rats suggest a difference in the proliferative dynamics of the midline and lateral cells of the floor plate; whereas some of the lateral cells are labeled, the midline cells are typically unlabeled (Figure 4-57). The possibility that the lateral region is the site of cell production and that some of the new cells move to the midline is not supported by observations made in sequential survival autoradiograms (Figure 4-58). There is no decrease in the concentration of labeled cells laterally 24 hours after the administration of ³H-thymidine, and since the medial cells are unlabeled, no lateral cells seem to have moved medially during this period. In an immunocytochemical study of the embryonic rat spinal cord, McKanna (1993) identified two compartments in the floor plate,

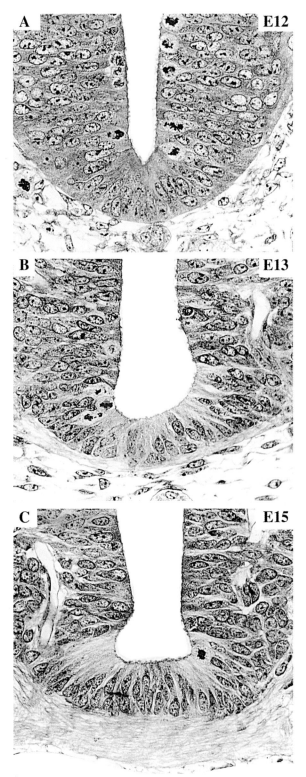

Figure 4-56. A. The floor plate and the notochord (bottom), with a "bridge" between the two, in an E12 rat. **B.** The first commissural fibers crossing beneath the floor plate, in an E13 rat. **C.** The components of the floor plate in an E15 rat: a medial compartment several cells deep and short fibers, and a lateral compartment with cells in a single file and longer fibers. Mitotic cells are rare in the lateral compartment and virtually absent medially. The ventral commissure has grown considerably. Methacrylate; hematoxylin-eosin.

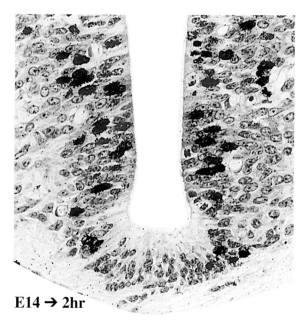

E14 → 2hr

Figure 4-57. The labeling pattern in this short survival autoradiogram from an E14 rat indicates low level of cell proliferation in the lateral compartment of the floor plate and its absence medially.

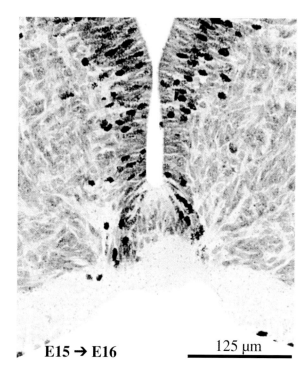

E15 → E16   125 µm

Figure 4-58. Labeling pattern in the floor plate of this E16 rat tagged with ^{3}H- thymidine on E15. The proliferating cells of the lateral floor plate have not moved medially within the available 24 hour period.

a median band that expresses lipocortin 1, and a paramedian band that expresses S100-beta. Since lipocortin 1 is also expressed by microglia, McKanna hypothesized that the median cells of the floor plate are progenitors of adult microglia. Our evidence that midline cells are mitotically inactive does not support (but does not necessarily rule out) that possibility.

According to a popular hypothesis, floor plate cells secrete chemoatractants that guide axons approaching the ventral midline to the opposite side (e.g., Kingsbury, 1930; Jessell et al., 1988; Bovolenta and Dodd, 1990, 1991; Yaginuma et al., 1991). Among the many candidates for these chemotropic factors, are netrin-1 (Kennedy et al., 1994; Tessier-Lavigne et al., 1988; Placzek et al., 1990); axonin-1 (Stoeckli et al., 1997); integrin, extracellular matrix molecules, transforming growth factor betas (Ohyama et al., 1997); and a factor recognized by the cell surface antigen, CARO 2 (Zhu et al., 1998). We question this chemotropic hypothesis as a principal function of the floor plate. On the basis of histological observations and the autoradiographic evidence, we propose instead that the floor plate has two other important morphogenetic functions.

As we have seen before, as early as E13 (Figure 3-45), vertically oriented, spindle-shaped cells line up in the sojourn zone of the neuroepi-

thelium and extrude axons that grow ventrally and cross in the ventral commissure to the opposite side. These vertically oriented interneurons are located between the neuroepithelium medially, and the primordial white matter and the incipient ventral horn laterally, at this stage of development. The population of vertically oriented interneurons increases on the following days, and so do the commissural axons that decussate ventrally between the floor plate and the pia of the spinal cord (e.g., Figures 3-47, 3-49). By E15, the trajectory of commissural axons is clearly constrained by two solid "walls" – the neuroepithelium medially and the gray matter laterally – within which, as in a river bed, they course. We have also seen, as summarized in Figure 3-82, that within the sojourn zone of the neuroepithelium, the vertically oriented contralaterally projecting interneurons form microsegments that alternate with microsegments containing horizontally oriented, ispilaterally projecting interneurons. Thus, before leaving the neuroepithelium, and presumably before any influence could be exerted on the prospective interneurons by attractants of the distant floor plate, their polarity has already been determined by some intrinsic mechanism so that cells in one microsegment extrude axons that grow ventrally and those in the adjacent microsegment extrude axons that grow laterally. If that is correct, the axons of the vertically oriented interneurons growing within the confines of a vertical channel will not encounter a choice point until after they have crossed to the opposite side above the floor plate (Figure 4-59). That is, mechanical constraints force the growing fibers to follow the path of least resistance and cross to the opposite side. Only after they have crossed to the opposite side, do these fibers encounter their first choice point, i.e., whether to grow rostrally, caudally, or in some other direction.

The hypothetical channel guiding the decussation of growing axons has to remain intact to fulfil its structural role. In mutants lacking a floor plate, the bulwark that forces the growing axons to cross to the oppsite side is absent; it is not surprising, therefore, that their decussation is perturbed (Bovolenta and Dodd, 1991). However, our morphogenetic evidence suggests that the floor plate, in cooperation with the the roof plate, has another structural role than hitherto considered. That role is the morphogenesis of the unique H shape of the spinal cord gray matter. We propose that from the outset of spinal cord develop-

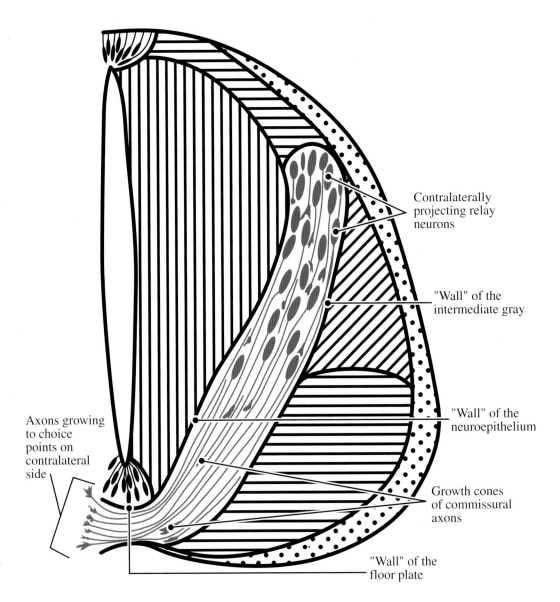

Figure 4-59. The hypothetical confining "walls" – composed of the neuroepithelium medially, the gray matter laterally, and the floor plate ventrally – that channel the growing commissural across the midline. The initial vertical orientation of interneurons within the commissural microsegment, and the presence of these walls during this stage of spinal cord development may by sufficient to ensure the unerring growth of these commissural fibers to the opposite side.

ment the fibers of the floor plate cells and the fibers of the roof plate cells anchor the dorsomedial and ventromedial lining of the spinal cord to the dorsal and ventral tips of the spinal canal. Then, as the elongated embryonic spinal canal starts to shrink to form the permanent central canal, the taut fibers of the regressing roof plate and floor plate pull the pia and the meninges surrounding the spinal cord centripetally to produce the dorsal and ventral invagination of the gray matter, and the dorsal median septum and the ventral median sulcus of the spinal cord as a whole.

We saw earlier the shrinkage of the ventral canal and dorsal canal between E16 and E19 (Figures 3-5 and 3-6). How does this morphogenetic process come about? A hint comes from the observation that the fibrous matrices of the roof plate and floor plate retreat conjointly with the shrinking spinal canal. As seen in Figure 4-60, the two matrices are associated with radial fibers that extend to the point where the dorsal median septum and the ventral median sulcus will later form (Figure 4-60). The progressive invaginations of the dorsal median septum and the ventral median sulcus in association with the shrinkage of the spinal canal is shown in tracings of the growing spinal cord in E16, E17, E18 and E19 rats (Figure 4-61). As the spinal canal shrinks, the meningeal lining of the incipient dorsal median septum dips downward and the incipient ventral median sulcus moves upward, as if pulled by the taut ropes. Where these constraining forces are absent, the expanding gray matter bulges outward. Thus, the ventral horn, containing the growing and segregating motoneurons expands in the ventrolateral direction, and the dorsal horn containing the migrating interneurons expands

Figure 4-60. A. Fibers of the roof plate that anchor the dorsomedial tip of the central gray to the dorsal tip of the receding spinal canal in the cervical spinal cord of an E17 rat. **B.** Fibers of the floor plate that anchor the tip of the shrinking ventral canal to the base of the spinal cord in an E18 rat. We postulate that these two anchoring sites play a pivotal role in the formation of the dorsal median septum and the ventral median sulcus (arrows). Methacrylate; hematoxylin-eosin.

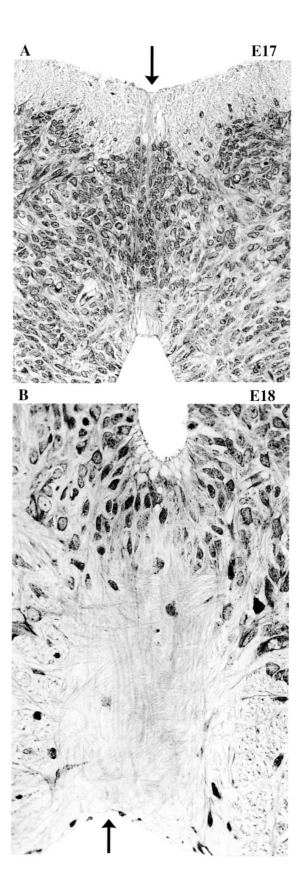

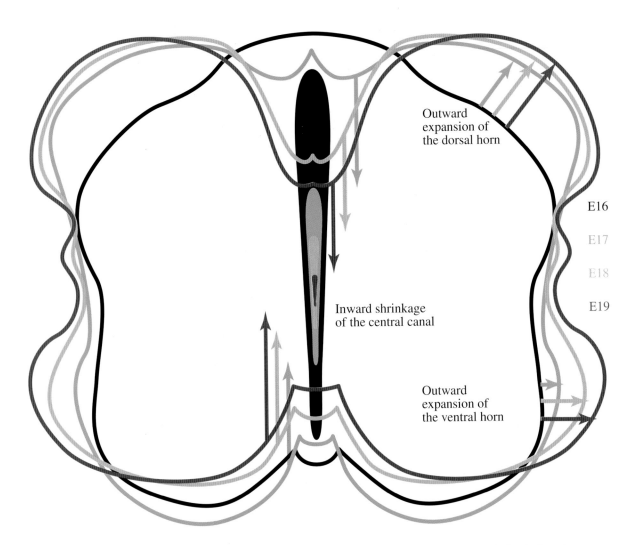

Figure 4-61. Superimposed outlines of the gray matter and the spinal canal in the cervical spinal cord of E16 (black), E17 (green), E18 (blue), and E19 (red) rats. In the E16 rat, the slit-shaped spinal canal extends all the way from the dorsal to the ventral surface of the cord. In the E17 rat, the regression of the spinal canal is associated with the shrinkage of the gray matter dorsomedially and ventromedially (green arrows). The ventral horn, and even more so the dorsal horn are expanding freely at the same time. In the E18 rat, the continuing shrinkage of the spinal canal (blue arrows) is associated with the invagination of the gray matter ventrally and dorsally (the space created dorsally is occupied by the expanding dorsal funiculus). In the E19 rat, the ventromedial and dorsomedial constriction of the gray matter continues in relation to the terminal shrinkage of the persisting central canal (red arrows).

in the dorsolateral direction. As the spinal cord continues to grow after E19, and in particular as the dorsal funiculus expands dorsomedially, the anchoring "ropes" of the roof plate and floor plate ensure that the central gray region surrounding the central canal does not expand. This is seen in the comparable widths of the central gray in the cervical spinal cord of an E19 and a P60 rat (Figure 4-62).

The necessity for this structural outcome is uncertain. It is possible that these mechanical con-

straining forces, which produce both the H-shape of the mature gray matter as well as the invagination of the dorsal median septum and ventral median sulcus, assure that the shrunken central canal and the surrounding central autonomic area of the gray matter remain in close proximity to the meninges of the spinal cord and its blood vessels. If it were not for this process, the great expansion of the ventral funiculus and, in particular, of the dorsal funiculus would place the fluid compartment of the central canal too far removed from the meningeal lining.

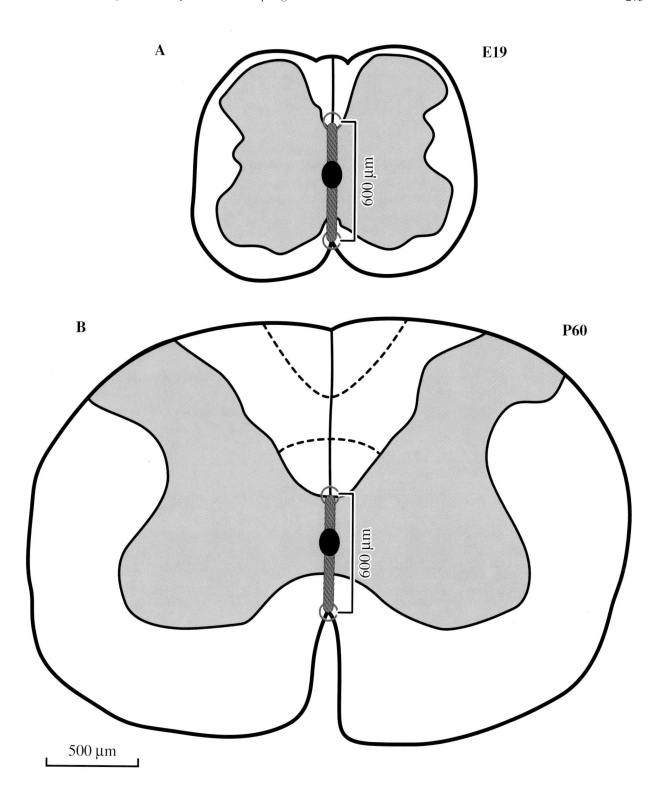

Figure 4-62. Outlines of the boundaries of the white matter (white) and the gray matter (gray) in the cervical spinal cord of an E19 rat fetus (**A**) and a 60-day-old adult rat (**B**). The width of the central gray region surrounding the central canal, and the distance between the tips of the dorsal median septum and the ventral median sulcus, remain roughly constant while elsewhere the gray matter has expanded considerably. It is hypothesized that the medial expansion of the gray matter was prevented by the taut fibers (red "ropes" and "rings") of the floor plate and the roof plate that anchor the tips of the central canal. This structural feature may ensure that the meningeal lining and the blood vessels of the spinal cord remain in the vicinity of the central canal.

4.4.5 Myelination in the Spinal Cord.

The histological study of myelination in the spinal cord was pioneered by Flechsig (1876) in conjunction with his investigation of human brain development. More recently, spinal cord myelination has been studied in several mammalian species, including the cat (Tilney and Casamajor, 1924; Langworthy, 1929; Windle et al., 1934), the dog (Fox et al., 1967), the rat (Samora-jski and Friede, 1968; Matthews and Duncan, 1971; Schwab and Schnell, 1989; Gorgels, 1990), and the opossum (Leblond and Cabana, 1997). Windle et al. (1934) reported that, in the cat cervical spinal cord, myelination begins in the ventral funiculus between the ages of E42 and E45 (80-90 mm body length). The earliest myelinating fiber tract is the medial longitudinal fasciculus but a few myelinating fibers are also seen in the cuneate fasciculus and in the ventral root (Figure 4-63A). In E50 (100 mm) cat fetuses, myelination spreads from the ventral funiculus to the lateral funiculus, expands in the cuneate fasciculus but has not yet begun in the gracile fasciculus (Figure 4-63B). At that age, the dorsal root fibers are myelinated inside the spinal cord but not peripherally. Fibers of the fasciculus gracilis are still unmyelinated at cervical levels of the spinal cord in E54 (120 mm) fetuses (Figure 4-63C) and in newborn kittens. Similarly, Langworthy (1929) reported that fibers of the cuneate fasciculus myelinate earlier in the cat than the fibers of the gracile fasciculus and the entire dorsal funiculus is not fully myelinated until P38. The rubrospinal and corticospinal fibers are still poorly myelinated about this age. In the lumbar spinal cord of the dog (Fox et al., 1967), the dorsal, lateral, and ventral funiculi myelinate rapidly during the first three weeks of postnatal life (Figure 4-64) but myelination of the the lateral corticospinal tract is not complete until after the fifth week. All these investigators related regional differences in myelination to the development of spinal reflexes and voluntary movements.

Matthews and Duncan (1971) counted glia in three components of the dorsal funiculus – the fasciculus gracilis, fasciculus cuneatus, and corticospinal tract – of the cervical spinal cord of rats between P3 and P120 (Figure 4-65) to correlate increases in glial concentration with the onset and progress of myelination. In the fasciculus gracilis, there was a sharp rise in glial concentration on P5, and that was followed there by the onset of myelination by P10. In the corticospinal tract, the concentration of glia steadily

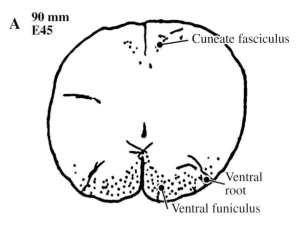

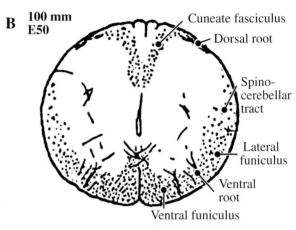

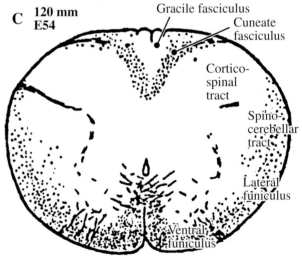

Figure 4-63. Sequence of myelination in the cervical spinal cord of fetal cats. **A.** At E45 (90 mm body length) myelination starts in the ventral funiculus and the ventral root; a few myelinated fibers are also present in the cuneate fasciculus. **B.** By E50 (100 mm), myelination has spread from the ventral funiculus to the lateral funiculus, and expands in the cuneate fasciculus. Myelination starts in the dorsal root. **C.** The lateral corticospinal tract and the gracile fasciculus are still unmyelinated on E54 (120 mm). After Windle et al. (1934).

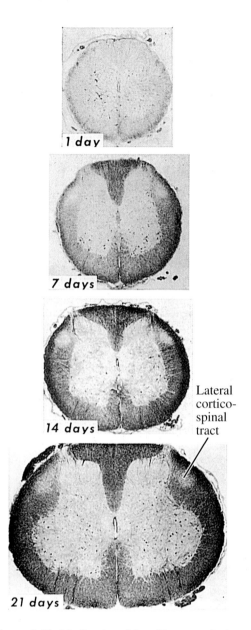

Figure 4-64. Myelination of the white matter in the lumbar spinal cord of the dog between days 1 and 21 of postnatal life. Myelination is well advanced in all regions of the white matter by P21, except in the lateral corticospinal tract. After Fox et al. (1967).

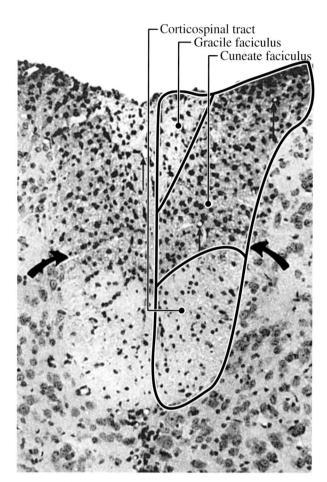

Figure 4-65. Myelination gliosis in the cuneate fasciculus in the cervical spinal cord of a P10 rat. Myelination gliosis is not yet evident in the gracile fasciculus and the medial corticospinal tract (region of dorsal funiculus underneath arrows). After Matthews and Duncan (1971).

increased from P3 to P20 but declined thereafter. Myelination of the corticospinal tract begins between P10 and P15, and peaks by P20. While the commencement of myelination lags behind the onset of "myelination gliosis" the two run parallel during the height of the myelination process. In an immunohistochemical study, Hartman et al. (1979) found that myelin basic protein first appeared in the brain of newborn rats in the soma of oligodendroglia cells and, but then the intensity of the chemical reaction decreased in the glial cell bodies and increased in the neighboring nerve fibers. The work of Collinson et al. (1998) suggests that neurofascin, a cell adhesion molecule, may play a role in the initiation of glial-axon contact when myelination starts. Neurofascin first appears in oligodendrocytes, then shifts to the surface of neurons, then stabilizes in both by adulthood. Using three antigens, Schwab and Schnell (1989) found regional differences in the appearance of myelin-specific glycolipids and myelin basic protein in fiber tracts of the rat cervical spinal cord (Figure 4-66). Some myelin constituents are present by birth in the ventral root and the dorsal root. Within the spinal cord, myelin constituents first appear in the ventral funiculus on P1, next in the fasciculus cuneatus and ventrolateral funiculus on P2-P3 and, finally, in the fasciculus gracilis and dorsolateral funiculus during the latter part of the first week of postnatal life. The myelin constituents begin to appear in the corticospinal tract towards the end of the second week and somewhat later in Lissauer's tract. In the gray matter, myelin constituents show up in a patchy manner around P11-P14. In the rat, the myelination of corticospinal axons proceeds from rostral to caudal and the process is not completed until about the fourth postnatal week (Gorgels, 1990). Electron microscopic observations in the rat corticospinal tract (Samorajski and Friede; 1968; Matthews and Duncan, 1971) indicate that the larger axons tend to myelinate first (Figure 4-67) and that there is a correlation between axon diameter and the number of myelin lamellae.

Considering the fact that two different cell types (Schwann cells and oligodendrocytes, respectively) are involved in the myelination of the peripheral and central branches of dorsal and ventral root fibers, are there differences in the onset and rate of

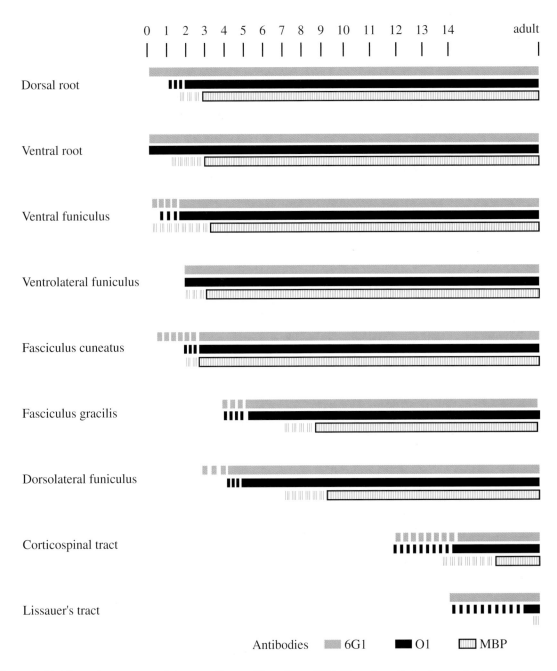

Figure 4-66. Time of appearance of three myelin specific antigens (6G1, 01, and myelin basic protein) in the white matter of the rat cervical spinal cord during the first 2 weeks of postnatal life, in relation to degree of myelination in adulthood. Interrupted lines indicate low levels of the particular antigen. Selected data from Schwab and Schnell (1989).

myelination at these two sites? According to Fraher (1976) the central and peripheral branches of ventral root axons in rats start to myelinate concurrently at birth (Fraher, 1976). Similarly, Berthold and Carlstedt (1982) found that, in the cat dorsal root myelination starts at about the same age (E53) centrally and peripherally some distance away from the entry zone. However, the dorsal root fibers remain unmyelinated near the dorsal root entry zone for about another 10 days. This is the site of the dorsal root boundary cap at the transitional region of the peripheral and central components of dorsal root axons. To the extent that impulse conduction is facilitated by myelination, this unmyelinated gap may represent a temporary obstacle in the transmission of sensory messages from the periphery to the spinal cord.

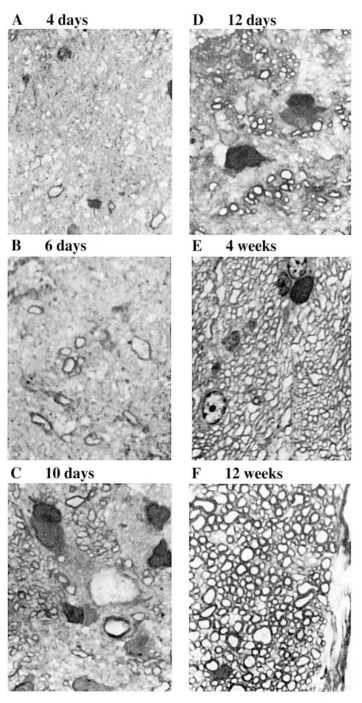

Figure 4-67. Myelination of individual fibers in the medial corticospinal tract of the rat cervical spinal cord between 4 days and 12 weeks of postnatal life. Electron microscopy. After Samorajski and Friede (1968).

5 DEVELOPMENT OF THE HUMAN SPINAL CORD DURING THE FIRST TRIMESTER: GESTATIONAL WEEKS 3.5 TO 13

5.1 The Problem of Dating and Staging Spinal Cord Development

5.1.1   The Dating of Human Embryos.
Embryonic development begins with fertilization of a female ovum by a male sperm during sexual intercourse. If time of fertilization is known, that date is designated as the first day of conception or gestation. Thus, in the experimental studies described in Chapters 3 and 4, we could specify the gestational age of rat embryos with an accuracy of about half a day. In those studies, estrous rats were mated with studs late in the afternoon. The females found next morning with vaginal sperm plugs were transferred to individual maternity cages and those that became pregnant were known to have conceived during the mating period. Accordingly, the age of their offspring was designated embryonic day 1 (E1). (Some investigators call the first day of gestation either day E0 or E0.5.)

But an accurate dating of conception is usually not possible in humans, except in the case of artificial insemination or a single instance of sexual intercourse (as in the case of rape). Normally, even when detailed clinical protocols are available about the course of pregnancy, there is some uncertainty about the exact date of conception. Recollection of the time of sexual intercourse is often unreliable, and in the case of sexually active couples, may be unknown. Obstetricians often use a pregnant woman's last period of menstruation to estimate gestational age. The rationale is that while the human female is sexually receptive through all phases of the estrous cycle, fertilization can take place only shortly after ovulation. Ovulation tends to occur midway during the monthly menstrual cycle, hence the embryo is estimated to be 2 weeks old relative to the mother's last menstruation. However, the period of ovulation during the menstrual cycle and the duration of fertility are highly variable (Hartman, 1936). Hence, the accuracy of estimates based on menstrual dating may be off by several days or more.

In spite of these problems, the wealth of data accumulated by the turn of the twentieth century about various indices of embryonic growth – such as crown-heel length, crown-rump length, sitting height, head size, foot length, body weight – in relation to estimates of gestational age enabled investigators to construct reliable timetables of embryonic development (Michaelis, 1906; Keibel and Elze, 1908; Mall, 1910, 1918; Streeter, 1920; Scammon, 1927). Figure 5-1 is a recent timetable that correlates crown-rump (CR) length with estimated age in gestational weeks (GW) during the first trimester. The timetable is in good agreement with many of the specimens used in this book for which information was available about both CR length and estimated age in GW. We used this timetable to correct the gestational age of embryos for which that information was either not available or was discrepant with the norms.

5.1.2   The Staging of Human Embryos.
Embryonic development is an orderly process that has been recognized for a long time. The different organs of the body, including the central nervous system, grow and mature in a precise temporal sequence. The regularity of embryonic development gave rise to the effort to establish *stages* of embryonic development (Mall, 1914; Streeter, 1942). Stage norms could circumvent the problem of unreliable dating of gestational age and individual variability in the tempo of development. In a series of papers, Streeter (1942, 1945, 1948; Streeter et al., 1951) described in some detail his proposed stages of human embryonic development from the time of appearance of a few somites (stage XI) until the onset of the fetal period (stage XXIII). Assignment of an embryo to a specific stage was based on "scoring points " in terms of development of selected organs, such as the cornea, optic nerve, cochlea, hypophysis, vomeronasal organ, submandibular gland, kidney, and others. For instance, embryos were assigned to stage XIX, irrespective of their estimated gestational age, if they had the following features: the cornea is recognizable as a thin layer of mesoderm; the optic nerve is slender; the cochlea has a short tip (no turns); the hypophysis has a thick stalk; the vomeronasal organ is merely a pit; the submandibular gland forms a short clublike duct; the kidney lacks renal vesicles; and the differentiation of cartilage cells has progressed to phase 3. The last stage described by Streeter, stage XXIII, was typically reached by about gestational age of 46-48 days (GW6.5). O'Rahilly and Müller (1987) later described the first 10 stages of human embryonic development that precede Streeter's stages XI to XXIII.

More recently, O'Rahilly and Müller (1994) applied Streeter's staging system to the development of the human brain. However, O'Rahilly and Müller's staging is based principally on overt features of neural development rather than detailed morphoge-

Body Growth During the First Trimester
(1-13 Weeks)

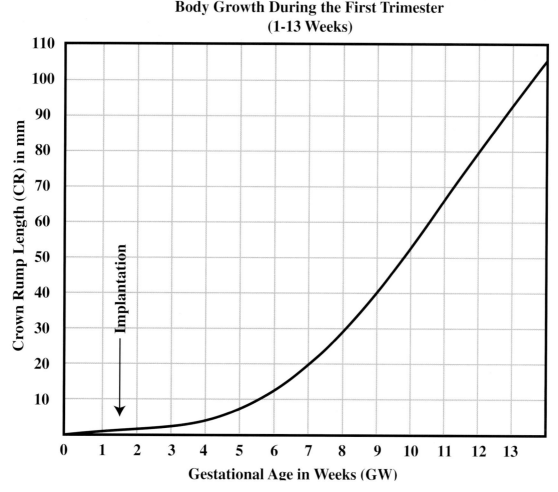

Figure 5-1. Estimated gestational age in weeks (GW) of human embryos and fetuses in relation to their crown-rump length (CR). Smoothed curve based on data collected by Mall (1910), Streeter (1920), and others. After Patten (1953).

netic, cytological, or maturational criteria. Thus, stage 8 of brain development is characterized by the formation of the neural groove; stage 9 by the appearance of the mesencephalic flexure; stage 10 by formation of the neural tube; stage 11 by the closure of the rostral neuropore; stage 12 by closure of the caudal neuropore; stage 13 by formation of the cervical flexure; stage 14 by the pontine flexure; stage 15 by the appearance of the cerebral vesicles; stage 16 by formation of the primordium of the hippocampus; stage 17 by the formation of the fourth ventricle choroid plexus; stage 18 by the formation of the choroid plexus of the lateral ventricles; stage 19 by "reflex responses," and so forth.

Although such gross staging of brain development may be useful to an obstetrician as a diagnostic tool, it is not very helpful to the developmental neurobiologist who is concerned with the details of brain development, such as neurogenesis, neuronal migra-

tion, axonal growth, dendritic development, synaptogenesis, transmitter maturation, myelogenesis, etc., of the central nervous system in general or of a selected brain region in particular. Little is gained, for instance, if the development of the spinal cord is lumped into stages defined by such gross features as the formation of the cervical or pontine flexure, such extraneous criteria as corneal growth, or hypophyseal development, or such irrelevant events as the development of the submandibular gland or the kidney. Each neural structure has its own timetable of development and that has to be independently determined before the question can be posed how a developmental stage in one brain region or system is linked to a developmental stage in some other brain region or system. For instance, there may be a causal link between the distribution of corticospinal tract fibers in the spinal cord and the timetable of neurogenesis, migration and maturation of lamina V neurons in the cerebral cortex; or between the segregation of different motoneuron columns in the ventral horn and the maturation of certain proximal and distal muscles of the forelimb. However, whether these are independent or interdependent events can only be usefully examined after the developmental stages of each structure or region have been separately determined. Indeed, the conceptualization of the continuous process of brain development in terms of discontinuous stages is useful only if that staging offers clues about the processes or mechanisms involved in the sequential emergence, differentiation, and maturation of the different brain structures or constituents.

5.1.3   The Dating and Staging of Spinal Cord Development.

Previous experimental studies with ^{3}H-thymidine autoradiography in rats have established that the early events in the development of the central nervous system – the birth of different classes of neurons, their sojourn, migration, and final settling in target structures – are precisely timed and sequentially ordered events (e.g., Altman and Bayer, 1982, 1984, 1997; Bayer and Altman, 1991). Undoubtedly, the sequential progression of later events in neural maturation – such as the outgrowth of axons. the trajectories that the axons follow, dendritic development, synaptogenesis, and myelination – are dependent on the precision of the early phases of neural development, although they may be somewhat more variable. The sequential order and chronology of the early landmark events can form the basis for staging the development of a particular neural system, such as the spinal cord.

In the two preceding chapters we have reviewed the sequential order of several facets of spinal cord development in animals, with particular reference to datings with ^{3}H thymidine autoradiography in the rat. Insofar as the autoradiographic technique cannot be used to date spinal cord development in man, we will rely heavily on the experimental evidence obtained in rats in describing and interpreting human spinal cord development. The histological evidence establishes that the sequence of events in the development of the human spinal cord is very similar to that in the rat, although the time course is longer in man. This offers some advantages. Because prenatal development is far more protracted in man (about 40 weeks) than in the rat (about 3 weeks), the successive stages of spinal cord development are often easier to discern in the developing human spinal cord than in the rat. An example of this is the easier identification of different compartments of the human spinal

cord neuroepithelium (the ventral, intermediate, and dorsal) that sequentially produce the neurons of the ventral horn, the intermediate gray, and the dorsal horn. Following a detailed analysis of the sequential order and chronology of spinal cord development in man, this chapter ends with a proposed schedule of 10 ontogenetic stages of spinal cord development during the first trimester (Section 5.9) The relationship between these stages to somatic and behavioral development during the first trimester is dealt with in Chapter 9 (Section 9.1.3).

5.1.4   Some Technical Notes.

The specimens used for investigating human spinal cord development during the first trimester come from three large collections in the National Museum of Health and Medicine (currently housed at the Armed Forces Institute of Pathology, Washington, DC). These are the Carnegie collection, the Minot collection, and the Yakovlev collection. To distinguish the specimens, we add the letters C, M, and Y to the numerical codes originally assigned to them in their respective collections. (In the case of the Yakovlev specimens, we omitted a string of letter and number combinations that refer to the details of different sources and projects.)

The specimens of the Minot collection, which to our knowledge, have never been described before, are of superior quality but lack detailed documentation. The only information available are the serial numbers of the slides, CR length of each embryo, the thickness of the serial sections (all sections have been saved in this material), and the histological stain used. Accordingly, all estimates of the gestational age of the specimens in the Minot collection are based on the timetable presented in Figure 5-1. Specimens from the Carnegie and Yakovlev collections have detailed protocols. However, there is variability in the methods used for estimating the age of the specimens (menstrual or gestational), in specifying their age (days, weeks, or months), and also in the survival time of some of the embryos or fetuses after abortion. Therefore, the gestational age given for each specimen was checked against the timetable in Figure 5-1 and was corrected if necessary.

Feldman (1920) divided prenatal development of the human nervous system into three periods: the germinal period (GW1.0–GW2.0), the embryonic period (GW3.0–GW6.0), and the fetal period (GW6.0 to birth). Unfortunately, Feldman's designated age for the germinal period is not valid. The period of neurogenesis is not only far more prolonged than the dates given, it also differs widely (though systematically) in different regions of the central nervous system. Indeed, there are regions of the central nervous system (such as the cerebellum and the hippocampus) in which neurogenesis peaks during the fetal period and extends well into early postnatal life. This leaves two prenatal periods to be distinguished, the embryonic and the fetal. Although this distinction is frequently made to this day, the separation between the two periods is difficult to define. There is no developmental transformation or event, either in terms of overall somatic development or overall neural development that unambiguously demarcates the embryonic period from the fetal period.

Coincidentally or not, the separation between the embryonic and fetal periods, if it has to be made, is easier to demarcate in the spinal cord than elsewhere in the central nervous system. As we shall see momentarily, it is about GW13 (the last week of the first trimester), that the spinal cord neuroepithelium disappears. This signals the end not only of spinal cord neurogenesis but also the neuroepithelial production of spinal cord neuroglia. Thus the dissolution of the neuroepithelium by GW13 could be said to end the embryonic period. The more protracted events during the second and third trimesters, associated with the arrival of many descending supraspinal fiber tracts, and the onset of myelination gliosis and myelination in the white matter of the spinal cord (the corticospinal tract excepted), could be assigned to the fetal stage. Accordingly, for the sake of convenience, this chapter deals with the "embryonic" growth of the spinal cord during the first trimester, and the next chapter deals with developments taking place during second and third trimesters, i.e., the "fetal" period.

The normal term of pregnancy is about 280 days (40 weeks), with an estimated range between 270 and 284 days (Williams, 1931). About 334 days is believed to be the longest period in which a fetus can survive in the uterus and be delivered alive. The first trimester was taken to last from GW1.0-GW13.0; the second trimester from GW14.0-GW26.0; the third trimester from GW27.0-GW40.0. Where gestational age was given in terms of days or months in the specimens used in this study, the age is always referred to in gestational weeks (GW). Throughout this study, we took an average month to consist of 30.5 days or 4.33 weeks.

To avoid repetitiveness, interpretations that are based on experimental work in animals summarized and documeted in Chapters 3 and 4, are not specifically mentioned again here.

5.2 Closure of the Neural Tube and the Early Growth of the Spinal Cord. GW3.0 to GW7.0

5.2.1 The Open and the Closed Neuroepithelium: Transformation of the Neural Plate into the Neural Tube. GW3.0 to GW3.5. The first histological sign of the development of a committed line of neural stem cells (neuroepithelial or NEP cells) is the appearance of the neural plate. The neural plate, or open neuroepithelium, is the elongated axial portion of the embryonic ectoderm that forms above the notochordal plate before GW3.0 (Figure 5-2A). The neural plate thickens in late presomite human embryos, then becomes depressed and forms the longitudinal neural groove. As more somites appear, the dorsolateral margins of the neural groove curve innward and fuse, forming the neural tube. This event – the formation of the closed neuroepithelium – coincides with the transformation of the notochordal plate into the notochord at about the 7-10 somite stage. The closure of the neuroepithelium begins at cervical levels of the future spinal cord on or about GW3.0 (Ingalls, 1918; Corner, 1929; Heuser, 1932) and proceeds concurrently both rostrally, where the brain vesicles will form, and caudally along the lengthening spinal cord (Figures 5-2B, C). The polar regions where the closure takes place last are the anterior and posterior neuropores. The posterior neuropore of the lumbosacral spinal cord closes at about the 25-somite stage (approximately GW3.5). The closure of the neuroepithelium creates the lumen of the spinal canal and cephalic vesicles. Henceforth, the NEP cells will undergo mitosis in the unique fluid-filled (humoral) milieu of the cerebrospinal ventricular system. The biochemical and morphogenetic significance of this transformation between GW3.0 and GW3.5 remains to be determined.

5.2.2 The Early Growth of the Spinal Cord in Relation to the Brain. GW3.5 to GW7.0. Figure 5-3 shows the immense growth of the spinal cord between GW3.5 and GW7.0. The length of the relatively straight spinal cord is about 2.5 mm in the GW3.0 embryo (*C5074*; CR 3 mm; 10 somites; Figure 5-3A). The cervical flexure is not present and the brain is narrow and short. Obviously, the growth

A

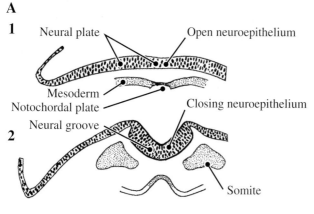

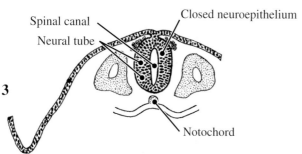

Figure 5-2. A. Three stages in the formation of the spinal cord neuroepithelium: 1. neural plate; 2, neural groove; 3, neural tube. The neuroepithelium is open during the first two stages and becomes closed during the third stage. The cell surfaces that form the *outer* lining of the open neuroepithelium come to form, after closure, the *inner* lining of the lumen of the spinal canal and cephalic ventricles. **B.** Fusion of the neuroepithelium (red outline) is limited to a few spinal segments in this less mature GW3.0 human embryo. After Payne; from Hamilton et al. (1964). **C.** Fusion at most spinal segments in this more mature GW3.0 human embryo. After Corner; from Hamilton et al. (1964).

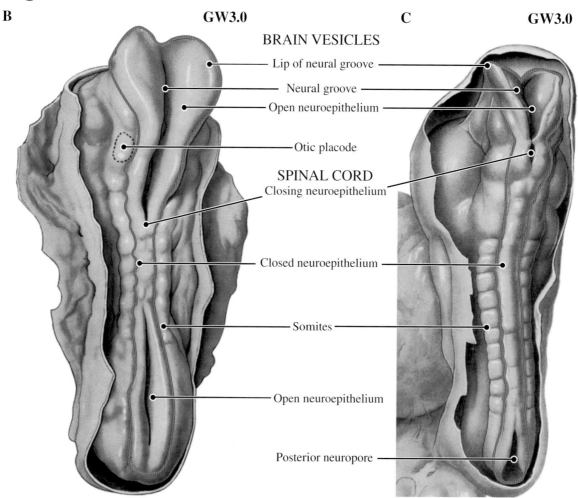

spurt of the spinal cord antedates that of the brain during this phase of central nervous system development. Several morphological changes are evident in the GW4.0 embryo (*C8066*; CR 5.3 mm; Figure 5-3B). The first of these is the lengthening and widening of the spinal cord and the formation of the cervical and the cephalic flexures in the brain. The formation of the cervical and cephalic flexures sig-

nals the onset of accelerated growth of the brain, roughly at a right angle to the body axis and the spinal cord. The second change is the upward curving of the caudal end of the spinal cord, what we shall call the transient sacral flexure. Whatever else may be the functional significance of these rostral and caudal foldings, the net effect is that the length of the growing spinal cord exceeds for a while the crown-rump

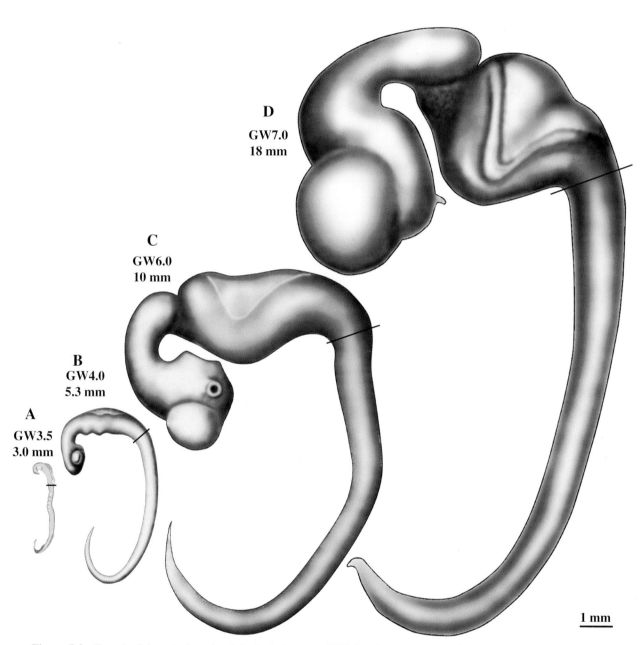

Figure 5-3. Growth of the spinal cord and the brain between GW3.5 and GW7.0. **A.** The relatively straight spinal cord is nearly as thick as the small brain (above the line) in a GW3.5 embryo (*C5074*; CR 3.0 mm; 10 somites). After Corner (1929). **B.** The lengthened spinal cord with its cervical (top) and sacral (bottom) flexure in a GW4.0 embryo (*C8066*; 5.3 mm). The growth spurt of the brain has begun rostrally. After Streeter (1945). **C.** The thickened spinal cord of a GW6.0 embryo (*C6517*; CR 10 mm). The expansion rate of the brain by now exceeds that of the spinal cord. After Streeter (1948). **D.** The spinal cord and the brain of a GW 7.0 embryo (*Hooker/Humphrey #142*; CR 18 mm). After Streeter et al. (1951).

length of the embryo. The growth of the spinal cord, both in terms of length and bulk, continues in the GW6.0 embryo (*C6517*; CR 10 mm; Figure 5-3C) and the GW7.0 embryo (Hooker-Humphrey #142; CR 18 mm; Figure 5-3D). A notable event at GW6 and GW7 is the accelerated growth of the brain stem relative to the spinal cord.

5.3 Development of the Cervical Spinal Cord During the First Trimester: An Overview

GW3.5. The histology of the cervical spinal cord in a GW3.5 embryo (*M714*; CR 4.0 mm) is illustrated in Figure 5-4A. This is the primordial spinal cord that consists of little else than a multiple-cell thick, pseudostratified germinal matrix of darkly staining cells that undergo mitosis near the lumen. The primordial spinal cord is cylindrical in shape and encases a slit-shaped spinal canal. Three "plates" may be distinguished in relation to the spinal canal: the roof plate and floor plate in the midline, and the lateral plates (the neuroepithelium) bilaterally. The roof and floor plates are much thinner than the lateral neuroepithelium. There are only a few scattered cells of unknown identity in the thin field that surrounds the lateral plates, indicating that the exodus of differentiating progeny of NEP cells has not yet begun to any significant extent at this age. The cells of the dorsal root ganglia are just beginning to assemble between the spinal cord and the segmental somite. This GW3.5 embryo illustrates the pre-exodus stage of spinal cord development, the stage that antedates the onset of neuronal differentiation.

GW4.5. Figure 5-4B shows both quantitative and a qualitative changes in the developing spinal cord of a GW4.5 embryo (*M2300*; CR 6.3 mm). The quantitative change is the growth of the lateral neuroepithelium, as judged by its increased height and thickness. This indicates that a major event between GW3.5 and 4.5 is the continuing proliferation and consequent increase in the stock of darkly staining NEP cells. But there is also a significant qualitative change in this embryo. This is the formation of a small cluster of lightly staining (differentiating) cells along the wall of the ventral portion of the lateral neuroepithelium. The neuroepithelial region flanked by these lightly staining cells will from now on be called the ventral neuroepithelium, and its cells the ventral NEP cells. The formation of this cluster of differentiating cells signals the beginning of the exodus of post-mitotic cells from the ventral neuroepithelium and the onset of differentiation of the earliest generated neurons of the spinal cord, the ventral horn motoneurons. In much smaller numbers, differentiating cells are also exiting from other parts of the neuroepithelium. Judging by the increase in the size of the dorsal root ganglion, cell proliferation has also become brisk at this peripheral site. Evidently, the primary sensory neurons and final motoneurons of the spinal cord are beginning to form by GW4.5

GW5.5. There are many developmental changes in the spinal cord of the GW5.5 embryo (*C8998*; CR 11.0 mm; Figure 5-5A). (1) As a whole the cylindrical spinal cord has become pear-shaped. This is due to the great increase in the motoneuron population in the expanding ventral horn. (2) The slit-shaped spinal canal now has three parts: a long recess ventrally, the ventral canal; an oval central region, the central canal; and a short recess dorsally, the dorsal canal. (3) The neuroepithelium surrounding the spinal canal has also changed its shape and now resembles an inverted vase. Three neuroepithelial compartments are now distinguishable: the dorsal neuroepithelium (alar plate), the intermediate neuroepithelium, and the ventral neuroepithelium (basal plate). (4) The ventral neuroepithelium is already becoming depleted of NEP cells. This feature, combined with the great increase in the population of differentiating motoneurons suggests that the peak of motoneuron production is ending in the cervical spinal cord by GW5.5. (5) Two new clusters of differentiating cells are beginning to form. One of these flanks the intermediate neuroepithelium, the other flanks the dorsal neuroepithelium. These two cell aggregates are the earliest differentiating interneurons of the incipient intermediate gray and the dorsal horn, respectively. (6) The dorsal root bifurcation zone (the oval bundle of His) appears dorsolaterally. Finally (7), the width of the ventral commissure has increased greatly, suggesting that the axons of early differentiating, contralaterally projecting interneurons are crossing to the opposite side in increasing numbers during GW5.5.

GW6.5. Most of the new features noted in the previous specimen have become more pronounced in the spinal cord of the GW6.5 embryo (*C7707*; CR 14.5 mm) shown in Figure 5-5B. But there are also some new developments. (1) The ventral neuroepithelium surrounding the receding ventral canal has become thinner, signaling the approaching

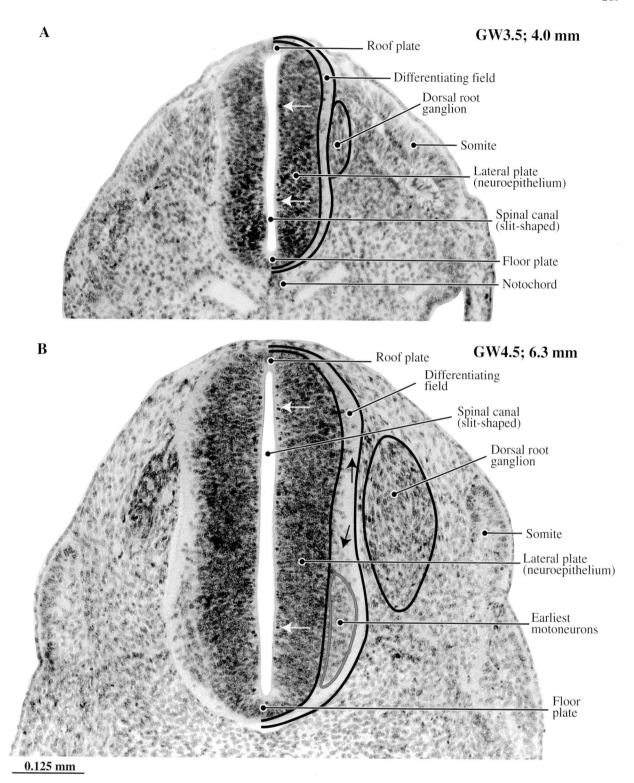

A GW3.5; 4.0 mm

Roof plate
Differentiating field
Dorsal root ganglion
Somite
Lateral plate (neuroepithelium)
Spinal canal (slit-shaped)
Floor plate
Notochord

B GW4.5; 6.3 mm

Roof plate
Differentiating field
Spinal canal (slit-shaped)
Dorsal root ganglion
Somite
Lateral plate (neuroepithelium)
Earliest motoneurons
Floor plate

0.125 mm

Figure 5-4. A. The cylindrical primordial spinal cord with its slit-shaped spinal canal in a GW3.5 embryo (*M714*; CR 4.0 mm). The spinal cord has three parts: the thin roof plate and floor plate medially, and the thick mitotically active (white arrows) lateral plates, or neuroepithelium, bilaterally. A few scattered lightly staining (differentiating) cells surrounds the neuroepithelium. **B.** The neuroepithelium has grown considerably in this GW4.5 embryo (*M2300*; CR 6.3 mm), indicating a great increase in the stock of NEP cells. The cluster of differentiating cells that flank the ventral neuroepithelium (red outline) are the earliest motoneurons of the incipient ventral horn. There is some increase in the population of other differentiating cells (black arrows) and the dorsal root ganglion has expanded considerably.

end of ventral NEP cell proliferation; i.e., the cessation of motoneuron production. (2) The diminishing ventral neuroepithelium is flanked by an enlarged field of ventral interneurons that displace the motoneurons ventrolaterally. (3) The motoneurons show incipient signs of segregation into clusters separated by cell-free surrounds. (4) The withdrawal of the ventral canal is coupled with the recession of the floor plate and the formation of the ventral median sulcus. (5) The differentiating field of intermediate interneurons flanking the massive intermediate neuroepithelium has increased in size. (6) The dorsal root bifurcation zone spreads mediodorsally over the differentiating field of dorsal interneurons. (7) Finally, the ventral funiculus and the lateral funiculus are beginning to expand.

GW7.0. The cervical spinal cord of the GW7.0 embryo (*C7254*; CR 22.5 mm) seen in Figure 5-6A illustrates the continuing development of the features noted in the previous specimen. These include: (1) further shrinkage of the ventral canal; (2) deepening of the ventral median sulcus; (3) thinning of the ventral neuroepithelium; (4) segregation of the medial and lateral motoneuronal clusters; (4) expansion of the ventral and intermediate fields of differentiating interneurons; (5) growth of the ventral and lateral funiculi; and (6) the expansion dorsomedially of the dorsal root bifurcation zone.

GW8.5. The GW8.5 embryo (*C609*; CR 32 mm) shown in Figure 5-6B illustrates some of the new developments that have occurred between GW7.0 and GW8.5. (1) The ventral canal has disappeared. (2) The ventral median sulcus has considerably deepened and its walls are occupied by the greatly enlarged ventromedial funiculus. (3) The segregation of sev-

eral motoneuron columns is in progress along the lateral wall of the ventral horn. (4) The central autonomic area has become identifiable. (5) The dorsal canal has retreated considerably and its site is occupied by (6) the dorsal median septum and (7) the fascicles of the developing dorsal funiculus. (8) The dorsal horn is expanding due to the arrival of a large population of small, densely packed neurons that will form the substantia gelatinosa.

GW10.4–GW14. The major morphogenetic change in the cervical spinal cord of the GW10.5 fetus (*Y380-62*; CR 56mm) reproduced in Figure 5-7A is the virtual disappearance of the dorsal canal. That signals the transformation of the embryonic spinal canal lined by NEP cells into the fetal central canal lined by specialized cells of the ependymal layer. Among other ongoing events are the increasing segregation of the lateral motor columns, the expansion of the intermediate interneuronal field, the deepening of the dorsal funiculus, and the growth of the dorsal horn. The gray matter of the spinal cord during the remaining 2-3 weeks of the first trimester, assumes in broad outlines its charactreristic configuration. This is suggested by the morphology of the spinal cord of the GW14 fetus (*Y68-65*; 108 mm) during the first week of the second trimester (Figure 5-7B).

Following this overview, we will now discuss in some detail (1) the sequential development of components of the spinal cord neuroepithelium, (2) the progressive segregation of motor columns in the ventral horn, and (3) the growth and distribution of branches of the dorsal root primary afferents during the first trimester in relation to body growth and skeletomuscular development.

Figure 5-5. A. The pear-shaped cervical spinal cord of a GW5.5 embryo (*C8998*; CR 11.0 mm). Three distinguishable neuroepithelial compartments surround the elongated slit-shaped ventral canal, the expanded central canal, and the incipient dorsal canal. The ventral neuroepithelium is thinning, as if depleted of NEP cells while the population of motoneurons is increasing ventrolaterally (red outline). This signals the large scale exodus of differentiating motoneurons (large red arrow) from the ventral neuroepithelium. The more modest exodus of interneurons from the ventral, intermediate, and dorsal neuroepithelia is also indicated (small red, green, and yellow arrows and outlines, respectively). **B.** The pear-shaped spinal cord of a GW6.5 embryo (*C7707*; CR 14.5 mm). The ventral canal and the surrounding ventral neuroepithelium are receding. The field of ventral interneurons has grown appreciably and has displaced the expanded field of motoneurons ventrolaterally. The exodus of differentiating interneurons from the intermediate neuroepithelium is pronounced but that is just beginning from the dorsal neuroepithelium. The ventral and lateral funiculi, and the dorsal root bifurcation zone are expanding.

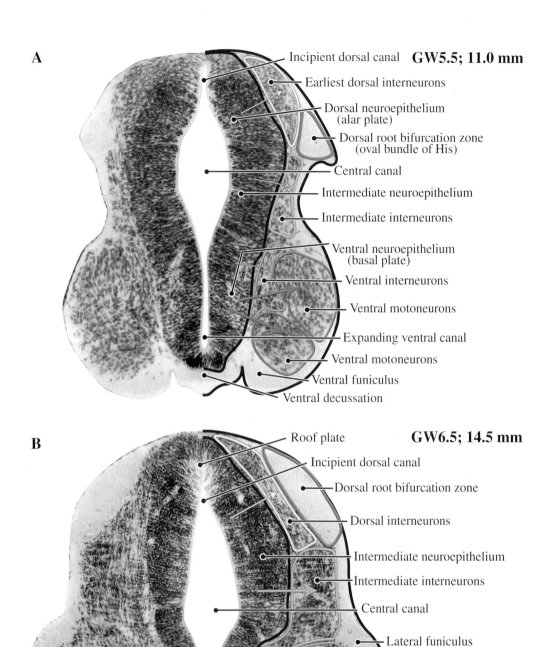

A Incipient dorsal canal **GW5.5; 11.0 mm**
Earliest dorsal interneurons
Dorsal neuroepithelium (alar plate)
Dorsal root bifurcation zone (oval bundle of His)
Central canal
Intermediate neuroepithelium
Intermediate interneurons
Ventral neuroepithelium (basal plate)
Ventral interneurons
Ventral motoneurons
Expanding ventral canal
Ventral motoneurons
Ventral funiculus
Ventral decussation

B Roof plate **GW6.5; 14.5 mm**
Incipient dorsal canal
Dorsal root bifurcation zone
Dorsal interneurons
Intermediate neuroepithelium
Intermediate interneurons
Central canal
Lateral funiculus
Ventral interneurons
Ventral neuroepithelium
Receding ventral canal
Ventral motoneurons
Floor plate
Ventral decussation
Ventral funiculus
Ventral median sulcus

0.25 mm

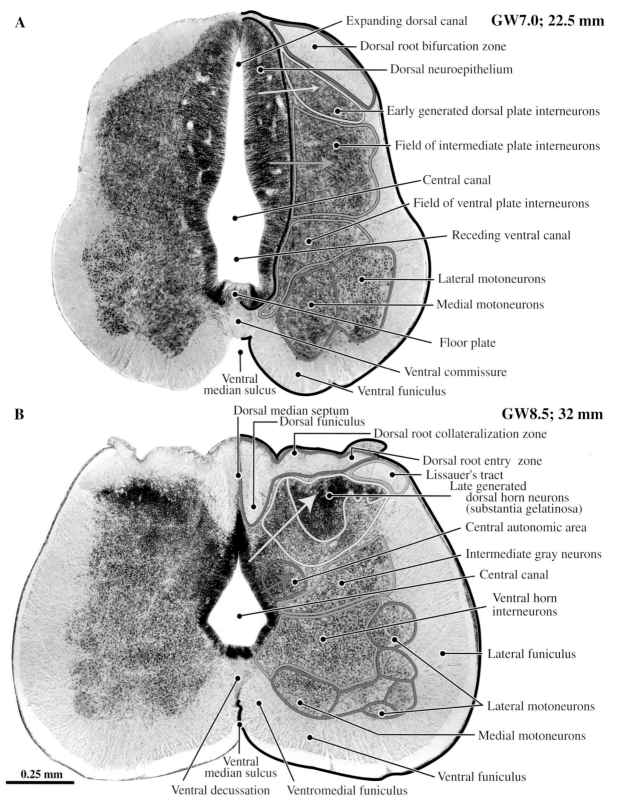

A. Expanding dorsal canal — **GW7.0; 22.5 mm**

Dorsal root bifurcation zone

Dorsal neuroepithelium

Early generated dorsal plate interneurons

Field of intermediate plate interneurons

Central canal

Field of ventral plate interneurons

Receding ventral canal

Lateral motoneurons

Medial motoneurons

Floor plate

Ventral commissure

Ventral median sulcus

Ventral funiculus

B. Dorsal median septum — **GW8.5; 32 mm**

Dorsal funiculus

Dorsal root collateralization zone

Dorsal root entry zone

Lissauer's tract

Late generated dorsal horn neurons (substantia gelatinosa)

Central autonomic area

Intermediate gray neurons

Central canal

Ventral horn interneurons

Lateral funiculus

Lateral motoneurons

Medial motoneurons

Ventral funiculus

0.25 mm

Ventral median sulcus

Ventral decussation   Ventromedial funiculus

Figure 5-6. A. The cervical spinal cord in a GW7.0 embryo (*C7254*; CR 22.5 mm). The ventral canal and the ventral neuroepithelium are disappearing, and the ventral horn motoneurons are segregating into a medial and a lateral cluster (red outlines). The field of ventral (red) and intermediate (green) interneurons has grown considerably but the population of dorsal interneurons (yellow) is still small. The dorsal root bifurcation zone is spreading dorsomedially. **B.** In the pumpkin-shaped spinal cord of this GW8.5 embryo (*C609*; CR 32 mm) the segregation of lateral motor columns is advanced, and the interneuronal fields are expanding. Darkly staining (young) cells outline the central autonomic area (purple). The dorsal neuroepithelium is in the process of dissolution and darkly staining cells are settling in the substantia gelatinosa (yellow inset) of the dorsal horn. The dorsal funiculus is developing.

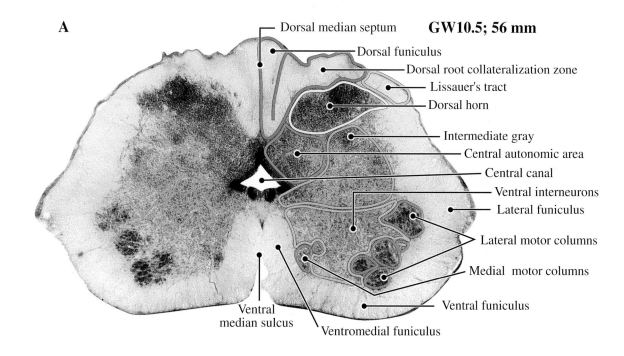

A. GW10.5; 56 mm

Dorsal median septum
Dorsal funiculus
Dorsal root collateralization zone
Lissauer's tract
Dorsal horn
Intermediate gray
Central autonomic area
Central canal
Ventral interneurons
Lateral funiculus
Lateral motor columns
Medial motor columns
Ventral funiculus
Ventromedial funiculus
Ventral median sulcus

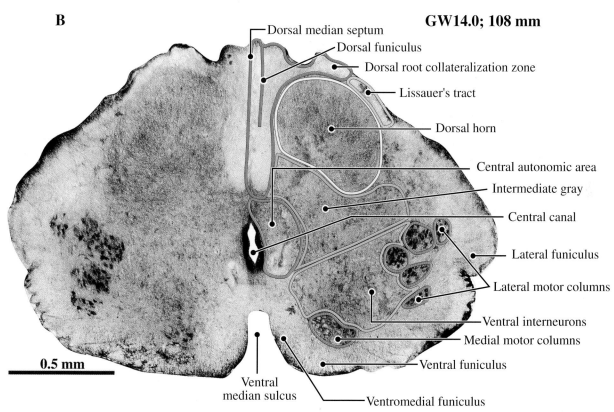

B. GW14.0; 108 mm

Dorsal median septum
Dorsal funiculus
Dorsal root collateralization zone
Lissauer's tract
Dorsal horn
Central autonomic area
Intermediate gray
Central canal
Lateral funiculus
Lateral motor columns
Ventral interneurons
Medial motor columns
Ventral funiculus
Ventromedial funiculus
Ventral median sulcus

0.5 mm

Figure 5-7. A. A major developmental event in the cervical spinal cord of this GW10.5 embryo (*Y380-62*; CR 56 mm) is the virtual disappearance of the dorsal canal and the dorsal neuroepithelium. That signals the end of spinal cord neurogenesis. The remaining active neuroepithelium probably generates the ependymal cells that line the enduring central canal. Among other developments are the ongoing maturation of motoneurons, the segregation of motor columns, the growth of the ventral and intermediate interneuronal fields, and the great expansion of the dorsal horn. **B.** These developments continue for several weeks, as seen in the GW14.0 fetus (*Y68-65*; CR 109 mm).

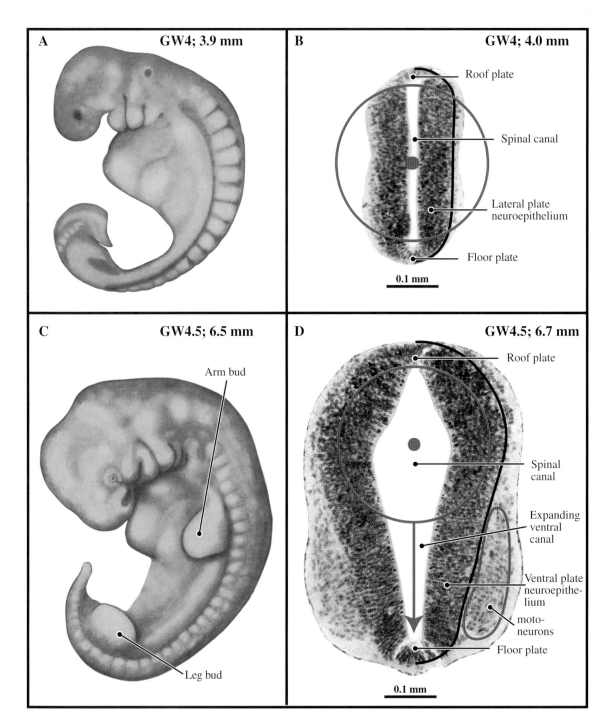

Figure 5-8. A. A GW 4.0 embryo (*C5923*; CR 3.9 mm). Limb buds have not yet formed at this age. **B.** The cervical spinal cord of another embryo of the same age (GW4.0; *M714*; CR 4.0 mm). At this stage, the spinal cord consists solely of NEP cells (the pre-exodus neuroepithelium). The inserted red dot indicates the center of the split-shaped spinal canal and the future location of the sulcus limitans; the red circle demarcates the dorsoventral extent of the lateral neuroepithelium. **C.** A major developmental event in this GW4.5 embryo (*C6502*; CR 6.5 mm) is the formation of the arm buds and leg buds. **D.** Several new developments are apparent in the spinal cord of another embryo of the same age (GW4.5; *M2285*; CR 6.7 mm). First, there is a great increase in the width and length of the neuroepithelium. Second, the shape of the spinal canal has changed. This is due to the expansion of the central canal and the disproportionate lengthening of the ventral canal (red arrow). Third, the exodus and differentiation of motoneurons has begun in the incipient ventral horn. These observations suggest a possible association between the onset of motoneuron differentiation and the formation of limb buds.

5.4 Development of the Cervical Spinal Cord Neuroepithelium in Relation to Somatic Development

5.4.1 The Pre-Exodus Spinal Cord Neuroepithelium. GW3.5 to GW4.0.

The neuroepithelium is virtually the sole neural component of the developing spinal cord in GW 3.5–GW4.0 embryos with CR lengths in the range of 3.5–5.5 mm (Figure 5-8B). That is, the primordial spinal cord (the neural tube) contains few differentiating neurons at this stage of development and the principal morphogenetic event is the continuing proliferation and great expansion of the pool of NEP cells. The thickness of the pre-exodus neuroepithelium is uniform over the slit-shaped spinal canal. If partitioning of the neuroepithelium into ventral, intermediate, and dorsal components has already begun in terms of cellular commitment, the boundaries of these presumptive components cannot be recognized in conventionally prepared histological sections. Since the exodus of differentiating motoneurons has not yet begun, it is probable that the outgrowth of motor fibers has not started either. As seen in another GW4 whole embryo (*C5923*; CR 3.9 mm) in Figure 5-8A, the limb buds, a major target of cervical motor fibers, have not yet formed at this stage of development.

We have placed a dot, roughly aligned with the invaginated "waist" of the spinal cord (the future site of the sulcus limitans), into the spinal canal of another GW4 embryo (*M714*; CR 4.0 mm) to mark the center of the split-shaped canal, and have drawn a circle that encompasses the spinal canal and most of the lateral neuroepithelium (Figure 5-8B). This circle will help us to gauge the changing polarity of the expansion and retraction of the spinal canal, and of the neuroepithelium surrounding it, during the following weeks of embryonic development.

5.4.2 The Ventral Neuroepithelium: Its Hypertrophy and the Peak of Motoneuron Production. GW4.5 to GW5.0.

A landmark somatic development at the beginning of this period, as seen in a GW4.5 embryo (*C6502*; CR 6.5 mm), is the outgrowth of the arm buds and leg buds (Figure 5-8C). In another embryo of a corresponding gestational age (*M2285*; CR 6.7 mm), a fair number of differentiating motoneurons have begun to settle in the incipient ventral horn. The marker circle with its center at the sulcus limitans indicates that by this stage the

spinal canal has expanded considerably in the ventral direction. Since the ventral canal is surrounded by a massive neuroepithelium, that selective expansion indicates that the ventral neuroepithelium is the most active proliferative compartment of the spinal cord during this period of embryonic development. We refer to this phenomenon as ventral neuroepithelial hypertrophy. With reference to somatic development, ventral neuroepithelial hypertrophy and the onset of motoneuron differentiation are associated with the sprouting of the limb buds at about GW4.0.

We have seen earlier in E13 rats, that shortly after their exodus from the ventral neuroepithelium, the differentiating motoneurons sprout axons that leave the spinal cord to form the ventral root. Figure 5-9 shows the drawing by Ramón y Cajal of the spinal cord of a mature GW4 human embryo. The axons of the differentiating motoneurons are exiting in large numbers and form the ventral rootlets of the spinal nerve. The decussation of the axons of the contralaterally projecting interneurons has also begun underneath the floor plate.

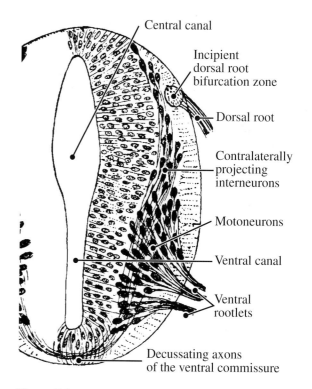

Central canal

Incipient dorsal root bifurcation zone

Dorsal root

Contralaterally projecting interneurons

Motoneurons

Ventral canal

Ventral rootlets

Decussating axons of the ventral commissure

Figure 5-9. Ramón y Cajal's (1909) drawing (after His) of the cytological organization of the spinal cord of a "4-week-old" human embryo. The accumulation of the earliest complement of motoneurons is associated with the outgrowth of motor fibers and the formation ventral rootlets. Some of the original labels have been modified.

5.4.3   The Ventral Neuroepithelium: Its Dissolution and the Cessation of Motoneuron Production. GW5.5 to GW6.0.

The GW5.5 embryo (CR 10 mm) reproduced in Figure 5-10A shows a new landmark in somatic development, the formation of the hand buds and foot buds. The spinal cord of a corresponding age embryo (GW5.5; *C8998*; CR 11 mm) shows a lengthening of the ventral neuroepithelium in association with reduction in the packing density of NEP cells in the midportion of the ventral neuroepithelium (Figure 5-10B). This suggests that ventral neuroepithelial production of motoneuron precursors may have just peaked. The settling of differentiating motoneurons is in progress in the ventral horn and there is a hint here for the segregation of medial (inferior) and lateral (superior) motoneuron clusters. In contrast, the accumulation of ventral, intermediate, and dorsal gray interneurons is modest. Thus, the formation of the hand and foot buds appears to be correlated with the imminent cessation of maximal motoneuron production and their settling in large numbers.

5.4.4   The Intermediate Neuroepithelium: Its Hypertrophy and the Peak of Interneuron Production. GW6.0 to GW7.0.

A major developmental event between GW6.0 and GW7.0 is the growth of the ventral and intermediate interneuronal fields. This is evident by comparing the size of these two fields in the GW5.5 embryo (Figure 5-10B) and the GW7.0 embryo (*C7254*; 22.5 mm; Figure 5-11B). This development can be related to a shift in NEP cell production along the spinal canal. While the neuroepithelium surrounding the receding ventral canal is in a process of dissolution by GW7.0, the upper portion of the intermediate neuroepithelium and, in particular, the dorsal neuroepithelium surrounding the elongating dorsal canal, in contrast, have expanded considerably. This indicates that the decline in ventral NEP cell production is immediately followed by an accelerated production of intermediate and dorsal NEP cells.

We assume that the intermediate and dorsal NEP cells are the precursors, respectively, of the developing interneurons of the intermediate gray and the dorsal horn. The origin of the ventral interneurons, however, is less certain. The ventral interneurons either come from a second wave of differentiating cells that leave the ventral neuroepithelium after the exodus of motoneurons or, what is more likely,

they are the progeny of NEP cells that flank the inferior bank of the central canal (Figure 5-11B). The high rate of production and differentiation of these interneurons is chronologically associated with the segregation of motoneurons into columns in the cervical spinal cord and, in relation to somatic development, with the formation of the finger buds (Figure 5-11A).

5.4.5   The Dorsal Neuroepithelium: Its Hypertrophy and the Production of Gelatinosal Microneurons. GW7.5 to GW8.5.

The last stage in spinal cord neurogenesis is the shift of NEP cell production from the intermediate neuroepithelium to the dorsal neuroepithelium. That change is associated with the production of the small sensory neurons of the substantia gelatinosa. This is illustrated in the thoracic spinal cord of a GW7.5 embryo (*M2042*; CR 25 mm) in Figure 5-12. (The plane of sectioning in this specimen does not provide coronal sections in the cervical cord.) There are indications in this specimen of the exodus of cells dorsolaterally and of the settling of a small contingent of cells in the formative substantia gelatinosa in the dorsal horn. The growing dorsal horn is capped by the expanding dorsal root bifurcation zone. The incipient dorsal funiculus, composed of fibers of the collateralization zone, is beginning to develop medially.

Figure 5-10.   A. Formation of the hand bud and foot bud in a GW5.5 embryo (CR 10 mm). After Patten (1974). **B.** The spinal cord of a corresponding age embryo (*C8998*; CR 11.0 mm). Among notable developments are the following. The neuroepithelium has grown considerably in width and length (compare the red marker circle and arrows with Figure 5-8D). The expansion of the ventral neuroepithelium has peaked and is now becoming depleted of NEP cells. These two developments are associated with an increase in the population of differentiating motoneurons in the expanding ventral horn. While the intermediate and dorsal neuroepithelia have grown considerably around the enlarged central canal and the lengthening dorsal canal, the growth of the ventral interneuronal field (orange), intermediate interneuronal field (green), and dorsal interneuronal field (yellow) is still minimal. Finally, the dorsal root bifurcation zone (the oval bundle of His) has formed. These observations suggests that the budding of the hand and foot is associated with the cessation of motoneuron production and the entrance of peripheral sensory fibers into the spinal cord.

⟶

A

GW5.5; 10 mm

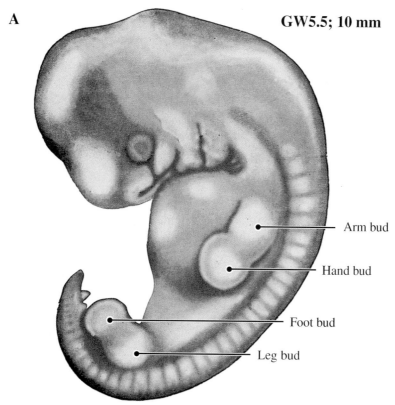

Arm bud

Hand bud

Foot bud

Leg bud

B

GW5.5; 11 mm

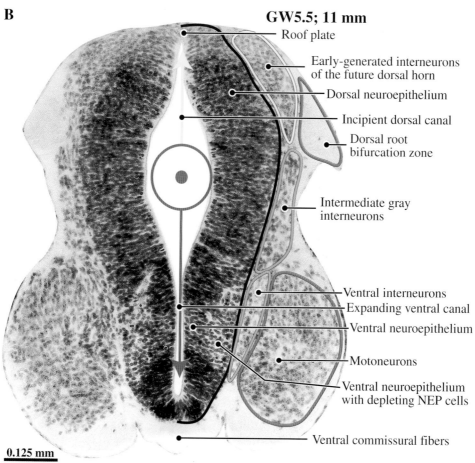

Roof plate

Early-generated interneurons
of the future dorsal horn

Dorsal neuroepithelium

Incipient dorsal canal

Dorsal root
bifurcation zone

Intermediate gray
interneurons

Ventral interneurons

Expanding ventral canal

Ventral neuroepithelium

Motoneurons

Ventral neuroepithelium
with depleting NEP cells

Ventral commissural fibers

0.125 mm

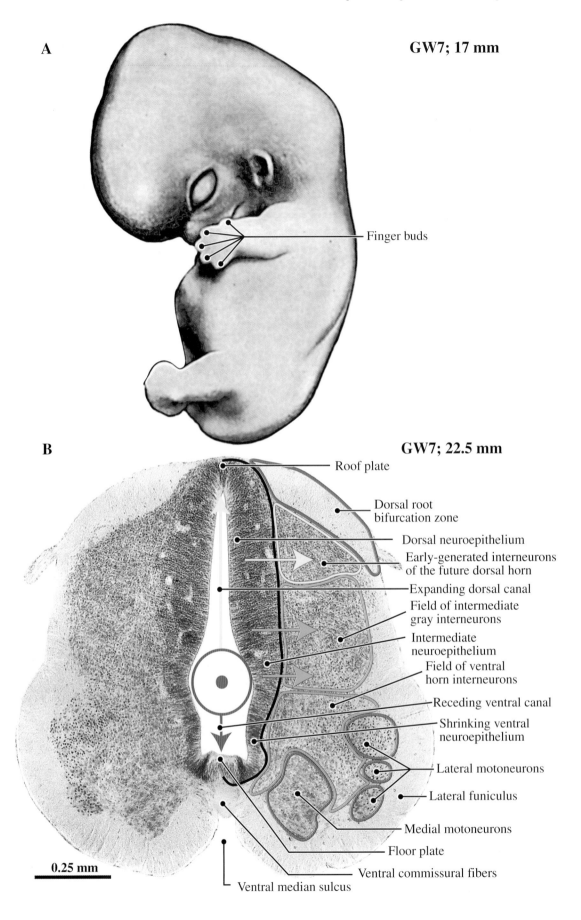

A   **GW7; 17 mm**

Finger buds

B   **GW7; 22.5 mm**

Roof plate

Dorsal root
bifurcation zone

Dorsal neuroepithelium

Early-generated interneurons
of the future dorsal horn

Expanding dorsal canal

Field of intermediate
gray interneurons

Intermediate
neuroepithelium

Field of ventral
horn interneurons

Receding ventral canal

Shrinking ventral
neuroepithelium

Lateral motoneurons

Lateral funiculus

Medial motoneurons

Floor plate

Ventral commissural fibers

Ventral median sulcus

0.25 mm

Figure 5-11. A. Formation of finger buds in a GW7 embryo (*C1324*; CR 17 mm). **B.** The spinal cord in a somewhat older GW7 embryo (*C7254*; CR 22.5 mm). Among noteworthy events in the development of the spinal cord are the following. The ventral canal has regressed (short red arrow) and the dissolution of the ventral neuroepithelium is in progress. The expansion of the ventral horn, in association with the segregation of the motor columns, has begun. The intermediate neuroepithelium remains prominent and the dorsal neuroepithelium is expanding with the lengthening dorsal canal (long yellow arrow). The ventral (orange), intermediate (green), and dorsal (yellow) interneuronal fields are becoming larger. Finally, the ventromedial, ventral, and lateral funiculi have grown considerably, and the dorsal root bifurcation zone is spreading dorsomedially.

The landmark developmental event in the GW8.5 embryo (*M2050*; CR 36 mm), as seen in Figure 5-13B, is the development of the dorsal horn. Two regions are by now distinguishable within the dorsal horn, the nucleus proprius (laminae IV-V) with its less darkly staining cells, and the substantia gelatinosa (laminae II-III) with its densely packed, more darkly staining cells. The settling of the late-generated microneurons of the substantia gelatinosa is associated with the dissolution of dorsal neuroepithelium and the formation of the dorsal funiculus. Other continuing events are the expansion of the ventral and intermediate interneuronal fields and the segregation of lateral motor columns. These developments in the spinal cord centrally are chronologically associated with the appearance of individual fingers and toes peripherally (Figure 5-13A).

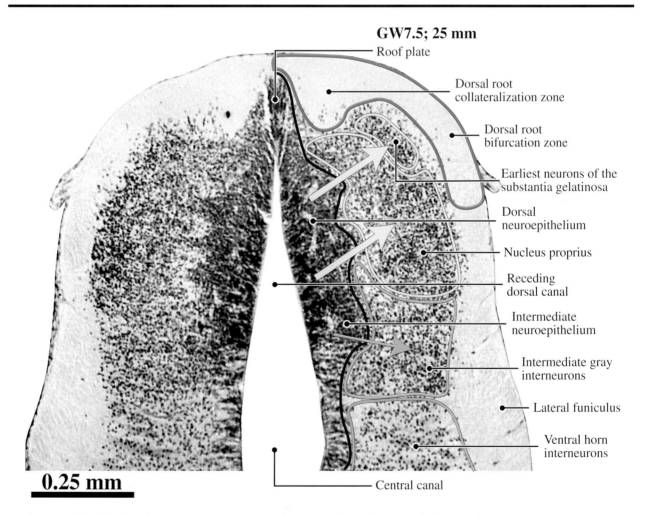

GW7.5; 25 mm

- Roof plate
- Dorsal root collateralization zone
- Dorsal root bifurcation zone
- Earliest neurons of the substantia gelatinosa
- Dorsal neuroepithelium
- Nucleus proprius
- Receding dorsal canal
- Intermediate neuroepithelium
- Intermediate gray interneurons
- Lateral funiculus
- Ventral horn interneurons
- Central canal

0.25 mm

Figure 5-12. The thoracic spinal cord of a GW7.5 embryo (*M2042*; CR 25 mm). The intermediate neuroepithelium has become thinner but the dorsal neuroepithelium remains bulky. The saw tooth pattern of the dorsal neuroepithelium suggests that the exiting late-generated neurons migrate in discrete batches (yellow arrows) to the expanding dorsal horn.

A   **GW8.5; 30.7 mm**

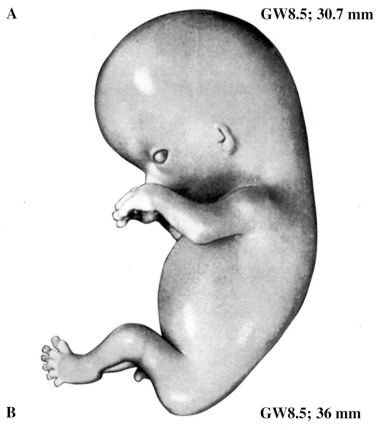

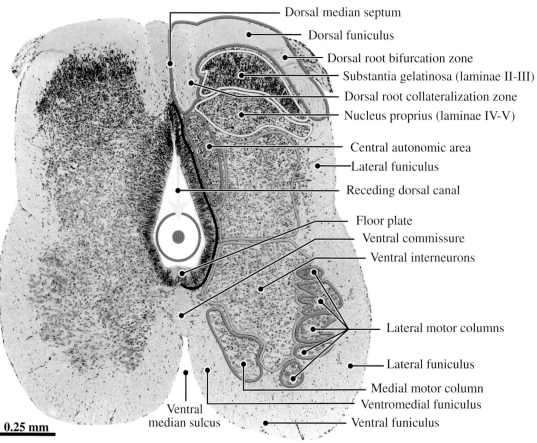

B   **GW8.5; 36 mm**

Dorsal median septum
Dorsal funiculus
Dorsal root bifurcation zone
Substantia gelatinosa (laminae II-III)
Dorsal root collateralization zone
Nucleus proprius (laminae IV-V)
Central autonomic area
Lateral funiculus
Receding dorsal canal
Floor plate
Ventral commissure
Ventral interneurons
Lateral motor columns
Lateral funiculus
Medial motor column
Ventromedial funiculus
Ventral funiculus
Ventral median sulcus

0.25 mm

Figure 5-13. A. A GW8.5 fetus (CR 30.7 mm) with well-formed fingers and toes. After Hamilton et al. (1964). **B.** The cervical spinal cord of another GW8.5 fetus (*M2050*; CR 36 mm). Among notable changes in the spinal cord at this age are the following. The dissolution of the dorsal neuroepithelium (short yellow arrow) is nearly complete. The young (darkly staining) neurons of the substantia gelatinosa have settled above the older (less darkly staining) neurons of the nucleus proprius. The dorsal funiculus is deepening and the latest forming central autonomic area is developing. The ventral and intermediate interneuronal fields have greatly expanded and the segregation of the lateral motor columns continues in the ventral horn.

5.4.6 Dissolution of the Neuroepithelium and the Cessation of Spinal Cord Neurogenesis. GW9.0 to GW10.5.

Following the shrinkage and subsequent fusion of the dorsal canal, the elongated embryonic spinal canal is transformed into the small but permanent central canal. This is illustrated in a GW10.5 specimen (*Y380-62*; CR 56 mm) in Figure 5-14. As we have seen, the transient branches of the embryonic tripartite spinal canal (the ventral, central and dorsal canals) sustain the corresponding compartments of the proliferative neuroepithelium (the ventral, intermediate and dorsal) that successively generate the motoneurons, interneurons, and sensory microneurons of the spinal cord. The disappearance of the dorsal canal sometimes around GW10 signals the completion of spinal cord neurogenesis. Significantly, the diamond-shaped central canal remains surrounded for some time by a proliferative matrix (Figures 5-14, 5-15). This germinal matrix may generate some glial cells and must be the source of the ependymal cells and tanycytes that will come to line the persisting central canal.

GW10.5; 56 mm

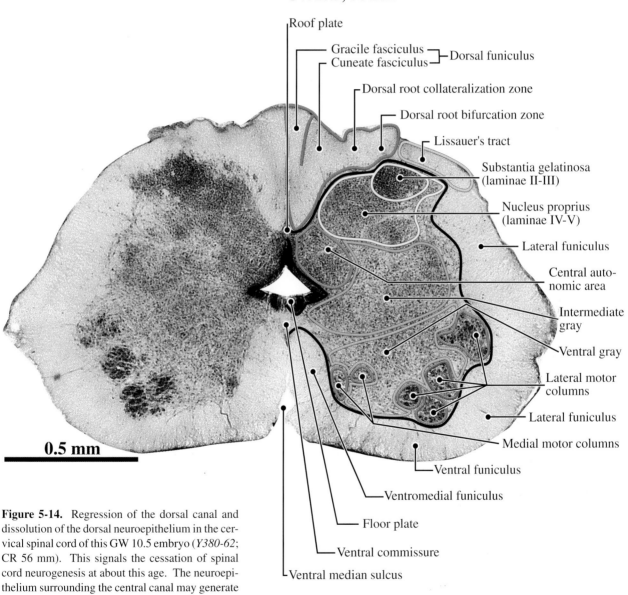

Figure 5-14. Regression of the dorsal canal and dissolution of the dorsal neuroepithelium in the cervical spinal cord of this GW 10.5 embryo (*Y380-62*; CR 56 mm). This signals the cessation of spinal cord neurogenesis at about this age. The neuroepithelium surrounding the central canal may generate glia and ependymal cells. With the expansion of the dorsal horn and the ventral horn the gray matter starts to assume its adult configuration.

5.4.7   Maturation of the Gray Matter Toward the End of the First Trimester. GW10.5 to GW14.0.

The continuing maturation and expansion of the gray matter between GW10.5 and GW14 can be seen by comparing the two specimens, *Y380-62* and *Y68-65,* in Figures 5-14 and 5-15. The segregation of the motor columns continues in the ventral horn, the ventral and intermediate interneuronal fields have expanded greatly, and the cells in of the substantia gelatinosa have lost their dark appearance. However, there is little indication of appreciable growth in the bulk of the ventral and lateral funiculi by the beginning of the second trimester, suggesting a lag in the growth of many of the fiber systems that interconnect the spinal cord with supraspinal structures and the brain. The expansion of the white matter relative to the gray matter is a slow process that takes place mostly during the second and third trimesters (the fetal period) and is coupled with two other developments, the proliferation of glia throughout the spinal cord and the myelination of the developing ascending and descending tracts.

GW14; 108 mm

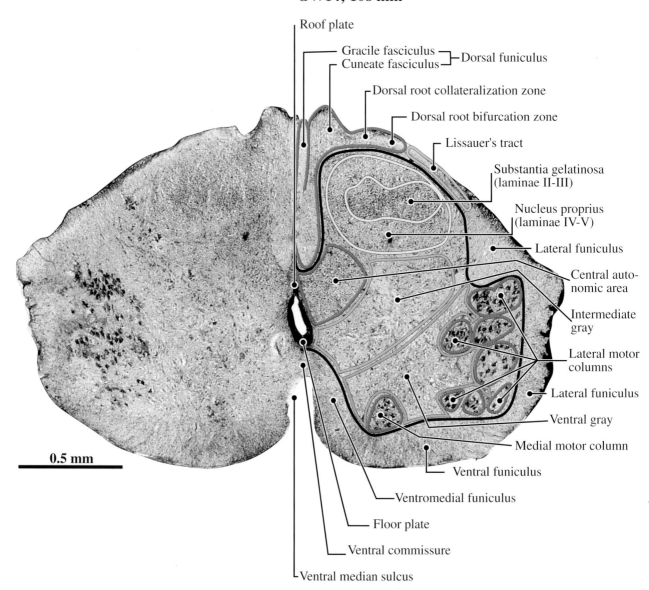

Figure 5-15. The cervical spinal cord of a GW14 fetus (*Y68-65*; CR 108 mm) at the transition period between the end of the first trimester and the beginning of the second trimester. All the structural components of the gray matter are recognizable and the segregation of motor columns resembles the adult pattern. What distinguishes the spinal cord at this age from the mature spinal cord is the relatively small size of the white matter. This indicates that both the ascending and descending supraspinal connections of the spinal cord are poorly developed during the embryonic period.

5.5 Development of Motoneurons in the Cervical Spinal Cord in Relation to Skeletomuscular Development

5.5.1 The Amorphous Field of Differentiating Motoneurons. GW4.5 to GW5.0.

The differentiating motoneurons that start to assemble outside the ventral neuroepithelium at about GW4.5 (Figure 5-16A) greatly increase in number by GW5.0 (Figure 5-16B). For a week or so the young motoneurons remain near the ventral neuroepithelium and form a seemingly amorphous (unsegregated) cell mass in the incipient ventral horn. According to Okado et al. (1979), no synapses are present in the cervical spinal cord at this stage of spinal cord development. The GW5.0 (9 mm) embryo dissected by Bardeen and Lewis (1901), reproduced in Figure 5-16C, indicates that while the arm and leg buds have already emerged by GW 5.0 (for comparison see the GW4.5 embryo in Figure 5-8C), the skeletal system is still in a precartilageous state and the immature muscular system is represented by the axial myotomes and mesenchymal limb primordia. The possibility that the outgrowing motor axons are already contacting the primordial muscle masses by GW5.0 is suggested by the presence of the lumbosacral plexus at this age (Figure 5-16 C).

5.5.2 Formation of the Inferior and Superior Motoneuron Masses. GW5.5 to GW6.0.

Two changes appear in the developing spinal cord by GW5.5 (Figure 5-17A). The first of these is the interdigitation of a small field of differentiating interneurons between the ventral neuroepithelium and the motoneurons. The second change is the partitioning of the amorphous motoneuron mass into an inferior and a superior compartment. Okado (1981) found that axodendritic synapses with asymmetrical membrane thickenings and round vesicles (presumably excitatory synapses) begin to appear in the ventral horn in GW5.5 (CR 10 mm) embryos. Furthermore, the dissected GW5.5 (CR 11 mm) embryo (Bardeen

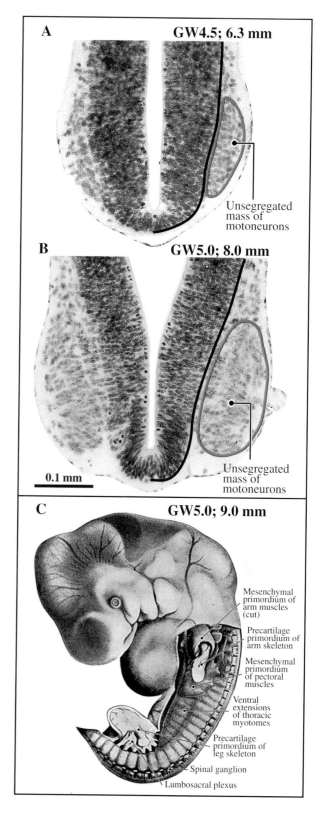

Figure 5-16. A. Accumulation of the earliest motoneurons (red outline) in a GW4.5 embryo (*M2300*; CR 6.3 mm). **B.** Expansion of the unsegregated mass of motoneurons in a GW5.0 embryo (*M2065*; CR 8.0 mm). **C.** Partial dissection of a GW5.0 embryo (CR 9.0 mm) by Bardeen and Lewis (1901). The future axial muscles are represented by primitive myotomes, the muscles of the extremities have a mesenchymal composition, and the bones of the arm and leg are present in a precartilagous state of development. The presence of the lumbosacral plexus suggests, however, that the innervation of the limbs is already in progress by GW5.0.

and Lewis,1901; Figure 5-17B), shows that by this age the trunk muscles and the muscles of the shoulder (levator scapulae, trapezius, deltoid, teres major) are recognizable, and the muscles of the arm and hand have started to develop. With reference to the skeletal system, the precartilagous primordia of the discrete forelimb bones and digits are separate by GW5.5 (Figure 5-17C) but the maturation of the hind limb skeleton, particularly the foot plate, is less advanced (Figure 5-17D).

5.5.3 Segregation of the Medial and Lateral Columns. GW6.5 to GW7.5.

The segregation of motoneurons progresses in the GW6.5 embryo (*C7707*; CR 14.5 mm; Figure 5-18A). The location of the medial panel of motoneurons corresponds to the inferior mass seen earlier in a younger embryo (Figure 5-17A). The lateral displacement of the original superior compartment is at least partly attributable to the immense enlargement of the field of ventral interneurons. Another development is the segre-

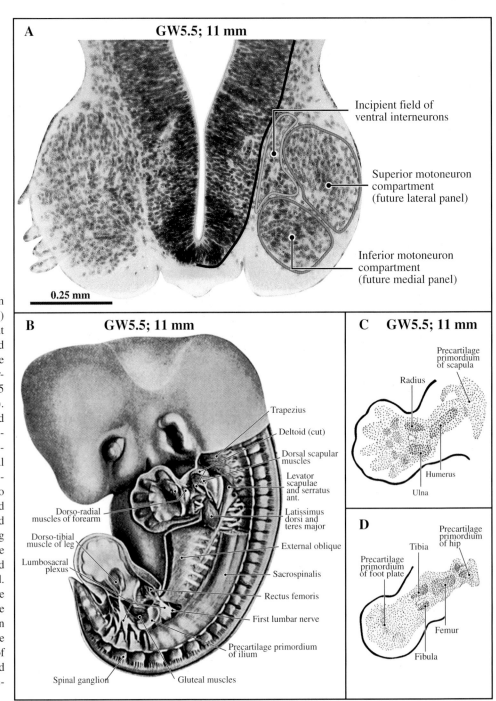

Figure 5-17. A. Segregation of motoneurons (red outline) into an inferior compartment (the future medial panel) and a superior compartment (the future lateral panel) in the cervical spinal cord of a GW5.5 embryo (*C8998*; CR 11 mm). This development is coupled with the settling of interneurons between the ventral neuroepithelium and the ventral horn (orange outline). **B.** Dissection of a GW5.5 embryo (CR 11 mm) by Bardeen and Lewis (1901). The axial and girdle muscles are maturing but the differentiation of the distal muscles of the hand and foot is less advanced. **C.** The individual bones of the shoulder, arm and hand are in a precartilageous state in this GW5.5 embryo. **D.** The development of the digits of the hind limb is less advanced than the digits of the forelimb.

gation of the lateral panel motoneurons into ventral and dorsal tiers (Figure 5-18A). Dissection of the forelimb (Figure 5-18B) and hind limb (Figure 5-18C) in two embryos of corresponding ages (GW6.5; CR 14.5 and CR 14.0, respectively) indicates considerable progress in the differentiation of the skeletal elements of the forelimb and hind limb.

Relating these observations to our scheme of motor column organization in the adult ventral horn (Figures 1-51 and 1-52) suggests that the first phase in the segregation of motoneurons is into a medial panel (inferior compartment) and a lateral panel (superior compartment). The second phase is the segregation of the lateral panel of motoneurons in a ventral and a dorsal tier. The next phase, as seen in the GW7.0 embryo (*C7254*; CR 22.5 mm; Figure 5-19), is the segregation of dorsal tier motoneurons into dorsal and a retrodorsal tiers. The dissected embryo of a corresponding stage of development (GW7.0; CR 22 mm),

reproduced in Figure 5-19B, indicates great strides made in the differentiation of the muscles of the shoulder and the upper limb, and the pelvis and lower limb.

5.5.4 Segregation of the Lateral and Far-Lateral Motor Columns. GW8.5 to GW13.0.

Whereas the panel of medial motoneurons undergoes little change during the next period, the segregation of the lateral motoneurons continues. In the GW8.5 embryo (*M2050*; CR 36 mm; Figure 5-20A), the lateral motoneurons are partitioned into three tiers: the ventral, dorsal, and retrodorsal. In the GW10.5 embryo (*Y380-62*; CR 56 mm; Figure 5-20B), motoneurons in the lateral panel are further partitioned into lateral and far-lateral panels. The pattern of progressive segregation continues into the beginning of the second trimester (GW14; *Y68-65*; CR 108 mm; Figure 5-20C). By this age, discrete motor columns have formed that occupy different sectors in the lat-

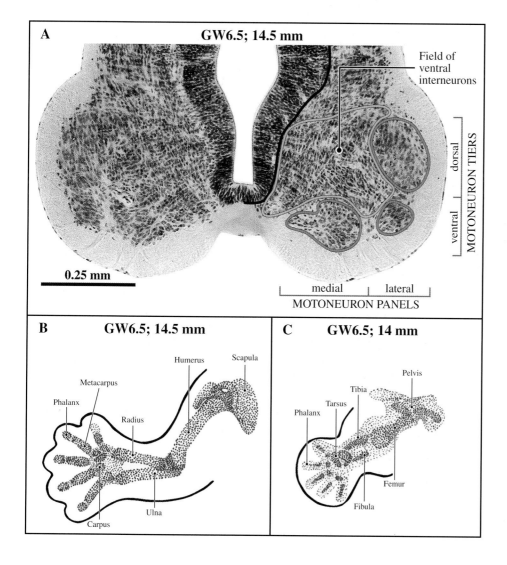

Figure 5-18. A. The ventral horn of the cervical spinal cord in a GW6.5 embryo (*C7707*; CR 14.5 mm). A notable event is the segregation of lateral cluster of motoneurons (the former superior compartment) into two horizontal tiers, the ventral and the dorsal (red outlines). Another development is the great expansion of the field of ventral interneurons (pink outline). **B.** Development of the forelimb skeleton in a GW6.5 embryo (CR 14.5 mm). **C.** Development of the hind limb skeleton is less advanced in another GW6.5 embryo (CR 14.0 mm). **B** and **C** after Bardeen and Lewis (1901).

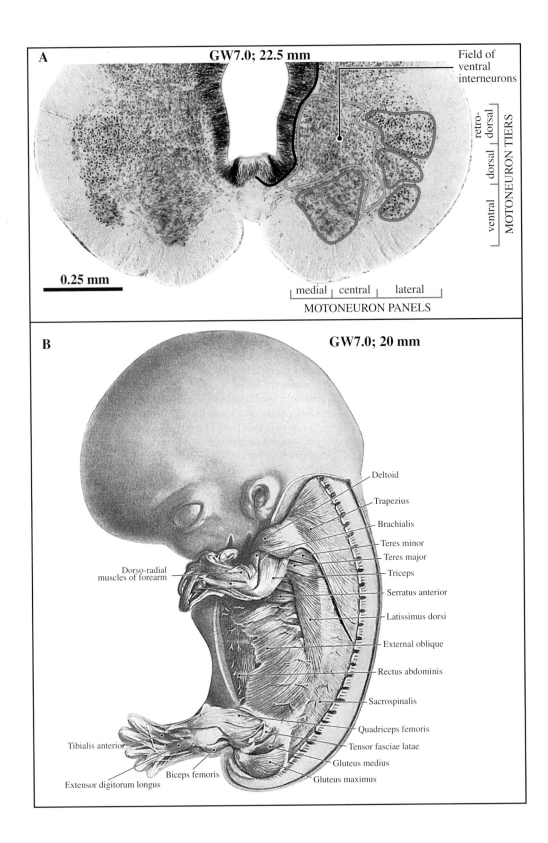

Figure 5-19. A. The ventral horn of the cervical spinal cord in a GW7.0 embryo (*C7254*; CR 22.5 mm). The lateral motoneurons are segregated in three tiers: the ventral, dorsal, and retrodorsal. **B.** In the dissected embryo of a corresponding age (GW7.0; CR 20 mm) considerable differentiation of the shoulder, arm, and forearm muscles (compare with Figure 5-17B). After Bardeen Cord Lewis (1901).

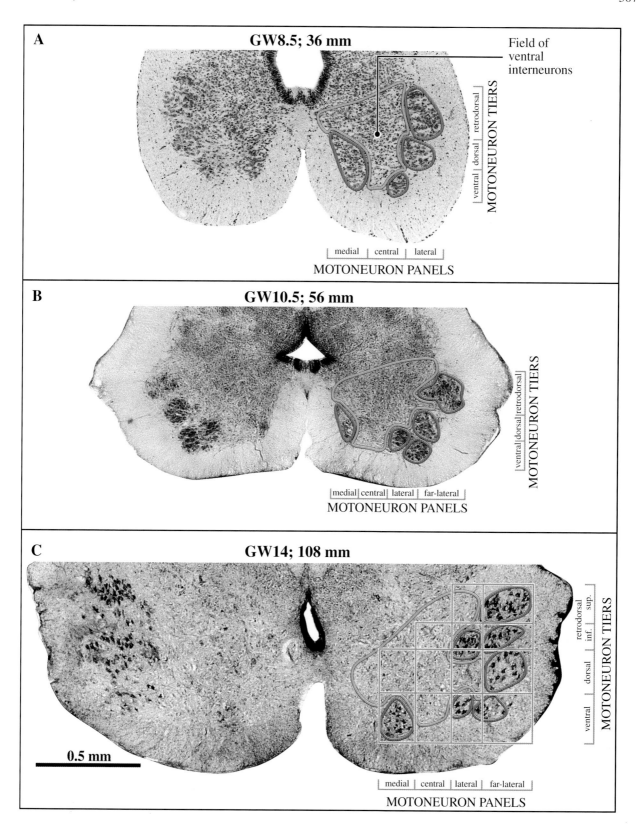

Figure 5-20. Progressive segregation of motor columns (red) and expansion of the field of ventral interneurons (orange) in the cervical spinal cord of **A**, a GW8.5 embryo (*M2050*; CR 36 mm), **B**, a GW10.5 embro (*Y380-62; CR 56 mm*), and **C**, a GW14.0 fetus (*Y68-65*; CR 108 mm). The motoneurons that occupy two panels in the GW8.5 embryo are segregated into three panels (medial, lateral, far-lateral) and three tiers (ventral, dorsal, retrodorsal) in the GW10.5 embryo, and become further segregated in the GW14.0 fetus. The motor columns in the retrodorsal sector laterally and far-laterally innervate the muscles of the distal wrist, hand, and fingers.

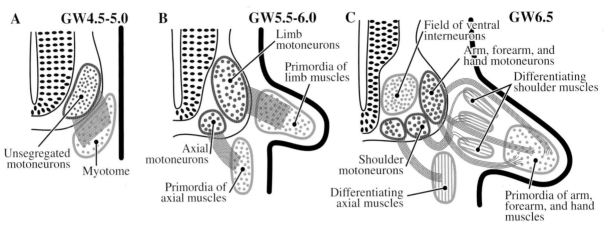

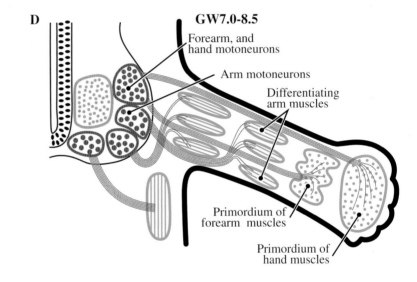

Figure 5-21. The hypothetical relationship between the progressive segregation of motoneurons in the cervical spinal cord and the successive innervation of the proximodistally developing forelimb muscles during the first trimester. **A.** At GW4.5-GW5.0, the motoneurons (red dots) form an amorphous mass and their axons (red lines) contact the myotomes (green dots). **B.** By GW5.5-GW6.0, the motoneurons are segregated into medial and the lateral compartments, and their axons begin to innervate, respectively, axial and limb muscle primordia (green dots). **C.** At about GW6.5, the partitioning of the lateral motoneurons into ventral and dorsal tiers is coupled with the innervation of differentiating axial and shoulder muscles (green stripes). The innervation of the primordia of the arm, forearm and hand muscles may have also begun. **D.** By GW7.0-GW8.5, the segregation of lateral motoneurons into dorsal and retrodorsal compartments is associated with the innervation of the differentiating arm muscles and the primordia of forearm muscles. **E.** Finally, by GW9-GW12, the partitioning of the retrodorsal motoneurons into inferior and superior columns is associated with the innervation of the wrist and the hand muscle primordia. Pink outlines indicate the concurrent expansion of the field of ventral interneurons.

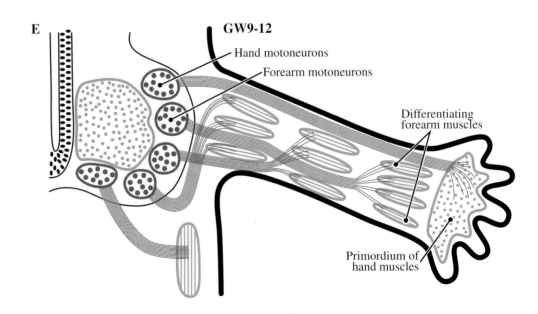

eral and far lateral panels and in the inferior and superior divisions of the retrodorsal tier. Motoneurons in these columns innervate principally the distal wrist and hand muscles.

In summary, the maturing motoneurons first form two separate compartments, the medial and the lateral. Then the motoneurons of the lateral compartment become segregated in two panels (the lateral and far-lateral) and three tiers (the ventral, dorsal, and restrodorsal. The hypothetical relationship between the sequential segregation of motoneuron columns in the cervical spinal cord between GW4.5 and GW12 and the sequential maturation of the proximal (trunk, arm) and distal (wrist and hand) muscles of the forelimb that they innervate is schematically summarized in Figure 5-21.

5.5.5 Synaptogenesis in the Ventral Horn.
Okado (1980) reported that the concentration of axodendritic synapses is very low, about 1.4/200 μm², in the lateral ventral horn of the human cervical spinal cord on GW6 and GW7. The concentration of synapses increases abruptly to 10/200 μm² by GW8, and more gradually to 13/ 200μm² by GW13 (Figure 5-22). During GW13, there is also an increase in the concentration of axosomatic synapses. The majority

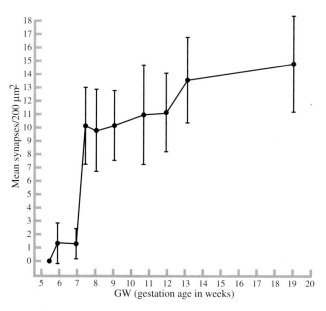

Figure 5-22. Concentration of axodendritic synapses in unit areas (200 μm²) of the ventral horn of the human cervical spinal cord in relation to gestational age. Note the sudden increase, from less than 2 synapses to over 10 synapses per unit area, at about GW8.0. The majority of synapses during the first trimester are axodendritic and of the asymmetrical (presumably excitatory) type. After Okado (1980).

of synapses that form in the first trimester are of the asymmetrical (presumably excitatory) type. Symmetrical (presumably inhibitory) synapses do not appear in appreciable numbers until the second trimester.

5.6 Development of the Dorsal Funicular Complex in the Cervical Spinal Cord

5.6.1 Arrival of Dorsal Root Fibers and Formation of the Dorsal Root Bifurcation Zone. GW5.0.
The boundary cap, which is the site of entry of dorsal root afferents, is first seen as a cap overlying the spinal ganglion in the GW4.5 embryo (*M2285*; CR 6.7 mm; Figure 5-23A). It is recognizable as a more distinct structure, together with traversing axons of the dorsal root ganglion, in the GW5.0 embryo (*M2065*; CR 8.0 mm; Figure 5-23B). The arrival and entry of the first complement of dorsal root fibers in this embryo is associated with the emergence of a distinctive fibrous structure, the oval bundle of His. Based on observations in rats, this is called the dorsal root bifurcation zone. The entering dorsal root axons bifurcate here into ascending and descending branches on or about GW5.0 as the first step in their successive branching within the spinal cord. Some of the earliest generated neurons of the future dorsal horn, presumably the early generated Waldeyer cells and related neurons of lamina I, are scattered in the vicinity of the dorsal root bifurcation.

5.6.2. Growth of the Dorsal Root Bifurcation Zone. GW5.5 to GW7.0.
In the GW5.5 embryo (*C8998*; CR 11.0 mm; Figure 5-24A) , the dorsal root bifurcation zone has become larger and expands dorsomedially over the band of early-generated neurons of the dorsal horn. In the GW6.5 embryo (*C7707*; CR 14.5 mm; Figure 5-24B), the bifurcation zone has spread farther dorsomedially. According to Okado (1981), the first synapses appear in the primordial dorsal horn at about this age. The progressive expansion of the bifurcation zone, which approximates the midline in the GW7.0 embryo (*C7254*; CR 22.5 mm; Figure 5-25A), reflects the arrival and bifurcation of more and more dorsal root afferents. However, the medial portion of this fiber band, as judged by subsequent developments (see below), is probably no longer the bifurcation zone but is composed of sprouting collaterals of the ascending and descending branches of dorsal root parent axons. Collateralization constitutes the second step in the branching of dorsal root sensory fibers.

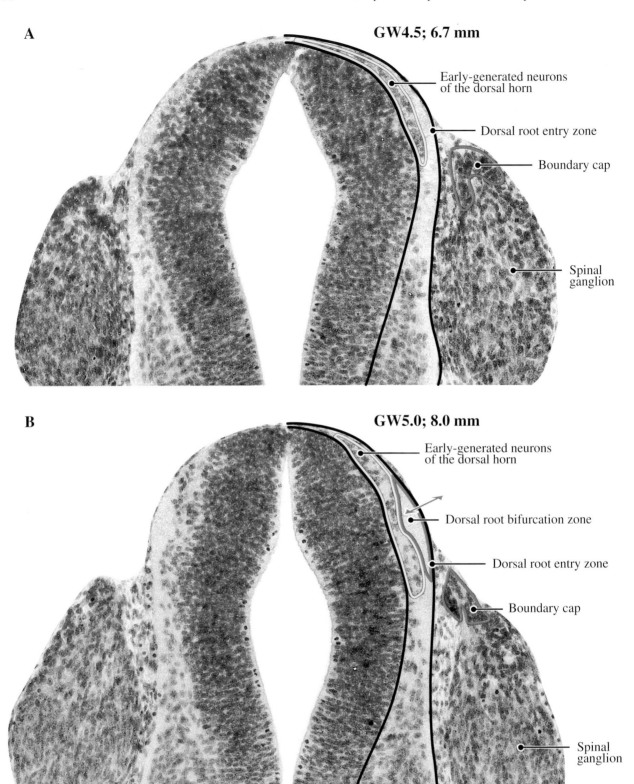

A   **GW4.5; 6.7 mm**

Early-generated neurons
of the dorsal horn

Dorsal root entry zone

Boundary cap

Spinal
ganglion

B   **GW5.0; 8.0 mm**

Early-generated neurons
of the dorsal horn

Dorsal root bifurcation zone

Dorsal root entry zone

Boundary cap

Spinal
ganglion

0.125 mm

Figure 5-23. A. The dorsal half of the cervical spinal cord in a GW4.5 embryo (*M2285*; CR 6.7 mm). There is as yet no indication of the entrance of dorsal root fibers into the spinal cord. **B.** Dorsal root fibers traverse the boundary cap (blue outline) in this GW5.0 embryo (*M2065*; CR 8.0 mm) and split into ascending and descending branches (double arrow) to form the bifurcation zone (oval bundle of His) upon entering the spinal cord.

5.6.3. Formation of the Dorsal Root Collateralization Zone. GW7.5 to GW8.0. The next event is the expansion of the dorsal funiculus in the GW7.5 embryo (*M2042*; CR 25 mm; Figure 5-25B), in the form of a ventromedial medial club-like extension. That region is identified as the proximal component of the collateralization zone, composed of locally terminating offshoots of the ascending and descending branches of dorsal root axons. As development proceeds, these collaterals will curve around the dorsal horn and penetrate the gray matter underneath it, and either proceed to the ventral horn and the intermediate gray, or recurve and terminate in the dorsal horn.

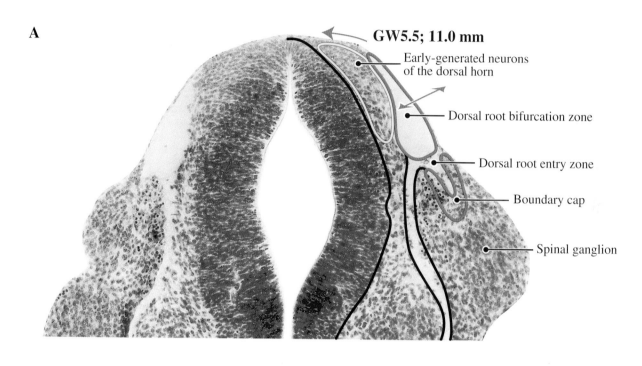

A **GW5.5; 11.0 mm**

Early-generated neurons of the dorsal horn

Dorsal root bifurcation zone

Dorsal root entry zone

Boundary cap

Spinal ganglion

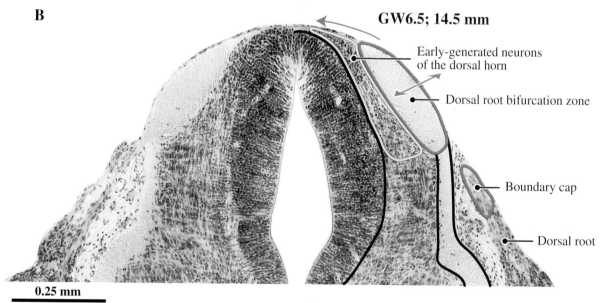

B **GW6.5; 14.5 mm**

Early-generated neurons of the dorsal horn

Dorsal root bifurcation zone

Boundary cap

Dorsal root

0.25 mm

Figure 5-24. A. The dorsal root bifurcation zone (double arrow) is expanding dorsomedially (top arrow) in this GW5.5 embryo (*C8998*; CR 11.0 mm). **B.** The expansion of the bifurcation zone (top arrow) continues in this GW6.5 embryo (*C7707*; CR 14.5 mm).

5.6.4 *Formation of the Core of the Dorsal Funiculus. GW8.5 to GW10.0.* Several new developments are discernible in the cervical spinal cord of the GW8.5 embryo (*M2050*; CR 36 mm; Figure 5-26A). The first of these is the dorsomedial shift of the boundary cap and the dorsal root entry zone.

That may be due to the arrival of a new contingent of afferents (the nociceptive fibers) and the formation of Lissauer's tract. The second is the emergence of a new "hump" alongside the dorsal median septum. The third development is the pronounced deepening of the dorsal funiculus that now appears to be com-

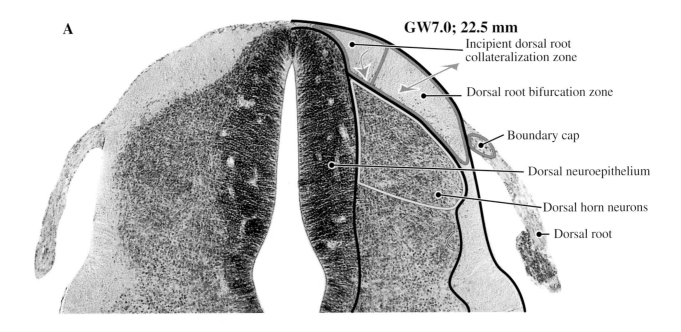

A   **GW7.0; 22.5 mm**

Incipient dorsal root collateralization zone

Dorsal root bifurcation zone

Boundary cap

Dorsal neuroepithelium

Dorsal horn neurons

Dorsal root

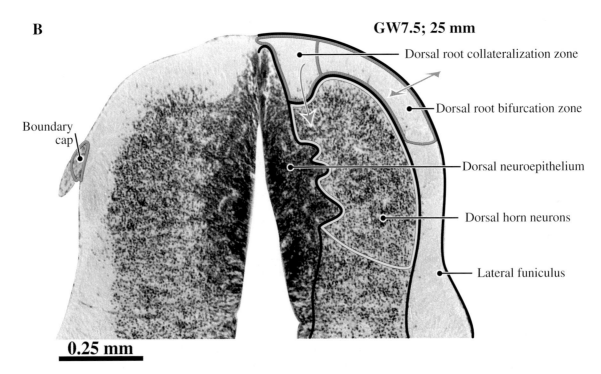

B   **GW7.5; 25 mm**

Dorsal root collateralization zone

Dorsal root bifurcation zone

Boundary cap

Dorsal neuroepithelium

Dorsal horn neurons

Lateral funiculus

0.25 mm

Figure 5-25. A. The dorsomedial expansion of the bifurcation zone in this GW7.0 embryo (*C7254*; CR 22.5 mm). Curved medial arrow points to the site where the ascending and descending fiber branches will sprout collaterals (the incipient dorsal root collateralization zone). **B.** The club-shaped, collateralization zone of the dorsal funiculus in this GW7.5 embryo (*M2042*; CR 25 mm) with putative downward growing collaterals (medial downward arrow).

posed of two discrete compartments. We propose that the new hump and medial compartment contains the long ascending fibers that proceed uninteruptedly to the dorsal column nuclei of the medulla. At this stage of development, the dorsal funiculus is composed of a single compartment, the cuneate fasciculus composed of dorsal root afferents from the neck and upper body. The other component of this system, the ascending fibers of the gracile funiculus from thoracic and lumbar levels, forms another "hump" in the developing cervical cord. This second hump and compartment in the core of the dorsal funiculus first appears in a GW10.0 embryo in the materal available to us (Figure 5-26B).

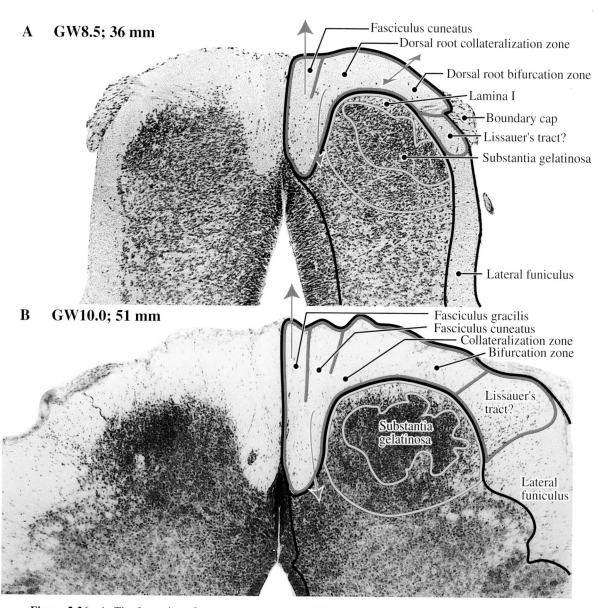

A   GW8.5; 36 mm

Fasciculus cuneatus
Dorsal root collateralization zone
Dorsal root bifurcation zone
Lamina I
Boundary cap
Lissauer's tract?
Substantia gelatinosa
Lateral funiculus

B   GW10.0; 51 mm

Fasciculus gracilis
Fasciculus cuneatus
Collateralization zone
Bifurcation zone
Lissauer's tract?
Substantia gelatinosa
Lateral funiculus

Figure 5-26. A. The formation of a new compartment medial to the collateralization zone, and a slight dorsal "hump," in the cervical spinal cord of this GW8.5 embryo (*M2050*; CR 36 mm). This compartment is identified as the cuneate fasciculus, composed of the ascending branch of dorsal root axons from the upper body that proceed uninterruptedly to the medulla (large vertical arrow). **B.** The formation of another medial compartment and a new "hump" in the cervical spinal cord of this GW10.0 fetus (*Y74-68*; CR 51 mm). This compartment, which displaces the cuneate fasciculus laterally, is identified as the gracile fasciculus. It is composed of newly arriving fibers from the lower body that proceed uninterruptedly to the medulla (large vertical arrow). The shift of the boundary cap dorsomedially may be due to the arrival of nociceptive fibers and the formation of Lissauer's tract.

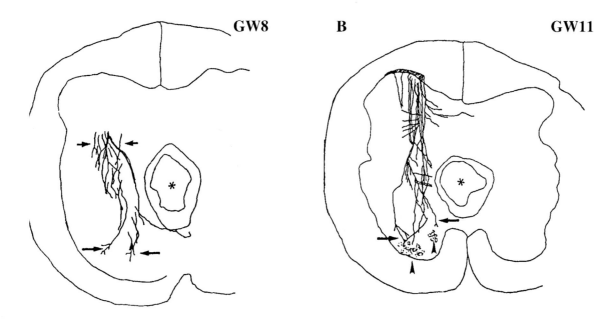

Figure 5-27. Growth of dorsal root fiber collaterals in a GW8.0 (**A**) and GW11.0 (**B**) human embryos, traced with carbocyanide DiI. A few collaterals reach the ventral horn by GW8.0. The collaterals increase in number and begin to arborize by GW11.0. From Konstantinidou et al. (1995)

In summary, these observations suggest that dorsal root axons traverse the boundary cap and penetrate the cervical spinal cord by GW5.0. Upon entering the cord, the axons split into longitudinally growing ascending and descending branches. Collectively, these branches form the dorsal root bifurcation zone. The budding of local collaterals of these branches starts at about GW7.0. By GW7.5, these collaterals start to grow downward and form the earliest maturing compartment of the dorsal funiculus, the dorsal root collateralization zone. The material available to us fails to provide infomation when the earliest developing collaterals, which are probably proprioceptive fibers, reach the ventral horn. Konstantinidou et al. (1995), who used carbocyanide DiI to trace dorsal root afferents in fixed human embryos, reported that a few afferents reach the ventral horn as early as GW8.0 (Figure 5-27). This would be within a few days after the formation of the collateralization zone. The number of collaterals and their length increases by GW11.0. The growth of the long ascending branch of the dorsal root axon, which form the cuneate and gracile fasciculi, is the last event. In the cervical cord, the fibers from the upper body that form the cuneate fasciculus are present by GW8.5, and the fibers from the lower body that form the gracile fasciculus are recognizable rostrally by GW10.0.

The early steps in the compartmental development of the dorsal funiculus in relation to our hypothesis of the branching of dorsal root afferents is summarized in Figure 5-28. (The subsequent growth of the dorsal funiculus through the addition of the cuneate fasciculus and the gracile funiculus is dealt with in greater detail in Section 5.7.3 and is summarized in Figure 5-49.)

Figure 5-28. An interpretation of the expansion of the dorsal root bifurcation zone and the growth of the collateralization zone in the human cervical spinal cord in terms of the branching of earlier arriving and later arriving dorsal root fibers (DR). **A.** The earliest entering DR fibers split into an ascending and descending branch between GW5.0 and GW5.5. These form the initial portion of the DR bifurcation zone ("oval bundle of His"). **B.** The increase in the number of bifurcating fibers results in the expansion of the bifurcation zone dorsomedially between GW6.0 and GW6.5. **C.** The next event is the sprouting of local collaterals between GW7.0 and GW7.5. **D.** The increase in the number of collaterals and their downward growth continues between GW8.0 and GW9.0. **E.** By GW9.5 to GW10.0 the local collaterals begin to enter the gray matter underneath the dorsal horn.

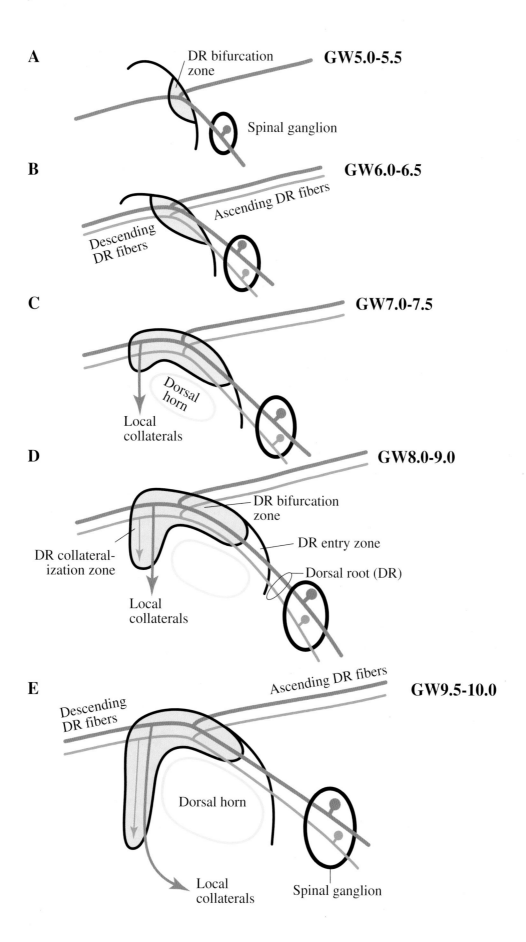

A DR bifurcation zone   **GW5.0-5.5**

Spinal ganglion

B   **GW6.0-6.5**

Ascending DR fibers

Descending DR fibers

C   **GW7.0-7.5**

Dorsal horn

Local collaterals

D   **GW8.0-9.0**

DR bifurcation zone

DR entry zone

Dorsal root (DR)

DR collateralization zone

Local collaterals

E   Ascending DR fibers   **GW9.5-10.0**

Descending DR fibers

Dorsal horn

Local collaterals

Spinal ganglion

5.7 Development of the Whole Spinal Cord During the First Trimester

5.7.1 Overview of Spinal Cord Development in a GW8.5 and a GW10.5 Embryo. Streeter's reconstruction of the spinal cord of a 30 mm (GW8), 67 mm (GW11), and a 111 mm (GW14) specimen (Figure 5-29) indicates that it lengthens over three-fold during the second half of the first trimester. The length of the spinal cord matches that of the vertebral column up to GW11, but by GW14 the length of spine exceeds that of the spinal cord. The greater growth rate of the bony vertebrae relative to the spinal cord continues henceforth until the elongation of the body stops during adolescence.

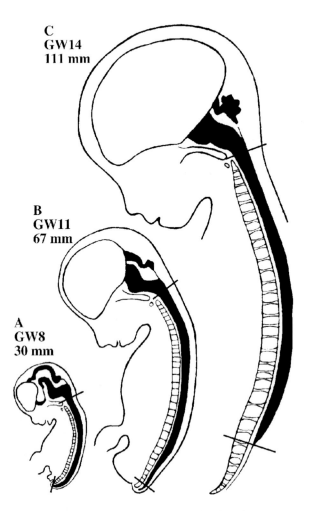

Figure 5-29. The spinal cord in a GW8 embryo (**A**) and a GW11.0 embryo (**B**), and a GW14.0 (**C**) fetus. By GW14, the vertebrae extend beyond the caudal tip (bottom line) of the spinal cord. After Streeter, from Hamilton et al. (1964).

The rapid lengthening of the spinal cord during the first trimester is paralleled by an increase in its width. We compare below eleven matched sections from upper cervical to coccygeal levels in two specimens – a GW8.5 embryo (*M2050*, CR 36 mm) an a GW10.5 fetus (*Y380-62*; CR 56 mm) – to determine what contributes cytologically to the lengthening and widening of the spinal cord. The segmental location of the analyzed histological sections in the two specimens is schematically indicated in Figure 5-30. For an easy comparison of the developmental changes between GW8.5 and GW10.5, the matched sections are shown at succeeding rostrocaudal levels on facing pages in Figures 5-31 to 5-38.

Upper Cervical Cord. The elongated dorsal canal and the dorsal neuroepithelium surrounding it are still present in the upper cervical cord (transition region to the medulla) in the GW8.5 embryo (Figure 5-31A); both are virtually absent at the same level of the cord in the GW10.5 embryo (Figure 5-32A). Among other noteworthy changes in the older specimen, representing two weeks' of growth, are the increase in the size of motoneuron perikarya in the ventral horn and the segregation of the larger motoneuron clusters into smaller columns. In the white matter, the dorsal funiculus is deeper, and the lateral and ventrolateral funiculi are larger in the older embryo. Except for an overall expansion, there is little difference in the appearance of the dorsal horn and the substantia gelatinosa in the two embryos.

Middle Cervical Cord. While the dorsal canal is receding in the midcervical spinal cord beneath the expanding dorsal funiculus in the GW8.5 embryo (Figure 5-31B), parts of the the dorsal neuro-epithelium and intermediate neuroepithelium remain bulky, suggesting that neurogenesis is still in progress at the latter sites at this age. In contrast, the dorsal canal and the neuroepithelium surrounding it have disappeared at a corresponding level in the GW10.5 embryo (Figure 5-32B). The diamond-shaped central canal pesists, and it is surrounded by a thin but darkly staining germinal zone, the presumptive ependyma. The dorsal horn and the central autonomic area have expanded greatly between GW8.5 and GW10.5. The considerable expansion of the ventral horn during the same period is associated with the segregation of motoneuron clusters into discrete motor columns and with the great expansion of the ventral interneuronal field.

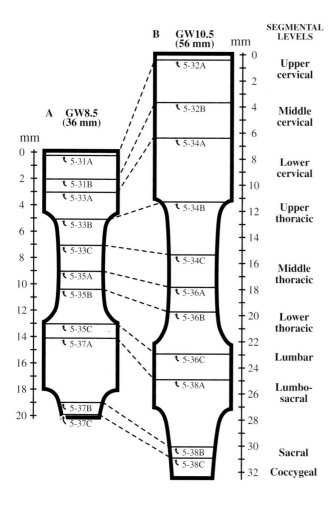

Figure 5-30. A, schematic reconstruction of the spinal cord of a GW8.5 embryo (*M2050*; CR 36 mm) and **B,** of a GW10.5 embryo (*Y380-62*; CR 56 mm). The estimated length of the spinal cord in the two embryos (20 mm and 32 mm, respectively) is based on the total number and nominal thickness of the serial sections. The width and shape of the spinal cord are exaggerated. Lines in the graphs and the figure numbers below the lines indicate the exact location of the sections illustrated in Figures 5-31 to 5-38.

From the Lower Cervical to the Midthoracic Cord. In the GW8.5 embryo, the neuroepithelium that surrounds the dorsal canal and the upper central canal is bulkier at low cervical (Figure 5-33A), upper thoracic (Figure 5-33B), and middle thoracic (Figure 5-33C) levels than more rostrally. This suggests that the production of gelatinosal neurons and neurons of the central autonomic area are still in progress in the caudal spinal cord at this age. That is only one indication of the rostral-to-caudal gradient in spinal cord development. But there is another. In the GW10.5 embryo (Figure 5-34A), the most obvious change is the appearance of "humps" on the surface of the dorsal funiculus. These transient humps are attrib-

uted to the rapid accumulation of ascending branches of dorsal root axons in the core portion of the dorsal funiculus. It is noteworthy that only the cuneate fasciculus (composed of afferents from the upper body parts) is recognizable in the cervical cord of the GW8.5 embryo (Figures 5-31B, 5-33A). In the GW10.5 embryo, in contrast, a pair of medial humps representing the gracile fasciculus (composed of afferents from the lower regions of the body) are also present (Figure 5-32B, 5-34A). This suggests that the distal fibers of the gracile fasciculus reach the cervical cord sometime between GW8.5 and GW10.5. As this happens, the fibers of he ascending gracile fasciculus displace the fibers of the cuneate fasciculus from medial to lateral.

From the Middle Thoracic to the Lumbar Cord. In the GW8.5 embryo, the spinal canal is more elongated and the neuroepithelium bulkier at the thoracic cord (Figures 5-35A, B) and the upper lumbar cord (Figure 5-35C) than more rostrally. As judged by the changes seen at the corresponding levels of the gray matter in the GW10.5 embryo (Figures 5-36A, B, C), the neuroepithelium is still generating neurons for the dorsal horn and the central autonomic area at these caudal levels of the cord in the GW8.5 embryo. Another indication of the caudal lag in spinal cord development is the immature, cap-like appearance of the dorsal funiculus in the GW8.5 embryo (Figure 5-35) relative to its greater depth in the GW10.5 embryo (Figure 5-36).

From the Lumbosacral to the Coccygeal Cord. The spinal cord of the GW8.5 embryo, as judged by the elongated spinal canal and the bulky neuroepithelium, is least developed at lumbosacral (Figure 5-37A), sacral (5-37B), and coccygeal (Figure 5-37C) levels. Indeed, in the sacral and coccygeal cord, the spinal canal retains its primitive tripartite configuration. Another indication of the immaturity of the spinal cord at these far-caudal levels is the absence of the gracile fasciculus. This suggests the the growth of the ascending branch of dorsal root axons has not yet begun from the lumbosacral spinal cord. At corresponding levels in the GW10.5 fetus (Figure 5-38A, B, C), the fasciculus gracilis is recognizable. However, the neuroepithelium remains prominent even at this late age around the central and ventral canals, indicating that some neurogenesis, and probably robust gliogenesis, are still in progress in the caudal spinal cord at GW10.5.

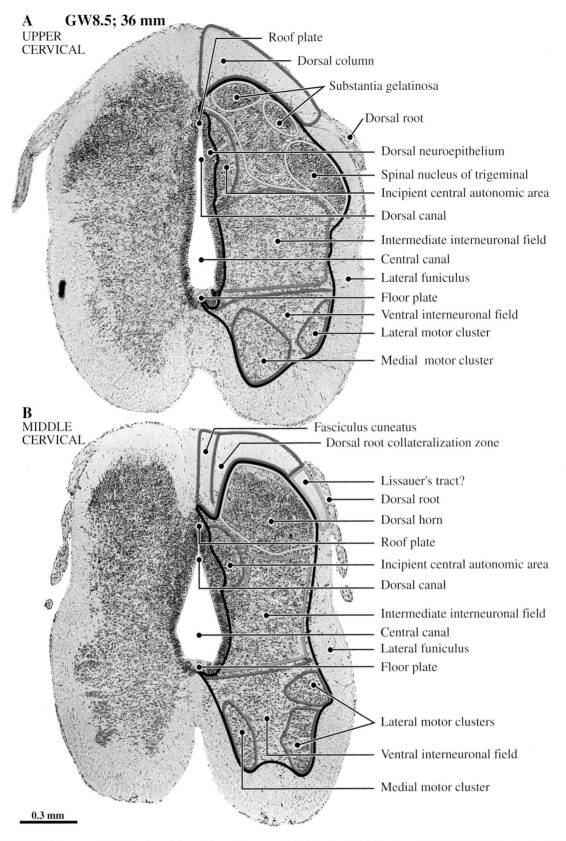

A   GW8.5; 36 mm
UPPER
CERVICAL

Roof plate

Dorsal column

Substantia gelatinosa

Dorsal root

Dorsal neuroepithelium

Spinal nucleus of trigeminal

Incipient central autonomic area

Dorsal canal

Intermediate interneuronal field

Central canal

Lateral funiculus

Floor plate

Ventral interneuronal field

Lateral motor cluster

Medial motor cluster

B
MIDDLE
CERVICAL

Fasciculus cuneatus

Dorsal root collateralization zone

Lissauer's tract?

Dorsal root

Dorsal horn

Roof plate

Incipient central autonomic area

Dorsal canal

Intermediate interneuronal field

Central canal

Lateral funiculus

Floor plate

Lateral motor clusters

Ventral interneuronal field

Medial motor cluster

0.3 mm

Figure 5-31. A. Upper cervical spinal cord (transition to lower medulla) in the GW 8.5 embryo (*M2050*; CR 36 mm). A thining
dorsal neuroepithelium is still present along the receding dorsal canal. **B.** At the midcervical level in the same embryo, the dorsal
canal has receded underneath the dorsal funiculus but the dorsal neuroepithelium is still present. The motoneurons are aggregated
in large clusters in the ventral horn. Color outlines in these and the following illustrations: blue, branches of dorsal root afferents;
yellow, dorsal horn; purple, central autonomic area; green, intermediate interneuronal field; red, motoneurons and ventral horn.

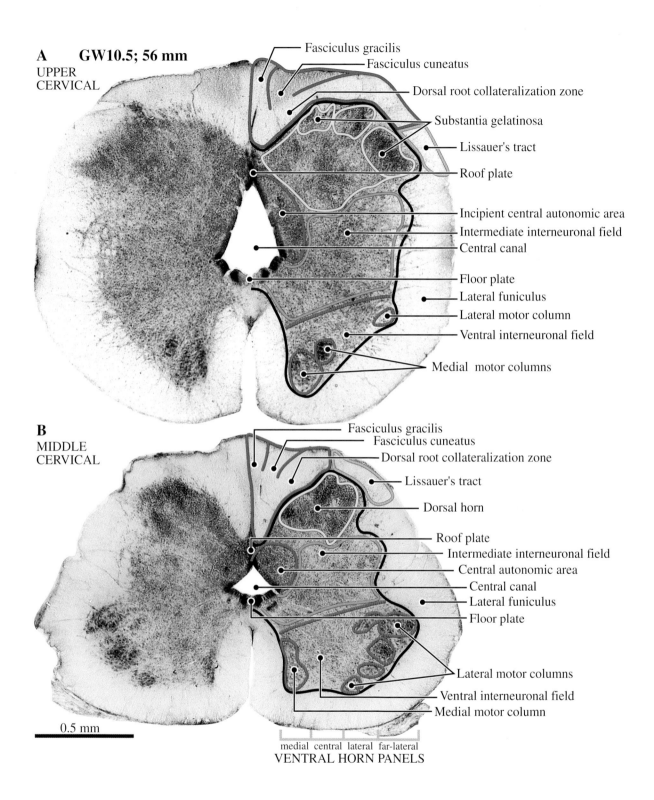

A. GW10.5; 56 mm
UPPER CERVICAL

- Fasciculus gracilis
- Fasciculus cuneatus
- Dorsal root collateralization zone
- Substantia gelatinosa
- Lissauer's tract
- Roof plate
- Incipient central autonomic area
- Intermediate interneuronal field
- Central canal
- Floor plate
- Lateral funiculus
- Lateral motor column
- Ventral interneuronal field
- Medial motor columns

B. MIDDLE CERVICAL

- Fasciculus gracilis
- Fasciculus cuneatus
- Dorsal root collateralization zone
- Lissauer's tract
- Dorsal horn
- Roof plate
- Intermediate interneuronal field
- Central autonomic area
- Central canal
- Lateral funiculus
- Floor plate
- Lateral motor columns
- Ventral interneuronal field
- Medial motor column

0.5 mm

medial central lateral far-lateral
VENTRAL HORN PANELS

Figure 5-32. A. Upper cervical spinal cord in the GW10.5 embryo (*Y380-62*; CR 56 mm). The site of the withdrawn dorsal canal and the dissolved dorsal neuroepithelium is occupied by the central autonomic area. **B.** In the midcervical cord of the same embryo, the large spinal canal has been reduced to the small central canal. Coupled with the shrinkage of the neuroepithelium and cessation of neurogenesis, the dorsal horn has expanded considerably. By this age, not only the fasciculus cuneatus but also the fasciculus gracilis is present in the widened dorsal funiculus. The motoneurons have become more prominent in the greatly enlarged ventral horn and their segregation into discrete columns is in progress. The spinal canal is now lined by the primitive ependyma.

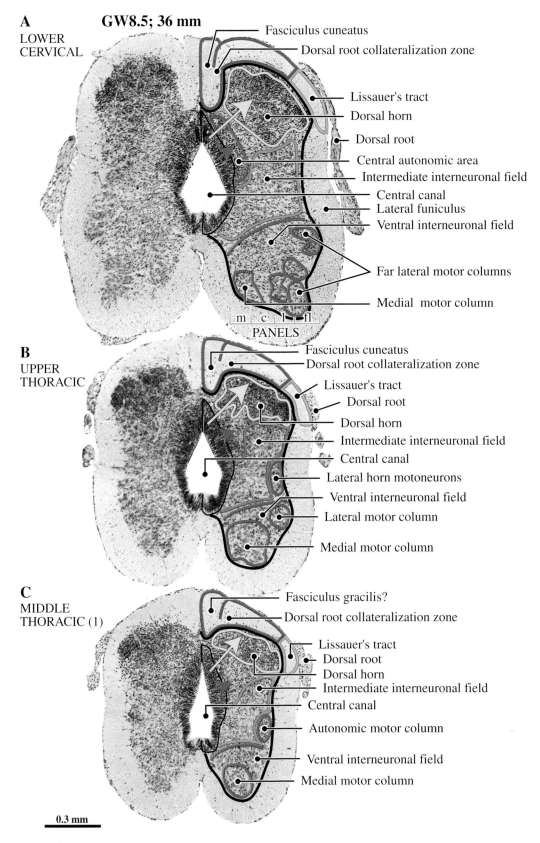

A
LOWER
CERVICAL

GW8.5; 36 mm

Fasciculus cuneatus
Dorsal root collateralization zone
Lissauer's tract
Dorsal horn
Dorsal root
Central autonomic area
Intermediate interneuronal field
Central canal
Lateral funiculus
Ventral interneuronal field
Far lateral motor columns
Medial motor column

m   c   l   fl
PANELS

B
UPPER
THORACIC

Fasciculus cuneatus
Dorsal root collateralization zone
Lissauer's tract
Dorsal root
Dorsal horn
Intermediate interneuronal field
Central canal
Lateral horn motoneurons
Ventral interneuronal field
Lateral motor column
Medial motor column

C
MIDDLE
THORACIC (1)

Fasciculus gracilis?
Dorsal root collateralization zone
Lissauer's tract
Dorsal root
Dorsal horn
Intermediate interneuronal field
Central canal
Autonomic motor column
Ventral interneuronal field
Medial motor column

0.3 mm

Figure 5-33. The spinal cord of the GW8.5 embryo *(M2050; CR 36 mm)* at low cervical (**A**), upper thoracic (**B**), and high middle thoracic (**C**) levels. The dorsal and intermediate neuroepithelia are thicker at these caudal levels than more rostrally (compare with Figure 5-31), suggesting ongoing production of gelatinosal and central autonomic neurons. Arrows indicate the presumed migration of late-generated neurons.

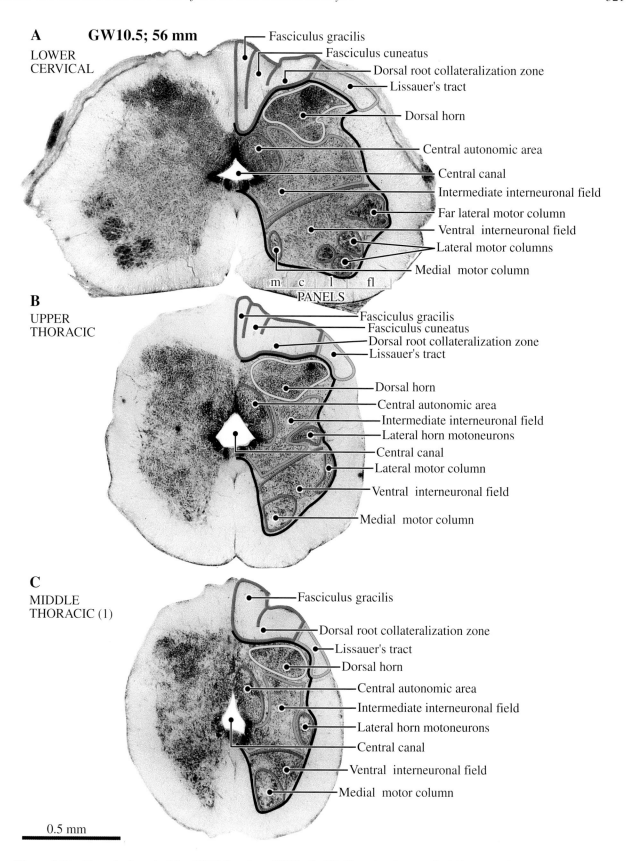

A   GW10.5; 56 mm
LOWER
CERVICAL

- Fasciculus gracilis
- Fasciculus cuneatus
- Dorsal root collateralization zone
- Lissauer's tract
- Dorsal horn
- Central autonomic area
- Central canal
- Intermediate interneuronal field
- Far lateral motor column
- Ventral interneuronal field
- Lateral motor columns
- Medial motor column

m   c   l   fl
PANELS

B
UPPER
THORACIC

- Fasciculus gracilis
- Fasciculus cuneatus
- Dorsal root collateralization zone
- Lissauer's tract
- Dorsal horn
- Central autonomic area
- Intermediate interneuronal field
- Lateral horn motoneurons
- Central canal
- Lateral motor column
- Ventral interneuronal field
- Medial motor column

C
MIDDLE
THORACIC (1)

- Fasciculus gracilis
- Dorsal root collateralization zone
- Lissauer's tract
- Dorsal horn
- Central autonomic area
- Intermediate interneuronal field
- Lateral horn motoneurons
- Central canal
- Ventral interneuronal field
- Medial motor column

0.5 mm

Figure 5-34. The spinal cord of the GW10.5 embryo (*Y380-62*; CR 56 mm) at low cervical (**A**), upper thoracic (**B**), and high middle thoracic (**C**) levels. The dorsal horn, the central autonomic area, and the ventral horn have expanded. The transient "humps" in the dorsal funiculus reflect the arrival of fibers of the fasciculus gracilis medially and the displacement of the fasciculus cuneatus laterally. Note the bulging of the gracile fasciculus in the upper portion of the middle thoracic cord in **C**.

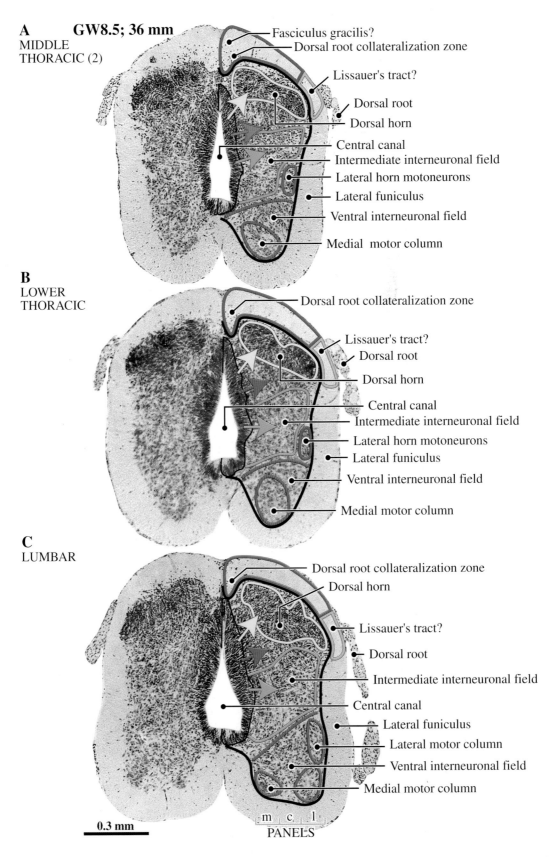

A **GW8.5; 36 mm**
MIDDLE
THORACIC (2)

— Fasciculus gracilis?
— Dorsal root collateralization zone
— Lissauer's tract?
— Dorsal root
— Dorsal horn
— Central canal
— Intermediate interneuronal field
— Lateral horn motoneurons
— Lateral funiculus
— Ventral interneuronal field
— Medial motor column

B
LOWER
THORACIC

— Dorsal root collateralization zone
— Lissauer's tract?
— Dorsal root
— Dorsal horn
— Central canal
— Intermediate interneuronal field
— Lateral horn motoneurons
— Lateral funiculus
— Ventral interneuronal field
— Medial motor column

C
LUMBAR

— Dorsal root collateralization zone
— Dorsal horn
— Lissauer's tract?
— Dorsal root
— Intermediate interneuronal field
— Central canal
— Lateral funiculus
— Lateral motor column
— Ventral interneuronal field
— Medial motor column

0.3 mm

m c l
PANELS

Figure 5-35. A, B, C. The spinal cordat middle thoracic to lumbar levels in the GW8.5 embryo (*M2050*; CR 36 mm). The spinal
canal is longer and the neuroepithelium is thicker than more rostrally. Another sign of the rostrocaudal gradient is the absence of the
fasciculus gracilis in **B** and **C**. (The fasciculus cuneatus is present in the cervical spinal cord; compare with Figures 5-31A, 5-33A).
Arrows indicate the presumed migration of neurons to the dorsal horn, the central autonomic area, and the intermediate gray.

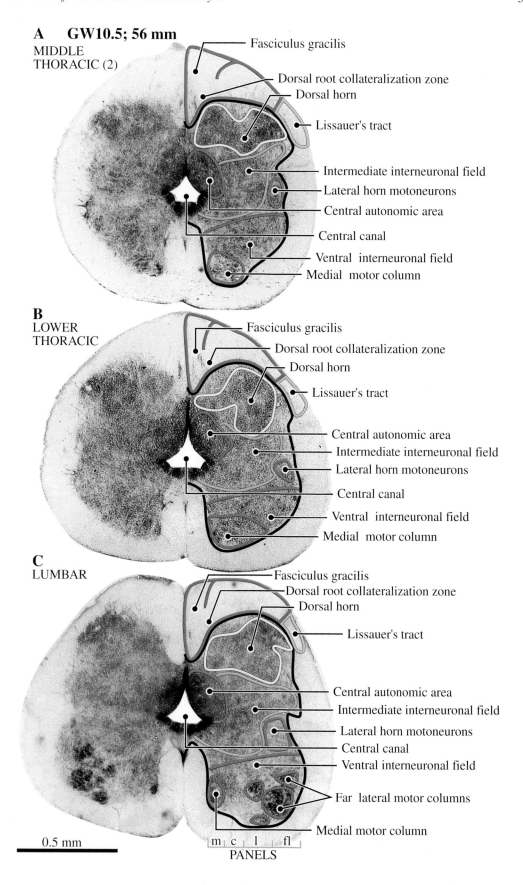

A   GW10.5; 56 mm
MIDDLE
THORACIC (2)

Fasciculus gracilis
Dorsal root collateralization zone
Dorsal horn
Lissauer's tract
Intermediate interneuronal field
Lateral horn motoneurons
Central autonomic area
Central canal
Ventral interneuronal field
Medial motor column

B
LOWER
THORACIC

Fasciculus gracilis
Dorsal root collateralization zone
Dorsal horn
Lissauer's tract
Central autonomic area
Intermediate interneuronal field
Lateral horn motoneurons
Central canal
Ventral interneuronal field
Medial motor column

C
LUMBAR

Fasciculus gracilis
Dorsal root collateralization zone
Dorsal horn
Lissauer's tract
Central autonomic area
Intermediate interneuronal field
Lateral horn motoneurons
Central canal
Ventral interneuronal field
Far lateral motor columns
Medial motor column

0.5 mm

m | c | l | fl
PANELS

Figure 5-36. A, **B**, **C.** The spinal cord at middle thoracic to lumbar levels in the GW10.5 embryo (*Y380-62*; CR 56 mm). Developments include the growth of the gracile fasciculus and Lissauer's tract, the expansion of the dorsal horn, the central autonomic area and the ventral horn, and the progressive segregation of motor columns in the lumbar cord.

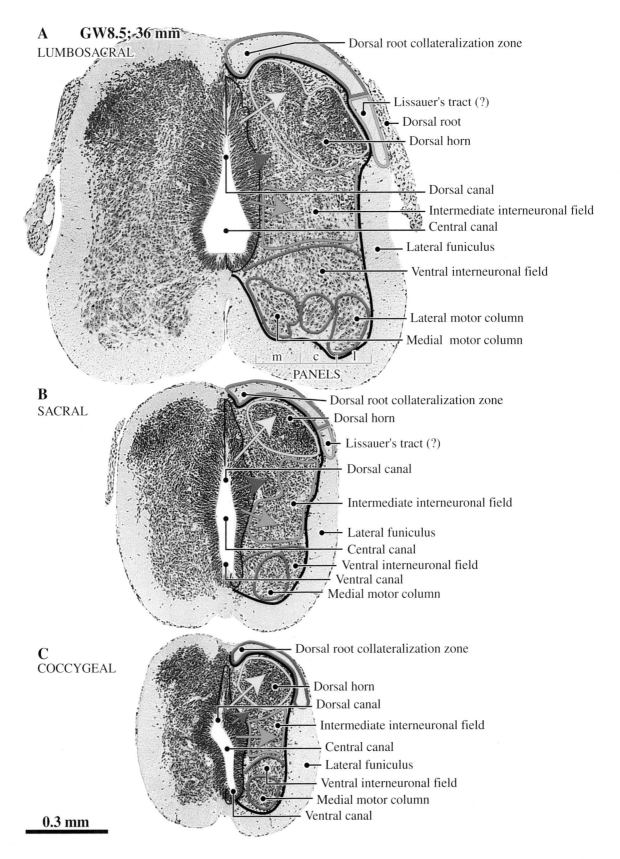

A   **GW8.5; 36 mm**
LUMBOSACRAL

— Dorsal root collateralization zone
— Lissauer's tract (?)
— Dorsal root
— Dorsal horn

— Dorsal canal
— Intermediate interneuronal field
— Central canal
— Lateral funiculus
— Ventral interneuronal field

— Lateral motor column
— Medial motor column

m   c   l
PANELS

B
SACRAL

— Dorsal root collateralization zone
— Dorsal horn
— Lissauer's tract (?)

— Dorsal canal

— Intermediate interneuronal field

— Lateral funiculus
— Central canal
— Ventral interneuronal field
— Ventral canal
— Medial motor column

C
COCCYGEAL

— Dorsal root collateralization zone

— Dorsal horn
— Dorsal canal
— Intermediate interneuronal field
— Central canal
— Lateral funiculus
— Ventral interneuronal field
— Medial motor column
— Ventral canal

0.3 mm

Figure 5-37. The spinal cord of the GW8.5 embryo (*M2050*; CR 36 mm) at lumbosacral (**A**), sacral (**B**), and coccygeal (**C**) levels. The spinal canal is becoming increasingly longer and the neuroepithelium more prominent at descending levels. The dorsal root collateralization zone is forming but the fasciculus gracilis is probably absent. Arrows indicate presumed migration of late-generated neurons to the dorsal horn, the central autonomic area, and the intermediate gray.

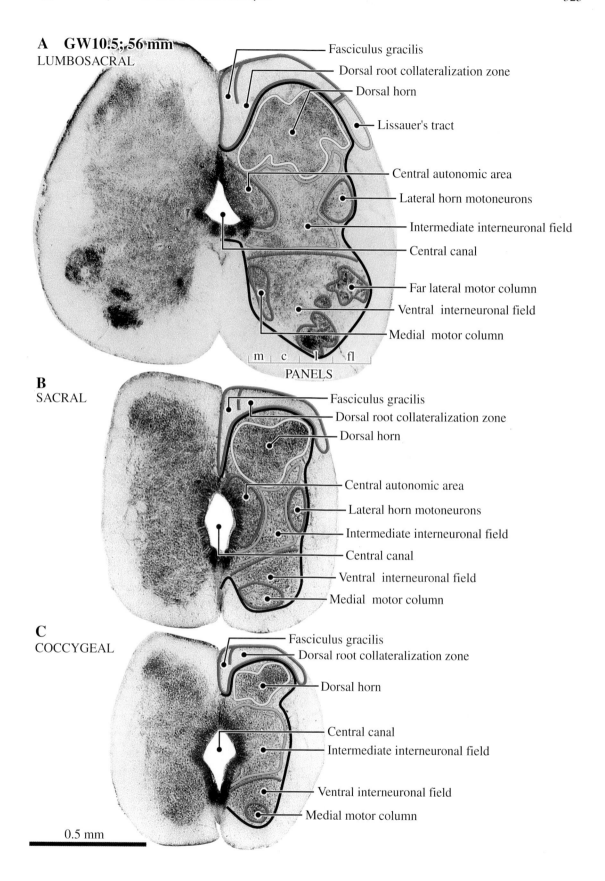

A GW10.5; 56 mm
LUMBOSACRAL

- Fasciculus gracilis
- Dorsal root collateralization zone
- Dorsal horn
- Lissauer's tract
- Central autonomic area
- Lateral horn motoneurons
- Intermediate interneuronal field
- Central canal
- Far lateral motor column
- Ventral interneuronal field
- Medial motor column

m | c | l | fl
PANELS

B
SACRAL

- Fasciculus gracilis
- Dorsal root collateralization zone
- Dorsal horn
- Central autonomic area
- Lateral horn motoneurons
- Intermediate interneuronal field
- Central canal
- Ventral interneuronal field
- Medial motor column

C
COCCYGEAL

- Fasciculus gracilis
- Dorsal root collateralization zone
- Dorsal horn
- Central canal
- Intermediate interneuronal field
- Ventral interneuronal field
- Medial motor column

0.5 mm

Figure 5-38. The spinal cord of the GW10.5 (*Y380-62*; CR 56 mm) embryo at lumbosacral (**A**), sacral (**B**), and coccygeal (**C**) levels. The spinal canal is shrinking but the neuroepithelium persists at these levels. The collateralization zone is evident but the fasciculus gracilis is still poorly developed in the sacral and coccygeal cord.

5.7.2 Development of Motoneurons Between GW8.5 and GW10.5.

The growth of motoneuron perikarya and their segregation into discrete motor columns between GW8.5 and GW10.5 is compared at higher magnification in Figures 5-39 to 5-42. On facing pages, roughly comparable levels are matched from the middle cervical to the sacral levels of the spinal cord. In the middle cervical cord of the GW8.5 embryo (Figure 5-39A), the perikarya of motoneurons are relatively small and only a medial and lateral panel of motor columns is recognizable (the central panel is filled with interneurons). At a corresponding level in the GW10.5 fetus (Figures 5-40A), the motoneurons have become much larger and they are segregated into smaller clusters. A similar growth of motoneuron perikarya and increased columnar segregation as a function of age is seen in the lower cervical cord (compare Figures 5-39B and 5-40B) the thoracic cord (compare Figures 5-41A and 5-42A), and the lumbar cord (compare Figures 5-41B

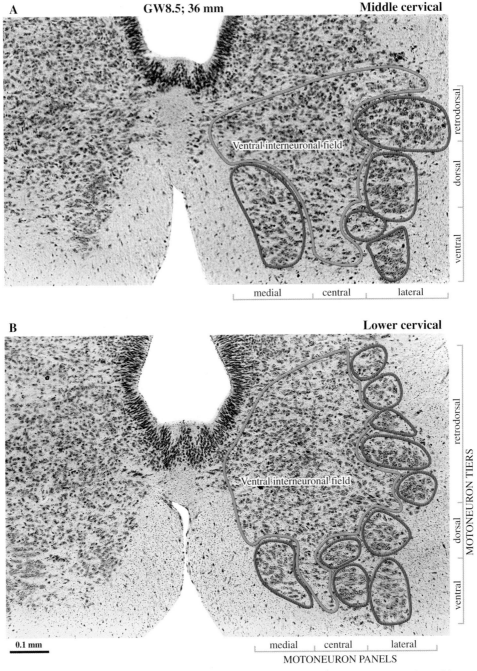

Figure 5-39. The ventral horn of the GW8.5 embryo (*M2050*; CR 36 mm) at midcervical (**A**) and low cervical (**B**) levels. The segregation of motor columns in the medial, central and lateral panels is in progress.

and 5-42B). This difference is least evident farthest caudally in the sacral cord (compare Figures 5-41C and 5-42C). The multipolar shapes of motoneurons in the older embryo (at all levels but the sacral cord) indicate that dendritic development is in progress by GW10.5.

Regrettably, an embryo exactly representing the last week of the first trimester (GW13) has not been available. To roughly gauge the development of the ventral horn at about this age, we show sections

from a GW14 fetus (*Y68-65*; CR 108 mm) from upper cervical to lumbosacral levels of the cord in Figures 5-43 and 5-44. Among the developmental achievements by the first week of the second trimester are the continuing growth of motoneuron perikarya, their segregation in discrete columns, further dispersal of motoneurons within the columns and, last but not least, the expansion of the ventral interneuronal field. Moreover, there is no longer any obvious difference in motoneuronal maturation between the rostral and caudal levels of the spinal cord.

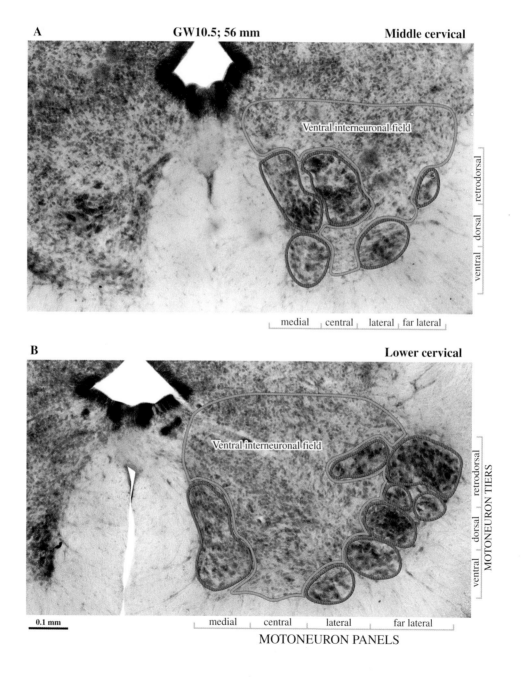

Figure 5-40. The ventral horn of the GW10.5 fetus (*Y380-62*; CR 56 mm) at midcervical (**A**) and low cervical (**B**) levels. The perikarya of motoneurons have grown appreciably and they are becoming segregated into smaller clusters.

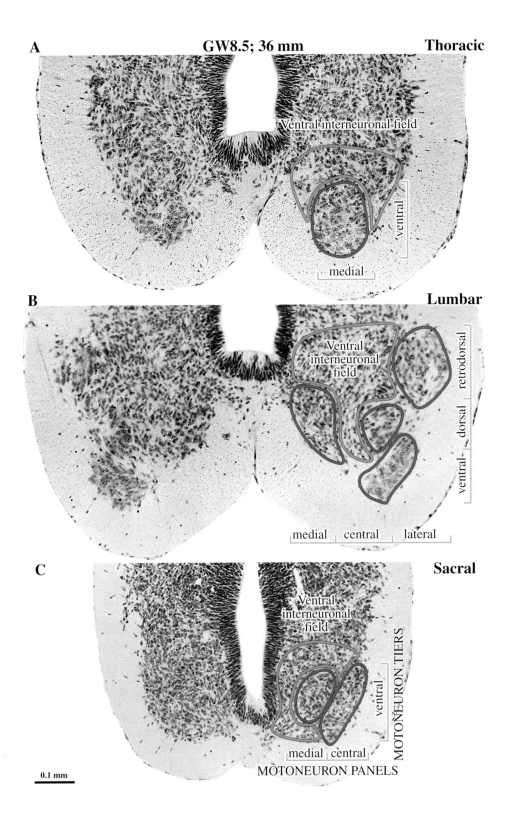

Figure 5-41. The ventral horn at thoracic (**A**), lumbar (**B**), and sacral (**C**) levels in the GW8.5 embryo (*M2050*; CR 36 mm). The segregation of motor columns and the growth of motoneuron perikarya are in progress.

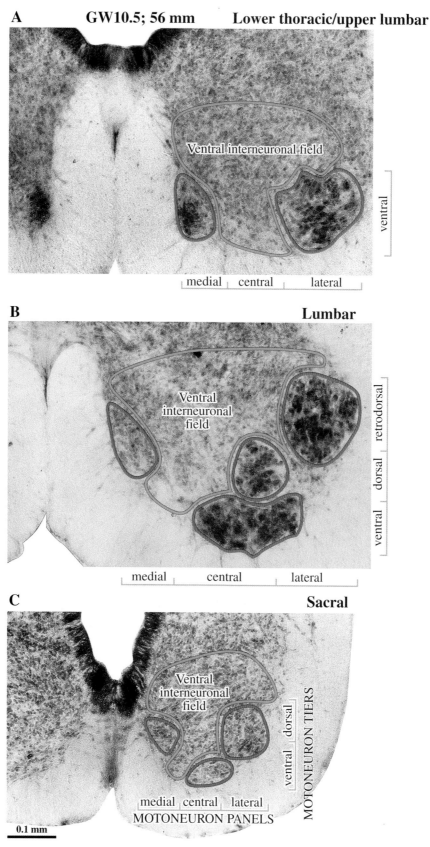

Figure 5-42. The ventral horn at thoracic (**A**), lumbar (**B**), and sacral (**C**) levels in the GW10.5 fetus (*Y380-62*; CR 56 mm). The growth of motoneuron perikarya is pronounced at thoracic and lumber levels but is less advanced in the sacral cord.

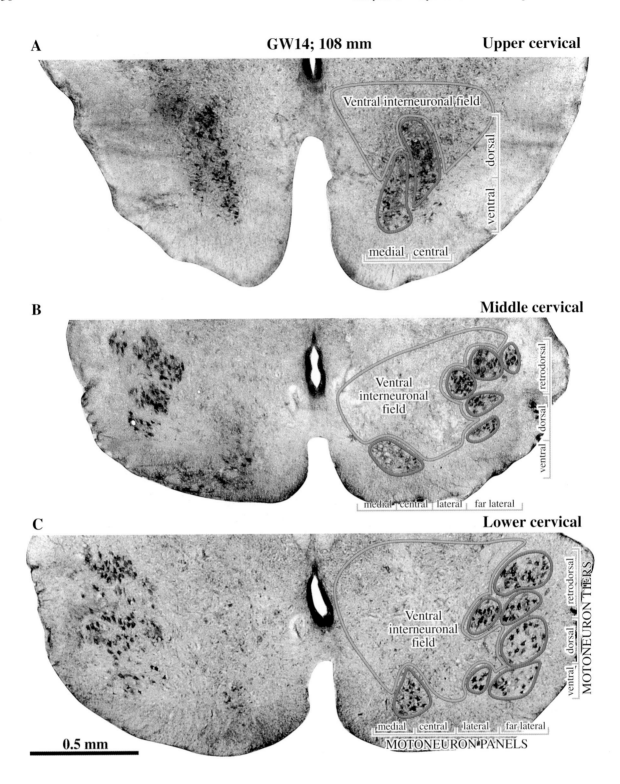

A **GW14; 108 mm** **Upper cervical**

Ventral interneuronal field

dorsal
ventral

medial   central

B **Middle cervical**

Ventral
interneuronal
field

retrodorsal
dorsal
ventral

medial   central   lateral   far lateral

C **Lower cervical**

Ventral
interneuronal
field

retrodorsal
dorsal
ventral

MOTONEURON TIERS

0.5 mm

medial   central   lateral   far lateral

MOTONEURON PANELS

Figure 5-43. The ventral horn in a GW14 fetus (*Y68-65*; CR 108 mm) at upper cervical (**A**), midcervical (**B**), and low cervical (**C**) levels. The most pronounced changes relative to earlier ages are the dispersal of motoneurons within the motor columns and the increase in the number of the lateral and far-lateral motor columns.

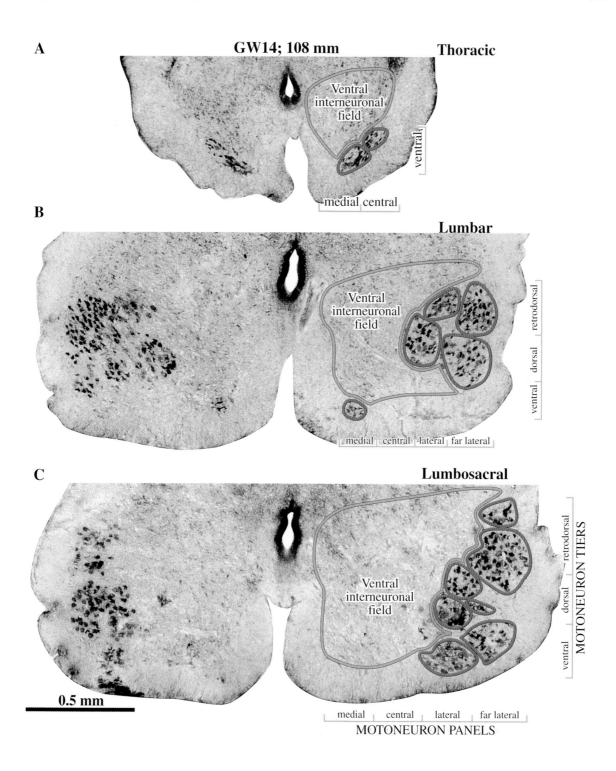

Figure 5-44. The ventral horn in the GW14 fetus (*Y68-65*; CR 108 mm) at thoracic (**A**), lumbar (**B**), and lumbosacral (**C**) levels. The developments seen more rostrally are also evident at these caudal levels of the spinal cord.

5.7.3 Development of the Dorsal Funiculus Between GW7.5 and GW14.
The dorsal funiculus undergoes profound changes between GW7.5 and GW14. We analyze these changes first in the cervical cord. The collateralization zone is absent in the less mature GW7.5 embryo (*M2314*; CR 23.8 mm; Figure 5-45A) and the neurons of the substantia gelatinosa, which will be among the targets of the dorsal root sensory fibers, are just beginning to settle in the incipient dorsal horn. In the larger and more mature GW7.5 embryo (*M2042*; CR 25 mm; Figure 5-45C), the collateralization zone is beginning to form; as indicated by the club-like fibrous mass that occupies the site vacated by the receding dorsal neuroepithelium. In the GW8.5 embryo (*C609*; CR 32 mm; Figure 5-45C), the place of the receding dorsal neuroepithelium is occupied by the greatly enlarged dorsal funiculus with its "humps." (The surface of the dorsal funiculus will become smooth again as the period of rapid fiber growth subsides.)

We use these transient "humps" to distinguish four successively developing compartments in the developing dorsal funiculus. Compartment 1, which forms at about GW5.0 dorsolaterally (Figure 5-23B) and expands dorsomedially during the next two weeks (Figures 5-24A,B; 5-25A) is the dorsal root bifurcation zone. Compartment 2, which forms at about GW7.5 (Figures 5-45A,B), is the dorsal root collateralization zone. The formation of the collateralization zone between GW7.5 and GW8.0 is the first step in the development of the dorsal funiculus. Compartment 3 appears on GW8.5 as a small wedge abutting the dorsal median septum; it is identified as the cuneate fasciculus (Figure 5-45C). The formation of the cuneate fasciculus in the cervical cord is the second step in the development of the dorsal funiculus. Finally, compartment 4, which displaces the cuneate fasciculus laterally by GW10.0 (Figure 5-46A) is identified as the gracile fasciculus. These fibers may be forming later than the fibers of the cuneate fasciculus and, in addition, have to grow some distance to reach the cervical cord. The appearance of the gracile fasciculus in the cervical cord is the third step in the development of the dorsal funiculus.

These developments suggest the following sequence of events when applied to the successive branching of a hypothetical early forming (proprioceptive or exteroceptive) dorsal root axon. The sprouting of local collaterals begins at about GW7.5, but the growth of the ascending long branch that proceeds to the dorsal column nuclei (which includes switching from the "local" to the "express" lanes) does not start until about GW8.5. In the case of a dorsal root axon from the lumbar level, the ascending fiber may not reach the cervical cord until GW10.0. As judged by the expansion of the cuneate and gracile fasciculi by GW14 (Figure 5-46B), the number of fibers ascending in the core of the dorsal funiculus increases greatly in the last few weeks of the first trimester.

Still another development, but one that is difficult to trace in the available material, is the formation of a fibrous sheet lateral to the bifurcation zone. This event, as we have seen earlier, is associated with the displacement of the boundary cap and dorsal root entry zome dorsomedially (Figures 4-28, 4-29). This fascicle is probably composed of the small caliber nociceptive fibers of Lissauer's tract. If this is correct, the nociceptive axons that arborize with cap terminals in the substantia gelatinosa are the latest sensory fibers to reach the dorsal horn.

The sequence of the compartmental development of the dorsal funiculus in the cervical spinal cord also holds for the midthoracic spinal cord but, in line with the rostrocaudal gradient in spinal cord development, there is a chronological delay in that sequence. The collateralization zone (compartment 2) is first seen in the thoracic cord in the GW8.5 embryo (*M2050*; CR 36 mm; Figure 5-47A); about one week later than in the cervical cord (GW7.5; Figure 5-45B). Like the branching of collaterals, the formation of the ascending branch of the dorsal root axons is also delayed. The gracile fasciculus in the thoracic cord corresponds to the cuneate fasciculus in the cervical cord in terms of distance from the spinal ganglion, where the parent axons originate. But in contrast to the cuneate fasciculus, which is present by GW8.5 in the cervical cord (Figure 5-45C), the gracile fasciculus is first seen in the thoracic cord in the GW10 embryo (Figure 5-47B). It should be noted, however, that in the same GW10 embryo (*Y74-68*), the gracile fasciculus is also recognizable more rostrally in the cervical cord (Figure 5-46A). This raises the possibility that the caudal component of the gracile fasciculus may form some time before GW10. The gracile fasciculus deepens appreciably in the ensuing weeks, as seen in the GW 14 fetus (Figure 5-47C). This suggests the continual addition of later forming ascending dorsal root fibers.

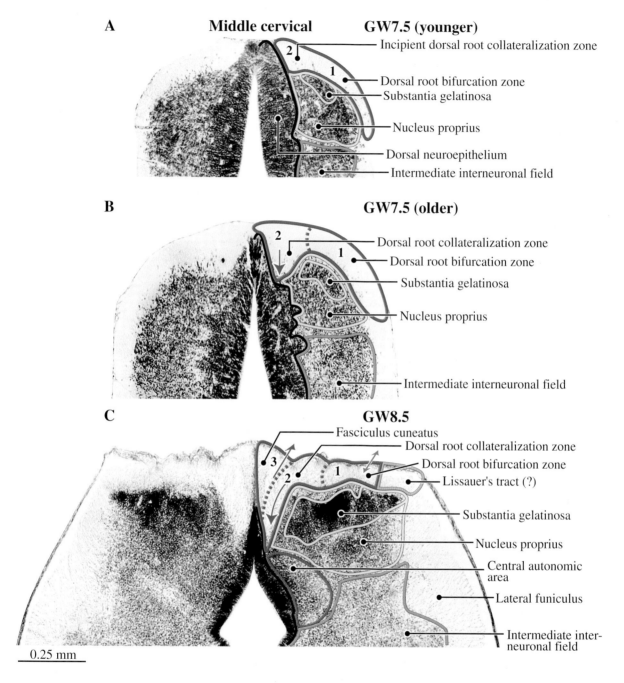

A   **Middle cervical**   **GW7.5 (younger)**

2 — Incipient dorsal root collateralization zone

1 — Dorsal root bifurcation zone
— Substantia gelatinosa

— Nucleus proprius

— Dorsal neuroepithelium
— Intermediate interneuronal field

B   **GW7.5 (older)**

2 — Dorsal root collateralization zone
1 — Dorsal root bifurcation zone

— Substantia gelatinosa

— Nucleus proprius

— Intermediate interneuronal field

C   **GW8.5**

— Fasciculus cuneatus
3 — Dorsal root collateralization zone
2 — Dorsal root bifurcation zone
1 — Lissauer's tract (?)

— Substantia gelatinosa

— Nucleus proprius

— Central autonomic area

— Lateral funiculus

— Intermediate inter-neuronal field

0.25 mm

Figure 5-45. Development of the dorsal funiculus in the midcervical region of the spinal cord between GW7.5 and GW8.5. **A.** In the less mature GW7.5 embryo (*M2314*; CR 23.8 mm), the dorsal gray matter is capped by the crescent-shaped fibrous tissue composed of the bifurcating branches of dorsal root afferents. This region is designated here as compartment 1. The widened medial region may be the site where the local collaterals begin to sprout. **B.** In this more mature GW7.5 embryo (*M2042*; CR 25 mm), the outgrowing collaterals form the club-shaped collateralization zone of the dorsal funiculus. This region is designated as compartment 2. **C.** In this GW8.5 embryo (*C609*; CR 32 mm), a new wedge-shaped band has formed dorsomedial to the lengthened collateralization zone. This is identified as the fasciculus cuneatus, composed of the earliest ascending branches of dorsal root axons from the upper body that terminate in the medulla. This region is designated as compartment 3.

The sequential development of the compartments of the dorsal funiculus in the lumbar cord is illustrated in Figure 5-48. The collateralization zone (compartment 2) is less well developed in the lumbar cord in the same GW8.5 fetus (*M2050*; Figure 5-48A) as it is in the thoracic cord (Figure 5-47A). This again indicates a rostral-to-caudal gradient in the successive branching of dorsal root axons. However, by GW10.0 (Figure 5-48B), the lag is less evident, and

by GW14.0 there is little difference in the maturation of the gracile fasciculus at GW10.0 (Figure 5-47C) and GW14.0 (Figure 5-48C). The successive emergence of the different compartments of the dorsal funiculus in relation to the hypothetical growth of different branches of individual dorsal root sensory axons – the bifurcating branches, their collaterals, and the principal ascending branch – is schematically summarized in Figure 5-49.

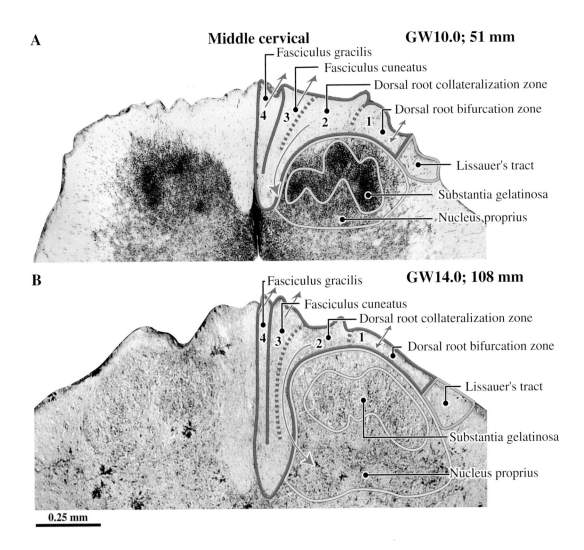

Figure 5-46. Growth of the dorsal funiculus in the midcervical region of the spinal cord between GW10.0 and GW14.0. **A.** In this GW10.0 fetus (*Y74-68*; CR 51 mm), a new compartment in the dorsal funiculus displaces the fasciculus cuneatus laterally. This is the fasciculus gracilis, designated here as compartment 4, composed of the ascending branches of dorsal root axons from the lower body. **B.** This GW14 fetus (*Y68-65*; CR 108 mm) shows deepening of both the cuneate and gracile fasiculi.

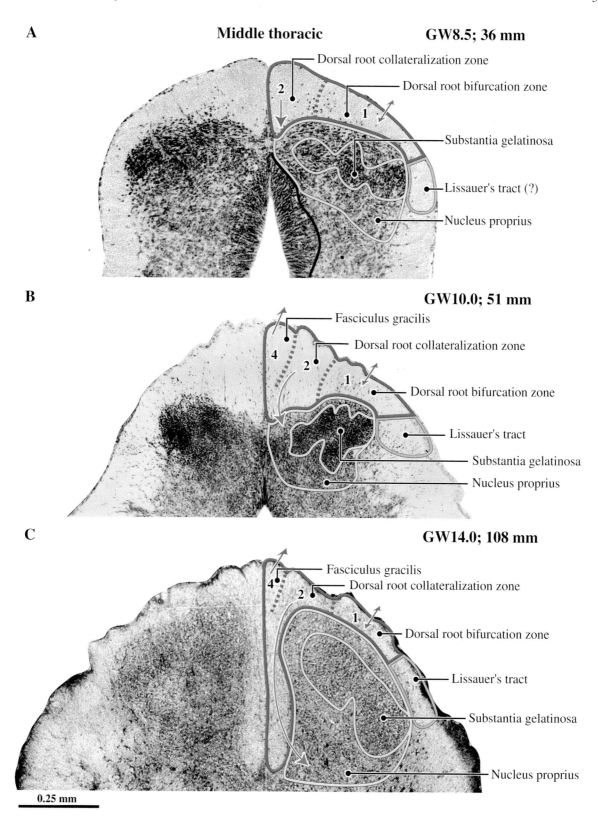

Figure 5-47. Growth of the dorsal funiculus in the middle thoracic spinal cord. **A.** The collateralization zone (compartment 2) is developing in the GW8.5 embryo (*M2050*; CR 36 mm). Lissauer's tract may also be present. **B.** Notable in the GW10.0 fetus (*Y74-68*; CR 51 mm) is the deepening of the collateralization zone and the growth of the fasciculus gracilis (compartment 4). **C.** The collateralization zone and the gracile fasciculus have expanded considerably in the GW14.0 fetus (*Y68-65*; CR 108 mm). Lissauer's tract is now more prominent over the lateral flank of the maturing dorsal horn.

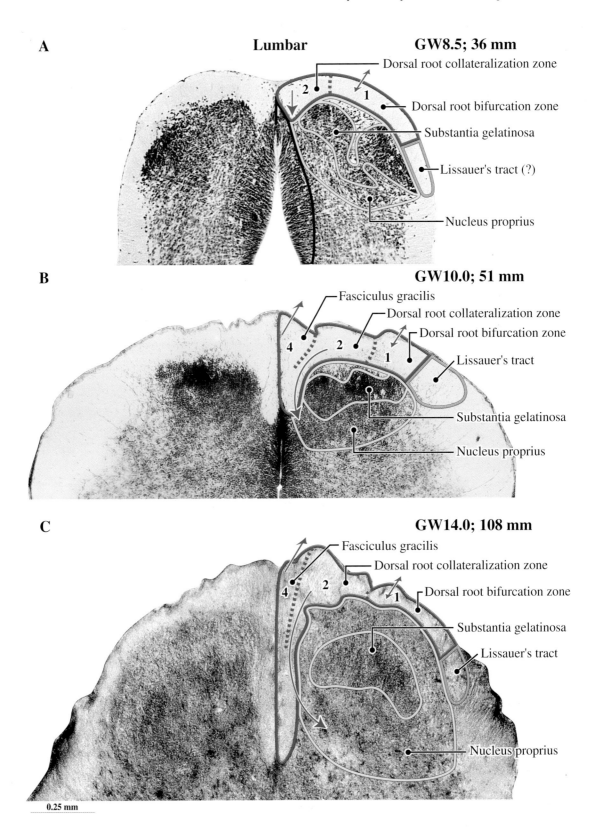

Figure 5-48. Growth of the dorsal funiculus in the lumbar spinal cord. **A.** The collateralization zone (compartment 2) is inconspicuous in the GW8.5 embryo (*M2050*; CR 36 mm). **B.** In the GW10 embryo (*Y74-68*; CR 51 mm), the collateralization zone has become deeper and is displaced laterally by the fasciculus gracilis (compartment 4). **C.** The collateralization zone and the gracile fasciculus have become deeper in this GW14 fetus (*Y68-65*; CR 108 mm). The cuneate fasciculus (compartment 3) is not present in the lumbar cord.

Figure 5-49. Hypothetical stages in the sequential branching of dorsal root axons in the cervical spinal cord in relation to the successive formation of the different compartments, and the development of the "local lanes" and "express lanes" of the dorsal funiculus. **A.** Following its entry into the spinal cord by about GW5.5, the dorsal root axon splits into an ascending and descending branch. This results in the formation of the bifurcation zone (outer gray band). **B.** By GW7.0, the ascending and descending branches begin to sprout local collaterals; these form the incipient collateralization zone dorsomedially. **C.** By GW7.5, the downward growing collaterals form the club-shaped collateralization zone (outer white band). **D.** By GW8.5, the continuing downward growth of the local collaterals results in the deepening of the collateralization zone. Concurrently, the cuneate fasciculus forms (inner gray band) and displaces the collateralization zone laterally. We hypothesize that, after issuing collaterals locally, the ascending branch of the dorsal root axon switches from the local lanes of the collateralization zone to the express lanes of the cuneate fasciculus. The core of the dorsal funiculus is composed of fibers in these express lanes. **E.** By GW10, the ascending axons from the caudal spinal cord arrive in the cervical cord and form the express lanes of the gracile fasciculus. The gracile fasciculus (inner white band) displaces the cuneate fasciculus laterally.

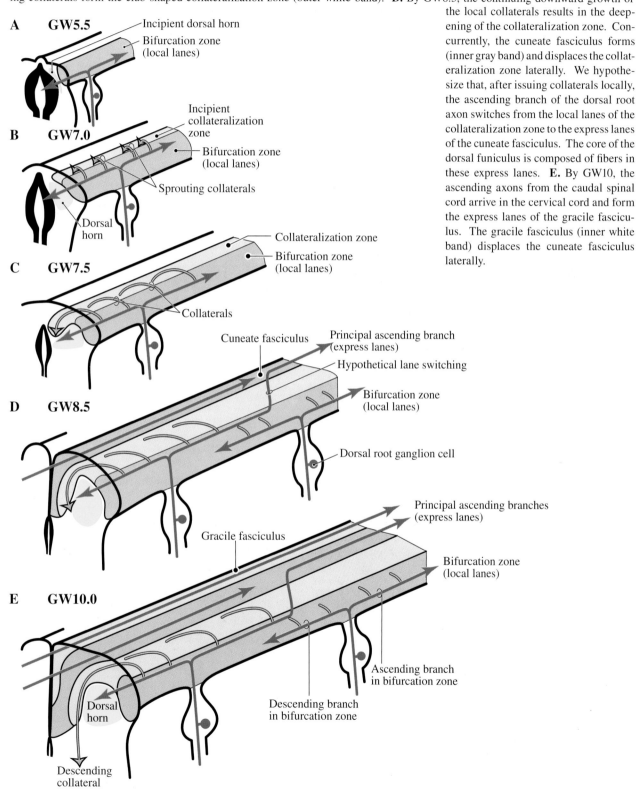

5.8 Development of the Preganglionic Motoneurons of the Lateral Horn

We trace the development of the autonomic motoneurons of the lateral horn in the thoracic spinal cord in Figures 5-50 and 5-51. As was described earlier (Section 4.3.3), autoradiographic and histochemical studies in animals indicate that the preganglionic motoneurons of the sympathetic nervous system orig-inate in the ventral neuroepithelium, the same site where the somatic motoneurons are produced. After their generation, the preganglionic sympathetic moto-neurons migrate dorsally to settle in the lateral horn of the intermediate gray. In the histological mate-rial available to us, we could not trace this migration with certainty in human embryos. The pregangli-onic motoneurons could only be definitively identi-fied after they have settled in the intermediate gray

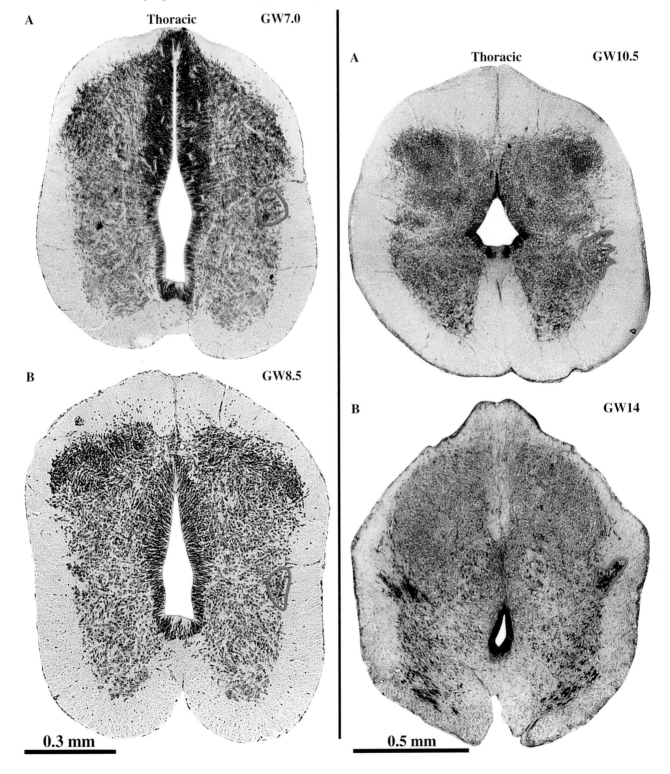

A   **Thoracic**   **GW7.0**

B   **GW8.5**

0.3 mm

A   **Thoracic**   **GW10.5**

B   **GW14**

0.5 mm

in a GW7.0 embryo (*M2304*; CR 21.7 mm; Figure 5-50A). Since the exodus of motoneurons begins as early as GW4.5 (Figure 5-4B,), and is in full progress by GW5.5 (Figure 5-5A), this suggests that another two weeks may elapse before all the differentiating autonomic motoneurons have settled in their final location. The maturation of autonomic motoneurons, as judged by their size and staining intensity, is also a protracted process. In the GW8.5 embryo (*M2050*; CR 36 mm; Figure 5.50B) and the GW10 fetus (*Y380-62*; CR 56 mm; Figure 5-51A), the lateral horn motoneurons are still small and do not stain intensely. It is in the GW14 fetus (*Y68-65*; CR 108 mm; Figure 5-51B) that, by virtue of their staining intensity, the lateral horn motoneurons become conspicuous elements of the intermediate gray.

5.9 Stages of Spinal Cord Development During the First Trimester

In the beginning of this chapter we have discussed the difficulty of dating the exact gestational age of human embryos, and referred to earlier attempts to partially overcome this difficulty by establishing "stages" of embryonic development. Embryonic staging requires the identification of sequential morphogenetic changes through which all embryos pass before their complete their embryonic development. Theoretically, staging can overcome the problem of individual differences in the tempo of embryonic development and, from a practical perspective, staging can be useful where adequate information about an embryo's gestational is not available. A staging system of early brain development was recently proposed by O'Rahilly and Müller (1994) and was briefly summarized in Section 5.1.2. Unfortunately, because that system is based on gross features of overall neural development, it is not helpful for us here where our concern is with the details of spinal cord development, such as the neurogenesis, dendritic development, gliogenesis, synaptogenesis, and the growth of the afferent and efferents connections of the spinal

cord in general, and of its structural and functional components in particular.

The staging of spinal cord development that we propose is limited to the cervical cord during the first trimester (Table 5-1). The staging begins at GW3.0, when the neural plate forms, and ends at GW13.0 when the neuroepithelium is dissolved. Neural plate formation is a landmark because that is the first time when a distinct tissue composed of dedicated NEP cells can be morphologically identified in the presumptive spinal cord. The dissolution of the neuroepithelium is another landmark because that signals the disappearance of the last identifiable spinal cord tissue which is exclusively composed of NEP cells.

We distinguish 10 morphogenetic stages in the development of the spinal cord during the first trimester, and assign these to 3 epochs. The principal event during the first epoch is the exuberant proliferation of NEP cells in the neuroepithelium. Neuroepithelial growth progresses through four stages: formation of the neural plate (stage 1), formation of the neural groove (stage 2), closure of the neural tube (stage 3), and the expansion of the closed neuroepithelium (stage 4). There is little or no cell exodus from the neuroepithelium during the first epoch. There are four stages in the second epoch, and these are described under separate headings in terms of the continued production of NEP cells, the differentiation and exodus of neurons and glia, the maturation of motoneurons, the growth of primary afferents, the growth of intraspinal and suprasipnal connections, and synaptogenesis. For instance, in terms of NEP cell production and neuronal differentiation, we distinguish the hypertrophy of the ventral neuroepithelium and peak period of motoneuron production as stage 5. The hypertrophy of the intermediate neuroepithelium and peak period of interneuron production is stage 6. The hypertophy of the dorsal neuroepithelium and peak of sensory microneuron production is stage 7. Finally, the cessation of neurogenesis is stage 8. The third epoch consists of two stages, the neuroepithelial production of glia (stage 9) and the dissolution of the neuroepithelium and the production of ependymal cells of the central canal (stage 10). The gestational ages assigned to these stages in Table 5-1 are based on the limited data of this study and are, therefore, provisional. Correlations of these stages of spinal cord development with somatic and behavioral development are summarized in Table 9-1.

Figure 5-50. Sympathetic preganglionic motoneurons of the lateral horn (purple outline) in **A**, a GW7.0 embryo (*M2304*; CR 21.7 mm) and **B**, a GW8.5 embryo (*M2050*; CR 36 mm). **Opposite page, left.**

Figure 5-51. Sympathetic preganglionic motoneurons of the lateral horn (purple outline) in **A**, a GW10.5 embryo (*Y380-62*; CR 56 mm) and **B**, a GW14 fetus (*Y68-65*; CR 108 mm). **Opposite page, right.**

Table 5-1
Stages of Cervical Spinal Cord Development
During the First Trimester (Part 1)

Epochs		Stage	Gestational Age (in weeks)	CELL GENERATION AND DIFFERENTIATION		
				NEP Cell Production	Neurogenesis	Gliogenesis
I	NEP CELL PRODUCTION	1	<GW3.0	Formation of the neural plate.		
		2	<GW3.0	Formation of the neural groove.		
		3	GW3.0 GW3.5	Closure of the neural tube.		
		4	GW3.5 GW4.5	Expansion of the pre-exodus neuroepithelium.		
II	NEUROGENESIS	5	GW4.5 GW5.5	Hypertrophy of the ventral neuroepithelium.	Peak period of motoneuron production, differentiation, and exodus.	
		6	GW5.5 GW6.5	Hypertrophy of the intermediate neuroepithelium.	Peak period of interneuron production, differentiation, and exodus.	
		7	GW6.5 GW7.5	Hypertropy of the dorsal neuroepithelium.	Peak period of gelatinosal microneuron production, differentiation, and exodus.	
		8	GW7.5 GW8.5	Dissolution of the dorsal neuroepithelium.	Production of visceral interneurons. Cessation of neurogenesis.	
III	GLIOGENESIS	9	GW8.5 GW11	Persistence of the central canal neuroepithelium.		Neuroepithelial glial production.
		10	GW11 GW13	Dissolution of the central canal neuroepithelium.		Production of ependymal cells.

Table 5-1
Stages of Cervical Spinal Cord Development
During the First Trimester (Part 2)

NEURAL GROWTH AND MATURATION				Stage
Motoneurons	Primary Afferents	Connections	Synaptogenesis	
				1
				2
				3
				4
Settling of moto-neurons. Exit of ventral root motor fibers.	Arrival of earliest dorsal root fibers. Onset of fiber bifur-cation and formation of oval bundle.	Formation of ventral funiculus. (Arrival of vestibulospinal tract?)	Earliest synapses in ventral horn (asymmetrical, axodendritic).	5
Segregation of inferior and superior motoneuron clusters.	Expansion of the DR bifurcation zone. Extension of ascending and descending branches.	Formation of lateral funiculus. (Growth of propriospinal fibers?)	?	6
Segregation of medial and lateral motoneuron clusters.	Formation of the DR collateralization zone. Sprouting of local collaterals.	Expansion of lateral funiculus. (Growth of spinocephalic tract?)	Earliest synapses in dorsal horn (?)	7
Segregation of lateral motor columns.	Expansion of the DR collateralization zone. (Branching of local collaterals?)	Expansion of lateral funiculus. (Growth of spinocerebellar tract?)	Increase in concentration of synapses.	8
Beginning of segregation of far-lateral and retro-dorsal motor columns.		Formation of cuneate fasciculus. (Growth of spinolemniscal tract from upper body.)	?	9
Continuing segregation of far-lateral and retro-dorsal motor columns.		Formation of gracile fasciculus. (Growth of spinolemniscal tract from lower body.)	?	10

6 DEVELOPMENT OF THE HUMAN SPINAL CORD DURING THE SECOND AND THIRD TRIMESTERS: GESTATIONAL WEEKS 14 TO 44

6.1 Overview of the Development of the Spinal Cord Between GW14 and GW44

6.1.1 Overview of the Development of the Cervical Spinal Cord. The development of the spinal cord at cervical levels from the beginning of the second trimester until birth is illustrated in photomicrographs at low magnification in sections stained for cell bodies and myelin (Figures 6-1 to 6-6).

GW14 to GW19. In the GW14 fetus (*Y68-65*; CR 108 mm; cell body stain), the gray matter is well developed (Figure 6-1A). In the ventral horn, discrete columns composed of prominent motoneurons are in evidence, and a high proportion of the small cells in the ventral horn, the intermediate gray, and the dorsal horn are probably maturing neurons. In contrast, the white matter is thin relative to the gray matter and the concentration of interfascicular glia is quite low in most fiber tracts. However, in the GW19 fetus (*Y52-61*; CR 130 mm; cell body stain), there is an abundance of glia in some components of the expanding white matter (Figure 6-1B). Glial concentration is increasing in the early developing ventral and lateral funiculi, and is highest in the cuneate fasciculus. In the gracile fasciculus and the lateral corticospinal tract glial concentration is low, and it is lowest in the relatively large ventral corticospinal tract of this fetus.

GW20. In the section of the cervical spinal cord of a GW20 fetus (*Y27-60*; CR 160 mm), processed with a sudanophilic stain (the Loyez technique) for the visualization of myelin ingredients, the inferior circumferential fasciculus (for nomenclature, see Figure 2-26) and the collateralization zone of the cuneate fasciculus show an intense fine-grained or punctate reaction (Figure 6-2). These glia, presumably oligodendrocytes, are assumed to have started to produce myelin ingredients and are henceforth referred to as reactive glia. There is a fair concentration of reactive glia (presumably Schwann cells) in the dorsal root and a much higher concentration in the ventral root. The coarse-grained clumps of stain in the ventral root suggest the onset of nerve fiber myelination at this site. There is a modest concentration of reactive glia in the thin lateral, ventromedial, and ventral funiculi. Only scattered reactive glia are present in the gracile funiculus, the upper portion of the cuneate funiculus, Lissauer's tract, and the late developing lateral and ventral corticospinal tracts. Few of the cells in the gray matter (most of

them neurons, some perhaps astrocytes) react with the sudanophilic stain.

GW26. The relationship in a GW26 fetus (*Y60-61*; CR 210 mm) between the increase in net glial concentration (as seen by cell body staining) and reactive glia concentration (as revealed by myelin staining) is illustrated in two neighoring sections of the cervical spinal cord in Figure 6-3. The section stained for cell bodies (Figure 6-3A) shows a high and roughly equal concentration of glia in both the cuneate and gracile fasciculi. However, the myelin stained section shows a different pattern: staining is intense in the collateralization zone of the cuneate fasciculus, but not in its apical portion or in the gracile fasciculus (Figure 6-3B). Similarly, the uniform concentration of glia in the cell body stained section throughout the lateral funiculus is not matched by the myelin stained section where two bands are visible: intense staining in the inferior circumferential fasciculus and weak staining in the rest of lateral funiculus. Changes in net glial concentration and reactive glial concentration are apparently different facets of myelination gliosis. In addition to the punctate staining in several of these regions reflecting reactive gliosis, there is clumpy staining in others. The latter is interpreted as the onset of the myelination of nerve fibers. That is evident in the ventral root peripherally (but not in the dorsal root), in the bifurcation zone and the collateralization zone, and the ventral commissure beneath the central canal.

GW32. In the GW32 fetus (*Y76-60*, CR 300 mm), the cell body stained section shows a relatively high concentration of glia in the lower three-fourths of the gracile and cuneate fasciculi, and a somewhat lower concentration superficially (Figure 6-4A). The staining pattern in the corresponding locations in the myelin-stained section (Figure 6-4B) is quite complex. Staining is intense in both the collateralization zone and the lower two-thirds of the cuneate fasciculus but the gracile fasciculus is devoid of reactive glia except for a disc-shaped region at its base. The massive staining at these sites suggests the onset of fiber myelination in a circumscribed component of the cuneate and gracile fasciculi. There is a similar lack of correspondence between the net concentration of glia in the lateral and ventral corticospinal tracts in the cell body stained section, and the virtual absence of reactive glia at the same sites in the myelin stained section. Finally, the high concentration of reactive glia in the inferior circumferential fasciculus (Figure

6-4B), and the growing concentration of reactive glia in the ventromedial and ventral funiculi, are not matched by any increase in net glial concentration at the same sites (Figure 6-4A).

GW37. There is little change in the net concentration of glia in the gracile and cuneate fasciculi in the cell body stained section of the GW37 neonate (*Y117-61*; CR 310 mm) illustrated in Figure 6-5A

(compare with Figure 6-4A). However, the matched myelin-stained section indicates a continued complex pattern of regionally distinct reactive gliosis and myelination (Figure 6-5B). The superficial regions of the cuneate and gracile fasciculi now contain a higher concentration of reactive glia (punctate staining), while myelination (coarse staining) is expanding in the depth of the cuneate fasciculus and the disc-shaped region of the gracile fasciculus. Myelination

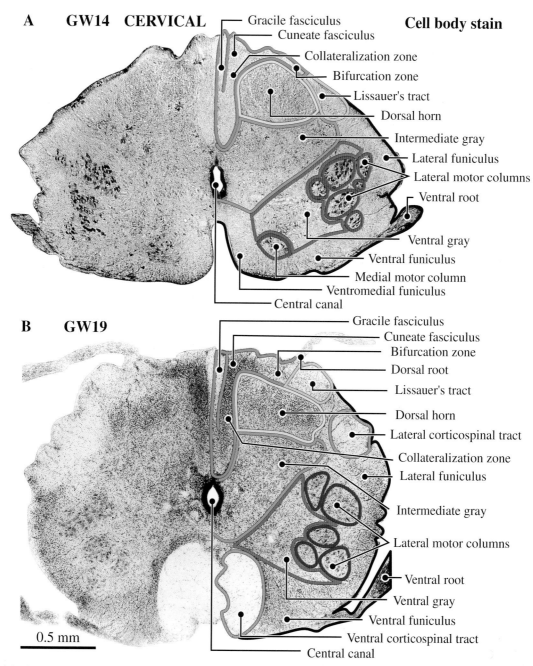

A GW14 CERVICAL — Gracile fasciculus — Cuneate fasciculus — Collateralization zone — Bifurcation zone — Lissauer's tract — Dorsal horn — Intermediate gray — Lateral funiculus — Lateral motor columns — Ventral root — Ventral gray — Ventral funiculus — Medial motor column — Ventromedial funiculus — Central canal **Cell body stain**

B GW19 — Gracile fasciculus — Cuneate fasciculus — Bifurcation zone — Dorsal root — Lissauer's tract — Dorsal horn — Lateral corticospinal tract — Collateralization zone — Lateral funiculus — Intermediate gray — Lateral motor columns — Ventral root — Ventral gray — Ventral funiculus — Ventral corticospinal tract — Central canal

0.5 mm

Figure 6-1. A. The cervical spinal cord in a GW14 fetus (*Y68-65*, CR 108 mm) in a cell body (Nissl) stained section. The gray matter is well developed but the white matter is small and contains relatively few glia. **B.** The cervical spinal cord in a GW19 fetus (*Y52-61*, CR 130 mm) in a similarly stained section. The concentration of glia has increased in the ventral funiculus, the lateral funiculus, and is highest in the collateralization zone and the cuneate fasciculus. Glial concentration is lowest in the lateral and ventral corticospinal tracts, and parts of the gracile fasciculus.

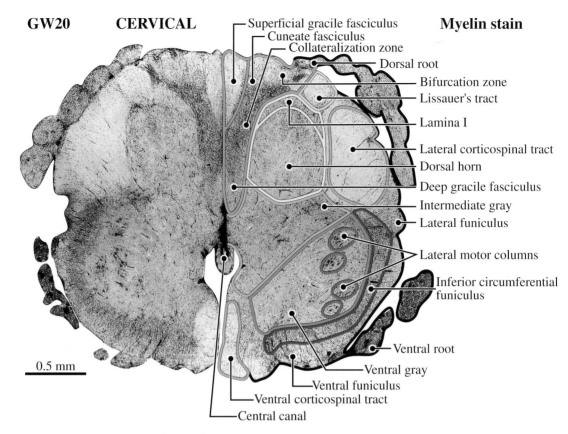

GW20   CERVICAL   **Myelin stain**

0.5 mm

Figure 6-2. The cervical spinal cord of GW20 fetus (*Y27-60*, CR 160 mm) stained for myelin constituents (Loyez stain). There is a fair concentration of reactive glia (punctate staining) in the collateralization zone and the inferior circumferential fasciculus, and a modest concentration in the ventral funiculus. The concentration of reactive glia is sparse in the gracile fasciculus, the superficial cuneate fasciculus, and the lateral and ventral corticospinal tracts. Peripherally, there is a high concentration of reactive Schwann cells in the ventral root, and a fair concentration in the dorsal root.

may have also begun in the inferior circumferential fasciculus and in the marginal fasciculus. Lissauer's tract, and the lateral and ventral corticospinal tracts remain devoid of reactive glia.

GW44. We complete this overview of the complex process of myelination in the different tracts of the white matter during the perinatal period by comparing two sections of the cervical spinal cord in a late delivered and unusually large GW44 neonate (*Y23-60*; CR 410 mm). Net glial concentration, as seen in the cell body stained section, is quite uniform throughout the white matter (Figure 6-6A). However, the corresponding myelin stained section shows considerable heterogeneity. Myelination has expanded to all parts of the dorsal funiculus and is in progress in the inferior circumferential fasciculus and the marginal fasciculus. Reactive gliosis is in progress in the far-lateral fasciculus. Two regions are devoid of reactive glia: Lissauer's tract (a region composed of unmyelinated fibers) and the late myelinating lateral and ventral corticospinal tracts.

In summary, two major events characterize the maturation of the cervical spinal cord during the second and third trimesters. One is the gradual expansion of the white matter relative to the gray matter, the other is the progressive myelination of the white matter. Myelination is characterized by two important features. First, its chronology varies in different fiber tracts and often in subdivisions of the same tract. Second, myelination occurs in three successive steps: (i) increase in net glial concentration, (ii) increase in the concentration of reactive glia, and (iii) myelination of the nerve fibers. The myelination of the white matter begins in the collateralization zone of the dorsal root and in the inferior circumferential fasciculus (which was earlier identified as the propriospinal or intraspinal tract; Figure 1-89). These two tracts contain the nerve fibers that "close" the segmental and intersegmental reflex circuits of the spinal cord. The next myelinating fiber tracts are the cuneate and gracile fasciculi, the ventromedial and ventral funiculi, and the marginal fasciculus. These tracts contain ascending exteroceptive and pro-

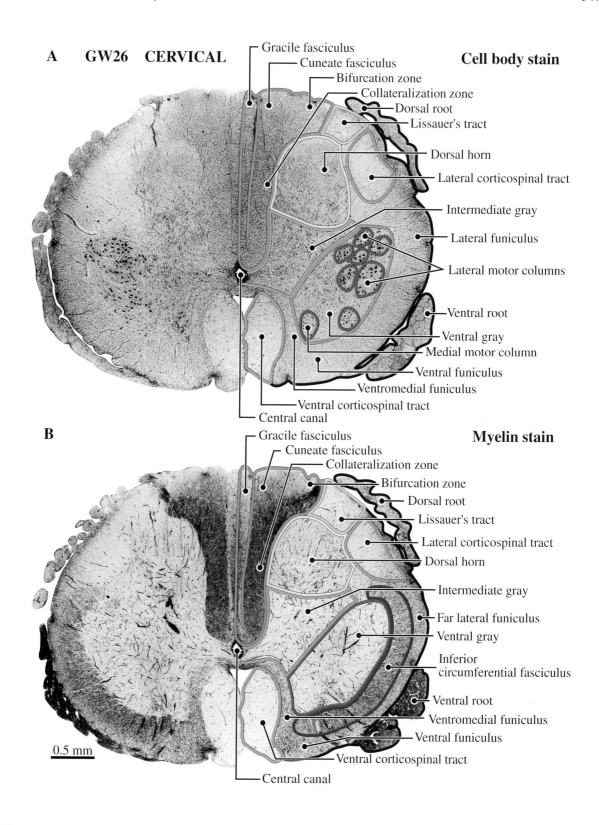

A   GW26   CERVICAL   **Cell body stain**

Gracile fasciculus
Cuneate fasciculus
Bifurcation zone
Collateralization zone
Dorsal root
Lissauer's tract
Dorsal horn
Lateral corticospinal tract
Intermediate gray
Lateral funiculus
Lateral motor columns
Ventral root
Ventral gray
Medial motor column
Ventral funiculus
Ventromedial funiculus
Ventral corticospinal tract
Central canal

B   **Myelin stain**

Gracile fasciculus
Cuneate fasciculus
Collateralization zone
Bifurcation zone
Dorsal root
Lissauer's tract
Lateral corticospinal tract
Dorsal horn
Intermediate gray
Far lateral funiculus
Ventral gray
Inferior circumferential fasciculus
Ventral root
Ventromedial funiculus
Ventral funiculus
Ventral corticospinal tract
Central canal

0.5 mm

Figure 6-3. Differences in net glial concentration, as revealed by cell body staining (**A**), and reactive glial concentration, as revealed by myelin staining (**B**), in different fiber tracts of the white matter in a GW26 fetus (*Y60-61*; CR 210 mm). In contrast to the uniform net glial concentration in different components of the dorsal funiculus, the concentration of reactive glia is very high in the collateralization zone (suggesting the onset of myelination) but low in the superficial portion of the cuneate fasciculus and the gracile fasciculus. Similarly, the high concentration of reactive glia in the inferior circumferential fasciculus is not matched by unusually high level of net glial concentration.

prioceptive axons and some descending paleospinal axons (tectospinal, vestibulospinal) responsible for the lower-level supraspinal control of the spinal cord. Two regions stand out by not showing signs of myelination at the time of birth: Lissauer's tract (which remains unmyelinated) and the postnatally myelinating lateral and ventral corticospinal tracts. The latter exerts a higher-level supraspinal control of the spinal cord.

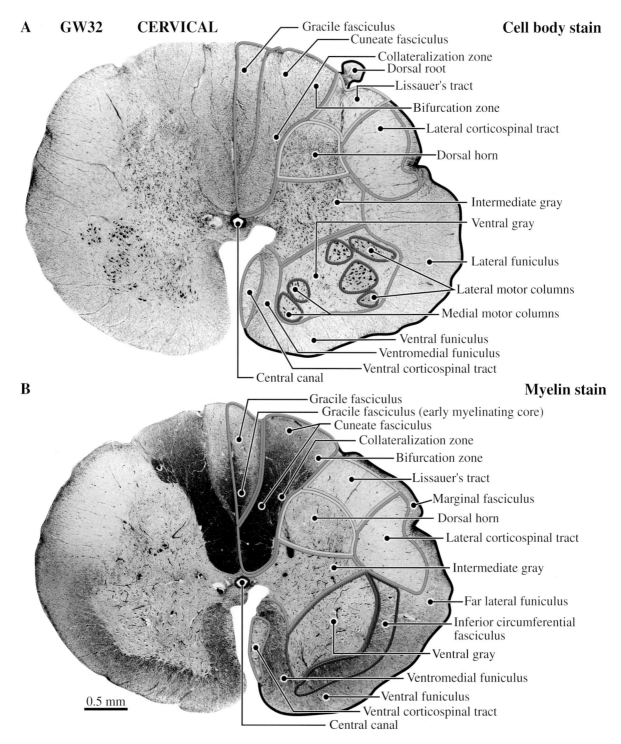

A   GW32   CERVICAL   **Cell body stain**

Gracile fasciculus
Cuneate fasciculus
Collateralization zone
Dorsal root
Lissauer's tract
Bifurcation zone
Lateral corticospinal tract
Dorsal horn
Intermediate gray
Ventral gray
Lateral funiculus
Lateral motor columns
Medial motor columns
Ventral funiculus
Ventromedial funiculus
Ventral corticospinal tract
Central canal

B   **Myelin stain**

Gracile fasciculus
Gracile fasciculus (early myelinating core)
Cuneate fasciculus
Collateralization zone
Bifurcation zone
Lissauer's tract
Marginal fasciculus
Dorsal horn
Lateral corticospinal tract
Intermediate gray
Far lateral funiculus
Inferior circumferential fasciculus
Ventral gray
Ventromedial funiculus
Ventral funiculus
Ventral corticospinal tract
Central canal

0.5 mm

Figure 6-4. The difference in the net concentration of glia in the cell body-stained section (**A**) and the concentration of reactive glia in a neighboring myelin-stained section (**B**) of the cervical spinal cord in a GW32 fetus (*Y76-60*, CR 300 mm). The ongoing myelination (coarse staining) at the base of the cuneate fasciculus and the gracile fasciculus, is not reflected by a substantial increase in net glial concentration. There is a similar lack of correspondence between net glia concentration and reactive glia concentration in the inferior circumferential fasciculus.

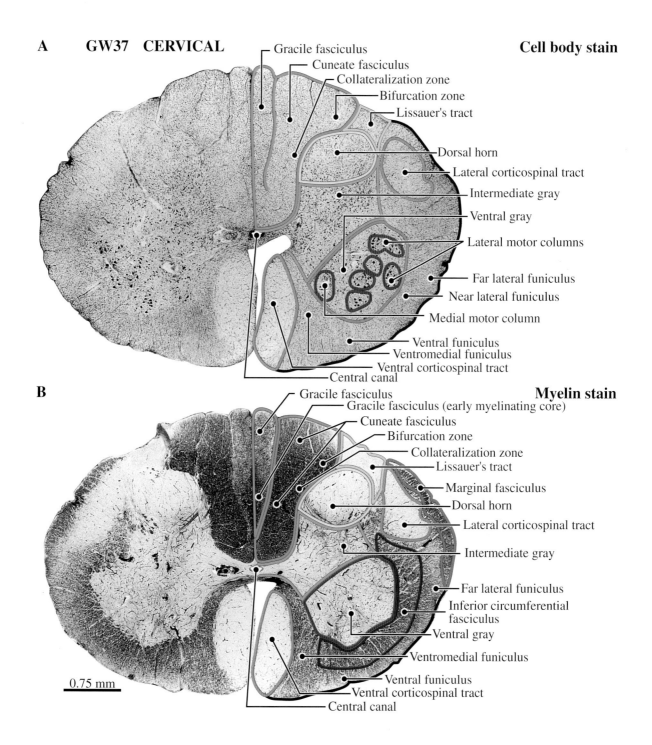

A GW37 CERVICAL **Cell body stain**

- Gracile fasciculus
- Cuneate fasciculus
- Collateralization zone
- Bifurcation zone
- Lissauer's tract
- Dorsal horn
- Lateral corticospinal tract
- Intermediate gray
- Ventral gray
- Lateral motor columns
- Far lateral funiculus
- Near lateral funiculus
- Medial motor column
- Ventral funiculus
- Ventromedial funiculus
- Ventral corticospinal tract
- Central canal

B **Myelin stain**

- Gracile fasciculus
- Gracile fasciculus (early myelinating core)
- Cuneate fasciculus
- Bifurcation zone
- Collateralization zone
- Lissauer's tract
- Marginal fasciculus
- Dorsal horn
- Lateral corticospinal tract
- Intermediate gray
- Far lateral funiculus
- Inferior circumferential fasciculus
- Ventral gray
- Ventromedial funiculus
- Ventral funiculus
- Ventral corticospinal tract
- Central canal

0.75 mm

Figure 6-5. The uniform concentration of glia in the cell body-stained section (**A**) and the complex pattern of ongoing reactive gliosis (punctate staining) and myelination (coarse staining) in a matched myelin stained section (**B**) of the cervical spinal cord of the GW37 newborn (*Y117-61*, CR 310 mm). Myelination is in progress in the depth of the cuneate and gracile fasciculi and in the inferior circumferential fasciculus.

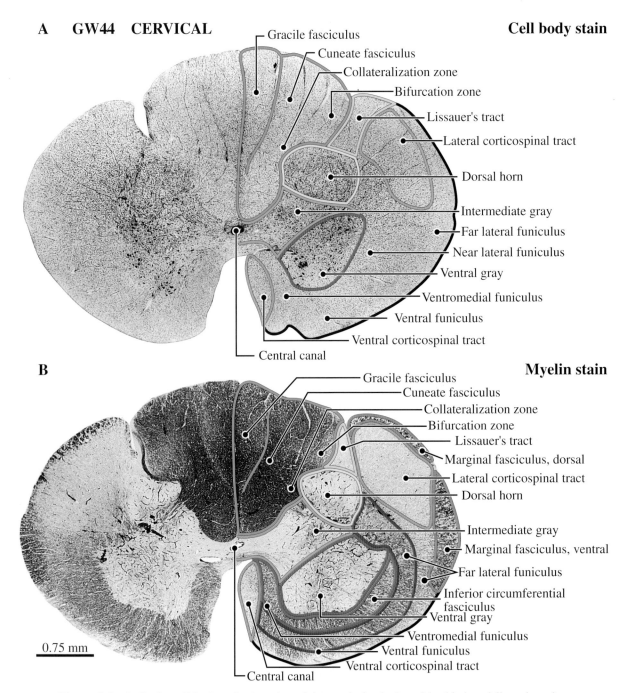

A   GW44   CERVICAL   **Cell body stain**

- Gracile fasciculus
- Cuneate fasciculus
- Collateralization zone
- Bifurcation zone
- Lissauer's tract
- Lateral corticospinal tract
- Dorsal horn
- Intermediate gray
- Far lateral funiculus
- Near lateral funiculus
- Ventral gray
- Ventromedial funiculus
- Ventral funiculus
- Ventral corticospinal tract
- Central canal

B   **Myelin stain**

- Gracile fasciculus
- Cuneate fasciculus
- Collateralization zone
- Bifurcation zone
- Lissauer's tract
- Marginal fasciculus, dorsal
- Lateral corticospinal tract
- Dorsal horn
- Intermediate gray
- Marginal fasciculus, ventral
- Far lateral funiculus
- Inferior circumferential fasciculus
- Ventral gray
- Ventromedial funiculus
- Ventral funiculus
- Ventral corticospinal tract
- Central canal

0.75 mm

Figure 6-6. A. In the cell body-stained section of the cervical spinal cord in this late delivered newborn (GW44, *Y23-60*, CR 410 mm), the distribution of glia is quite uniform throughout the white matter. **B.** The neighboring myelin-stained section, in contrast, shows a complex pattern of reactive gliosis (punctate staining) and myelination (coarse staining). Myelination is advanced in all compartments of the dorsal funiculus and is in progress, with an inside-out gradient, in the different components of the lateral funiculus. The concentration of reactive glia is low in the large lateral corticospinal tract and in the small ventral corticospinal tract.

Figure 6-7. The thoracic spinal cord in cell body-stained sections of **(A)** a GW14 fetus (*Y68-65*; CR 108 mm) and **(B)** a GW19 fetus (*Y52-61*; CR 130 mm). The concentration of glia is low in the thin white matter of the younger fetus but is increasing in some parts of the expanding white matter in the older fetus. The ventral and lateral corticospinal tracts contain few glia.

6.1.2 Overview of the Development of the Thoracic Spinal Cord. The development of the thoracic spinal cord from the beginning of the second trimester until birth is illustrated in Figures 6-7 to 6-10.

GW14 and *GW19.* The gray matter is well developed in the thoracic spinal cord of the GW14 (*Y68-65*, CR 108 mm) fetus. As seen in a cell body-stained section, the dorsal horn is large, the interme-diate gray contains the maturing neurons of Clarke's column, the preganglionic motoneurons are settled in the lateral horn, and somatic motoneurons are prominent in the ventral horn (Figure 6-7A). In contrast, the white matter is thin relative to the gray matter and contains few glia. In the similarly processed GW19 fetus (*Y52-61*, CR 130 mm), the white matter is somewhat larger and interfascicular glia are abundant in several regions, including the collateralization zone,

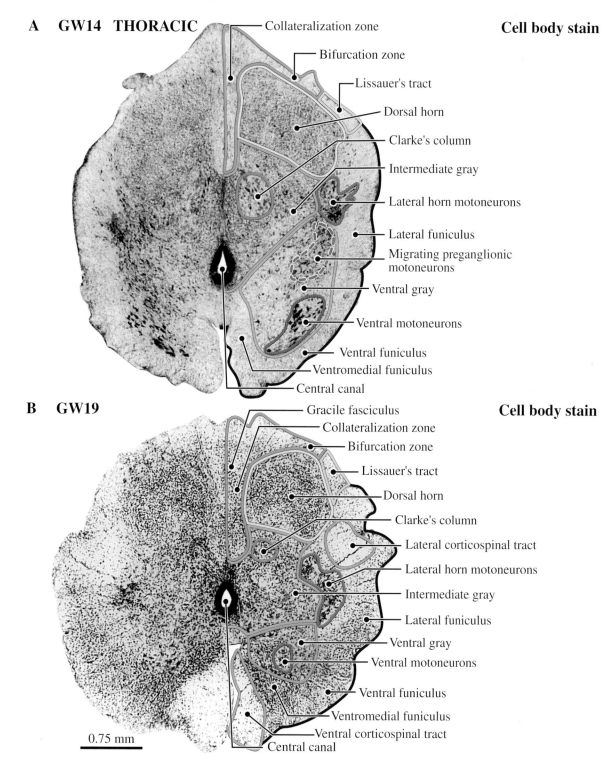

A GW14 THORACIC — Collateralization zone
— Bifurcation zone
— Lissauer's tract
— Dorsal horn
— Clarke's column
— Intermediate gray
— Lateral horn motoneurons
— Lateral funiculus
— Migrating preganglionic motoneurons
— Ventral gray
— Ventral motoneurons
— Ventral funiculus
— Ventromedial funiculus
— Central canal

Cell body stain

B GW19 — Gracile fasciculus
— Collateralization zone
— Bifurcation zone
— Lissauer's tract
— Dorsal horn
— Clarke's column
— Lateral corticospinal tract
— Lateral horn motoneurons
— Intermediate gray
— Lateral funiculus
— Ventral gray
— Ventral motoneurons
— Ventral funiculus
— Ventromedial funiculus
— Ventral corticospinal tract
— Central canal

Cell body stain

0.75 mm

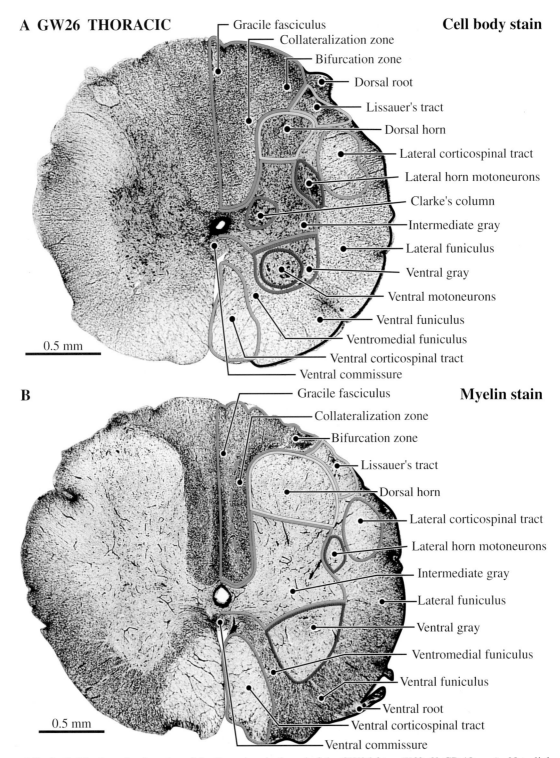

A GW26 THORACIC   **Cell body stain**

- Gracile fasciculus
- Collateralization zone
- Bifurcation zone
- Dorsal root
- Lissauer's tract
- Dorsal horn
- Lateral corticospinal tract
- Lateral horn motoneurons
- Clarke's column
- Intermediate gray
- Lateral funiculus
- Ventral gray
- Ventral motoneurons
- Ventral funiculus
- Ventromedial funiculus
- Ventral corticospinal tract
- Ventral commissure

0.5 mm

B   **Myelin stain**

- Gracile fasciculus
- Collateralization zone
- Bifurcation zone
- Lissauer's tract
- Dorsal horn
- Lateral corticospinal tract
- Lateral horn motoneurons
- Intermediate gray
- Lateral funiculus
- Ventral gray
- Ventromedial funiculus
- Ventral funiculus
- Ventral root
- Ventral corticospinal tract
- Ventral commissure

0.5 mm

Figure 6-8. A. Cell body-stained section of the thoracic spinal cord of the GW26 fetus (*Y60-61*, CR 10 mm). Net glial concentration is highest in the core of the dorsal funiculus, slightly lower in the collateralization zone, and still lower elsewhere in the white matter. **B.** In the myelin-stained section of the same fetus the pattern is different. Coarse staining is seen in the dorsal root bifurcation zone and the collateralization zone, suggesting the onset of myelination. Reactive gliosis (punctate staining) is high in the dorsal funiculus, and in the lateral, ventral, and ventromedial funiculi.

the lower portion of the gracile fasciculus, and the ventral and lateral funiculi (Figure 6-7B). That indicates the onset of the proliferative phase of myelination gliosis. Some other regions contain fewer glia, and the paucity of glia is most obvious in the small

lateral corticospinal tract and the large ventral corticospinal tract of this fetus.

GW26. The white matter has grown relative to the gray matter in the GW26 fetus (*Y60-61*, CR

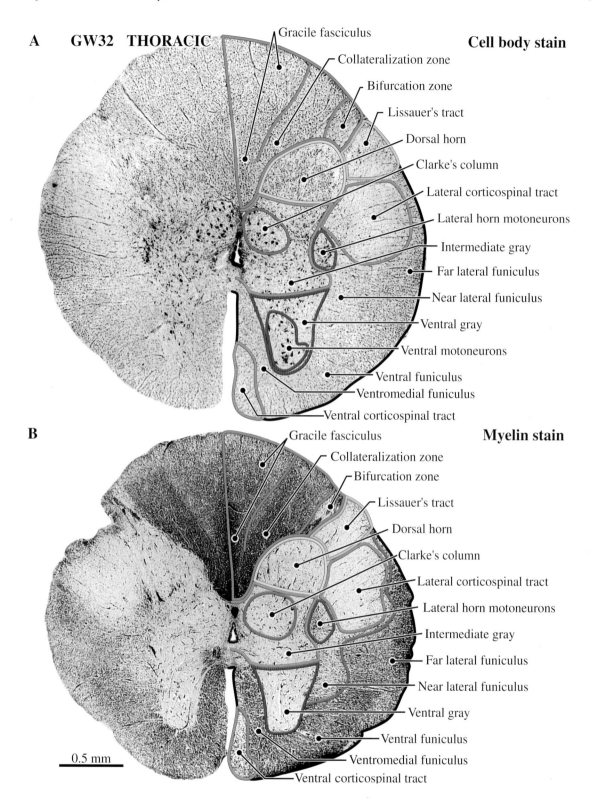

A **GW32** **THORACIC** **Cell body stain**

Gracile fasciculus
Collateralization zone
Bifurcation zone
Lissauer's tract
Dorsal horn
Clarke's column
Lateral corticospinal tract
Lateral horn motoneurons
Intermediate gray
Far lateral funiculus
Near lateral funiculus
Ventral gray
Ventral motoneurons
Ventral funiculus
Ventromedial funiculus
Ventral corticospinal tract

B **Myelin stain**

Gracile fasciculus
Collateralization zone
Bifurcation zone
Lissauer's tract
Dorsal horn
Clarke's column
Lateral corticospinal tract
Lateral horn motoneurons
Intermediate gray
Far lateral funiculus
Near lateral funiculus
Ventral gray
Ventral funiculus
Ventromedial funiculus
Ventral corticospinal tract

0.5 mm

Figure 6-9. A. Cell body-stained section of the thoracic spinal cord of the GW32 fetus (*Y76-60*, CR 300 mm). The distribution of glia is high throughout the entire dorsal funiculus and somewhat lower and less uniform elsewhere in the white matter. **B.** This matched myelin-stained section indicates that myelination (coarse staining) is in progress in the collateralization zone and in the depth of the gracile fasciculus. Reactive gliosis (punctate staining) is high in the core of the dorsal funiculus and is in progress in most other regions of the white matter, except the large lateral corticospinal tract and the small ventral corticospinal tract.

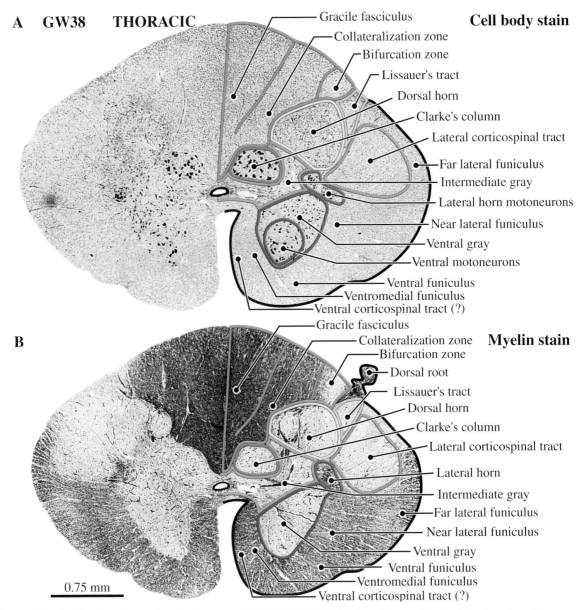

A   GW38   THORACIC

Gracile fasciculus
Collateralization zone
Bifurcation zone
Lissauer's tract
Dorsal horn
Clarke's column
Lateral corticospinal tract
Far lateral funiculus
Intermediate gray
Lateral horn motoneurons
Near lateral funiculus
Ventral gray
Ventral motoneurons
Ventral funiculus
Ventromedial funiculus
Ventral corticospinal tract (?)

Cell body stain

B

Gracile fasciculus
Collateralization zone
Bifurcation zone
Dorsal root
Lissauer's tract
Dorsal horn
Clarke's column
Lateral corticospinal tract
Lateral horn
Intermediate gray
Far lateral funiculus
Near lateral funiculus
Ventral gray
Ventral funiculus
Ventromedial funiculus
Ventral corticospinal tract (?)

Myelin stain

0.75 mm

Figure 6-10. A. The thoracic spinal cord of a neonate (*Y163-61*, GW38, CR 320 mm) in a cell body-stained section. There is a moderate concentration of glia in the greatly expanded white matter. **B.** An adjacent myelin-stained section indicates that all compartments of the dorsal funiculus are well myelinated (coarse staining), and reactive gliosis (punctate staining) is in progress in other regions of the white matter, except Lissauer's tract and the lateral corticospinal tract.

210 mm), and the cell body-stained section shows increasing glial concentration in the core of the dorsal funciculus but not, paradoxically, in the collateralization where the net concentration of glia has decreased (Figure 6-8A). The rest of the white matter shows variable glial concentration, with lowest concentration in the lateral and ventral corticospinal tracts. The myelin-stained section reveals a complex pattern (Figure 6-8B). In the collateralization zone – where net glial concentration is decreasing– the intense sudanophilic staining indicates the onset of myelination. Reactive glia concentration, in contrast to net glial concentration, is low in the gracile fasciculus, except for the ventral wedge. While net glial concen-

tration is high in the ventromedial and ventral funiculi in the GW19 fetus (Figure 6-7B) and low in the GW26 fetus (Figure 6-8A), the intense myelin staining in the latter suggests the onset of myelination. Apparently, reactive gliosis and myelination is preceded by a rise then a fall in glial proliferation.

GW32. The complex relationship between the net concentration of glia and myelin staining continues in the GW32 fetus (*Y76-60*, CR 300 mm; Figure 6-9). The dorsal funiculus contains a moderate and uniform concentration of glial cell bodies throughout the dorsal funiculus. The concentration is somewhat lower and less uniform in the rest of the white matter (Figure 6-9A). In the matched myelin-stained section (Figure 6-9B) myelination is in progress in the collateralization zone and the depth of the gracile fasciculus. Dense to moderate staining characterizes the rest of the white matter with the exception of the unstained lateral corticospinal tract.

GW38. Several developments characterize the thoracic spinal cord of the neonate (GW38, *Y163-61*; CR 320 mm; Figure 6-10). The first of these is the continuing growth of white matter relative to gray matter. Second, the cell body-stained section shows a reduction in the concentration of glia throughout the white matter (Figure 6-10A). Third,

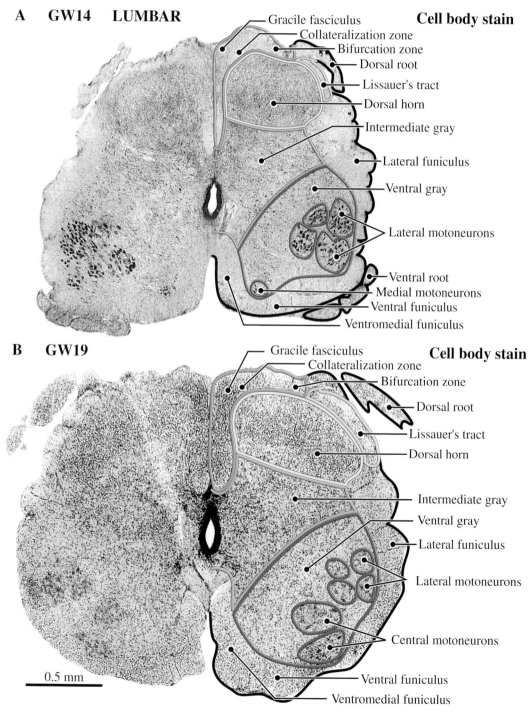

Figure 6-11. A. A cell body-stained section of the lumbar spinal cord of a GW14 fetus (*Y68-65*, CR 108 mm). The white matter is small relative to the gray matter and contains few glia. **B.** There is some increase in the concentration of glia in the white matter in the GW19 fetus (*Y52-61*, CR 130 mm). This suggests the onset of glial proliferation, the first phase of myelination gliosis.

the dense staining of the entire dorsal funiculus suggests that myelination is in progress throughout the lateral, ventral, and ventromedial funiculi (Figure 6-10B). Myelination may also have begun in the rest of the white matter but there is no indication in this neonate of the onset of reactive gliosis in the large lateral corticospinal tract.

6.1.3 Overview of the Development of the Lumbar Spinal Cord.
The development of the lumbar spinal cord from the beginning of the second trimester until birth is illustrated in Figures 6-11 to 6-15.

GW14 and *GW19*. The dorsal horn, intermediate gray and ventral horn are well developed in the lumbar spinal cord of the GW14 fetus (*Y68-65*, CR 108 mm; Figure 6-11A on previous page). In contrast, the white matter is quite narrow and mostly devoid of interfascicular glia. The white matter is still small in the GW19 fetus (*Y52-61*, CR 130 mm) but by now it is densely populated with glia in many regions, with the highest concentration in the collateralization zone (Figure 6-11B), suggesting a high rate of glial proliferation.

GW21. In the myelin-stained section of the lumbar spinal cord of a GW21 fetus (*Y390-62*, CR 200 mm, Figure 6-12), the concentration of reactive glia is highest in the collateralization zone and is evident in most other regions of the white matter, with the exception of the lateral corticospinal tract. The entering axons in the bifurcation zone and the exiting axons of the ventral root are myelinated.

GW29. The cell body-stained section of the GW29 fetus (*Y222-65*, CR 235 mm, Figure 6-13A) shows a high and uniform concentration of glia in the collateralization zone and gracile fasciculus, and it is also evident in other parts of the white matter. The matched myelin-stained section (Figure 6-13B) shows a fair concentration of reactive glia throughout the white matter, and the onset of myelination in the collateralization zone. Lissauer's tract and the small lateral corticospinal tract contain few reactive glia.

GW32. There is an apparent *reduction* in the concentration of glia in the white matter in the cell body-stained section of the lumbar cord in GW32 fetus (*Y76-60*, CR 300 mm, Figure 6-14A). The matched myelin-stained section (Figure 6-14B) indi-

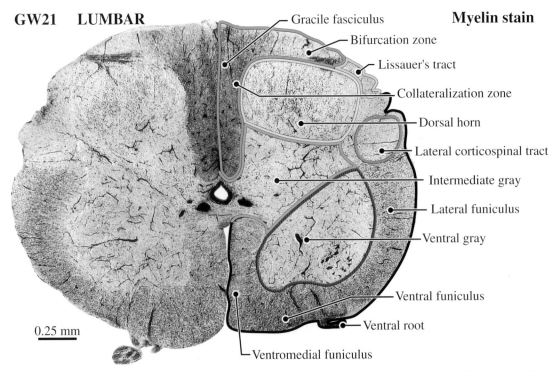

GW21   LUMBAR   **Myelin stain**

- Gracile fasciculus
- Bifurcation zone
- Lissauer's tract
- Collateralization zone
- Dorsal horn
- Lateral corticospinal tract
- Intermediate gray
- Lateral funiculus
- Ventral gray
- Ventral funiculus
- Ventral root
- Ventromedial funiculus

0.25 mm

Figure 6-12. A myelin-stained section of the lumbar spinal cord from a GW21 fetus (*Y390-62*, CR 200 mm). The concentration of reactive glia is highest in the dorsal funiculus. Staining intensity is also high in the circumferential band around the ventral horn, and in the ventral and ventromedial funiculi; it is lowest in the lateral corticospinal tract. Dorsal root fibers in the bifurcation zone and motor fibers of the ventral horn and ventral root are myelinating.

cates the onset of myelination of the collaterals that penetrate the gray matter. Some of these traverse the dorsal horn and end at its base, others curve around the dorsal horn and penetrate the gray matter from beneath. Myelination of motor fibers in the ventral horn continues. Lissauer's tract and the lateral corticospinal tract contain few reactive glia.

GW44. There is little obvious change in the concentration of glia in the white matter of the lumbar spinal cord in the late GW44 neonate (*Y23-60*; CR 410 mm), as seen in a cell body stained section (Figure 6-15A). The matching myelin-stained section (Figure 6-15B) indicates that myelination has progressed considerably throughout most of the white

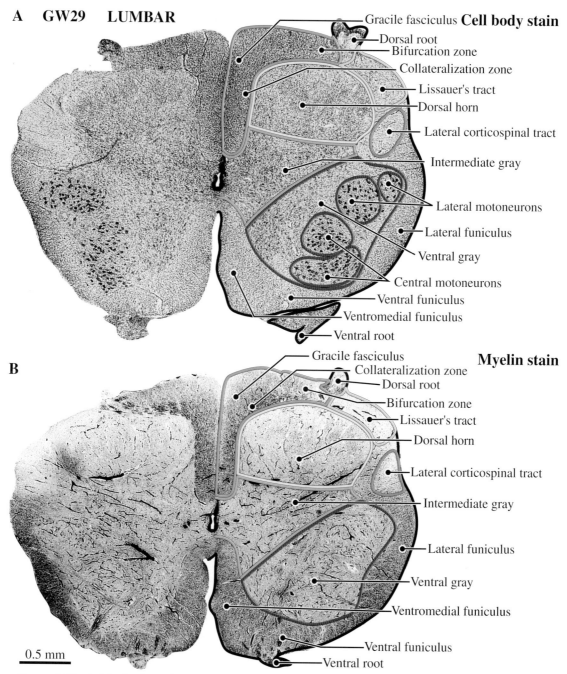

Figure 6-13. A. The lumbar spinal cord of a GW29 fetus (*Y22-65*, CR 235 mm) in a section stained for cell bodies. The gracile fasciculus contains the highest concentration of glia, the lateral corticospinal tract the lowest. **B.** In the matched myelin-stained section, the concentration of reactive glia (punctate staining) is high in the collateralization zone and throughout the lateral and ventral funiculi. Myelinated sensory fibers begin to appear in the collateralization zone, and bundles of myelinated motor fibers are traversing the ventral funiculus. There are few reactive glia in Lissauer's tract and in the lateral corticospinal tract.

matter. The number of myelinated collaterals that traverse or arc around the dorsal horn has increased greatly as have the myelinated axons of ventral horn motoneurons . However, the lateral corticospinal tract remains devoid of reactive glia and is unmyelinated. The same holds for Lissauer's tract.

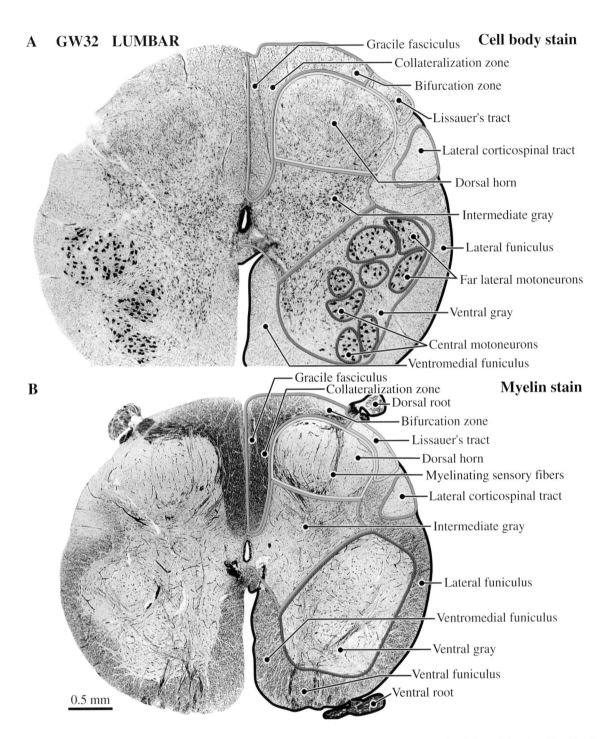

A   GW32   LUMBAR   **Cell body stain**

Gracile fasciculus
Collateralization zone
Bifurcation zone
Lissauer's tract
Lateral corticospinal tract
Dorsal horn
Intermediate gray
Lateral funiculus
Far lateral motoneurons
Ventral gray
Central motoneurons
Ventromedial funiculus

B   **Myelin stain**

Gracile fasciculus
Collateralization zone
Dorsal root
Bifurcation zone
Lissauer's tract
Dorsal horn
Myelinating sensory fibers
Lateral corticospinal tract
Intermediate gray
Lateral funiculus
Ventromedial funiculus
Ventral gray
Ventral funiculus
Ventral root

0.5 mm

Figure 6-14. A. The lumbar spinal cord of a GW32 fetus (*Y76-60*, CR 300 mm) in a section stained for cell bodies. The distribution of glia is greatly reduced in the dorsal funiculus (compare with Figure 6-13A) and in the rest of the white matter. This indicates that myelination gliosis is ending here. **B.** The matching myelin-stained section reveals that myelination is in progress in the collateralization zone and the core of the gracile fasciculus. The distal strands of some collaterals that penetrate the gray matter are also myelinating. There is a high concentration of reactive glia (punctate staining) spin most regions of the white trimatter, except in Lissauer's tract and the lateral corticospinal tract. Myelinated motor fibers in the ventral horn form ventral rootlets.

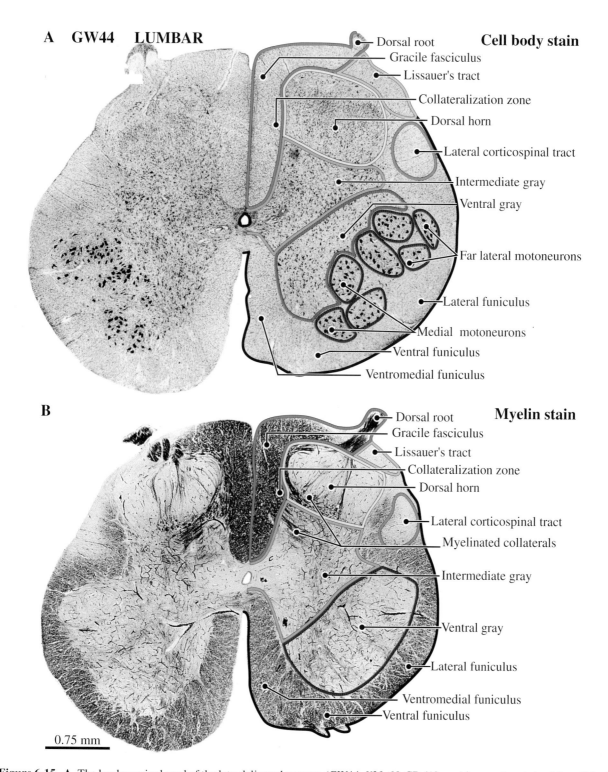

A **GW44** **LUMBAR**   **Cell body stain**

- Dorsal root
- Gracile fasciculus
- Lissauer's tract
- Collateralization zone
- Dorsal horn
- Lateral corticospinal tract
- Intermediate gray
- Ventral gray
- Far lateral motoneurons
- Lateral funiculus
- Medial motoneurons
- Ventral funiculus
- Ventromedial funiculus

B   **Myelin stain**

- Dorsal root
- Gracile fasciculus
- Lissauer's tract
- Collateralization zone
- Dorsal horn
- Lateral corticospinal tract
- Myelinated collaterals
- Intermediate gray
- Ventral gray
- Lateral funiculus
- Ventromedial funiculus
- Ventral funiculus

0.75 mm

Figure 6-15. A. The lumbar spinal cord of the late-delivered neonate (GW44, *Y23-60*, CR 410 mm) in a section stained for cell bodies. The concentration of glia is moderate and quite uniform throughout much of the white matter. **B.** The matching myelin-stained section indicates advanced myelination of the dorsal funiculus and the onset of myelination in most areas of the white matter, except Lissauer's tract and the lateral corticospinal tract. The concentration of myelinated sensory collaterals in the gray matter has increased.

6.2 Growth of the Ascending and Descending Fiber Tracts of the White Matter

6.2.1 The Problem of Identifying Fiber Tracts in the Human Spinal Cord.

The definitive identification of a particular fiber tract requires the use of experimental tracer techniques. Degeneration tracer techniques (like the Gudden, Marchi, and Nauta procedures) have been used occasionally in the analysis of pathological samples of the adult spinal cord (see, for instance, Figures 1-83, 1-93) but rarely in the developing spinal cord. Because the use of physiological tracers in live human fetuses is not done for ethical and legal considerations, we have to rely on descriptive histological evidence, such as the absence of a certain fiber tract at a particular stage of development and its incremental growth at later stages, to draw inferences about the development of that fiber tract. For instance, the absence of the dorsal funiculus is obvious at early stages of spinal cord development, and it is not difficult to follow its growth and changing shape at later stages. However, the identification of a particular fiber tract that is surrounded by or interdigitated with other fiber tracts is difficult and may be impossible.

The challenge of identifying, if only tentatively, the development of some of the fiber tracts in the fetal human spinal cord has been aided by the circumstance that different traditionally recognized fibers tracts (see Figure 1-80) undergo myelination gliosis and subsequent myelination at different stages of fetal development. Thus, as we have seen, the lateral corticospinal tract remains devoid of reactive glia and does not become myelinated for some time after the adjacent tracts of the lateral funiculus have been myelinated. This procedure, of course, has its shortcomings. First, it does not allow the identification of the early arriving fibers of a particular tract at an age when the neighboring fiber tracts are themselves devoid of reactive glia and/or are unmyelinated. Second, it makes the delineation of the boundaries of a fiber tract difficult after it has become myelinated to the same extent as the neighboring tracts.

6.2.2 Growth of the Large Ascending and Descending Fiber Tracts in the Cervical Spinal Cord.

We trace the emergence and growth of fiber tracts and their progressive myelination in the cervical spinal cord in myelin-stained sections from GW14 until birth in Figures 6-16 to 6-20.

GW14. There are several fiber tracts that can be identified with some confidence in the thin white matter of the cervical spinal cord in the GW14 fetus (*Y68-65*; CR 108 mm) by virtue of their topographic location (Figure 6-16A). These are, in addition to the compartments of the dorsal funiculus already discussed: the intraspinal (propriospinal) tracts of the inferior circumferential fasciculus; the medial longitudinal fasciculus and tectospinal tract in the ventromedial fasciculus; and the ventral vestibulospinal tract in the ventral funiculus. The lateral corticospinal tract may be present but, if so, it is quite small. As yet none of these tracts contain many glia, indicating that myelination gliosis has not yet begun at this stage of development.

GW20. In the cervical spinal cord of the GW20 fetus (*Y27-60*; CR 160 mm) all the fiber tracts identified in the younger fetus have grown considerably and some new ones have emerged (Figure 6-16B). Some of these tracts contain a high concentration of reactive glia, others are virtually devoid of them. Among the fiber tracts with most reactive glia are the greatly expanded collateralization zone dorsally and the circumferential intraspinal tracts ventrally. The concentration of reactive glia is low in the medial longitudinal fasciculus, the tectospinal tract, and the vestibulospinal tract. Among the newly emerged fiber tracts are the dorsal spinocerebellar tract and the lateral spinocephalic tract. They are thin and contain few reactive glia. The large lateral corticospinal tract and the smaller ventral corticospinal tract contain few, if any, reactive glia.

GW26. Practically all the fiber tracts seen in the younger fetus have greatly expanded by the end of the second trimester, as seen in the GW26 fetus (*Y60-61*; CR 210 mm; Figure 6-17). The myelination of dorsal root fibers in the collateralization zone is in progress and a few faintly myelinated collaterals appear in the gray matter beneath the dorsal horn. Judging by the intense staining in the depth (but not the apex) of the cuneate fasciculus, some ascending fibers are also myelinating. In contrast, the gracile fasciculus with ascending fibers from the lumbar cord (except for a deep wedge) contains a low concentration of reactive glia. The large lateral and ventral corticospinal tracts are virtually devoid of reactive glia. The myelination of the ventral rootlets is in progress, and the myelination of the ventral root is far more advanced than that of the dorsal root.

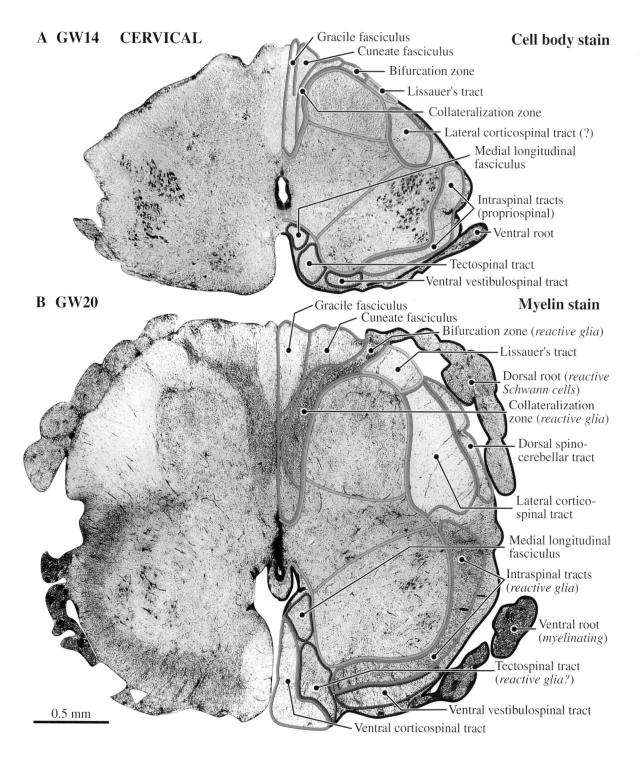

A GW14   CERVICAL   **Cell body stain**

Gracile fasciculus
Cuneate fasciculus
Bifurcation zone
Lissauer's tract
Collateralization zone
Lateral corticospinal tract (?)
Medial longitudinal fasciculus
Intraspinal tracts (propriospinal)
Ventral root
Tectospinal tract
Ventral vestibulospinal tract

B GW20   **Myelin stain**

Gracile fasciculus
Cuneate fasciculus
Bifurcation zone (*reactive glia*)
Lissauer's tract
Dorsal root (*reactive Schwann cells*)
Collateralization zone (*reactive glia*)
Dorsal spino-cerebellar tract
Lateral cortico-spinal tract
Medial longitudinal fasciculus
Intraspinal tracts (*reactive glia*)
Ventral root (*myelinating*)
Tectospinal tract (*reactive glia?*)
Ventral vestibulospinal tract
Ventral corticospinal tract

0.5 mm

Figure 6-16. A. The major identifiable fiber tracts in a cell body-stained section of the cervical spinal cord of a GW14 fetus (*Y68-65*, CR 108 mm). There is a paucity of glia throughout the white matter at the beginning of the second trimester. **B.** The white matter has greatly expanded in this GW20 fetus (*Y27-60*, CR 160 mm) and the onset of reactive gliosis (punctate staining) is indicated in some fiber tracts. There is a high concentration of reactive glia in the collateralization zone dorsally and the intraspinal (propriospinal) tracts ventrally. Reactive glia are present in lower concentration in the medial longitudinal fasciculus and the tectospinal tract. The newly formed dorsal spinocerebellar tract contains few reactive glia. The apical gracile and cuneate fasciculi contain few reactive glia, and there are virtually none in the lateral and ventral corticospinal tracts.

GW26   CERVICAL   **Myelin stain**

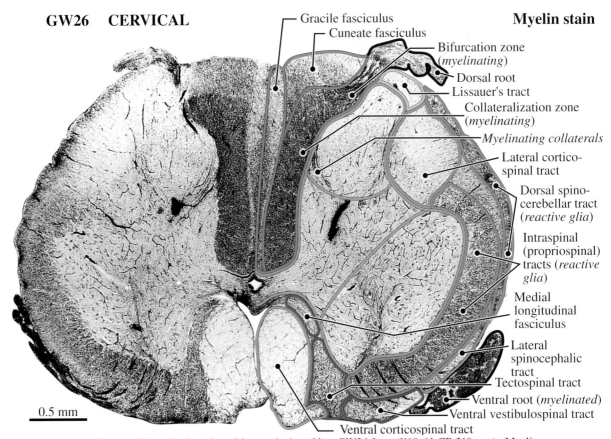

- Gracile fasciculus
- Cuneate fasciculus
- Bifurcation zone (*myelinating*)
- Dorsal root
- Lissauer's tract
- Collateralization zone (*myelinating*)
- *Myelinating collaterals*
- Lateral cortico-spinal tract
- Dorsal spino-cerebellar tract (*reactive glia*)
- Intraspinal (propriospinal) tracts (*reactive glia*)
- Medial longitudinal fasciculus
- Lateral spinocephalic tract
- Tectospinal tract
- Ventral root (*myelinated*)
- Ventral vestibulospinal tract
- Ventral corticospinal tract

0.5 mm

Figure 6-17. A myelin-stained section of the cervical cord in a GW26 fetus (*Y60-61*, CR 210 mm). Myelination in the collateralization zone and the depth of the dorsal funiculus is in progress. Collaterals entering the gray matter are myelinating. The concentration of reactive glia has increased in the superficial portion of the cuneate and gracile fasciculi. Reactive gliosis is high in the intraspinal tracts and has started in the spinocerebellar tract. The lateral and ventral corticospinal tracts are still devoid of reactive glia.

GW33. Myelination in the white matter continues in the GW33 fetus (*Y36-60*; CR 315 mm; Figure 6-18). The entire cuneate fasciculus is well myelinated, indicating that myelination has spread from the collateralizing branches (the local lanes) of dorsal root afferents to their long ascending branches (the express lanes). The concentration of reactive glia is high in the expanding gracile fasciculus, and myelination may have started in its midline wedge. The myelination of the spinocerebellar tract has begun and the spinocephalic tract contains many reactive glia. However, the lateral corticospinal tract is devoid of reactive glia (the ventral corticospinal tract appears to be absent in this fetus).

GW37 and GW44. Developmental advances are not remarkable in the white matter of the cervical spinal cord in the small, preterm newborn (GW37; *Y117-61*; CR 310 mm) seen in Figure 6-19. However, there are notable advances in the cervical spinal cord of the large, late-delivered neonate (GW44; *Y23-60*; 410 mm; Figure 6-20). To begin with, the white matter as a whole has expanded greatly relative to the

gray matter. That is attributable to the expansion of many fiber tracts, including the gracile fasciculus, and the emergence of some new tracts, such as the ventral spinocerebellar tract. In both the lateral funiculus and the ventral funiculus three bands may be distinguished with an inside-earlier and an outside-later myelination gradient. The large lateral corticospinal tract and the small ventral corticospinal tract remain virually devoid of reactive glia.

In summary, reactive gliosis and myelination in the different fiber tracts of the cervical spinal cord during the second and third trimesters is a sequential process that parallels the preceding outgrowth of the same fiber tracts. The earliest myelinating fascicles are the collateralization zone and the circumferential intraspinal tracts. These fibers are part of the local circuitry of the spinal cord. Next in line are a heterogeneous system of tracts that interconnect the spinal cord with lower-level brain structures (medulla and brain stem). Significantly, the descending efferents from the cerebral cortex remain unmyelinated at the time of birth.

GW33　CERVICAL　　Gracile fasciculus (*reactive glia*)　**Myelin stain**

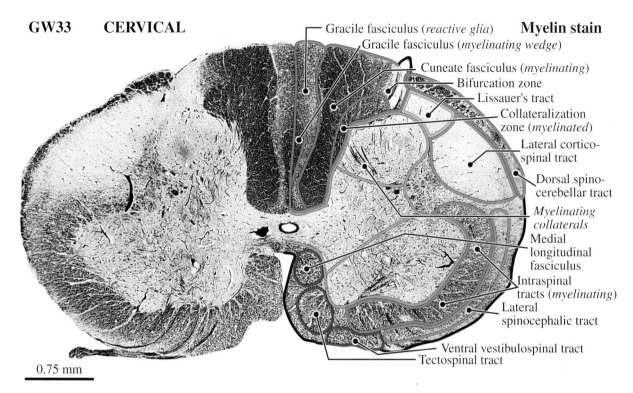

Gracile fasciculus (*myelinating wedge*)
Cuneate fasciculus (*myelinating*)
Bifurcation zone
Lissauer's tract
Collateralization zone (*myelinated*)
Lateral cortico-spinal tract
Dorsal spino-cerebellar tract
Myelinating collaterals
Medial longitudinal fasciculus
Intraspinal tracts (*myelinating*)
Lateral spinocephalic tract
Ventral vestibulospinal tract
Tectospinal tract

0.75 mm

Figure 6-18. A myelin-stained section of cervical spinal cord in a GW33 fetus (*Y36-60*, CR 315 mm). The expansion of the white matter relative to the gray matter continues. Myelination (coarse staining) has spread through the entire cuneate fasciculus and there is an increase in the concentration of reactive glia (punctate staining) in the apical portion of the gracile fasciculus. Myelination of the dorsal spinocerebellar tract is in progress. Reactive gliosis is high in the lateral spinocephalic tract. The lateral corticospinal tract is devoid of reactive glia. Note the absence of a ventral corticospinal tract in this fetus.

GW37 Newborn　CERVICAL　　Gracile fasciculus (*reactive glia*)　**Myelin stain**

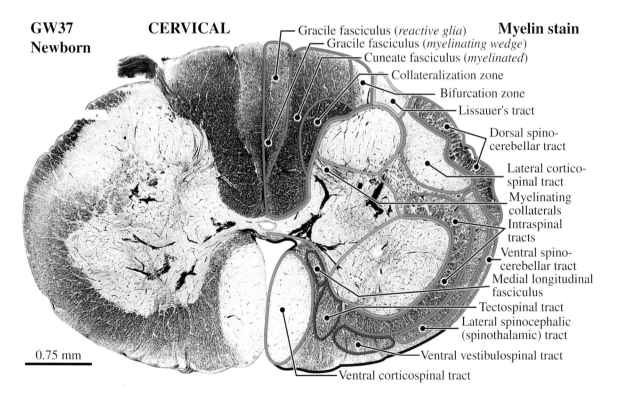

Gracile fasciculus (*myelinating wedge*)
Cuneate fasciculus (*myelinated*)
Collateralization zone
Bifurcation zone
Lissauer's tract
Dorsal spino-cerebellar tract
Lateral cortico-spinal tract
Myelinating collaterals
Intraspinal tracts
Ventral spino-cerebellar tract
Medial longitudinal fasciculus
Tectospinal tract
Lateral spinocephalic (spinothalamic) tract
Ventral vestibulospinal tract
Ventral corticospinal tract

0.75 mm

Figure 6-19. A myelin-stained section of cervical spinal cord in a GW37 newborn (*Y117-61*, CR 310 mm). There are few obvious developmental advances in myelination in this small, preterm newborn. But note the presence of a large ventral corticospinal tract in this neonate.

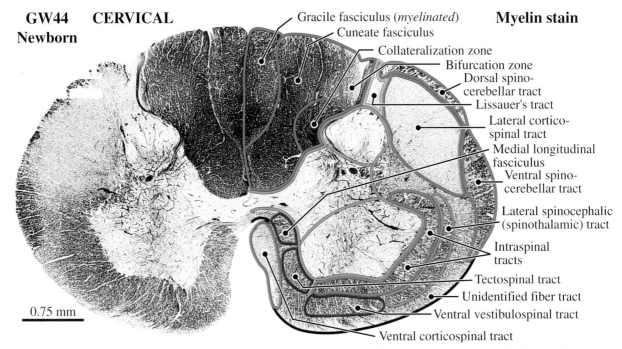

GW44   CERVICAL   Gracile fasciculus (*myelinated*)   **Myelin stain**
Newborn   Cuneate fasciculus
                                          Collateralization zone
                                          Bifurcation zone
                                          Dorsal spino-
                                             cerebellar tract
                                          Lissauer's tract
                                          Lateral cortico-
                                             spinal tract
                                          Medial longitudinal
                                             fasciculus
                                          Ventral spino-
                                             cerebellar tract
                                          Lateral spinocephalic
                                             (spinothalamic) tract
                                          Intraspinal
                                             tracts
0.75 mm   Tectospinal tract
                                          Unidentified fiber tract
                                          Ventral vestibulospinal tract
                              Ventral corticospinal tract

Figure 6-20. A myelin-stained section of cervical spinal cord in a large, late-delivered neonate (GW44; *Y23-60*, CR 410 mm). Among notable developmental advances are the spread of myelination (coarse staining) over the entire dorsal funiculus, and the ongoing myelination of the the ventral spinocerebellar tract and the lateral spinocephalic tract. An unidentified ventrolateral (far-lateral) tract remains unmyelinated. The lateral and ventral corticospinal tracts are still devoid of reactive glia.

6.2.3 Growth of the Large Ascending and Descending Fiber Tracts in the Lumbar Spinal Cord. The growth, glial proliferation, reactive gliosis, and myelination of some of the fiber tracts of the lumbar spinal cord during the second and third trimesters are illustrated in selected sections reproduced in Figures 6-21 to 6-23.

GW14 and *GW19.* The white matter is very small relative to the gray matter in the lumbar spinal cord of the GW14 fetus (*Y68-65*; CR 108 mm) and there is no hint in this cell body-stained section of the onset of myelination gliosis (Figure 6-21A). There is only modest gain in the relative size of the white matter in the GW19 fetus (*Y52-61*; CR 130 mm) but myelination gliosis is in progress in the collateralization zone and the intraspinal tracts (Figure 6-21B). There is as yet no clear indication of the arrival of fibers of the corticospinal tract. (The presence of glia in the fiber tract occupying the same location indicates that it is a different tract.)

GW29. Reactive gliosis and myelination in the white matter of the lumbar spinal cord is somewhat delayed when compared with the cervical spinal cord. That is suggested by the low intensity of myelin

staining in the collateralization zone, and particularly in the gracile fasciculus in the GW29 fetus (*Y22-65*; CR 235 mm; Figure 6-22A) when compared with the intense staining of the cuneate fasciculus in the cervical cord of a younger fetus (GW26; Figure 6-17). Notable, however in this GW29 fetus is the intense staining of the circumferential intraspinal tracts, and of the medial longitudinal fasciculus and ventral vestibulospinal tract. The first contingent of lateral corticospinal tract fibers have apparently reached the lumbar spinal cord in this fetus.

GW32. Myelination is in progress in the collateralization zone and deep gracile fasciculus in this GW32 fetus (*Y76-60*; CR 300 mm) but not yet in the apical portion of the gracile fasciculus (Figure 6-22B). The collaterals penetrating the gray matter are also myelinating. Some of these myelinated fibers enter the dorsal horn superficially and terminate at its base, others penetrate the cord underneath the dorsal horn and proceed ventrally. The descending lateral corticospinal tract has become more prominent but it is still devoid of glia.

GW40 and *GW44.* There is a marked increase in the area of the white matter in the lumbar spinal cord by birth, as seen in the smaller GW40 neonate (*Y115-61*; CR 330 mm; Figure 6-23A) and the late-delivered and larger GW44 neonate (*Y23-60*; CR 410 mm; Figure 6-23B). Particularly noteworthy is the expansion of the gracile fasciculus and the lateral funiculus. In the younger neonate, the apical portion of the gracile fasciculus is still at the stage of reactive gliosis, whereas in the older neonate the entire dorsal funiculus is characterized by advanced myelination. This is associated with an increase in the number of myelinated collaterals that penetrate the gray matter in the older neonate. The same increase in myelin staining intensity is seen in the intraspinal and spinocephalic tracts in the GW44 neonate. However, in both neonates reactive glia are still absent in the lateral corticospinal tract.

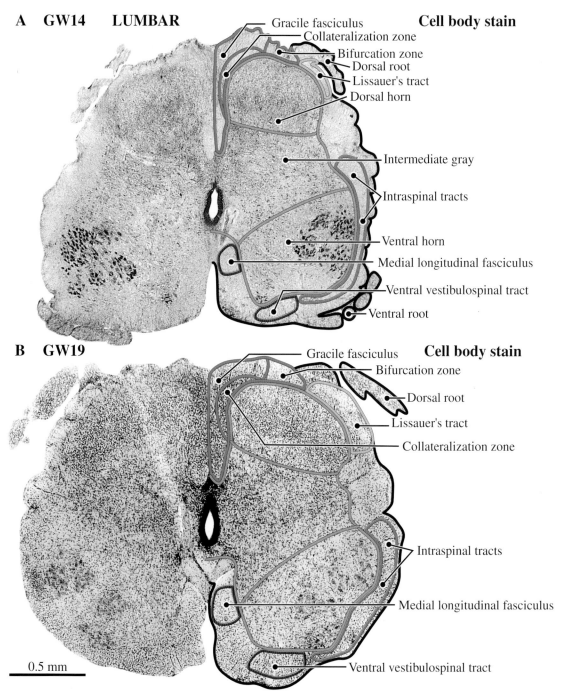

Figure 6-21. A. Cell body-stained section of the lumbar spinal cord of a GW14 fetus (*Y68-65*, 108 mm). The white matter is small relative to the gray matter and the few fiber tracts already present contain few glia. **B.** There is little increase in the relative size of the white matter in the cell body-stained section of the lumbar spinal cord of this GW19 fetus (*Y52-61*, CR 130 mm) but by now the fiber tracts present contain interfascicular glia in varying concentrations. High level of glial proliferation is indicated for the collateralization zone.

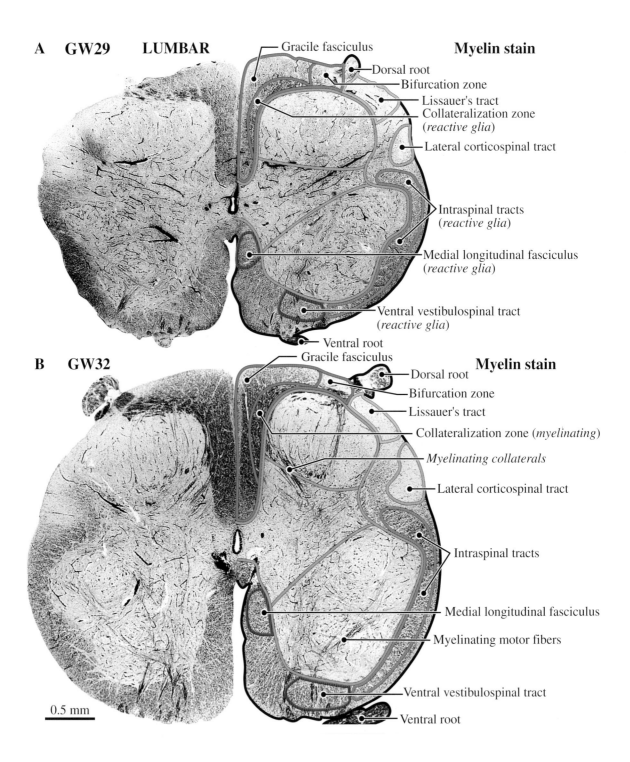

A GW29 LUMBAR　　　　　　　　　　　　　　　　　　　　　　**Myelin stain**

Gracile fasciculus
Dorsal root
Bifurcation zone
Lissauer's tract
Collateralization zone
(*reactive glia*)
Lateral corticospinal tract
Intraspinal tracts
(*reactive glia*)
Medial longitudinal fasciculus
(*reactive glia*)
Ventral vestibulospinal tract
(*reactive glia*)
Ventral root

B GW32　　　　　　　　　　　　　　　　　　　　　　　　**Myelin stain**

Gracile fasciculus
Dorsal root
Bifurcation zone
Lissauer's tract
Collateralization zone (*myelinating*)
Myelinating collaterals
Lateral corticospinal tract
Intraspinal tracts
Medial longitudinal fasciculus
Myelinating motor fibers
Ventral vestibulospinal tract
Ventral root

0.5 mm

Figure 6-22. A. Myelin-stained section of the lumbar spinal cord in a GW29 fetus (*Y222-65*, CR 235 mm). The myelination of fibers has begun in the collateralization zone. Reactive gliosis (punctate staining) is high in the depth of the gracile fasciculus but low superficially. Reactive glia abound in the intraspinal tracts, the medial longitudinal fasciculus, and the ventral vestibulospinal tract. **B.** Myelination has spread through the entire collateralization zone in this GW32 fetus (*Y76-60*; CR 300 mm), and reactive glia are scattered throughout the superficial gracile fasciculus. The myelination of distal strands of the collaterals is in progress in the gray matter.

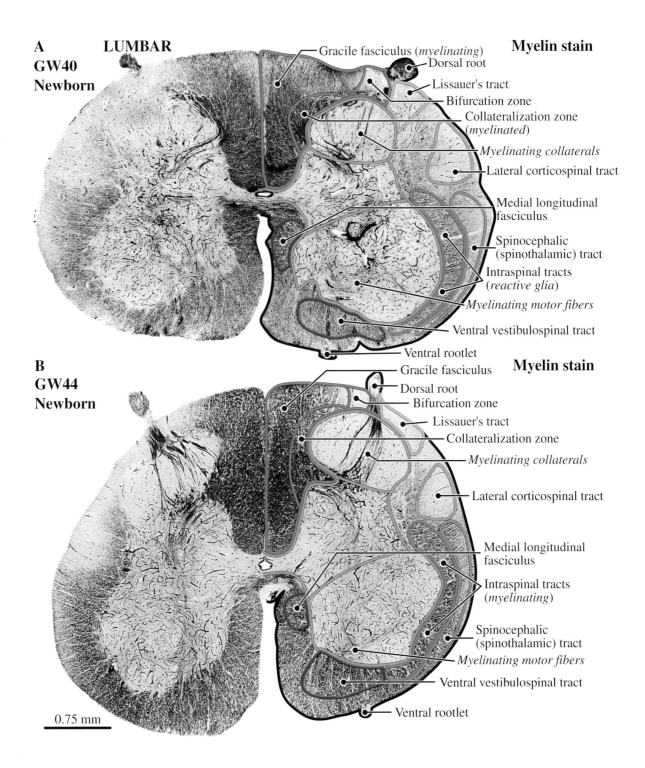

A
GW40
Newborn

LUMBAR

Myelin stain

Gracile fasciculus (*myelinating*)
Dorsal root
Lissauer's tract
Bifurcation zone
Collateralization zone (*myelinated*)
Myelinating collaterals
Lateral corticospinal tract
Medial longitudinal fasciculus
Spinocephalic (spinothalamic) tract
Intraspinal tracts (*reactive glia*)
Myelinating motor fibers
Ventral vestibulospinal tract
Ventral rootlet

B
GW44
Newborn

Myelin stain

Gracile fasciculus
Dorsal root
Bifurcation zone
Lissauer's tract
Collateralization zone
Myelinating collaterals
Lateral corticospinal tract
Medial longitudinal fasciculus
Intraspinal tracts (*myelinating*)
Spinocephalic (spinothalamic) tract
Myelinating motor fibers
Ventral vestibulospinal tract
Ventral rootlet

0.75 mm

Figure 6-23. A. Myelin-stained section of the lumbar spinal cord in a GW40 neonate (*Y115-61*; CR 330 mm). The collateralization zone and the depth of the gracile fasciculus are well-myelinated (dense staining) but the superficial gracile fasciculus is still at the stage of reactive gliosis (punctate staining). **B.** The myelination of the entire dorsal funiculus appears to be completed in this late-delivered GW44 neonate (*Y23-60*; CR 410 mm) and there is an increase in the number of myelinated collaterals in the gray matter. Notable also is the advance in the myelination of the intraspinal and ventral vestibulospinal tracts. The lateral corticospinal tract is still devoid of reactive glia.

6.3 Some Features of Myelination Gliosis and Myelination in the Spinal Cord

6.3.1 The Independence of Peripheral and Central Myelination Gliosis and Myelination. Schwann cells myelinate the peripheral branches of dorsal root axons and oligodendroglia myelinate their central branches. The observations described below suggest that myelination follows a different time table centrally and peripherally. In the cell-stained section of the cervical spinal cord of the GW11 embryo (*Y74-68*; CR 51 mm; Figure 6-24A), there are more interfascicular Schwann cells in the the dorsal root peripherally than there are interfascicular glia in the bifurcation and collateralization zones centrally. This pattern changes in the ensuing weeks, as seen in the myelin-stained section of the cervical spinal cord in the GW20 fetus (*Y27-60*; CR 160 mm; Figure 6-24B).

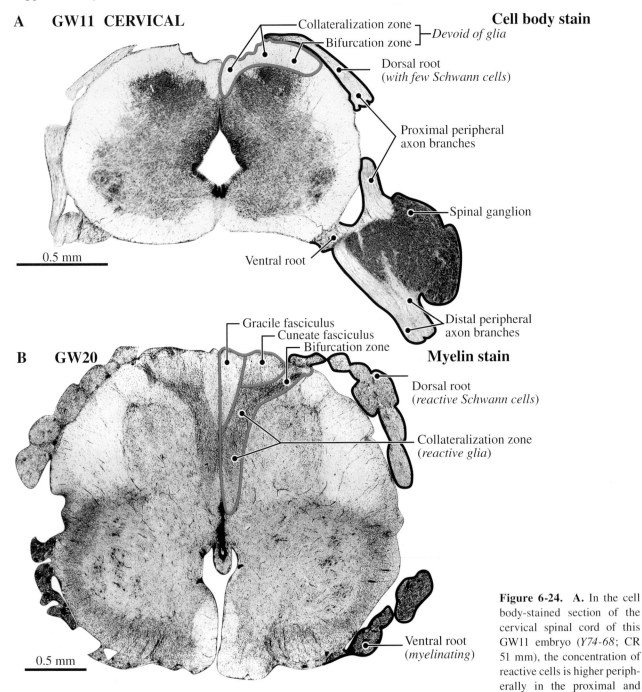

Figure 6-24. A. In the cell body-stained section of the cervical spinal cord of this GW11 embryo (*Y74-68*; CR 51 mm), the concentration of reactive cells is higher peripherally in the proximal and distal dorsal root than centrally in the collateralization and bifurcation zones. This suggests an earlier onset of the proliferation of Schwann cells than oligodendrocytes. **B.** In contrast, in this myelin-stained section from a GW20 fetus (*Y27-60*; CR 160 mm), the concentration of reactive cells is higher centrally in the bifurcation and collateralization zones than peripherally in the dorsal root. These two observations suggest a later onset but an accelerated tempo in the myelination of dorsal root fibers within the spinal cord.

By this age, the concentration of reactive glia is higher in the bifurcation and collateralization zones centrally than it is in the dorsal root peripherally. Thus, while its onset may be delayed, the myelination process progresses faster in the dorsal root fiber branches centrally than it does peripherally. Importantly, there are fewer reactive glia in the cuneate fasciculus and even fewer in the gracile fasciculus than in the collateralization zone. This suggests that the myelination of the local branches of dorsal root axons (those forming the bifurcation and collateralization zones) precedes the myelination of the ascending branches that project to

the medulla. Myelination of the motor fibers in the ventral root is far more advanced than is the myelination of the sensory fibers in the dorsal root.

Reactive gliosis in the bifurcation and collateralization zones, as seen in the GW20 fetus, is followed there several weeks later by the onset of myelination. This is illustrated in the myelin-stained section of the cervical spinal cord of the GW26 fetus (*Y60-61*; CR 210 mm) in Figure 6-25A. There is a high concentration of myelinated fibers in the bifurcation zone and a lesser concentration in the collat-

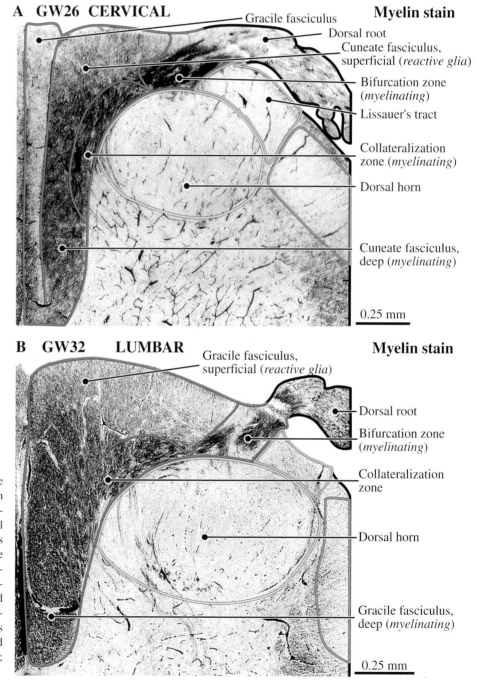

Figure 6-25. **A.** While myelination is in progress in the bifurcation and collateralization zones in the cervical spinal cord of this GW26 fetus (*Y60-61*; CR 210 mm), the earlier stage of reactive gliosis characterizes the superficial cuneate fasciculus and much of the gracile fasciculus. **B.** A similar pattern is seen in the lumbar spinal cord of an older fetus (GW32 fetus; *Y76-60*; CR 300 mm)

eralization zone. Dense patches in the depth of the cuneate fasciculus indicate that myelination may have begun here, but the punctate staining in the apex of the cuneate fasciculus and in the thin gracile fasciculus suggest that myelination has not yet expanded to the ascending branches of dorsal root axons. A similar pattern is seen in the myelin-stained section of the lumbar spinal cord of an older fetus (GW32; Y76-60; CR 300 mm; Figure 6-25B). In this specimen, the myelination of dorsal root fibers is advanced in the bifurcation and collateralization zones but the apical

portion of the gracile fasciculus contains only reactive glia. There is a break in the myelination of dorsal root axons where they enter the spinal cord in the dorsal root entry zone.

6.3.2 The Relationship Between Glial Proliferation, Reactive Gliosis, and Myelination. The material examined so far provides sufficient evidence that myelination is preceded by glial proliferation in the various fiber tracts of the spinal cord white matter. This phenomenon has been described in the literature

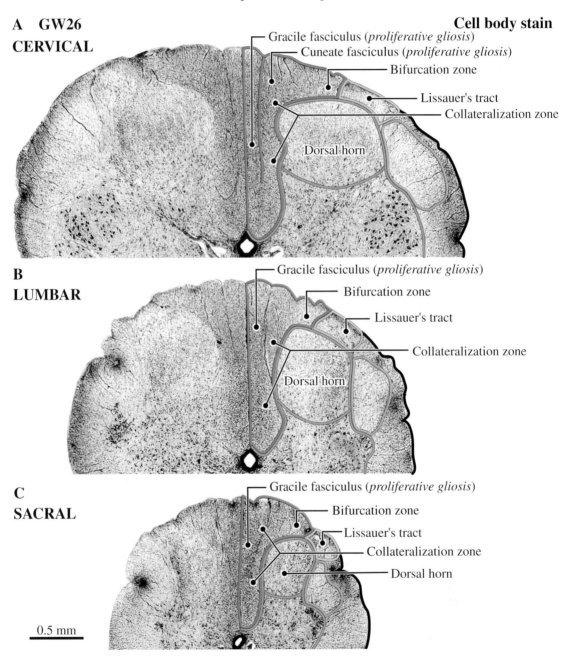

Figure 6-26. The dorsal funiculus in cell body-stained sections of a GW26 fetus (*Y60-61*; CR 210 mm) at cervical (**A**), lumbar (**B**), and sacral (**C**) levels of the spinal cord. The concentration of glia (reflecting proliferative gliosis) is high and uniform in all components of the dorsal funiculus at all segmental levels.

as "myelination gliosis" (see Section 4.4.1). Now we wish to make an additional point, based on repeated observations and to which we have alluded earlier. This is the fact that the initial increase in the concentration of glia in a particular fiber tract (as visualized with cell body staining) does not mean either that the same cells contain myelin constituents (as visualized with myelin staining) or that fiber myelinaion has begun in these locations. We illustrate this point by comparing the dorsal funiculus in the same GW26 fetus (*Y60-61*; 210 mm) at three levels of the spinal

cord, in matched sections stained for cell bodies (Figure 6-26) and for myelin constituents (Figure 6-27).

The cell body-stained section of the cervical spinal cord shows that oligodendroglia are distributed uniformly throughout the entire dorsal funiculus (Figure 6-26A). However, the matched cervical section stained for myelin constituents reveals a complex pattern with different phases of reactivity within the dorsal funiculus (Figure 6-27A). (i) Much of the grac-

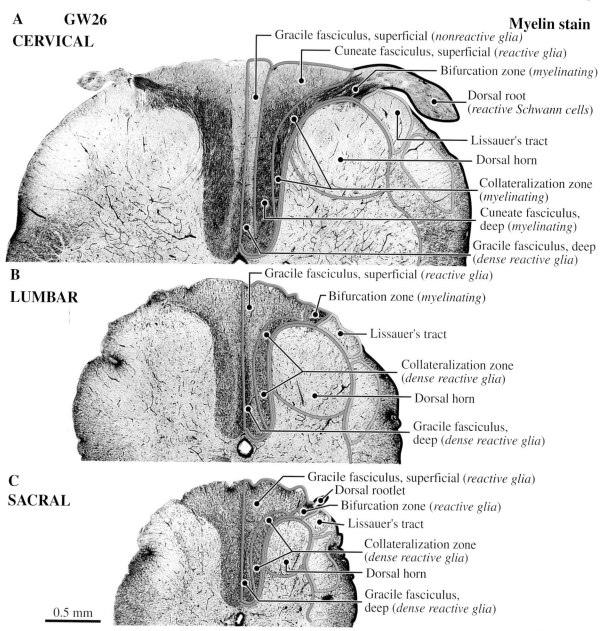

A GW26 CERVICAL   **Myelin stain**

- Gracile fasciculus, superficial (*nonreactive glia*)
- Cuneate fasciculus, superficial (*reactive glia*)
- Bifurcation zone (*myelinating*)
- Dorsal root (*reactive Schwann cells*)
- Lissauer's tract
- Dorsal horn
- Collateralization zone (*myelinating*)
- Cuneate fasciculus, deep (*myelinating*)
- Gracile fasciculus, deep (*dense reactive glia*)

B LUMBAR

- Gracile fasciculus, superficial (*reactive glia*)
- Bifurcation zone (*myelinating*)
- Lissauer's tract
- Collateralization zone (*dense reactive glia*)
- Dorsal horn
- Gracile fasciculus, deep (*dense reactive glia*)

C SACRAL

- Gracile fasciculus, superficial (*reactive glia*)
- Dorsal rootlet
- Bifurcation zone (*reactive glia*)
- Lissauer's tract
- Collateralization zone (*dense reactive glia*)
- Dorsal horn
- Gracile fasciculus, deep (*dense reactive glia*)

0.5 mm

Figure 6-27. The dorsal funiculus in matched myelin-stained sections of the GW26 fetus (*Y60-61*; CR 210 mm) at cervical (**A**), lumbar (**B**), and sacral (**C**) levels. In the cervical cord, the collateralization zone is myelinating, the lower portion of the gracile fasciculus is filled with reactive glia, the apical portion of cuneate fasciculus has fewer reactive glia, and the superficial gracile fasciculus is devoid of reactive glia. The regional differences are less obvious in this fetus at lumbar and sacral levels of the spinal cord.

ile fasciculus contains few reactive glia and the concentration of reactive glia is low in the apical portion of the cuneate fasciculus. (ii) There is a very high concentration of reactive glia in the depth of the cuneate fasciculus and in a narrow wedge in the depth of the gracile fasciculus. (iii) The bifurcation zone and the collateralization zone contain an appreciable concentration of myelinated fibers.

This complex relationship between glial concentration (as revealed by cell body staining) and reactive gliosis (as shown by myelin staining) also holds for the lumbar and sacral cord. Although glial concentration is uniform at both of these levels (Figures 6-26B, C) and comparable to that seen in the cervical cord, the myelin staining (Figures 6-27B, C) shows again a complex pattern and a lag in the myelination process at these c audal levels. The collateralization zone is characterized by a high concentration of reactive glia with few visible myelinated fibers. With respect to the gracile fasciculus, that relationship is reversed because reactive gliosis is more dense in the lumbar and sacral cord than in the cervical cord.

The interpretation of these patterns is that the developing white matter contains three types of oligodendroglia that correlate with three stages in the advance of "myelination gliosis" in the different fiber tracts, each tract following its own time table. The process begins with glia proliferating in high numbers that are not yet producing those lipids and proteins that react with the sudanophilic myelin stain (Mickel and Gilles, 1970; Chi et al., 1976). These nonreactive glia may represent the O-2A precursor cells described in Section 4.4.1. The second stage is represented by the glia with punctate myelin staining. These are the oligodendroglia that are producing myelin constituents but have not yet begun to form the myelin lamellae that wrap around neighboring axons. Finally, the fiber tracts with intense and coarse myelin staining contain oligodendroglia that have started to myelinate the axons in their neighborhood; this is the final stage in the myelination process. This sequence is easiest to follow during fetal development in the dorsal funiculus but is discernible in several other tracts. (A similar sequence in the myelination of the lateral corticospinal tract during the early postnatal period will be described in Chapter 8.)

6.3.3 Local Gradients in Myelination of the Dorsal Funiculus.

We have referred repeatedly to the observation that the dorsal funiculus, which appears homogeneous in the mature spinal cord, has in fact discrete components that develop at different times. To analyze the development of the heterogeneous dorsal funiculus, we begin caudally in the lumbar spinal cord, where the dorsal funiculus is usually described as being composed solely of the gracile fasciculus. The myelogenesis of the dorsal funiculus at this level suggests that it has several components. Early during development, as seen in the myelin-stained section of a GW21 fetus (Y390-62; CR 200 mm; Figure 6-28A), much of the dorsal funiculus is filled with reactive glia. But even at this stage, there is some indication of regional maturational differences, because myelination has already begun in the bifurcation zone. Later, additional regional differences emerge. As seen in the lumbar spinal cord of a GW31 fetus (Y162-61; CR 270 mm; Figure 6-28B), myelination spreads from the bifurcation zone to the collateralization zone abutting the dorsal horn. Myelination may have also started (judged by some of the clumpy staining) in the deep gracile fasciculus. While the upper dorsomedial gracile fasciculus contains many reactive glia there is as yet no indication of the onset of myelination. By GW32 (Y76-60; CR 300 mm; Figure 6-29A), myelination has advanced from the base of the gracile fasciculus dorsomedially, and by GW33 (Y36-60; CR 315 mm; Figure 6-29B) to the apical region of the gracile fasciculus. This gradient in the myelination of the dorsal funiculus in the caudal spinal cord is summarized in Figure 6-30. Myelination progresses from the collateralization zone to the depth of the gracile fasciculus, and from there dorsomedially and, finally, to the apical portion of the gracile fasciculus.

6.3.4 The Proximal-to-Distal Gradient in Myelination.

Our observations indicate that myelination of the dorsal root axon proceeds from proximal to distal: the bifurcation zone containing the local ascending and descending branches myelinate first, the local collaterals next, and the principal branch ascending to the medulla last. That hypothesis is illustrated in Figure 6-31. Heralding the start of the myelination process, the proliferating nonreactive glia distributed throughout the dorsal funiculus become reactive, i.e., competent to produce myelin constituents (Figure 6-31A; compare with Figure 6-28A). At this stage, the myelin constituents must be localized in the perikaryal cytoplasm of the differentiating oli-

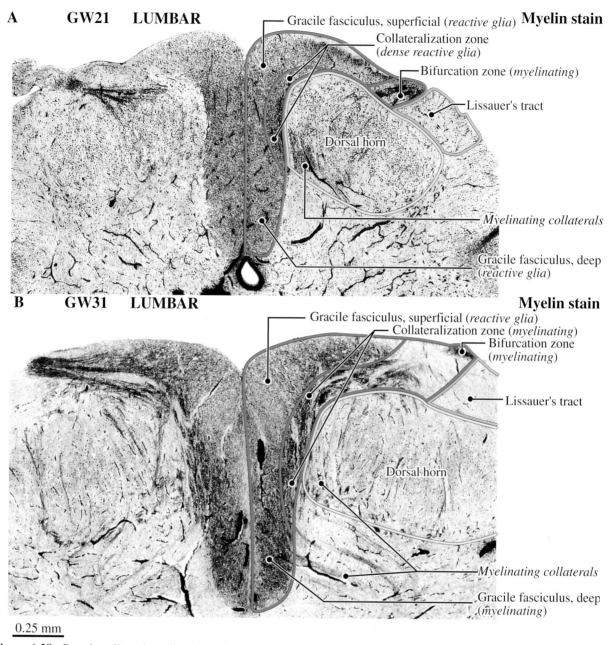

A GW21 LUMBAR **Myelin stain**

Gracile fasciculus, superficial (*reactive glia*)

Collateralization zone (*dense reactive glia*)

Bifurcation zone (*myelinating*)

Lissauer's tract

Dorsal horn

Myelinating collaterals

Gracile fasciculus, deep (*reactive glia*)

B GW31 LUMBAR **Myelin stain**

Gracile fasciculus, superficial (*reactive glia*)

Collateralization zone (*myelinating*)

Bifurcation zone (*myelinating*)

Lissauer's tract

Dorsal horn

Myelinating collaterals

Gracile fasciculus, deep (*myelinating*)

0.25 mm

Figure 6-28. Reactive glia and myelination in the lumbar spinal cord of **A**, a GW21 fetus (*Y390-62*; CR 200 mm) and **B**, a GW31 fetus (*Y162-61*; CR 270 mm). In the younger fetus, reactive glia fill the core of the dorsal funiculus. The onset of myelination is evident in the bifurcation zone, and patchy coarse staining in the collateralization zone and the deep gracile fasciculus suggests imminent myelination. In the older fetus, myelination is well advanced in the collateralization zone and is in progress in the depth the gracile fasciculus. The superficial gracile fasciculus is still in the reactive glia stage of development.

godendroglia. In the next stage of development, the oligodendroglia processes begin to wrap around the proximal branches of dorsal root fibers – the ascending and descending branches in the bifurcation zone and the local collaterals in the collateralization zone – and they become gradually myelinated (Figure 6-31B; compare with Figure 6-28B). The onset of myelination could be due to signals received from the early-maturing proximal branches of dorsal root axons.

These myelinating branches, as we saw earlier, constitute the "local" lanes of the dorsal funiculus afferent system. During the next stage of development myelination spreads to the distal branch of the dorsal root axon that proceeds toward the medulla of the core of the gracile fasciculus (Figure 6-31C; compare with Figures 6-28B, 6-29A). These late-myelinating branches constitute the "express" lanes of the dorsal funiculus.

A   GW32   LUMBAR   **Myelin stain**

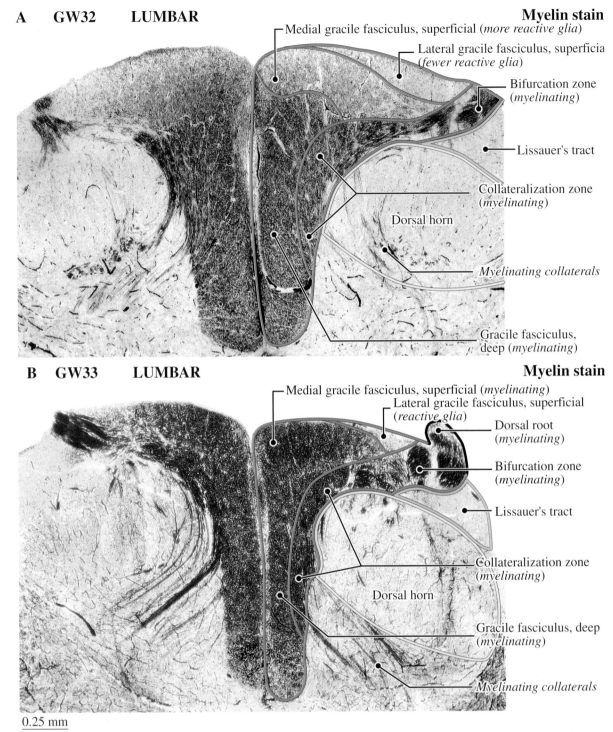

Medial gracile fasciculus, superficial (*more reactive glia*)

Lateral gracile fasciculus, superficia (*fewer reactive glia*)

Bifurcation zone (*myelinating*)

Lissauer's tract

Collateralization zone (*myelinating*)

Dorsal horn

Myelinating collaterals

Gracile fasciculus, deep (*myelinating*)

B   GW33   LUMBAR   **Myelin stain**

Medial gracile fasciculus, superficial (*myelinating*)

Lateral gracile fasciculus, superficial (*reactive glia*)

Dorsal root (*myelinating*)

Bifurcation zone (*myelinating*)

Lissauer's tract

Collateralization zone (*myelinating*)

Dorsal horn

Gracile fasciculus, deep (*myelinating*)

Myelinating collaterals

0.25 mm

Figure 6-29. Reactive glia and myelination in the lumbar spinal cord of **A**, a GW32 fetus (*Y76-60*; CR 300 mm) and **B**, a GW33 fetus (*Y36-60*; CR 315 mm). In the somewhat younger and smaller fetus, the wave of myelination has spread through the entire base of the gracile fasciculus and is spreading upward. The superficial gracile fasciculus is still in the reactive glia stage of development. In the somewhat older fetus, the fibers in the superficial gracile fasciculus are also myelinated.

If our interpretation is correct, it follows that the local and express lanes of the dorsal root afferent system myelinate in the same sequence as they were originally formed during the earlier stage of axonogenesis (see Figure 5-49). Since the dorsal root fibers in the local lanes (those that mediate segmen-

tal and intersegmental reflexes) myelinate first and the branches in the express lanes (those that transmit somatosensory input to the brain) myelinate later, it follows that the intraspinal reflex component of the dorsal root fiber system myelinates ahead of its supraspinal component. But the identity of the early

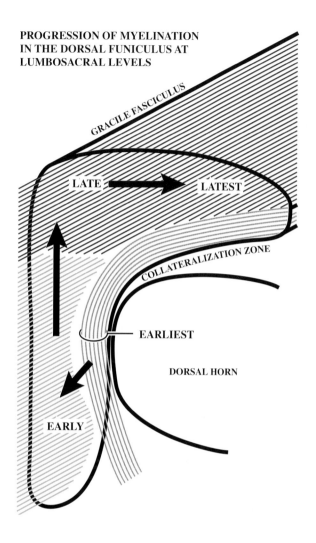

**PROGRESSION OF MYELINATION
IN THE DORSAL FUNICULUS AT
LUMBOSACRAL LEVELS**

GRACILE FASCICULUS

LATE → LATEST

COLLATERALIZATION ZONE

EARLIEST

DORSAL HORN

EARLY

Figure 6-30. Schematic summary of the gradient of myelination (arrows) in the dorsal funiculus of the lumbosacral spinal cord. The branches of dorsal root axons first myelinate in the bifurcation zone (not shown) and the collateralization zone. Myelination then spreads to the branches that occupy the depth of gracile fasciculus. The branches that occupy the dorsal portion of the superficial gracile fasciculus are the next to myelinate. The last myelinating branches are in the lateral portion of the superficial gracile fasciculus Due to lack of information, the diagram ignores the myelination of nonprimary (postsynaptic) fibers in the dorsal funiculus.

myelinating fibers in the depth of the gracile fasciculus is still a problem. If they, too, represent ascending express lane fibers, then the gracile fasciculus proper is divisible into two parts, an earlier myelinating deep region and a late myelinating apical region. We shall return to this question later.

6.3.5 The Complex Pattern of Myelination in the Gracile and Cuneate Fasciculi. We can now proceed and interpret the more complex organization of the dorsal funiculus in the cervical spinal cord. We begin this by comparing the staining pattern of the dorsal funiculus in cell body-stained sections at cervical and lumbar levels in a GW19 fetus (*Y52-61*; CR

130 mm; Figure 6-32). While in the gracile fasciculus glial concentration is high through much of the lumbar cord (Figure 6-32B); it is low in the cervical cord (Figure 6-32A). This apparent caudal-to-rostral gradient is paradoxical because all the other maturational gradients in the spinal cord are in the opposite direction. The paradox is resolved if this gradient is interpreted as a proximal-to-distal one. That is, glial proliferation (myelination gliosis) progresses in the gracile fasciculus along the ascending branches of dorsal root fibers from lumbar levels to cervcial levels, paralleling the initial growth of these ascending fibers in the same direction. That also explains the high concentration of glia in the cuneate fascicu-

lus, a site closer to the proximal portion of the ascending axons in the cervical cord. We noted previously a similar pattern in the distribution of reactive glia in myelin stained sections of an older fetus (GW26; *Y60-61*; CR 210 mm; Figure 6-27). Since, in the cer-

vical spinal cord, the dorsal root fibers in the cuneate fasciculus are closer to their origins while those in the gracile fasciculus are farther from their origin, both glial proliferation and reactive gliosis can be said to follow the same proximal-to-distal gradient.

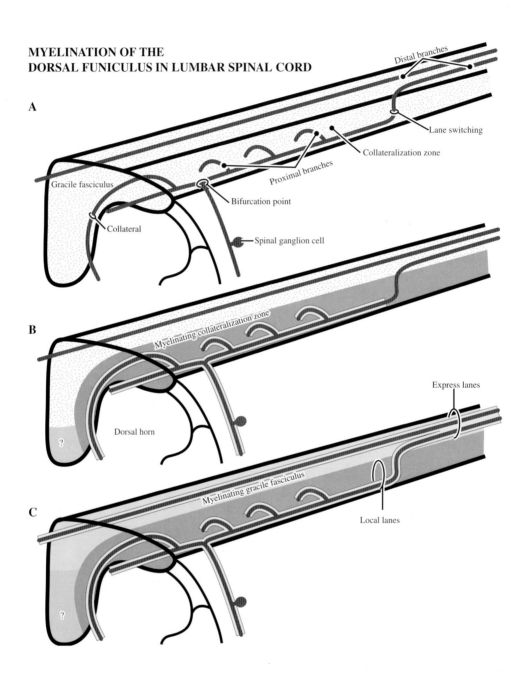

MYELINATION OF THE DORSAL FUNICULUS IN LUMBAR SPINAL CORD

Figure 6-31. Diagram illustrating the hypothesis that myelination of the branches of dorsal root fibers progresses in a proximal-to-distal order in the lumbar spinal cord. **A.** Unmyelinated ascending and descending branches, local collaterals, and the ascending distal branch of dorsal root axons (red lines) in a bed of reactive glia (fine dots) at the end of the second trimester. **B.** Myelination (yellow border) starts in the proximal branches and their collaterals in the "local lanes" (dark gray) responsible for the mediation of spinal reflexes early during the third trimester. **C.** Myelination then spreads to the distal ascending branches of dorsal root fibers in the "express lanes" (light gray).

We now turn to the more complex pattern of progressive myelination of the gracile fasciculus in the lumbar and cervical spinal cord of an older fetus (GW32; *Y76-60*; CR 300 mm). In the lumbar spinal cord (Figure 6-33B), the fibers occupying the lower three-fourths of the gracile fasciculus (including the collateralization zone) are myelinating while the superficial region of the gracile fasciculus is filled with reactive glia but devoid of myelinating fibers. Correspondingly, in the cervical cord of the same fetus (Figure 6-33A), fibers in the lower three-fourths of the cuneate fasciculus (including the collateralization zone) are myelinating while the superficial region is filled with reactive glia. In sharp contrast (but in line with the progression of reactive gliosis in younger fetuses), the bulk of the gracile fasciculus is filled

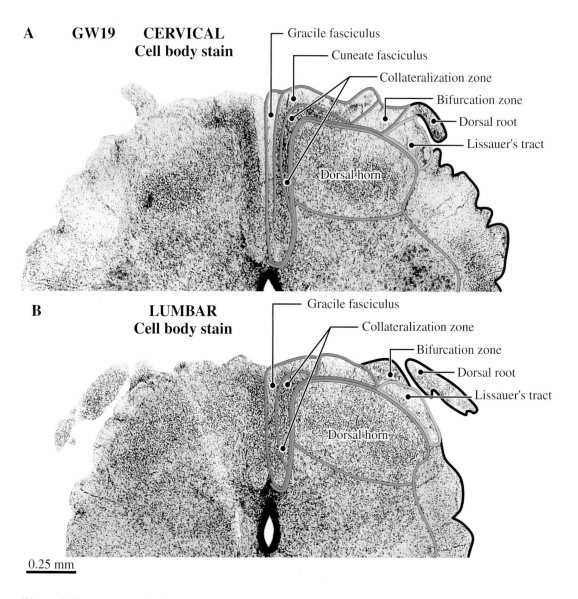

A   GW19   CERVICAL
Cell body stain

Gracile fasciculus
Cuneate fasciculus
Collateralization zone
Bifurcation zone
Dorsal root
Lissauer's tract
Dorsal horn

B   LUMBAR
Cell body stain

Gracile fasciculus
Collateralization zone
Bifurcation zone
Dorsal root
Lissauer's tract
Dorsal horn

0.25 mm

Figure 6-32. The dorsal funiculus in cell body-stained sections of a GW19 fetus (*Y52-61*; CR 130 mm) at cervical (**A**) and lumbar (**B**) levels of the spinal cord. While the gracile fasciculus in the lumbar cord and the cuneate fasciculus in the cervical cord are filled with glia, the gracile fasciculus contains few glia in the cervical cord. This suggests a proximal-to-distal (orthograde) gradient in glial proliferation (myelination gliosis) in relation to the ascending dorsal root fibers of the gracile fasciculus.

with reactive glia but is as yet unmyelinated in the cervical cord. It seems that myelination, like glial proliferation and reactive gliosis, progresses in a proximal-to-distal order in the dorsal funiculus. But there is one exception to this generalization; namely, the early myelinating medial wedge-shaped region in the

gracile fasciculus. The identity of this compartment of the gracile fasciculus remains to be determined.

This complex pattern persists in a modified form in the cervical spinal cord of an older fetus (GW33; *Y36-60*; CR 315 mm; Figure 6-34). In this

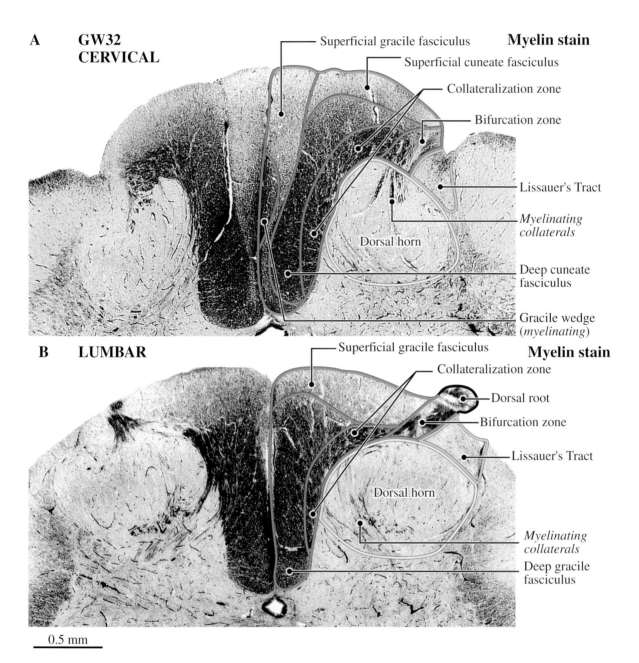

A   GW32 CERVICAL

- Superficial gracile fasciculus — **Myelin stain**
- Superficial cuneate fasciculus
- Collateralization zone
- Bifurcation zone
- Lissauer's Tract
- *Myelinating collaterals*
- Dorsal horn
- Deep cuneate fasciculus
- Gracile wedge (*myelinating*)

B   LUMBAR

- Superficial gracile fasciculus — **Myelin stain**
- Collateralization zone
- Dorsal root
- Bifurcation zone
- Lissauer's Tract
- Dorsal horn
- *Myelinating collaterals*
- Deep gracile fasciculus

0.5 mm

Figure 6-33. The dorsal funiculus in myelin-stained sections of a GW32 fetus (*Y76-60*; CR 300 mm) at cervical (**A**) and lumbar (**B**) levels of the spinal cord. The proximal fibers in the collateralization zone of both the lumbar cord and the cervical cord are myelinating. Similarly, the fibers in the depth of the gracile fasciculus in the lumbar cord, and in the depth of the cuneate fasciculus in the cervical cord, both of which are presumably composed of ascending fibers of local origin, are myelinating. However, the distal ascending fibers in the core of the gracile fasciculus in the cervical cord are unmyelinated. The exception is the myelinating gracile wedge in the cervical cord.

fetus the myelination of both the gracile fasciculus in the lumbar cord (Figure 6-34B) and of the cuneate fasciculus in the cervical cord (Figure 6-34A) is nearing completion. That is, both caudally and rostrally the proximal portion of the ascending dorsal root fibers are myelinated. However, in the cervical cord there are still two distinct regions within the gracile

fasciculus: the bulk of the gracile fasciculus is in the reactive gliosis phase but the gracile wedge is myelinating. The late myelination of the distal branch of ascending dorsal root fibers in the cervical spinal cord is in line with the proximal-to-distal gradient, or the othrograde process of myelination. But why are the fibers in the gracile wedge myelinating so early?

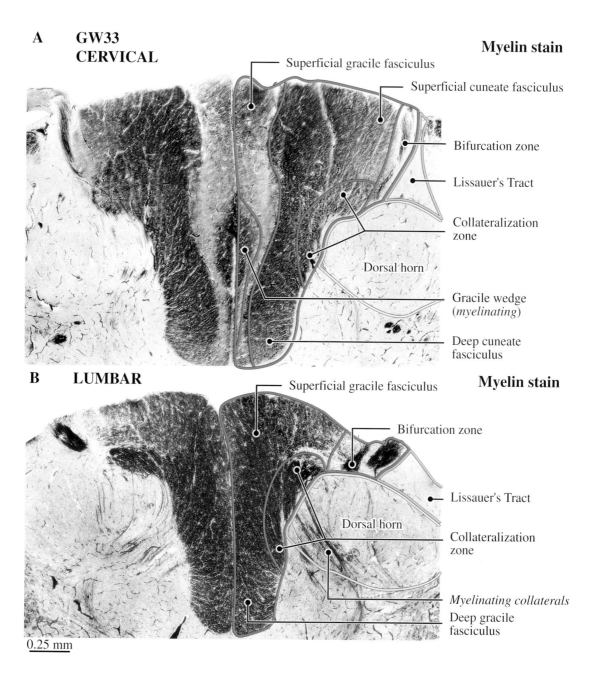

Figure 6-34. The dorsal funiculus in myelin-stained sections of a GW33 fetus (*Y36-60*; CR 315 mm) at cervical **(A)** and lumbar **(B)** levels of the spinal cord. Myelination has spread through the entire gracile fasciculus in the lumbar cord, and the entire cuneate fasciculus in the cervical cord. However, the distal ascending of the gracile fasciculus in the cervical cord are unmyelinated. The exception is the myelinating gracile wedge.

MYELINATION THROUGHOUT THE DORSAL FUNICULUS

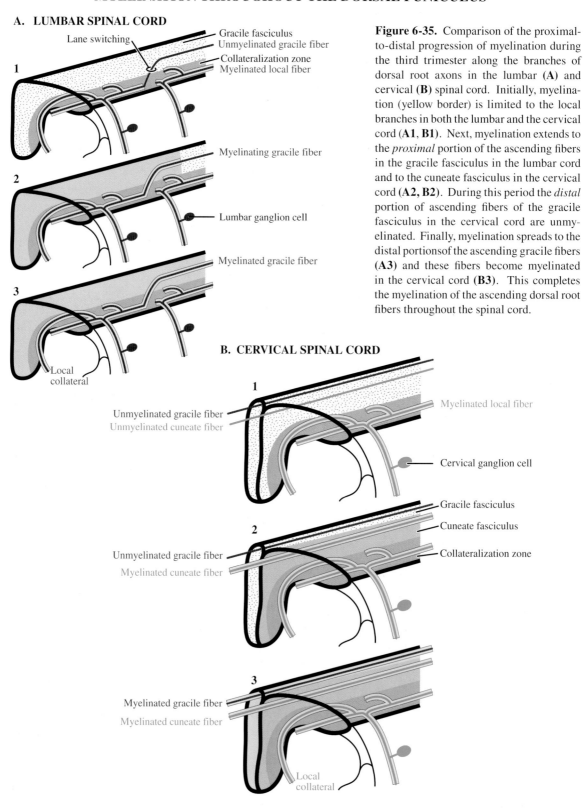

A. LUMBAR SPINAL CORD

Lane switching

Gracile fasciculus
Unmyelinated gracile fiber
Collateralization zone
Myelinated local fiber

Myelinating gracile fiber

Lumbar ganglion cell

Myelinated gracile fiber

Local collateral

Unmyelinated gracile fiber
Unmyelinated cuneate fiber

Myelinated local fiber

Cervical ganglion cell

Gracile fasciculus
Cuneate fasciculus
Collateralization zone

Unmyelinated gracile fiber
Myelinated cuneate fiber

Myelinated gracile fiber
Myelinated cuneate fiber

Local collateral

B. CERVICAL SPINAL CORD

Figure 6-35. Comparison of the proximal-to-distal progression of myelination during the third trimester along the branches of dorsal root axons in the lumbar (**A**) and cervical (**B**) spinal cord. Initially, myelination (yellow border) is limited to the local branches in both the lumbar and the cervical cord (**A1, B1**). Next, myelination extends to the *proximal* portion of the ascending fibers in the gracile fasciculus in the lumbar cord and to the cuneate fasciculus in the cervical cord (**A2, B2**). During this period the *distal* portion of ascending fibers of the gracile fasciculus in the cervical cord are unmyelinated. Finally, myelination spreads to the distal portionsof the ascending gracile fibers (**A3**) and these fibers become myelinated in the cervical cord (**B3**). This completes the myelination of the ascending dorsal root fibers throughout the spinal cord.

There are several possibilities but, due to lack of empirical evidence, they must all remain speculative. One possibility is that the fibers of the gracile wedge in the cervical cord originate at thoracic rather than lumbosacral levels, that is, they are closer to their point of entry into the spinal cord. This implies a ventral-to-dorsal gradient in the distribution of fibers in the gracile fasciculus: those occupying its deeper parts (i.e., the gracile wedge) originate rostrally while those situated more superficially originate progressively more caudally. The second possibility is that the gracile wedge is a distinct region composed of a unique set of fibers. The early myelinating dorsal root fibers may mediate some particular sensory modality or they may not be primary dorsal root afferents but postsynaptic fibers.

The pronounced proximal-to-distal gradient in myelination is illustrated in sections from the cervical, lumbar, sacral and coccygeal levels of the spinal cord in a single newborn (GW37; *Y117-61*; 310 mm; Figure 6-36). The extent of myelination, as judged by staining intensity, is similar in the collateralization zone at all levels of the cord. Indeed, the concentration of myelinated collaterals that enter the gray matter is similar in the lumbar cord (Figure 6-36B) to that seen in the cervical cord (Figure 6-36A). If this pattern is compared with what we saw in a fetus at the end of the second trimester (Figure 6-27), which showed a pronounced rostral-to-caudal gradient of maturation during the early phases of the myelination process, it becomes evident that by the time of birth the myelination of the local branches of dorsal fibers reached the same stage at all levels of the spinal cord. In sharp contrast, the myelination of the ascending fibers of the gracile fasciculus still displays a pronounced rostral-to-caudal gradient. The ascending fibers that appear to be well myelinated medially in the coccygeal and sacral cord (Figures 6-36 C, D), are joined by unmyelinated fibers in the apical portion of the lumbar spinal cord (Figure 6-36B), and at cervical level (Figure 6-36A) most of the gracile fasciculus, excepting the gracile wedge, is still at the reactive-glia stage of development.

In summary, myelination of the branches of dorsal root axons, with the exception of the gracile wedge in the cervical spinal cord, progresses in a proximal-to-distal order: from the branches in the collateralization zone (proximal) to the ascending branch in the core of the dorsal funiculus (distal), and within the ascending branch from lumbosacral (proximal) to

cervical (distal). This pattern of myelination of dorsal root fibers is schematically summarized in relation to the myelination of the different compartments of the dorsal funiculus in Figure 6-35.

We complete this survey of the myelination of dorsal root fibers by illustrating the distribution of the ascending fibers of the gracile and cuneate fasciculi near their terminus in the medulla of two GW30 fetuses. In one specimen (*Y180-64*; CR 295 mm; Figure 6-37A), the nucleus cuneatus is seen to be capped by myelinating fibers but not the nucleus gracilis. Many of the internal arcuate fibers of the decussating medial lemniscus (composed of higher-order ascending fibers that relay somatosensory information to the thalamus) are also myelinated. As yet, the fibers of the descending corticospinal tract in the pyramids are unmyelinated. In the other GW30 fetus (*Y219-65*; Figure 6-37B), the ascending fibers in the cuneate fasciculus are well myelinated but myelination in the gracile fasciculus is much less advanced. Again, the decussating fibers of the lateral corticospinal tract are unmyelinated.

6.3.6 *Myelination of Some of the Sensory Fibers that Penetrate the Gray Matter.* The dorsal root contains several classes of sensory fibers from the skin, muscle, joints and viscera, and we have presented evidence before that some of these follow a different trajectory and terminate in different regions of the gray matter (Section 1.4). Are there chronological differences in the growth and myelination of these different classes of afferents and, if so, what is their exact timetable? We do not currently have the necessary data to answer these questions. Below we present some material that bears on this issue and suggests some tentative hypotheses.

Two lumbar sections, one from a GW29 fetus (*Y20-60*, CR 270 mm;) and the other from a late-term neonate (GW44; *Y23-60*; CR 410 mm) are reproduced in Figure 6-38. They were prepared with Bielschowsky's silver staining technique that reacts somewhat indiscriminately and capriciously with both myelinated and unmyelinated fibers and also the perikarya of large neurons. In the GW29 fetus (Figure 6-38A), a few stained axons enter the gray matter underneath the dorsal horn. These fibers seem to follow a ventral trajectory, suggesting that their target is not the dorsal horn but rather the intermediate gray and/or the ventral horn. That is, they are probably proprioceptive rather than exteroceptive affer-

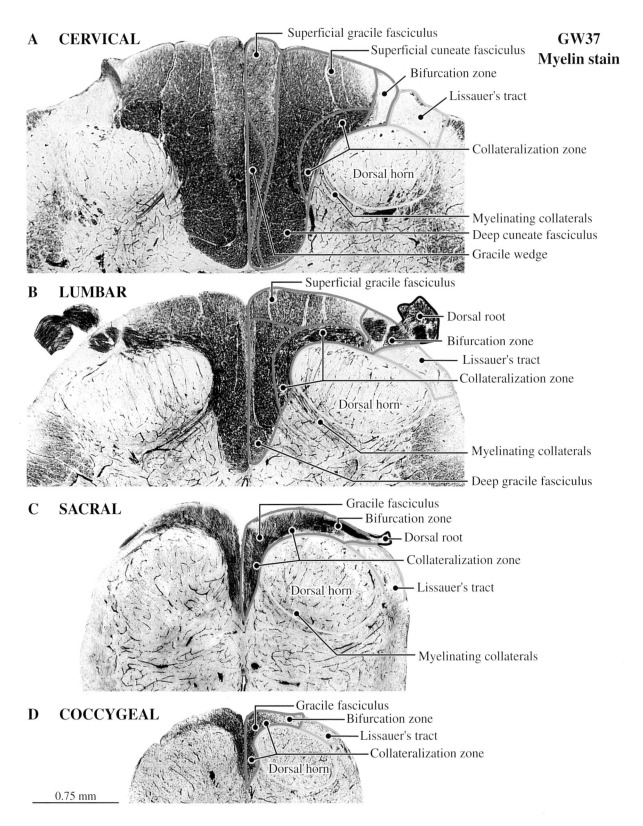

A   CERVICAL

Superficial gracile fasciculus
Superficial cuneate fasciculus
Bifurcation zone
Lissauer's tract
Collateralization zone
Dorsal horn
Myelinating collaterals
Deep cuneate fasciculus
Gracile wedge

**GW37
Myelin stain**

B   LUMBAR

Superficial gracile fasciculus
Dorsal root
Bifurcation zone
Lissauer's tract
Collateralization zone
Dorsal horn
Myelinating collaterals
Deep gracile fasciculus

C   SACRAL

Gracile fasciculus
Bifurcation zone
Dorsal root
Collateralization zone
Lissauer's tract
Dorsal horn
Myelinating collaterals

D   COCCYGEAL

Gracile fasciculus
Bifurcation zone
Lissauer's tract
Collateralization zone
Dorsal horn

0.75 mm

Figure 6-36. The dorsal funiculus in a newborn (GW37; *Y117-61*; 310 mm) at cervical (**A**), lumbar (**B**), sacral (**C**), and coccygeal (**D**) levels of the spinal cord. Myelination, as judged by staining intensity, is comparable at all levels of the spinal cord in the collateralization zone. However, myelination gradually decreases in the core and the apex of the expanding gracile fasciculus at lumbar and cervical levels, suggesting a proximal-to-distal gradient in the myelination of the ascending dorsal root fibers.

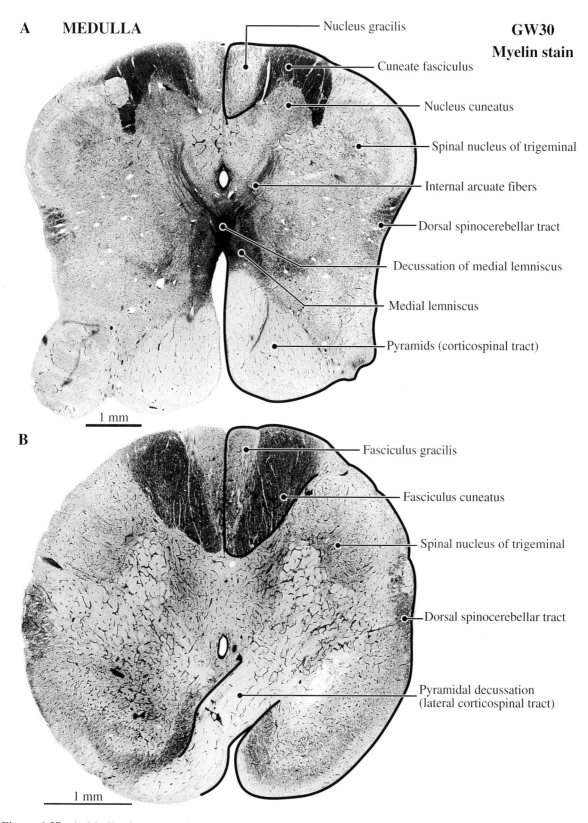

A MEDULLA   **GW30**
Myelin stain

- Nucleus gracilis
- Cuneate fasciculus
- Nucleus cuneatus
- Spinal nucleus of trigeminal
- Internal arcuate fibers
- Dorsal spinocerebellar tract
- Decussation of medial lemniscus
- Medial lemniscus
- Pyramids (corticospinal tract)

1 mm

B

- Fasciculus gracilis
- Fasciculus cuneatus
- Spinal nucleus of trigeminal
- Dorsal spinocerebellar tract
- Pyramidal decussation (lateral corticospinal tract)

1 mm

Figure 6-37. A. Myelination pattern in the medulla at the level of the decussation of the medial lemniscus in a GW30 fetus (*Y180-64*; CR 295 mm). The nucleus cuneatus is surrounded by myelinated fibers but not the nucleus gracilis. Many of the ascending arcuate fibers and the decussating fibers of the medial lemniscus are myelinated. **B.** In the lower medulla of another GW30 fetus (*Y219-65*; CR unknown), at the level of the pyramidal decussation, the concentration of myelinated fibers is high in the cuneate fasciculus but still low or absent in the gracile fasciculus. In both fetuses the corticospinal fibers (in the pyramids or the pyramidal decussation) are unmyelinated.

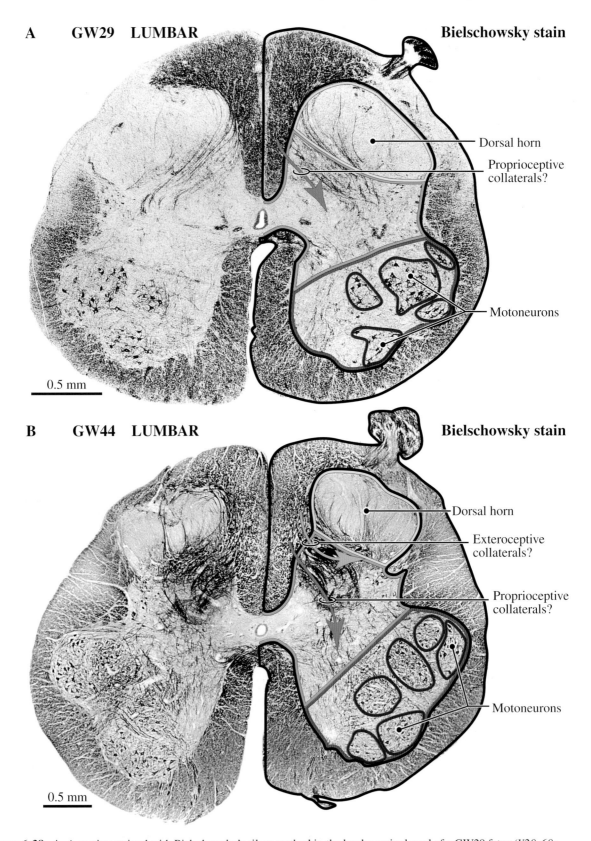

A   GW29   LUMBAR   **Bielschowsky stain**

Dorsal horn

Proprioceptive
collaterals?

Motoneurons

0.5 mm

B   GW44   LUMBAR   **Bielschowsky stain**

Dorsal horn

Exteroceptive
collaterals?

Proprioceptive
collaterals?

Motoneurons

0.5 mm

Figure 6-38. A. A section stained with Bielschowsky's silver method in the lumbar spinal cord of a GW29 fetus (*Y20-60*; CR 270 mm). Fine dorsal root collaterals, with an apparent ventral trajectory (arrow), enter the gray matter beneath the dorsal horn. These are putative proprioceptive fibers (dark blue). **B.** A similarly prepared section of the lumbar spinal cord of a late-term neonate (GW44; *Y23-60*; CR 410 mm). The fibers with a ventral trajectory have increased in number and staining intensity. In addition, there is a large plexus of fibers at the base of the dorsal horn (light blue). This subgelatinosal plexus may be composed of recurring exteroceptive collaterals (compare with Figure 4-40).

ents. In the older GW44 neonate (Figure 6-38B), presumed proprioceptive collaterals form a massive bundle heading downward. In addition, a prominent crescent-shaped plexus of fibers now appears beneath the substantia gelatinosa. Since only a few stained fibers traverse the dorsal horn from its dorsal aspect, the subgelatinosal plexus may contain the exteroceptive endings of recurving collaterals that form the flame terminals (Figures 1-26, 1-27). The subgelatinosal plexus and the ventrally oriented proprioceptive afferents underneath it in the GW44 newborn, are reproduced at higher magnification in Figure 6-39. By now, a few stained fibers traversing the dorsal horn from its surface appear. These fragmentary observations suggest that the myelination of proprioceptive collaterals, whose principal target is the ventral horn, precedes the myelination of exteroceptive terminals that end in the dorsal horn. The last terminals to enter the gray matter may be those of the nociceptive afferents.

The presence of other types of developing afferents is suggested by additional observations. In the myelin-stained section of the lumbar spinal cord of a GW32 fetus (*Y76-60*; CR 300 mm; Figure 6-40A), faintly stained dorsal root collaterals are visible that enter the dorsal horn from its surface. These fibers are stained more intensely and are present in larger numbers in the thoracic spinal cord of the late-term newborn (GW44; *Y23-60*; CR 410 mm; Figure 6-40B). While the exact identity of these collaterals that enter the substantia gelatinosa from its surface is unkown, they are likely to be exteroceptive afferents. Another class of afferents is made visible in a myelin-stained section of the same GW44 neonate. This is a compact bundle of fibers that leaves the lateral "spur" of the collateralization zone to enter Clarke's column (Figure 6-41). These are in all probability proprioceptive fibers that synapse with neurons of Clarke's column that are the source of the ascending dorsal spinocerebellar tract.

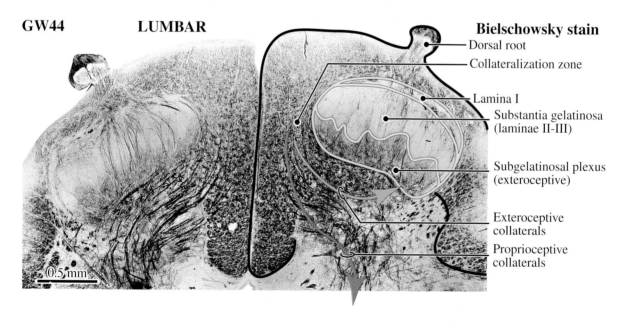

GW44 **LUMBAR** **Bielschowsky stain**

- Dorsal root
- Collateralization zone
- Lamina I
- Substantia gelatinosa (laminae II-III)
- Subgelatinosal plexus (exteroceptive)
- Exteroceptive collaterals
- Proprioceptive collaterals

0.5 mm

Figure 6-39. Fascicles of afferent collaterals and the subgelatinosal plexus in a section of the lumbar spinal cord of the GW44 neonate (*Y23-60*; CR 410 mm) stained with Bielschowsky's silver method. The collaterals with a ventral trajectory (dark blue arrow) are probably proprioceptive fibers. The subcallosal plexus may be the target of recurving exteroceptive collaterals (light blue arrow). A few lightly staining afferents penetrate the dorsal horn from its surface.

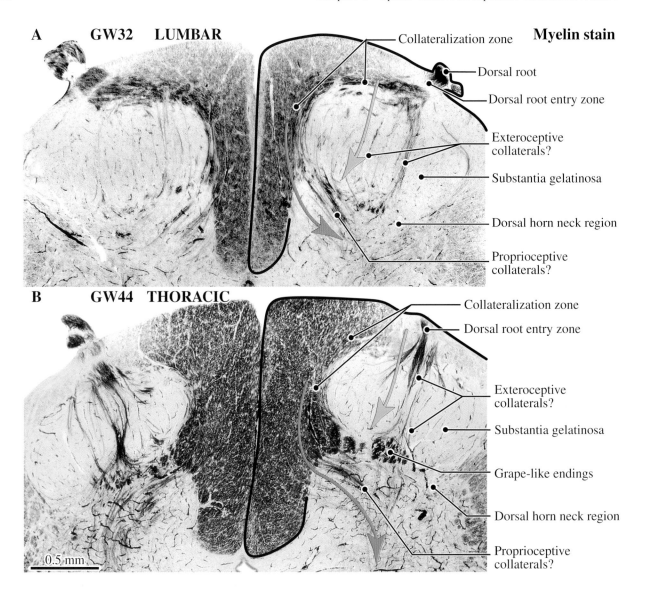

A. GW32 LUMBAR

Collateralization zone

Dorsal root

Dorsal root entry zone

Exteroceptive collaterals?

Substantia gelatinosa

Dorsal horn neck region

Proprioceptive collaterals?

Myelin stain

B. GW44 THORACIC

Collateralization zone

Dorsal root entry zone

Exteroceptive collaterals?

Substantia gelatinosa

Grape-like endings

Dorsal horn neck region

Proprioceptive collaterals?

0.5 mm

Figure 6-40. A. Myelin-stained section of the lumbar spinal cord from a GW32 fetus (*Y76-60*; CR 300 mm). A few faintly stained collaterals enter the substantia gelatinosa from its surface (light blue arrow). Other myelinating collaterals (presumably proprioceptive fibers) leave the collateralization zone and enter the gray matter beneath the dorsal horn (dark blue arrow). **B.** Myelin-stained section of the thoracic spinal cord from the GW44 neonate (*Y23-60*; CR 410 mm). The more heavily myelinated super-ficial collaterals (light blue arrow) terminate with grape-like endings at the base of the dorsal horn. Some of the fibers exiting from "spur" of the collateralization zone (dark blue arrow) proceed ventrally.

GW44   THORACIC

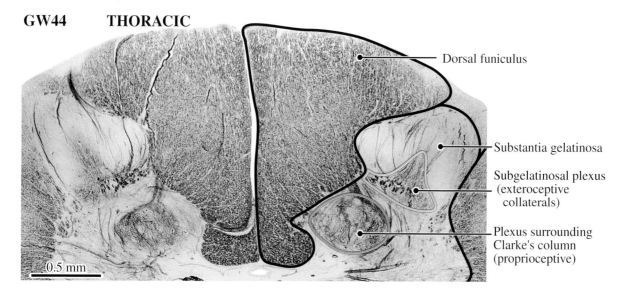

Dorsal funiculus

Substantia gelatinosa

Subgelatinosal plexus
(exteroceptive
collaterals)

Plexus surrounding
Clarke's column
(proprioceptive)

0.5 mm

Figure 6-41. Myelin-stained section of the thoracic spinal cord in the GW44 neonate (*Y32-60*; CR 410 mm). Some dorsal root collaterals leave the "spur" of the collateralization zone and seemingly end at two sites, the subgelatinosal plexus in the dorsal horn (light blue) and the spherical shell around Clarke's column (dark blue). The fibers arborizing in Clarke's column are undoubtedly proprioceptive terminals. The fibers contributing to the subgelatinosal plexus may be exteroceptive terminals.

6.4 Development of Clarke's Column Neurons

6.4.1 Site of Origin and Development of Neurons of Clarke's Column. Clarke's column is first identifiable in the thoracic cord of the spinal cord at the beginning of the second trimester. To trace the possible neuroepithelial origin of its neurons, we start by examining two first trimester embryos. In the thoracic spinal cord of a GW8.5 embryo (*M2050*; CR 36 mm; Figure 6-42A), there is a distinctive neuroepithelial locus and sojourn zone underneath the dorsal horn and above the central canal. The same aggregate of cells, now farther removed from the dorsal horn, is still present in a GW10 fetus (*Y74-68*; CR 51 mm; Figure 6-42B). After withdrawal of this neuroepithelial region and the formation of the dorsal funiculus, the Clarke's column neurons appear in the same location in the GW14 fetus (*Y58-65*; CR 108 mm; Figure 6-43A). The neurons of Clarke's column have grown in size and are more dispersed in a GW17.5 fetus (*Y50-60*; CR 155 mm; Figure 6-43B). Perikaryal growth and dispersion continues for a while, as seen in the GW31 fetus (*Y162-61*; CR 270 mm; Figure 6-44A). This dispersion may be completed by the time of birth, as indicated in the late-term GW44 neonate (*Y23-60*; CR 410 mm; Figure 6-44B).

6.4.2 Maturation of Neurons of Clarke's Column. The maturation of neurons of Clarke's column during the third trimester is a prolonged process. Several observations support this inference. As seen at higher magnification (Figure 6-45), the increase in the perikaryal size of Clarke's column is a gradual process between GW31 and GW44, and so is the expansion of the fibrous shell that surrounds the perikaryal core of the column. We saw earlier in a Bielschowsky-stained preparation of the GW44 neonate (Figure 6-41) that this fibrous shell contains dorsal root collaterals that enter the gray matter from the lateral "spur" of the collateralization zone. As seen at higher magnification in the same specimen (Figure 6-46), this expansion of the fibrous shell of Clarke's column is associated with the dendritic development of its large multipolar neurons. Another facet of the prolonged maturation of Clarke's column is the slow myelination of its afferents. That is illustrated in the matched cell body-stained and myelin-stained sections of the thoracic cord in the GW37 (*Y117-61*; CR 310 mm; Figure 6-47A), GW 38 (*Y163-61*; CR 320 mm; Figure 6-47B), and GW44 (*Y23-60*; CR 410 mm; Figure 6-47C) neonates.

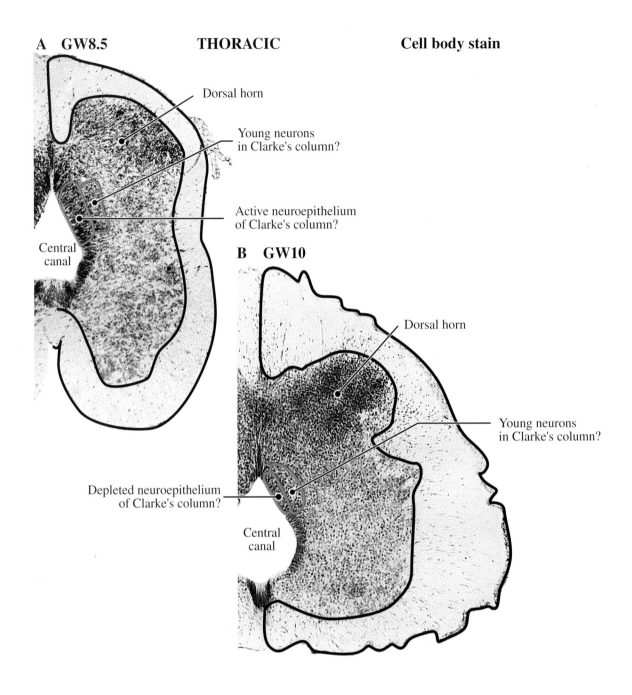

A GW8.5   **THORACIC**   **Cell body stain**

Dorsal horn

Young neurons
in Clarke's column?

Active neuroepithelium
of Clarke's column?

B GW10

Central
canal

Dorsal horn

Young neurons
in Clarke's column?

Depleted neuroepithelium
of Clarke's column?

Central
canal

Figure 6-42. Cell body-stained sections of the thoracic spinal cord in **A**, a GW8.5 embryo (*M2050*; CR 36 mm) and **B**, a GW10 embryo (*Y74-68*; CR 51 mm). The presumed neuro-epithelial source and settling area of young Clarke's column neurons are outlined.

THORACIC **Cell body stain**

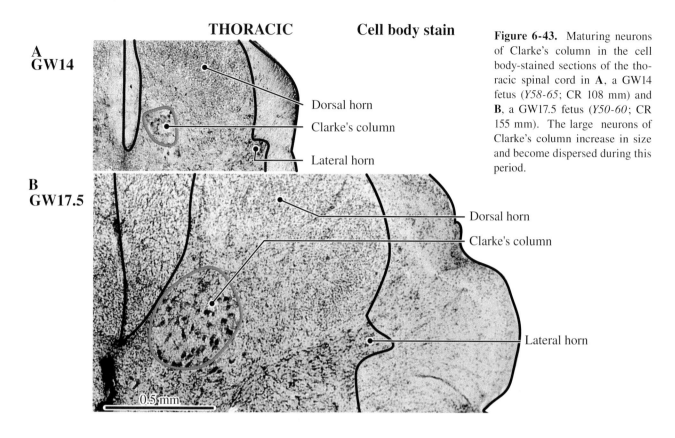

A
GW14

B
GW17.5

Dorsal horn

Clarke's column

Lateral horn

Dorsal horn

Clarke's column

Lateral horn

0.5 mm

Figure 6-43. Maturing neurons of Clarke's column in the cell body-stained sections of the thoracic spinal cord in **A**, a GW14 fetus (*Y58-65*; CR 108 mm) and **B**, a GW17.5 fetus (*Y50-60*; CR 155 mm). The large neurons of Clarke's column increase in size and become dispersed during this period.

THORACIC **Cell body stain**

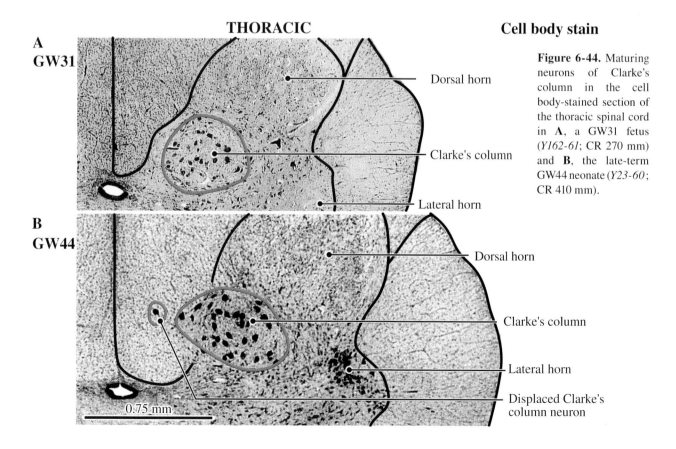

A
GW31

B
GW44

Dorsal horn

Clarke's column

Lateral horn

Dorsal horn

Clarke's column

Lateral horn

Displaced Clarke's column neuron

0.75 mm

Figure 6-44. Maturing neurons of Clarke's column in the cell body-stained section of the thoracic spinal cord in **A**, a GW31 fetus (*Y162-61*; CR 270 mm) and **B**, the late-term GW44 neonate (*Y23-60*; CR 410 mm).

THORACIC   Cell body stain

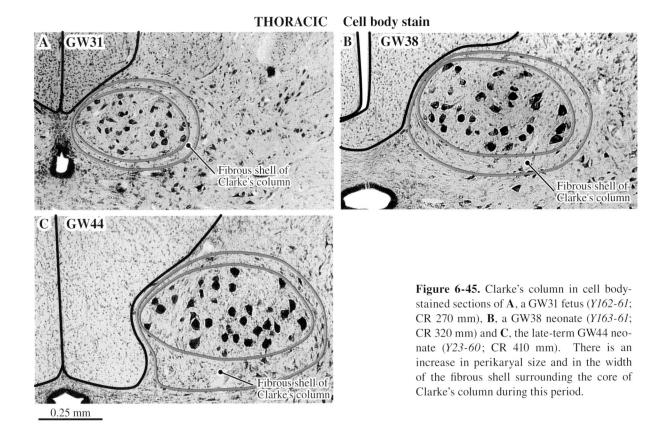

Figure 6-45. Clarke's column in cell body-stained sections of **A**, a GW31 fetus (*Y162-61*; CR 270 mm), **B**, a GW38 neonate (*Y163-61*; CR 320 mm) and **C**, the late-term GW44 neonate (*Y23-60*; CR 410 mm). There is an increase in perikaryal size and in the width of the fibrous shell surrounding the core of Clarke's column during this period.

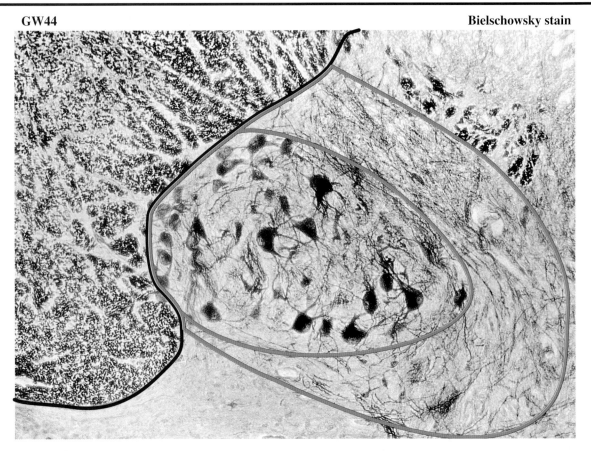

Figure 6-46. Dendritic development of the multipolar Clarke's column neurons and the fibrous shell of the column, as seen in a Bielschowsky-stained section of the thoracic spinal cord in the late-term GW44 neonate (*Y23-60*; CR 410 mm).

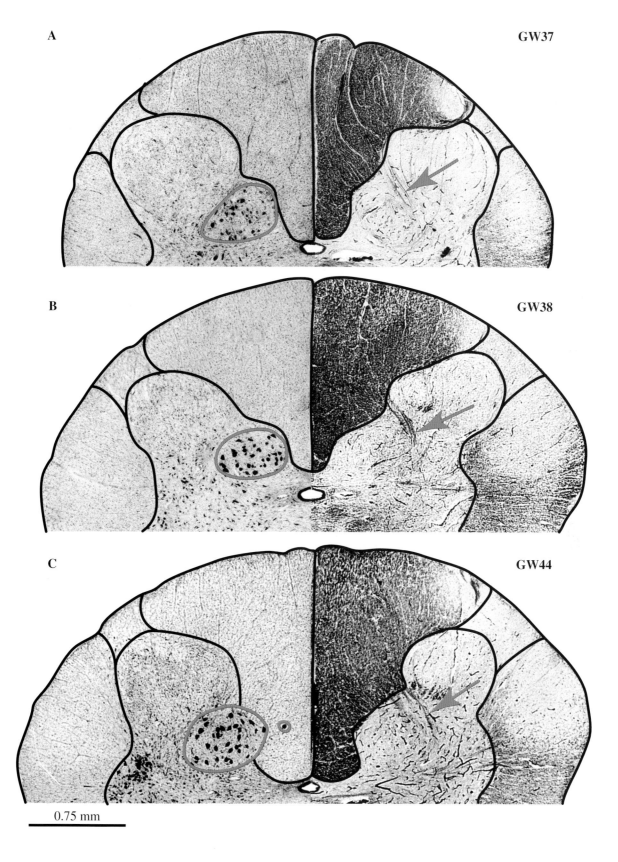

0.75 mm

Figure 6-47. The slow myelination of the dorsal root collaterals (arrow) that contribute to the shell around Clarke's column, as seen in **A**, a GW37 preterm neonate (*Y117-61*; CR 310 mm), **B**, a GW38 term neonate (*Y163-61*; CR 320 mm), and **C**, the late-term GW44 neonate (*Y23-60*; CR 410 mm). Matched sections stained for perikarya (**left**) and for myelin (**right**).

6.4.3 Individual Differences in the Size and Length of Clarke's Column. We have made so far only passing reference to individual differences in the development of various components of the spinal cord. We illustrate this important factor by comparing the length and the area of Clarke's column in two pairs of neonates. We begin with one pair of neonates closely matched for gestational age and body size. In the *Y117-61* neonate (GW37; 310 mm; Figure 6-48),

Clarke's column is not present at a low cervical level, has its maximal size but with relatively few cells at the middle thoracic level, and tapers off in the upper lumbar cord. In contrast, in the *Y163-61* neonate (GW38; 320 mm; Figure 6-49), Clarke's column begins in the low cervical cord, has a much higher concentration of cells at the middle thoracic cord, and it is still prominent in the upper lumbar cord. The other comparison is between two neonates of dif-

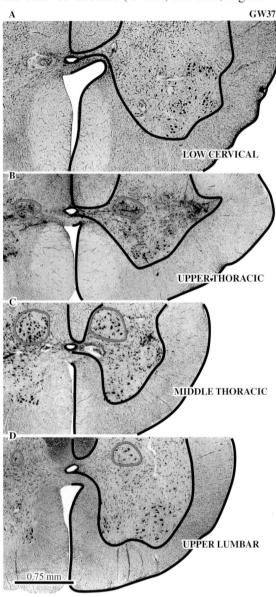

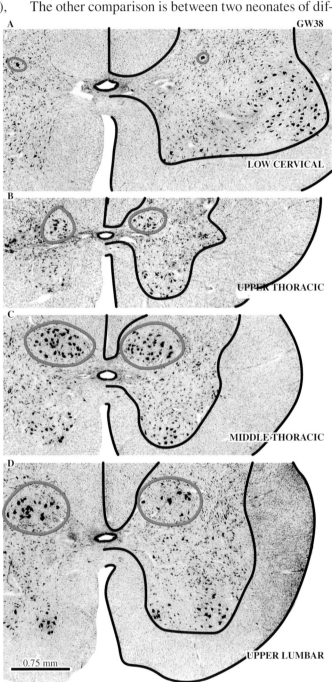

Figure 6-48. The length of Clarke's column in the spinal cord of one neonate (*Y117-61;* GW37; CR 310 mm). Clarke's column is absent in the low cervical cord (**A**), contains relatively few and smaller cells in the upper thoracic cord (**B**) and the middle thoracic cord (**C**), and tapers off in the upper lumbar cord (**D**).

Figure 6-49. The length of Clarke's column in the spinal cord of another neonate (*Y163-61;* GW38; CR 320 mm), matched in age and size with the previous specimen. Clarke's column begins in the low cervical cord (**A**), contains more and larger neurons in the upper thoracic cord (**B**) and middle thoracic cord (**C**), and is still of appreciable size in the upper lumbar cord (**D**).

ferent gestational age and size. In the younger and smaller neonate (*Y115-61*; GW40; 330 mm), Clarke's column is extensive in the upper and middle thoracic cord, and diminishes at lower thoracic levels (Figure 6-50). In contrast, in the older and larger neonate (*Y23-60*; GW44; 410 mm), Clarke's column is absent in the upper thoracic cord, well developed in the middle thoracic cord but small again in the low thoracic cord (Figure 6-51). The fact that Clarke's column is longer and larger in the smaller and younger neonate than in the larger and older neonate speaks against a simple correlation between gestational age and body size, on the one hand, and the size of Clarke's column, on the other. It suggests instead individual differences in Clarke's column, with possible functional implications.

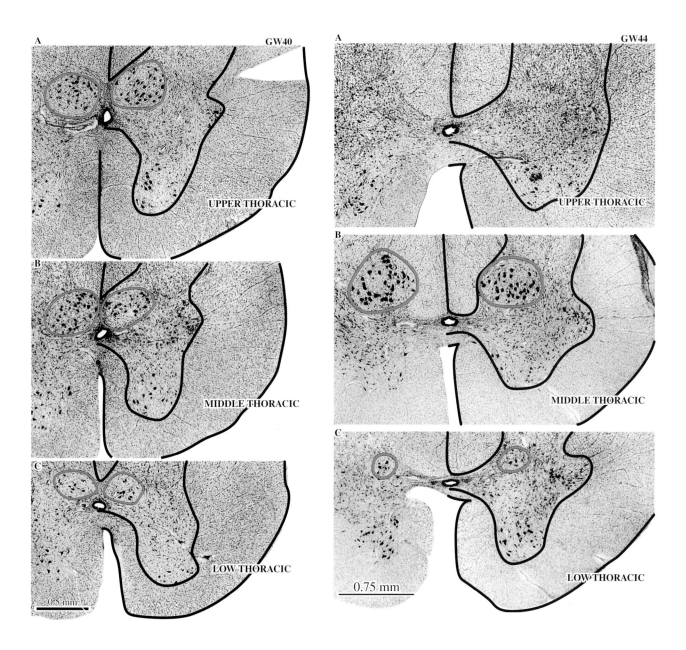

Figure 6-50. The length of Clarke's column in the spinal cord of the smaller and younger *Y115-6* neonate (GW40; CR 330 mm). Clarke's column is large in the upper thoracic cord (**A**) and middle thoracic cord (**B**) but tapers off in the low thoracic cord (**C**).

Figure 6-51. The length of Clarke's column in the spinal cord of the larger and older *Y23-60* neonate (GW44; CR 410 mm). In this specimen, Clarke's column is absent in the upper thoracic cord (**A**), is well developed in the middle thoracic cord (**B**), but tapers off in the low thoracic cord (**C**).

6.5   Development of Ventral Horn Motoneurons, Interneurons, and Interstitial Glia

6.5.1   Development of Motoneurons, the Segregation of Motoneuron Columns, and the Expansion of the Ventral Interneuronal Field. The growth of motoneuron perikarya, the segregation of motor columns, and the maturation of the ventral

interneuronal field are compared in two fetuses at several levels of the cervical and thoracic spinal cord in Figures 6-52 to 6-57. One of these specimens is an early second trimester fetus (GW14; *Y68-65*; CR 108 mm), the other a late second trimester fetus (GW26; *Y60-61*; CR 210 mm). (The ventral horn of the older fetus is reproduced at a lower magnification.)

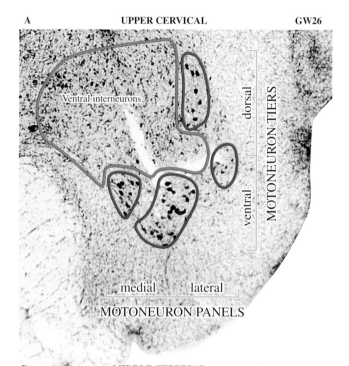

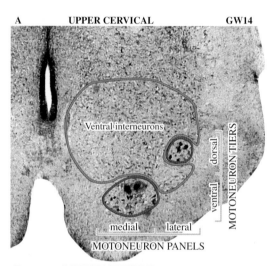

Figure 6-52. Contiguous motor clusters and an indistinct field of ventral interneurons in an early second trimester fetus (*Y68-65*; GW14; CR 108 mm) in the upper cervical (**A**) and middle cervical (**B**) ventral horn.

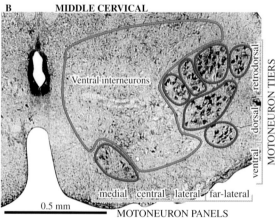

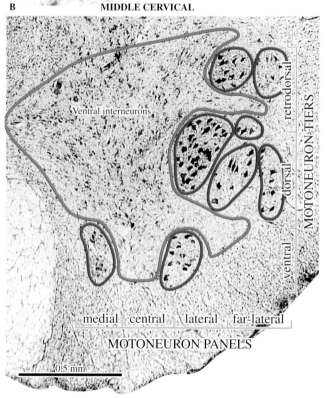

Figure 6-53. Segregation of motor columns, greater prominence of interneurons, and expansion of the ventral interneuronal field in a late second trimester fetus (GW26; *Y60-61*; CR 210 mm) in the upper cervical (**A**) and midcervical (**B**) ventral horn.

In the upper cervical cord of the GW14 fetus (Figure 6-52A), the motoneurons of the ventral horn form two clusters, one medially, the other laterally. At the corresponding level in the GW26 fetus (Figure 6-53A), there are four columns and there is reduction in the packing density of motoneurons within the columns. Also noteworthy is the greater prominence of interneurons in the ventral horn in the older fetus.

The segregation of motor columns in the lateral and far-lateral panels is more pronounced in the older fetus in the middle cervical cord. In the GW14 fetus (Figure 6-52B), the motoneurons are tightly

Figure 6-54. Contiguous motor clusters and an indistinct field of ventral interneurons in the early second trimester fetus (GW14; *Y68-65*; CR 108 mm) at two successive levels (**A, B**) in the lower cervical ventral horn.

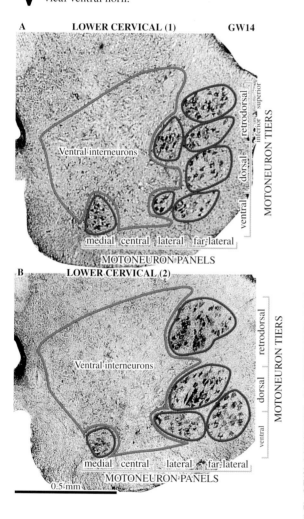

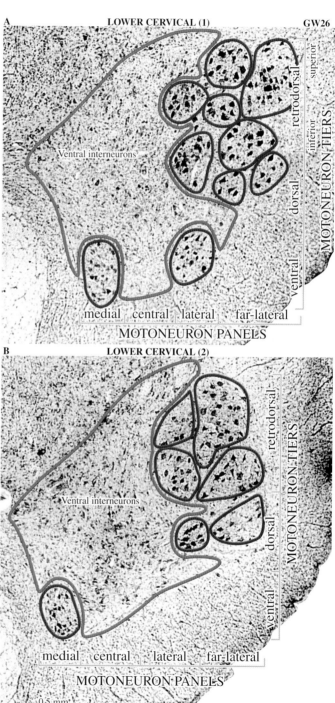

Figure 6-55. Segregation and increased number of motor columns, greater prominence of ventral interneurons, and expansion of the ventral interneuronal field in the late second trimester fetus (GW26; *Y60-61*; CR 210 mm) at two successive levels (**A, B**) in the lower cervical ventral horn.

packed and the segregating motor columns are contiguous; however, they can be assigned to three tiers (the ventral, dorsal, and retrodorsal) and two panels (the lateral and far-lateral). In the GW26 fetus (Figure 6-53B), the packing density of motoneurons is reduced and the spatial separation between the motor columns has increased. In association with these changes, the field of ventral interneurons has expanded and, due to their more intense staining, the interneurons have become more prominent. These developments suggest great advances in the cytologi-

cal maturation of the cervical ventral horn by the end of the second trimester.

The progressive segregation of larger motoneuron clusters into smaller motor columns between the beginning and the end of the second trimester is even more obvious in the lower cervical cord where, in addition, there is also an increase in the total number of separate motor columns (compare Figures 6-54 and 6-55). These changes are associated with the reduction in the packing density of motoneurons

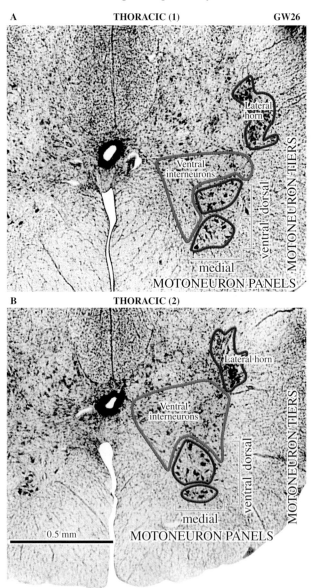

Figure 6-57. Modest increase in the segregation of motor columns and expansion of the ventral interneuronal field in the late second trimester fetus (GW26; *Y60-61*; CR 210 mm) at two levels (**A, B**) of the thoracic spinal cord.

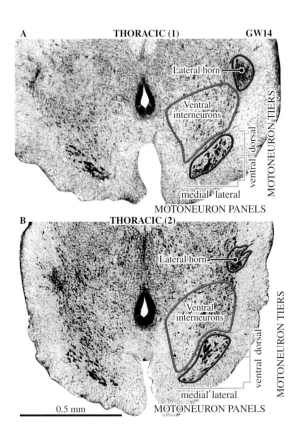

Figure 6-56. Motor columns and the field of ventral interneurons in the early second trimester fetus (GW14; *Y68-65*; CR 108 mm) at two levels (**A, B**) of the thoracic spinal cord.

within the columns. The segregated motor columns, which are gradually moving apart in particular in the far-lateral panel of the retrodorsal tier, contain fewer but larger motoneurons in the older fetus. We may recall that the lower cervical motoneuros innervate the distal muscles of the forearm and hand. The perikaryal growth of interneurons and the expansion of the ventral interneuronal field is also evident in the older fetus. In contrast to the lower cervical cord, the segregation of motor columns and the growth of the interneuronal field is modest in the thoracic cord

between GW14 and a GW26 (compare Figures 6-56 and 6-57). This region of the ventral horn, which innervates the axial muscles of the trunk, has no lateral, far-lateral, and retrodorsal motor columns.

The lumbar cord was not available in the GW26 fetus; hence the comparison is made at this level of the cord between the GW14 fetus and an early third trimester fetus (GW29; Y22-65; CR235 mm). The differences between the two specimens in the upper lumbar cord are obvious (compare Figures 6-58

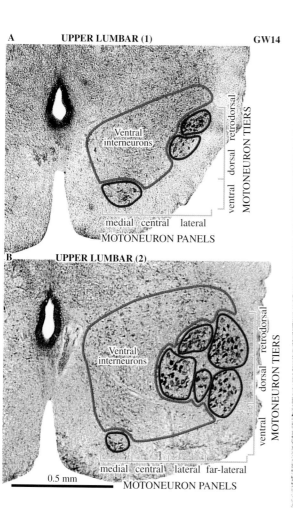

Figure 6-58. Contiguous motor clusters and an indistinct field of ventral interneurons in the early second trimester fetus (GW14; *Y68-65*; CR 108 mm) at two successive levels (**A, B**) in the upper lumbar ventral horn.

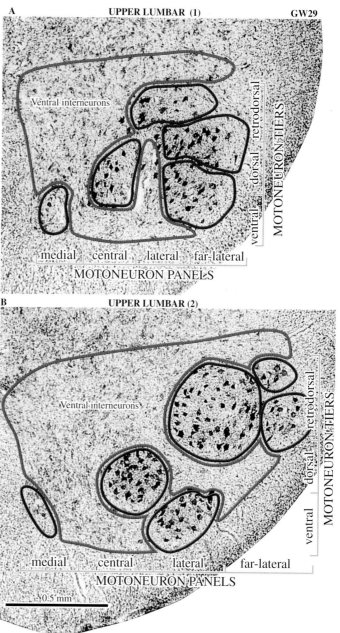

Figure 6-59. Segregation of motor columns, dispersion of motoneurons within the columns, greater prominence of interneurons, and the expansion of the field of ventral interneurons in the early third trimester fetus (GW29; *Y222-65*; CR 235 mm) at two successive levels (**A, B**) of the upper lumbar ventral horn.

and 6-59). Even more pronounced in the older fetus is the reduction in the packing density of motoneurons, the segregation of motor columns, and the growing prominence of ventral horn interneurons in the lower lumbar cord (compare Figures 6-60 and 6-61). This is the region of the lumbar cord that controls the distal muscles of the lower limb (ankle and toes). The great increase in the size and complexity of motoneurons during and after the second trimester is discussed in the next section.

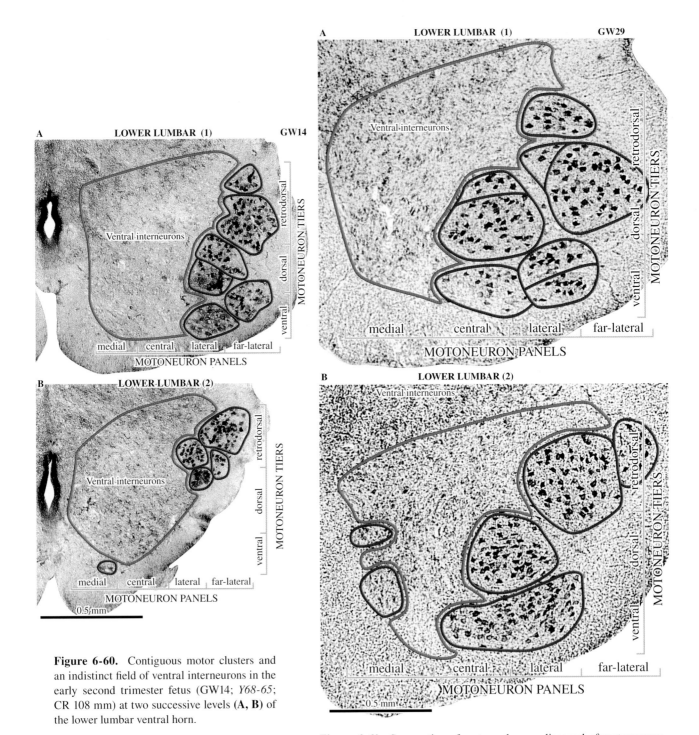

Figure 6-60. Contiguous motor clusters and an indistinct field of ventral interneurons in the early second trimester fetus (GW14; *Y68-65*; CR 108 mm) at two successive levels (**A, B**) of the lower lumbar ventral horn.

Figure 6-61. Segregation of motor columns, dispersal of motoneurons within the columns, greater prominence of interneurons, and the expansion of the field of ventral interneurons in an early third trimester fetus (GW29; *Y222-65*; CR 235 mm) at two successive levels (**A, B**) of the lower lumbar ventral horn.

6.5.2 Growth of Motoneurons and Ventral Interneurons, and the Increase in Glial Concentration Through the Fetal Period.

The perikaryal growth of ventral horn motoneurons and interneurons, and the concurremt increase in glial concentration in the lumbar spinal cord during the second and third trimesters, are illustrated in four specimens in Figures 6-62 and 6-63.

While the perikarya of motoneurons are easy to distinguish by virtue of their large size and intense staining from other ventral horn cells in the younger second trimester fetus (GW19; *Y52-61*; CR 130 mm; Figure 6-62A), they have not yet acquired their mature multipolar shape. In contrast, in the older second trimester fetus (GW21; *Y390-62*; CR 200 mm; Figure 6-62B), the perikarya of motoneurons have grown considerably and their multipolar shape is obvious. This suggests that the second stage of the dendritic development of motoneurons, signaling the outgrowth of multiple dendrites (compare with Figure 3-37/V), begins at about the middle of the second trimester.

Small spherical glia are clearly present within and between the motor columns in the GW19 fetus (Figure 6-62A). The concentration of these interstitial glia (presumably astrocytes) is comparable to the concentration of interfascicular glia (presumably oligodendroglia) in the neighboring ventral and lateral funiculi. The presence of glia is less clear in this specimen in the ventral interneuronal field because the glia are difficult to distinguish from the small, immature interneurons. However, in the older and much larger GW21 fetus (Figure 6-62B), the small spherical glia that are present are easy to distinguish from the larger, spindle-shaped ventral interneurons.

These limited observations suggest that the proliferation of interstitial glia in the ventral horn parallels the proliferation of interfascicular glia in the adjacent white matter.

The perikaryal growth of the multipolar motoneurons continues through the third trimester in association with the progressive dispersal of motoneurons within the motor columns, as seen in the GW29 fetus (*Y222-65*; CR 235 mm; Figure 6-63A) and the GW40 neonate (*Y115-61*; CR 330 mm: Figure 6-63B). This may reflect both ongoing dendritic development and the growth of the surrounding neuropil. There is no obvious increase in the concentration of glia within the same unit area in these specimens. However, since the motor columns are expanding considerably during this period, there must be a proportional increase in the ventral horn glial population. The progressive growth of motoneuron perikarya and their dispersion within the motor columns, and the inferred increase in the total glial population (which does not decrease as the motor columns expand) are illustrated at higher magnification in cell body-stained sections of the lumbar spinal cord in a GW21 (*Y390-62*; CR 200 mm; Figure 6-64A), GW29 (*Y222-65*; CR 235 mm; Figure 6-64B), and a GW33 (*Y36-60*; CR 315 mm; Figure 6-64C) fetus.

The inference that the progressive dispersal of motoneurons and expansion of motor columns are due to the growth of motoneuron dendrites and the increased complexity of the motor column neuropil, is supported by comparing the ventral horn in Bielschowsky-stained sections of a GW29 fetus (*Y20-60*; CR 270 mm; Figure 6-65A) and a late-term neonate (GW44; *Y23-60*; CR 410 mm; Figure 6-65B).

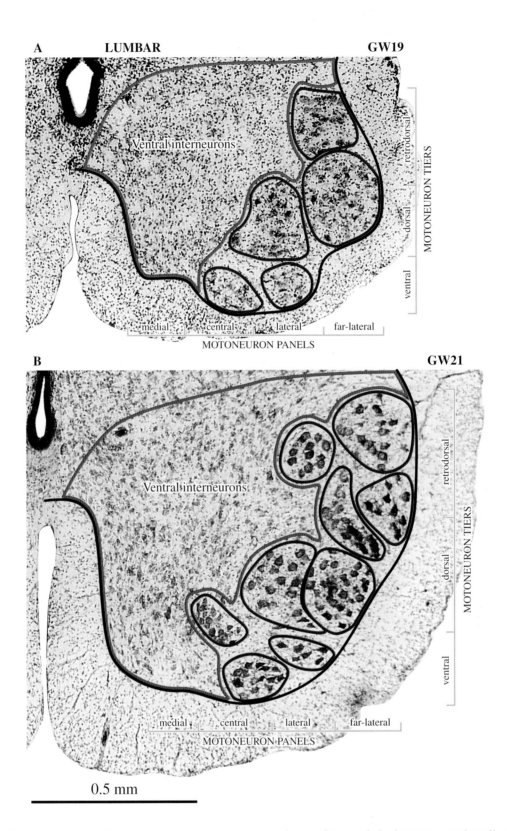

Figure 6-62. The ventral horn of the lumbar spinal cord in two second trimester fetuses. **A.** In the younger and smaller fetus (GW19, *Y52-61*; CR 130 mm) the motoneurons have not yet acquired their mature multipolar shape, The presence of small glia is evident within and between the motor columns but is less obvious in the adjacent field of immature interneurons. **B.** In the older and much larger fetus (GW21, *Y390-62;* CR 200 mm) the greatly enlarged motoneuron perikaryas have become distinctly multipolar, suggesting the onset of their second stage of dendritic development. (Compare with Figure 3-37/V.) Also notable is the perikaryal growth of ventral interneurons and the presence of glia among them.

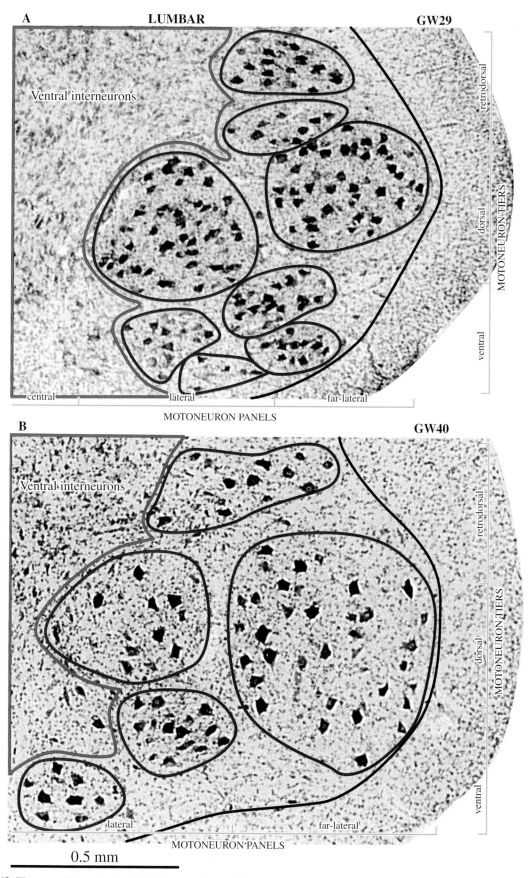

Figure 6-63. The ventral horn in **A**, a third trimester fetus (GW29; *Y222-65*; CR 235 mm), and **B**, a neonate (GW40; *Y115-61*; CR 330 mm). Noteworthy during this period is the progressive growth of motoneuron perikarya, their dispersion within the motor columns, and the high concentration of ventral horn glia.

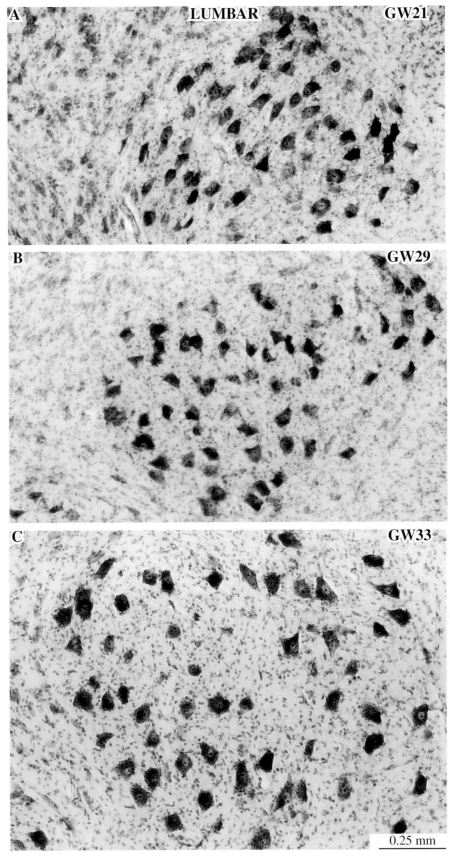

Figure 6-64. Motoneurons in a lateral motor column, visualized with cell body-staining, in the lumbar spinal cord of **A**, a GW21 (*Y390-62*; CR 200 mm), **B**, a GW29 (*Y222-65*; CR 235 mm), and **C**, a GW33 (*Y36-60*; CR 315 mm) fetus. Notable developments are the progressive dispersal of motoneurons, their perikaryal growth and more pronounced multipolarity, and the sustained high concentration of interstitial glia (suggesting continuing cell proliferation).

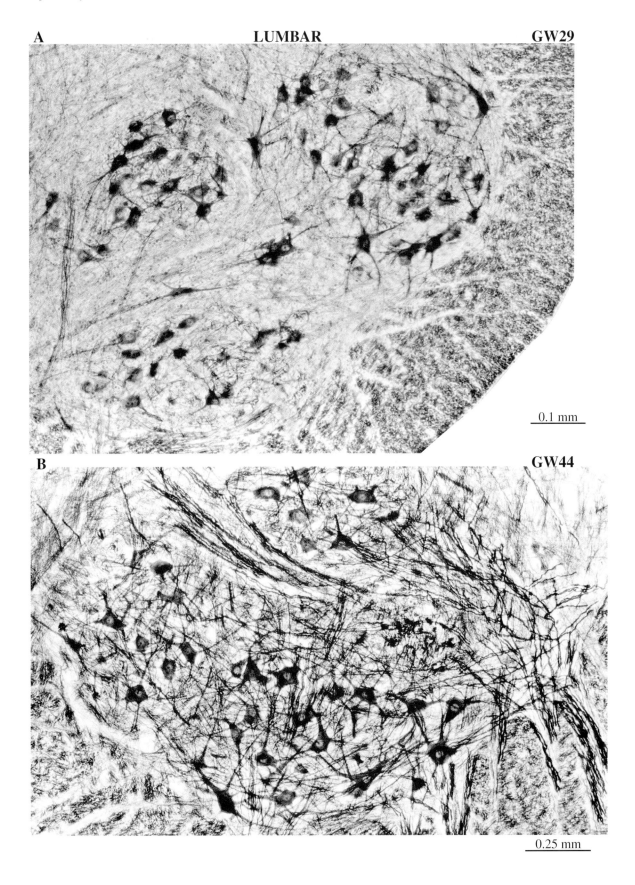

A **LUMBAR** **GW29**

0.1 mm

B **GW44**

0.25 mm

Figure 6-65. Dendritic development of motoneurons, visualized with the Bielschowsky staining technique, in the lumbar spinal cord of **A**, a GW29 fetus (*Y20-60*; CR 270 mm), and **B**, a late-term neonate (GW44; *Y23-60*; CR 410 mm). The dendritic development of motoneurons in the neonate is associated with an increased complexity of the ventral horn neuropil.

7 GROWTH OF THE HUMAN CORTICOSPINAL TRACTS DURING THE PRENATAL PERIOD

7.1 Growth of the Upper, Middle, and Lower Corticofugal Tracts

7.1.1 The Great Corticofugal System and the Lateral and Ventral Corticospinal Tracts. The descending axons and collaterals of the cerebral cortex terminate widely throughout the subcortical telencephalon (such as the basal ganglia), diencephalon (thalamus and hypothalamus), midbrain (tectum and tegmentum), pons, and medulla before they reach the spinal cord (Figure 7-1). The entire efferent system constitutes the great corticofugal tract, and it may be divided into four components. The first three compo-

nents terminate or give off collaterals at supraspinal levels: (1) the upper corticofugal tract (traditonally known as the internal capsule) traverses and gives off collaterals in the basal telencephalon; (2) the middle corticofugal tract (the cerebral peduncle or crus cerebri) collateralizes in the diencephalon and midbrain; and (3) the lower corticofugal tract (sometimes called the corticobulbar tract) collateralizes in the pons and the medulla.

The fibers of the lower corticofugal tract traverse the pontine gray as discrete fascicles. Collaterals of transpontine corticofugal axons synapse with

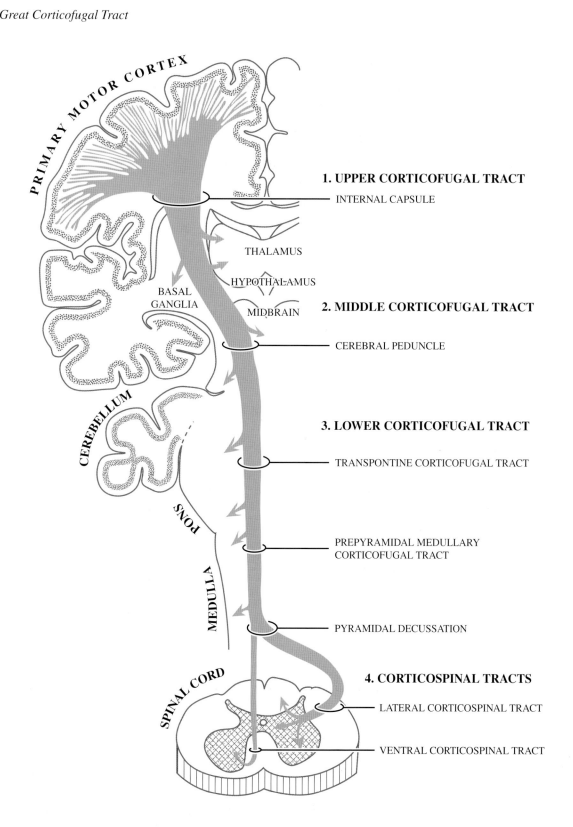

Figure 7-1. Four components of the great corticofugal tract. (**1**) The upper portion of the corticofugal tract, known as the internal capsule, converges upon and traverses the basal ganglia (striatum). (**2**) Its middle portion, known as the cerebral peduncle, descends along the lateral wall of the diencephalon and midbrain. (**3**) The lower corticofugal tract, known as the corticobulbar tract and the transpontine corticofugal tract, funnels through the pontine gray. At all these levels, collaterals of the descending axons terminate in various supraspinal brain structures. (**4**) The last component of the descending corticofugal tract forms the pyramids in the lower medulla. This is the corticospinal tract proper, and it has two components. The contralaterally terminating component, which crosses to the opposite side in the pyramidal decussation, forms the lateral corticospinal tract. The ipsilateral component is the ventral (or anterior) corticospinal tract. Illustration modified after Phillips and Porter (1977).

the neurons of the pontine gray, the source of the massive pontocerebellar fiber system, which reaches the cerebellum by way of the middle cerebellar peduncle (brachium pontis). Other fibers of the lower corticofugal system are distributed to various nuclei of the medulla, including the dorsal column nuclei. The fourth component of the descending corticofugal tract is the corticospinal tract proper. Fibers of the corticospinal tract form the medullary pyramids, where most of them cross to the opposite side in the pyramidal decussation. Other fibers continue uncrossed. The crossed (contralateral) fibers form the lateral corticospinal tract in the lateral funiculus of the spinal cord. The uncrossed (ipsilateral) fibers form the ventral corticospinal tract in the ventromedial funiculus.

7.1.2 Growth of the Upper, Middle, and Lower Corticofugal Tracts. Age: GW8.5 to GW19.

The fibers of the corticofugal tract are axons of lamina V neurons of the cerebral cortex (Section 2.2.6). The neurons of the cerebral cortex originate in the cortical neuroepithelium (Bayer and Altman, 1991). After their exodus, the differentiating cortical neurons sojourn in the intermediate zone and then settle in the cortex as a compact sheet of immature neurons, known as the cortical plate. Cell body-stained sections from specimens ranging between GW7.5 and GW19 reveal the growth of the corticofugal tract through the brain.

GW7.5. The neuroepithelium is prominent but the cortical plate is absent in the GW7.5 embryo (*M2314*; CR 23.8 mm) illustrated in Figure 7-2A. The fiber bundle in the lateral thalamus is the initial portion of the thalamocortical radiation (tract) which has yet to cross into and invade the telencephalon. There is no fiber bridge between the telencephalon and diencephalon, and the existence of a corticofugal tract can be ruled out at this stage of development.

GW8.5 to GW11. The cortical plate is well developed in a GW8.5 embryo (*C609*; CR 32 mm;

A   **GW7.5**
— Cortical neuroepithelium
— Striatal neuroepithelium
— Thalamocortical radiation (local)
— Thalamus
— Hypothalamus

B   **GW8.5**
Cortical neuroepithelium
Cortical intermediate zone
Cortical plate
Striatal neuroepithelium
Internal capsule
Thalamus
Cerebral peduncle (?)
Basal ganglia
Striatal neuroepithelium
Thalamocortical radiation
Hypothalamus

C   **GW9.5**
Striatal neuroepithelium
Thalamus
Internal capsule
Basal ganglia
Cerebral peduncle
Hypothalamus
1 mm

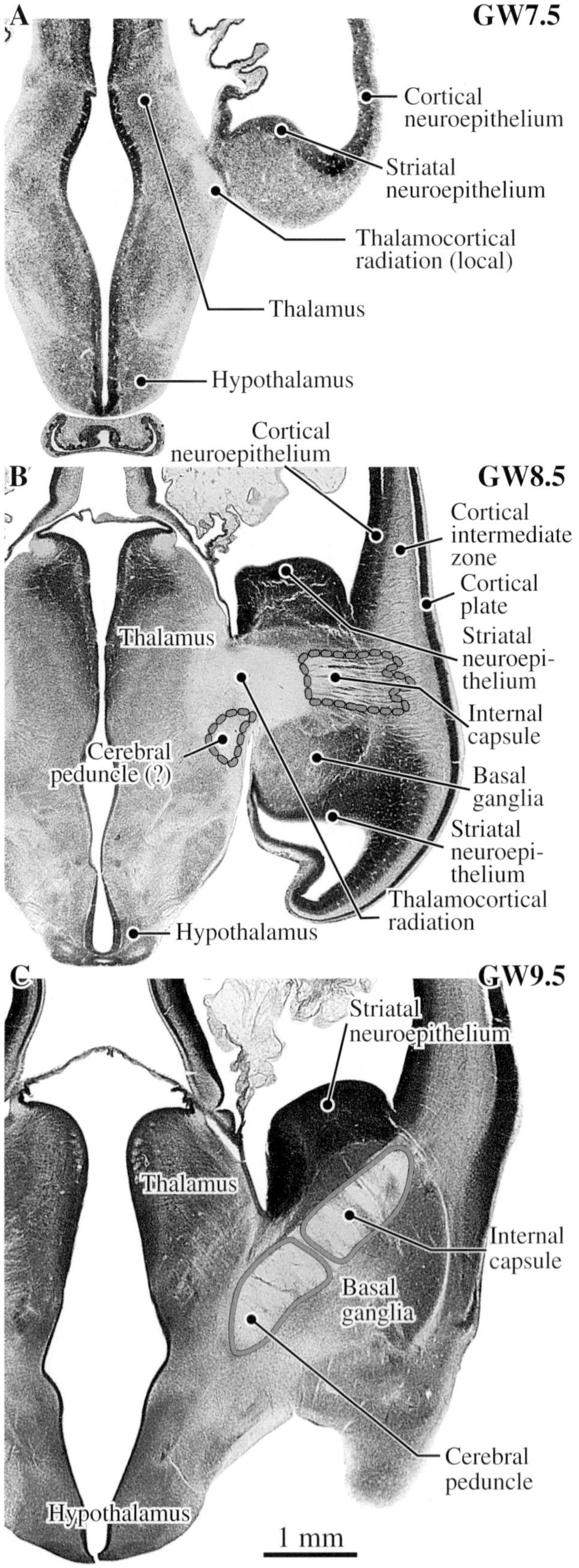

Figure 7-2. Maturation of the cerebral cortex in relation to the emergence and expansion of the corticofugal tract in cell body-stained coronal sections of human embryos. **A.** In this GW7.5 embryo (*M2314*; CR 23.8 mm), the primitive cerebral cortex consists solely of the proliferative neuroepithelium; the intermediate zone and the cortical plate are not yet present. **B.** In this GW8.5 embryo (*C609*; CR 32 mm), there is an active migration of differentiating neurons and many have settled in the cortical plate. Concurrently, ascending thalamocortical fibers begin to radiate en masse into the telencephalon. The presence of descending corticofugal fibers is less certain, although a small cerebral peduncle seems to be present. **C.** In this GW9.5 fetus (*C3699*; CR 47 mm), the internal capsule is well developed and the descending corticofugal fibers form a small cerebral peduncle along the wall of the diencephalon.

GW9.5 Cell body stain

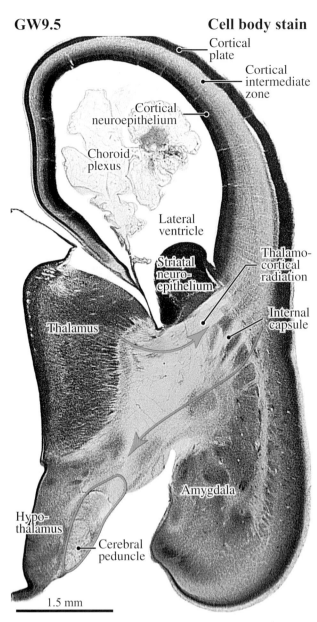

Figure 7-3. The ascending thalamocortical radiation (blue arrow) and the descending corticofugal tract (orange arrow) in the GW9.5 embryo (*C3699*; CR 47 mm) more rostrally and at a higher magnification. The cerebral peduncle, though small, is clearly delineated.

A GW11 Cell body stain

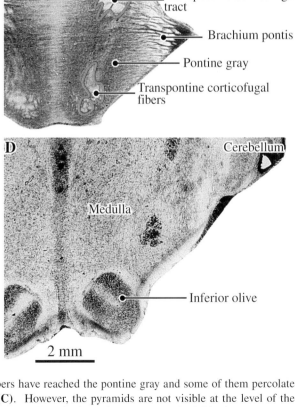

Figure 7-4. Growth of the descending corticofugal tract in a GW11 embryo (*Y1-59*; CR 60 mm). The internal capsule has expanded at the level of the anterior thalamus (**A**), and so has the cerebral peduncle at the level of the posterior thalamus (**B**). Farther caudally, the descending fibers have reached the pontine gray and some of them percolate through it to form the transpontine corticofugal tract (**C**). However, the pyramids are not visible at the level of the developing inferior olive in the medulla (**D**), indicating that corticospinal tract has not yet reached this site.

Figure 7-2B). In this specimen, many thalamocortical fibers traverse the striatum and radiate into the intermediate zone of the cerebral cortex. It is possible that the ventral portion of the incipient internal capsule contains the earliest corticofugal fibers. There is a hint of the formation of the cerebral peduncle in the lateral wall of the diencephalon but that identification is uncertain. In a GW9.5 fetus (*C3699*; CR 47 mm; Figure 7-2C), the internal capsule is evident as a prominent fibrous mass bisecting the basal ganglia, and the cerebral peduncle is recognizable beneath it. Since the cerebral peduncle is not visible at lower midbrain levels in this embryo (not illustrated), this may be the age (roughly between GW9 to GW10) when the earliest corticofugal fibers begin their descent into the brainstem. The trajectory of the ascending thalamocortical fibers and of the descending corticofugal fibers in the GW9.5 fetus is shown at higher magnification at another coronal level in Figure 7-3.

We can follow the descent of the corticofugal tract in a GW11 embryo (*Y1-59*; CR 60 mm) from the cerebral cortex, through the basal ganglia (Figure 7-4A), and along the wall of the diencephalon (Figure 7-4B) to the pontine gray (Figure 7-4C). In the pontine gray, some of the descending fibers have begun to percolate through the bed of transversely oriented fibers of the brachium pontis (Figure 7-4C). However, none of the descending fibers have reached the medulla at the level of the developing inferior olive (Figure 7-4D).

GW19. The development of the corticofugal fiber system continues during the early weeks of the second trimester. We follow this growth in a GW19 fetus (*Y15-63*; CR 150 mm) in seven rostral-to-caudal sections in Figures 7-5, 7-6 and 7-7. The internal capsule and the cerebral peduncle are massive at the level of the rostral diencephalon (Figures 7-5A, B). The cerebral peduncle is extensive in the transitional region between the diencephalon and the midbrain (Figure 7-6A) and the fascicles that traverse the pontine gray (Figure 7-6B) are bulkier than those seen toward the end of the first trimester (Figure 7-4C). Many of these transpontine fibers leave the pontine gray, pass the upper medulla ventromedial to the inferior olive, and form the pyramids in the lower medulla (Figures 7-7A, B, C). We could not determine in this fetus what proportion of these corticospinal fibers decussate and grow into the spinal cord.

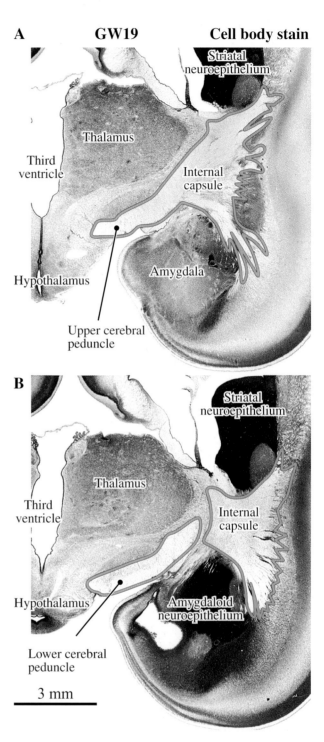

Figure 7-5. Corticofugal tract fibers in the expanding internal capsule and cerebral peduncle in a GW19 fetus (*Y15-63*; CR 150 mm) at the level of the anterior (**A**) and posterior (**B**) diencephalon.

In summary, the foregoing observations suggest that fibers of the outgrowing corticofugal tract reach the diencephalon by about GW9.5 and begin to percolate through the pontine gray by GW11. However, they do not reach the medulla until some time around GW19, that is, the middle of the second trimester. As we shall see below, the pyramids (corticospinal tract) form some time about GW20.

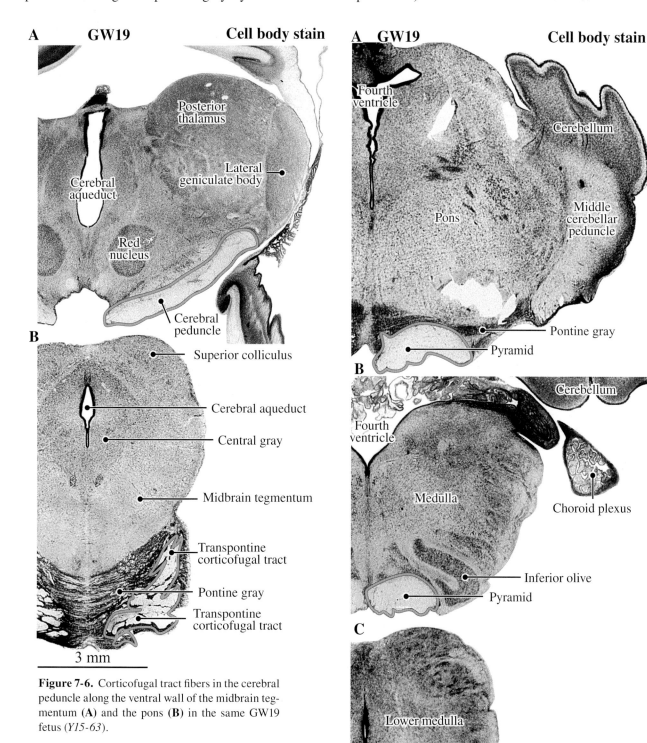

Figure 7-6. Corticofugal tract fibers in the cerebral peduncle along the ventral wall of the midbrain tegmentum (**A**) and the pons (**B**) in the same GW19 fetus (*Y15-63*).

Figure 7-7. Corticospinal tract fibers in the pyramids of the same fetus GW19 (*Y15-63*) at the level of the pons (**A**), the inferior olive (**B**), and lower medulla (**C**).

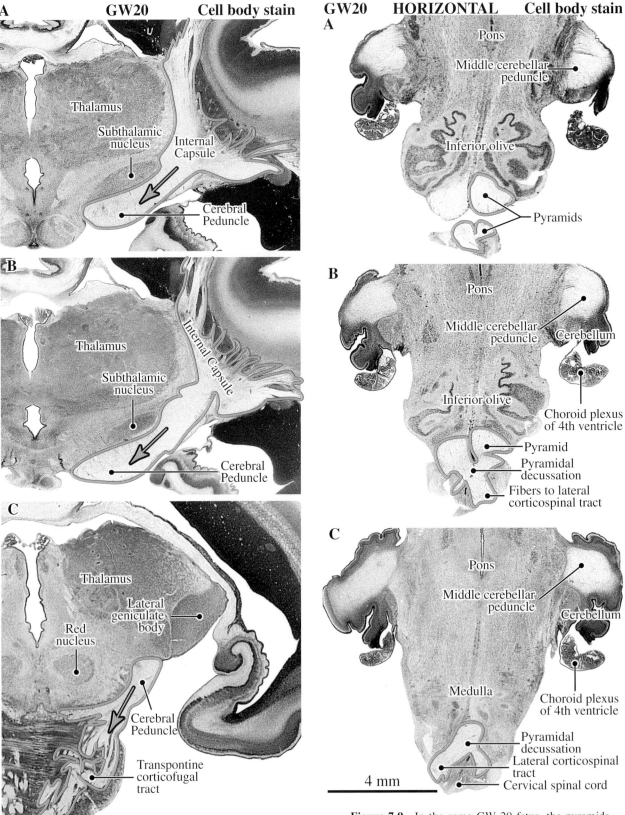

A   **GW20**   **Cell body stain**

Thalamus

Subthalamic nucleus

Internal Capsule

Cerebral Peduncle

B

Thalamus

Subthalamic nucleus

Internal Capsule

Cerebral Peduncle

C

Thalamus

Lateral geniculate body

Red nucleus

Cerebral Peduncle

Transpontine corticofugal tract

Pontine gray

4 mm

Figure 7-8. The corticofugal tract in a GW20 fetus (*Y17-63*; CM 165 mm) at rostral (**A**) and caudal (**B**) levels of the diencephalon. **C.** Fibers penetrate the pontine gray and form the transpontine portion of the corticofugal tract.

GW20   HORIZONTAL   Cell body stain
A

Pons

Middle cerebellar peduncle

Inferior olive

Pyramids

B

Pons

Middle cerebellar peduncle

Cerebellum

Inferior olive

Choroid plexus of 4th ventricle

Pyramid

Pyramidal decussation

Fibers to lateral corticospinal tract

C

Pons

Middle cerebellar peduncle

Cerebellum

Medulla

Choroid plexus of 4th ventricle

Pyramidal decussation

Lateral corticospinal tract

Cervical spinal cord

4 mm

Figure 7-9. In the same GW 20 fetus, the pyramids have grown appreciably in the upper medulla at the level of the inferior olive (**A**). Farther caudally in the lower medulla, the pyramidal tract decussates to form the lateral corticospinal tract (**B, C**).

7.1.3 Decussation of Corticospinal Fibers in the Medulla. Age: GW20 to GW28.

We follow the growth of the farthest component of the corticofugal system, the decussating corticospinal tract, in oblique horizontal and frontal sections in GW20, GW23, and GW28 fetuses in Figures 7-8 to 7-12.

GW20. In the GW20 fetus (*Y17-63*; CR 165 mm; Figures 7-8A, B), the internal capsule and cerebral peduncle are quite prominent in the rostral diencephalon and farther caudally the descending corticofugal fibers traverse the pontine gray in appreciable numbers (Figure 7-8C). In the same fetus, the pyramids are well developed in the upper medulla (Figure 7-9A) and a smaller complement of corticospinal tract fibers decussate farther caudally in the lower medulla (Figures 7-9B, C).

GW23. In the upper medulla, the pyramids are divisible into a dorsomedial and a ventrolateral component in the GW23 fetus (*Y197-65*; CR 190 mm; Figure 7-10A). In the lower medulla, the fibers of the dorsomedial component cross to the opposite side (Figures 7-10B, C). These fibers, as we shall see momentarily, form the contralateral corticospinal tract. The smaller complement of fibers of the ventrolateral pyramids do not change their position; they will form the ipsilateral ventral corticospinal tract.

GW28. The two components of the pyramids are more evident in frontal sections of the GW28 fetus (*Y183-64*; CR 225 mm). In this early third trimester fetus, the pyramids are elliptical in shape in the upper medulla beneath the inferior olive (Figures 7-11A, B) and become club-like farther caudally (Figure 7-11A). In the lower medulla, the "stem" of the club (the dorsomedial component of the pyramid) crosses to the opposite side underneath the central canal (Figures 7-11C, 712A). Finally, in the upper cervical cord, the stem becomes circular in shape; that is, it forms a longitudinally oriented fiber bundle (Figures 7-12B, C, D), the lateral corticospinal tract. In contrast, the "club" portion of the pyramid (its ventrolateral component) remains in that position in the lower medulla (Figures 7-12A, B), then shifts ventromedially in the upper cervical cord (Figure 7-12C, D) to form the ipsilateral ventral corticospinal tract.

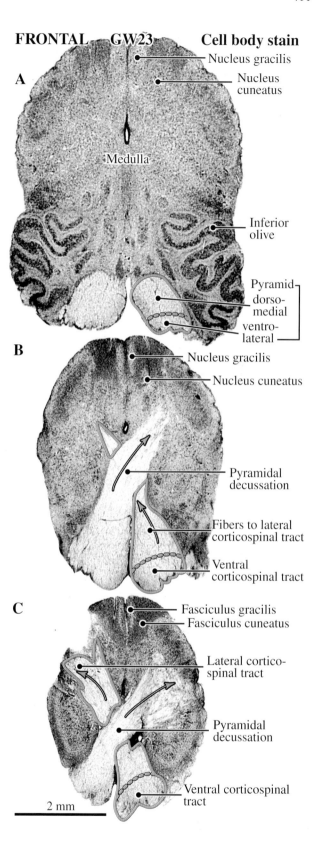

FRONTAL GW23 Cell body stain

A
Nucleus gracilis
Nucleus cuneatus
Medulla
Inferior olive
Pyramid—
dorso-medial
ventro-lateral

B
Nucleus gracilis
Nucleus cuneatus
Pyramidal decussation
Fibers to lateral corticospinal tract
Ventral corticospinal tract

C
Fasciculus gracilis
Fasciculus cuneatus
Lateral cortico-spinal tract
Pyramidal decussation
Ventral corticospinal tract

2 mm

Figure 7-10. In this GW23 fetus (*Y197-65*; CR 190 mm), the pyramids in the upper medulla are divisible into a dorso-medial and a ventrolateral component (**A**). The dorsomedial component decussates in the lower medulla (**B**) and ends in the upper cervical cord on the opposite side dorsolaterally (arrows) to form the lateral corticospinal tract (**C**).

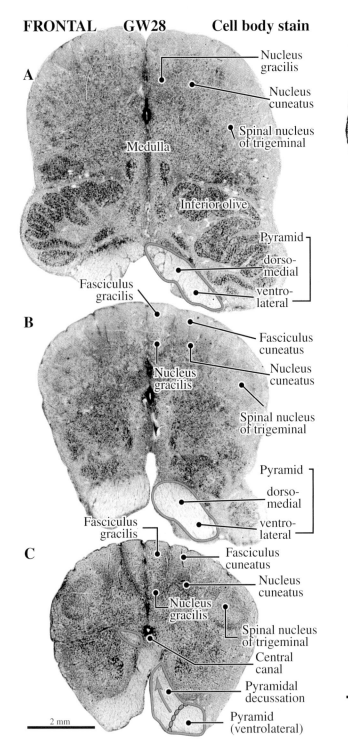

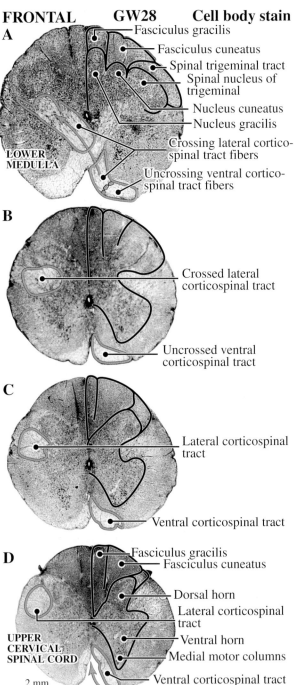

Figure 7-11. The segregation of the dorsomedial and ventrolateral portions of the corticospinal tract rostral to the pyramidal decussation in a GW28 fetus (*Y183-64*; CR 225 mm). In the upper medulla, the pyramids are elliptical in shape (**A, B**) while in the lower medulla they become club-shaped (**C**). The "stems" of the club-shaped pyramids cross to the opposite side beneath the central canal (arrow).

Figure 7-12. Decussation of the corticospinal fibers composing the "stems" (dorsomedial portion) of the pyramids in the same GW28 fetus (*Y183-64*) farther caudally in the lower medulla (**A**). Final position of the crossed lateral corticospinal tract in the upper cervical spinal cord (**B, C, D**). In contrast, the fibers in the "club" portion of the pyramids remain in a ventral position in the lower medulla, then shift farther medially in the cervical spinal cord (arrow). This is the ipsilateral ventral corticospinal tract.

7.1.4 The Incremental Growth of the Corticofugal Tract During the Second Trimester.

There is a great increase in the bulk of the corticofugal tract during the second trimester. That is shown in the midbrains of fetuses ranging in age from GW13.5 and GW28 (Figures 7-13 and 7-14) at the level of the red nucleus and underneath the substantia nigra. The cerebral peduncle is quite small in the GW13.5 fetus (*Y144-63*; CR 100 mm; Figure 7-13A). Its length and width doubles at the same level in one GW19 fetus (*Y15-63*; CR 150 mm; Figure 7-13B), and expands even more in another larger fetus of the same age (GW19; *Y17-63*; CR 165 mm; Figure 7-14A). Finally, in the GW28 fetus (*Y194-65*; CR 220 mm; Figure 7-14B) the length of the cerebral peduncle has more than tripled with respect to the GW13.5 fetus and its width has grown about fivefold.

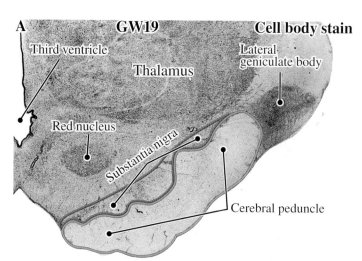

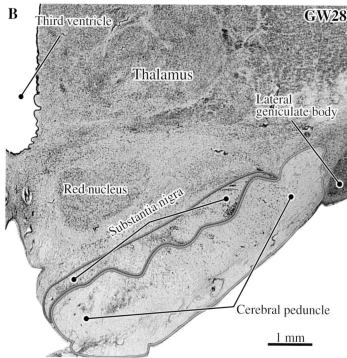

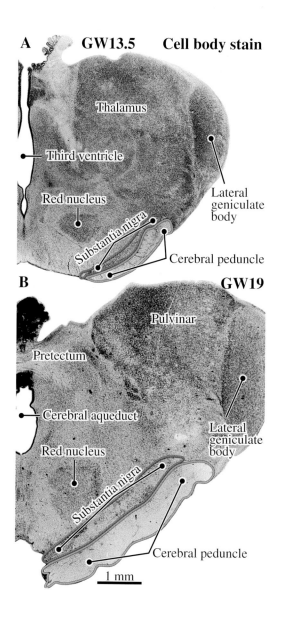

Figure 7-13. Growth of the descending corticospinal tract, as judged by the expansion of the cerebral peduncle at the level of the substantia nigra, in **A**, a GW13.5 fetus (*Y144-63*; CR 100 mm) and **B**, a GW19 fetus (*Y15-63*; CR 150 mm).

Figure 7-14. Continuing growth of the corticofugal tract, as judged by the expansion of the cerebral peduncle in **A**, a GW19 fetus (*Y17-63*; CR 165 mm) and **B**, a GW28 fetus (*Y194-65*; CR 220 mm).

We do not know what contributes to this great expansion. It is possible that some of it is due to the thickening of the corticofugal axons; but notably, myelination gliosis has not yet begun even in the oldest fetus. It is more likely that much of this expansion is due to the successive outgrowth of corticofugal fibers from different areas of the cereberal cortex. If that is correct, the question arises as to which areas of the cerebral cortex are the source of the early and the late descending corticofugal fibers.

7.1.5 The Onset of Myelination Gliosis in the Lower Corticofugal Tract During the Third Trimester.

High magnification microphotographs of cell body-stained sections are used to examine the onset of myelination gliosis (defined as the presence of and increase in the concentration of interfascicular glia) in the lower corticofugal tract at the level of the pontine gray (Figures 7-15 to 7-20), and in the corticospinal tract in the upper medulla at the level of the inferior olive (Figures 7-21 to 7-22).

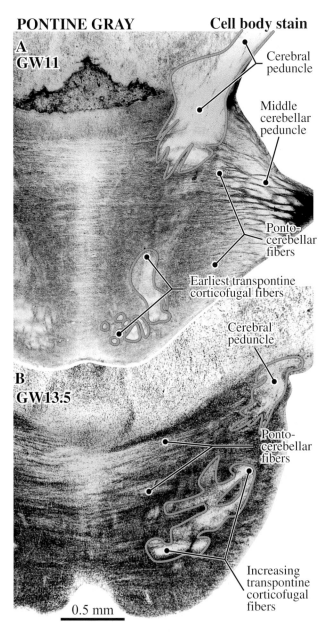

Figure 7-15. A. Absence of interfascicular glia in the cerebral peduncle that begins to penetrate the pontine gray in a GW11 embryo (*Y01-59*; CR 60 mm). **B.** While there are cells in the transpontine corticofugal tract in the GW13.5 fetus (*Y144-63*; CR 100 mm), observations in older embryos indicate that these are not glia but pontine gray neurons.

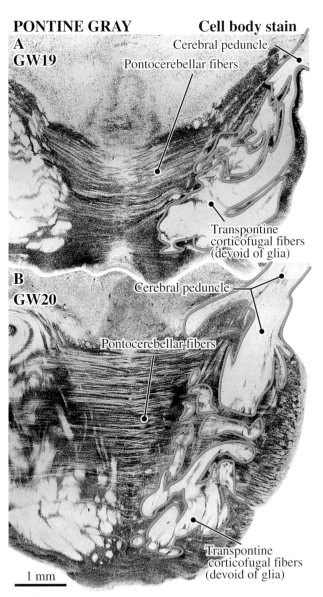

Figure 7-16. The expanding transpontine corticofugal tract is virtually devoid of interfascicular glia in **A**, a GW19 fetus (*Y15-63*; CR 150 mm) and **B**, a GW20 fetus (*Y17-63*; CR 165 mm).

In the GW11 embryo (*Y01-59*; CR 60 mm), the large corticofugal tract that starts to penetrate the pontine gray is devoid of interfascicular glia (Figure 7-15A). In the GW13.5 fetus (*Y144-63*; CR 100 mm; Figure 7-15B), a few fascicles of corticofugal fibers descend in the pons at a right angle to the transversely oriented fibers of the middle cerebellar peduncle (brachium pontis) that are embedded in a matrix of densely packed and darkly staining small cells. As we shall see below, an undetermined proportion of these small cells are young pontine gray neurons. Although there are some small cells within the transpontine tract in the GW13.5 fetus, these are prob-

ably not proliferating glia because there are no glia present in the expanding transpontine tract in several of the older specimens: the GW19 fetus (*Y15-63*; 150 mm; Figure 7-16A); the GW20 fetus (*Y17-63*; 165 mm; Figure 7-16B); and the GW22 fetus (*Y22-59*; 190 mm; Figure 7-17A). There is a hint of glia appearing

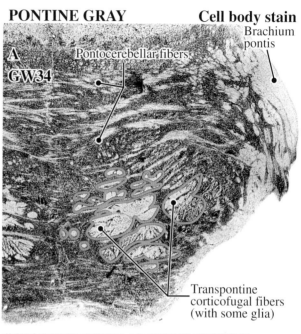

PONTINE GRAY **Cell body stain**

A GW34

Pontocerebellar fibers

Brachium pontis

Transpontine corticofugal fibers (with some glia)

PONTINE GRAY **Cell body stain**

A GW22

Pontocerebellar fibers

Transpontine corticofugal fibers (devoid of glia)

1 mm

B GW28

Pontocerebellar fibers

Cerebral peduncle

Brachium pontis

Transpontine corticofugal fibers (devoid of glia)

1 mm

Figure 7-17. Most of the fascicles of the massive transpontine corticofugal tract are still devoid of interfascicular glia in **A**, a GW22 fetus (*Y22-59*; CR 190 mm) and **B**, a GW28 fetus (*Y194-65*; CR 220 mm).

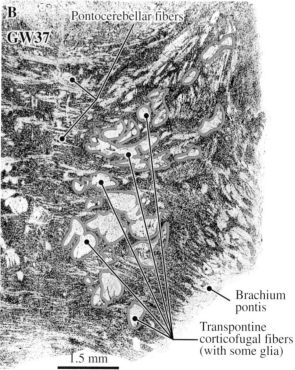

B GW37

Pontocerebellar fibers

Brachium pontis

Transpontine corticofugal fibers (with some glia)

1.5 mm

Figure 7-18. Moderate increase in the concentration of interfascicular glia in the thinning fascicles of the transpontine corticofugal tract in **A**, a late third trimester fetus (GW34; *Y232-66*; CR 295 mm) and **B**, a preterm neonate (GW37; *Y217-65*; CR 350 mm).

in increasing numbers in the GW28 fetus (*Y194-65*; 220 mm; Figure 7-17B). More glia are present in the late third trimester GW34 fetus (*Y232-66*; 295 mm; Figure 7-18A) and the newborn (GW37; *Y217-65*; 350 mm; Figure 7-18B). That may be the beginning of myelination gliosis in the transpontine corticofugal tract.

During the third trimester, the onset of myelination gliosis appears to be associated with (a) the partitioning of the large transpontine corticofugal bundles into smaller fascicles and (b) with the maturation of pontine gray neurons. Thus, the large bundles of transpontine fibers in the younger fetuses (GW19, GW22, GW28) contain few interfascicular

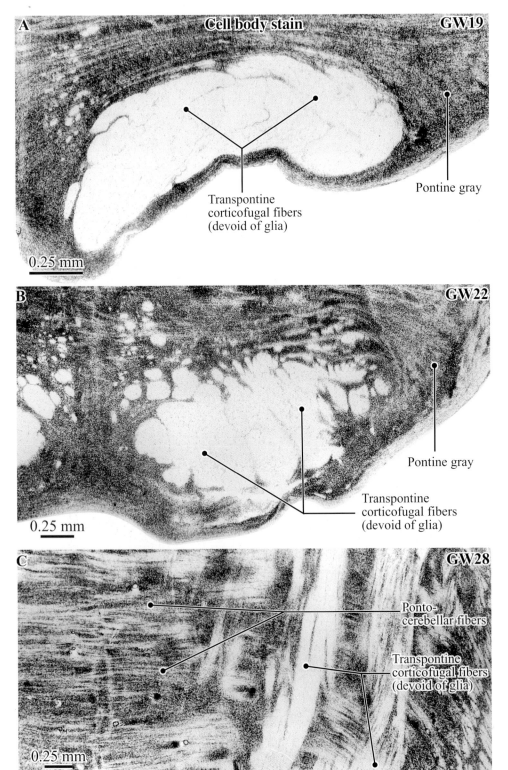

A Cell body stain   GW19

Transpontine
corticofugal fibers
(devoid of glia)

Pontine gray

0.25 mm

B   GW22

Pontine gray

Transpontine
corticofugal fibers
(devoid of glia)

0.25 mm

C   GW28

Ponto-
cerebellar fibers

Transpontine
corticofugal fibers
(devoid of glia)

0.25 mm

Figure 7-19. The transpontine corticofugal tract with few or no interfascicular glia in **A**, the GW19 fetus (*Y15-63*; CR 150 mm), **B**, the GW22 fetus (*Y22-59*; CR 190 mm) and **C**, the GW28 fetus (*Y194-65*; CR 220 mm).

glia (Figures 7-19A-C). The onset of myelination gliosis in the late third trimester fetus (GW34; Figure 7-20A) and in the neonate (GW37; Figure 7-20B) is associated with the formation of smaller transpontine fascicles, the enlargement of pontine gray neurons, and the appearance of many interfascicular glia.

The concentration of glia in the pyramids of the upper medulla is illustrated at higher magnification in Figures 7-21 and 7-22. The miniscule corticospinal tract of the GW13.5 fetus (*Y144-63*; CR 100 mm; Figure 7-21A) contains few glia. There is a small concentration of glia in the larger corticospi-

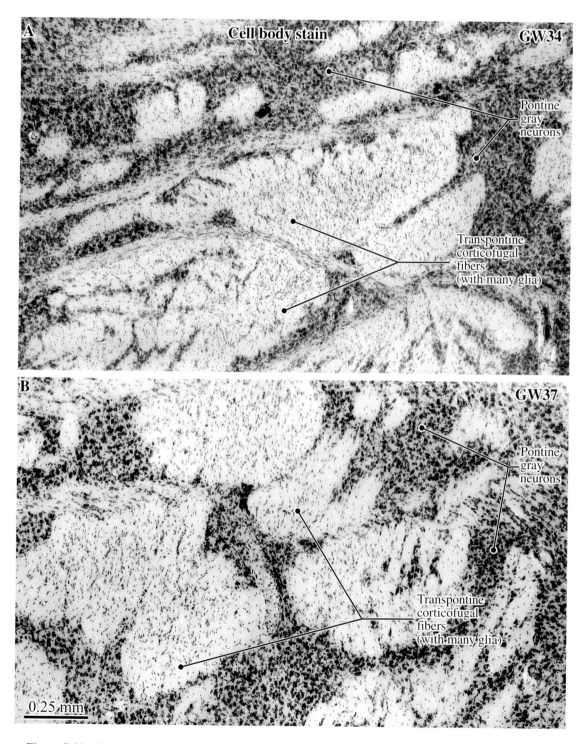

Figure 7-20. Great increase in the concentration of glia in the partitioning transpontine corticofugal tract of **A**, the late third trimester fetus (GW34, *Y232-66*; CR 295 mm) and **B**, the GW37 preterm neonate (*Y217-65*; CR 350 mm).

nal tract of the GW19 fetus (*Y15-63*; CR 150 mm; Figure 7-21B) but that concentration is far below what is in the fibrous capsule of the adjacent inferior olive. There is little change (perhaps a reduction) in glial concentration in the GW22 fetus (*Y22-59*; CR 190 mm; Figure 7-22A) and only a slight increase in the late third trimester (GW34; *Y232-66*; CR 295 mm; Figure 7-22B). These observations suggest that myelination gliosis in the corticospinal tract has not yet begun during the perinatal period.

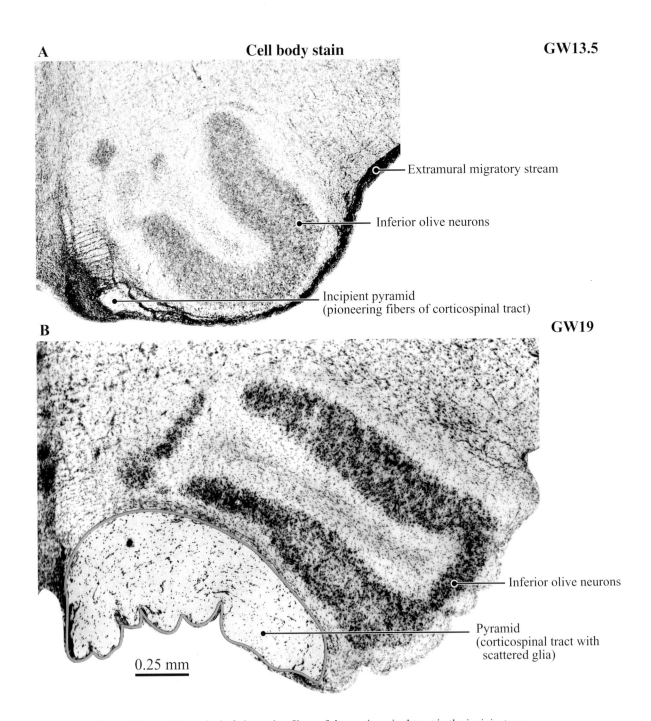

A   **Cell body stain**   **GW13.5**

— Extramural migratory stream

— Inferior olive neurons

Incipient pyramid
(pioneering fibers of corticospinal tract)

B   **GW19**

— Inferior olive neurons

Pyramid
(corticospinal tract with
scattered glia)

0.25 mm

Figure 7-21. A. The arrival of pioneering fibers of the corticospinal tract in the incipient pyramid of the GW13.5 fetus (*Y144-63*; CR 100 mm). **B.** The growing pyramid in the GW19 fetus (*Y15-63*; CR 150 mm). The concentration of interfascicular glia is quite low.

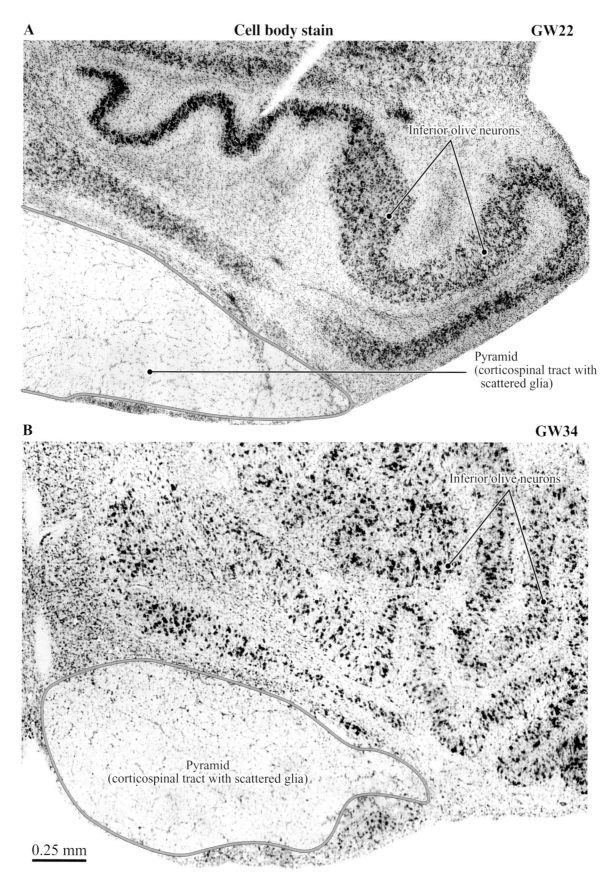

Figure 7-22. The concentration of glia remains low in **A**, the pyramid of the GW22 fetus (*Y22-59*; CR 190 mm) and **B**, the GW34 fetus (*Y232-66*; CR 295 mm).

We summarize the growth of the corticofugal tract in Figures 7-23 and 7-24. Because this summary is based on a small sample, the gestational ages given are necessarily tentative. The descent of the earliest corticofugal fibers begins in the upper portion of the corticofugal tract in the internal capsule between GW8.5 and GW9.5 (Figure 7-23A). As new fibers join the tract between GW9.5 and GW13 (note the expansion of the internal capsule), a small complement of fibers forms the corticofugal tract in the cerebral peduncle (Figure 7-23B). By the end of this period, some of the descending axons reach the pontine gray. The transpontine corticofugal tract lengthens between GW13 and GW18. Some of the fibers form the pyramids, which are composed exclusively of corticospinal fibers (Figure 7-24A). After GW18, an increasing proportion of descending fibers decussate in the medullary pyramids (Figure 7-24B). These crossed fibers form the lateral corticospinal tract in the cervical spinal cord; the uncrossed fibers form the ventral corticospinal tract.

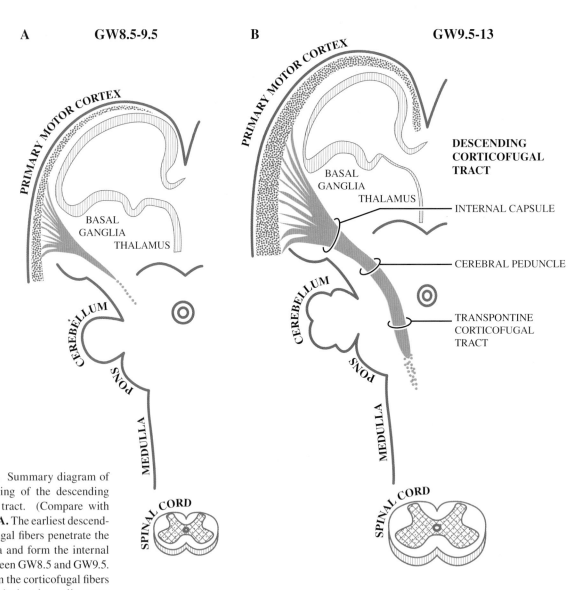

Figure 7-23. Summary diagram of the lengthening of the descending corticofugal tract. (Compare with Figure 7-1.) **A.** The earliest descending corticofugal fibers penetrate the basal ganglia and form the internal capsule between GW8.5 and GW9.5. **B.** Increase in the corticofugal fibers that traverse the basal ganglia, some of which reach the midbrain between GW9.5 and GW 13 where they form the internal capsule. Some pioneering fibers penetrate the pontine gray to form the transpontine corticospinal tract.

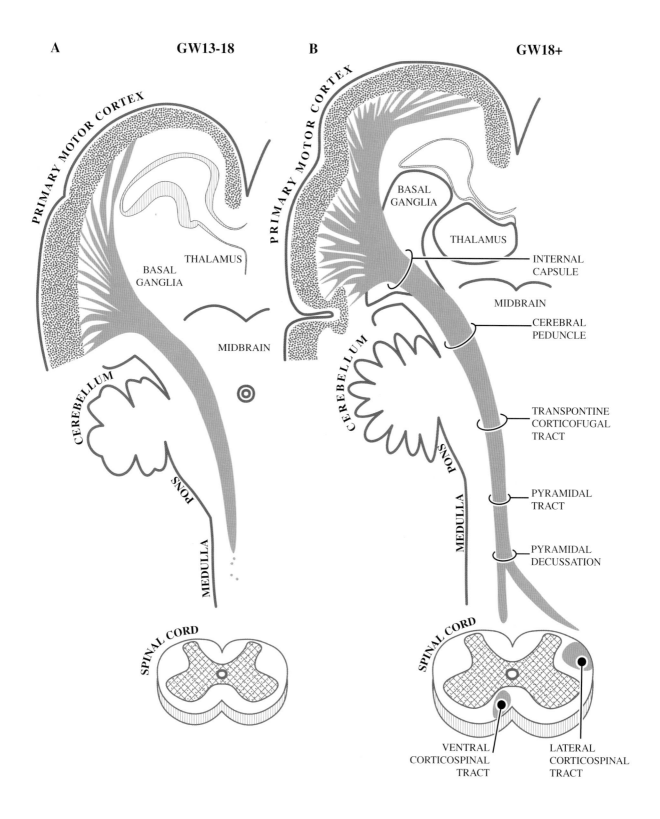

A GW13-18

B GW18+

PRIMARY MOTOR CORTEX

THALAMUS

BASAL GANGLIA

CEREBELLUM

MIDBRAIN

PONS

MEDULLA

SPINAL CORD

BASAL GANGLIA

THALAMUS

INTERNAL CAPSULE

MIDBRAIN

CEREBRAL PEDUNCLE

TRANSPONTINE CORTICOFUGAL TRACT

PYRAMIDAL TRACT

PYRAMIDAL DECUSSATION

VENTRAL CORTICOSPINAL TRACT

LATERAL CORTICOSPINAL TRACT

Figure 7-24. Summary diagram of the lengthening of the descending corticofugal tract (*continued from Figure 7-23*). **A.** The volume of the corticofugal tract increases greatly between GW 13 and GW18 and many of the fibers traversing the pontine gray reach the medulla where they form the pyramids. **B.** At about GW18, or shortly thereafter, the fibers of the corticospinal tract that form the pyramids split into two descending components, the larger contralaterally projecting lateral corticospinal tract, and the smaller ipsilaterally projecting ventral corticospinal tract.

7.2 Descent of the Lateral and Ventral Corticospinal Tracts in the Spinal Cord

7.2.1 Growth of the Lateral and Ventral Corticospinal Tracts From Cervical to Sacral Levels.
We trace the emergence and descent of the lateral and ventral corticospinal tracts in fetuses ranging in age from GW14 to GW31, and in newborns in Figures 7-25 to 7-34.

GW14 to GW19. There is no indication of the presence of a fibrous mass in the upper cervical cord of the early second trimester fetus (GW14; *Y68-65*; 108 mm) at the site where the lateral corticospinal tract and the ventral corticospinal tract will later be situated (Figure 7-25). However, in the spinal cord of the middle second trimester fetus (GW19; *Y52-61*; 130 mm), a glia-sparse, small lateral corticospinal tract is clearly present in the white matter lateral

to the dorsal horn, and even more prominent is the glia-sparse ventral corticospinal tract (Figure 7-26). The same GW19 fetus shows the descent of the two corticospinal tracts caudally. The lateral corticospinal tract may be present in the upper thoracic cord (Figure 7-27A) but it has certainly not reached the middle thoracic cord (Figure 7-27B). The larger ventral corticospinal tract is clearly present in the upper thoracic cord (Figure 7-27A) and just as clearly it is absent in the middle thoracic cord (Figure 7-27B).

GW26. The growth of the lateral and ventral corticospinal tracts from rostral to caudal is traced in older fetuses in sections stained for myelin, using the sparseness or absence of reactive glia as a marker of the boundaries of these two late-developing fiber tracts. In a late second trimester fetus (GW26; *Y60-61*; 210 mm), the lateral and ventral corticospinal tracts can be followed from the cervical cord

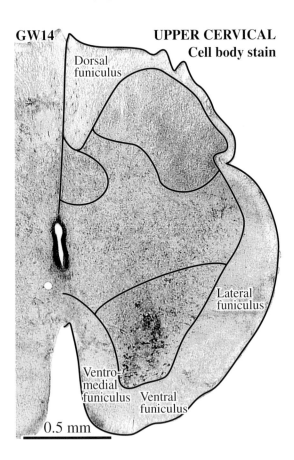

Figure 7-25. Cell body-stained section of the upper cervical spinal cord in a GW14 fetus (*Y68-65*; CR 108 mm). There is no indication of the presence of the lateral corticospinal tract in the lateral funiculus, or of the ventral corticospinal tract in the ventromedial funiculus in this early second trimester fetus.

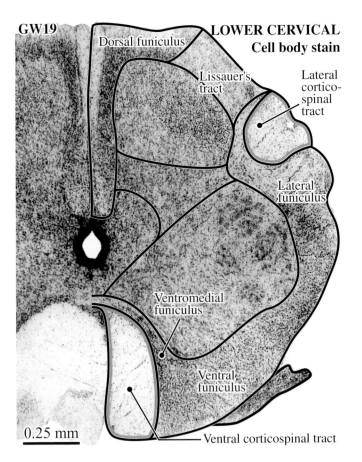

Figure 7-26. Cell body-stained section of the lower cervical spinal cord in a GW19 fetus (*Y52-61*; CR 130 mm). A small cell-sparse lateral corticospinal tract is present in the lateral funiculus, and a larger ventral corticospinal tract in the ventromedial funiculus in this specimen.

(Figure 7-28) through the upper thoracic cord (Figure 7-29A), and the middle thoracic cord (Figure 7-29B). Both tracts diminish in size from rostral to caudal and neither is recognizable at low thoracic levels (not shown).

GW29 to GW31. The youngest specimen in which we could follow the lateral corticospinal tract through the thoracic cord (Figure 7-30A) into the lumbar cord was a GW29 fetus (*Y222-65; 235 mm*; Figure 7-30B). In this specimen a ventral corticospinal tract could not be identified at any level by the criteria used (absence or sparseness of reactive glia). In a somewhat older and larger third trimester fetus (GW31; *Y162-61*; 270 mm) the growth of the lateral corticospinal tract can be followed from the upper lumbar cord (Figure 7-31A) to the lumbosacral cord (Figure 7-31B). However, the ventral corticospinal tract cannot be followed farther than the thoracic cord in this fetus.

GW37 to GW44. In Figures 7-32 to 7-34 we track the entire course of the corticospinal tract is traced in two neonates: one younger and smaller

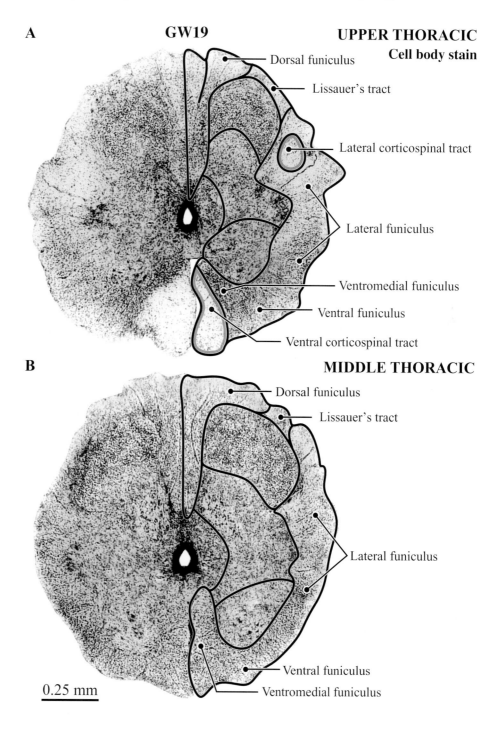

Figure 7-27. A. A small lateral corticospinal tract and a small ventral corticospinal tract are present in the same GW19 fetus (*Y52-61*) in the upper thoracic cord. **B.** However, neither of these tracts is recognizable in the midthoracic cord. Apparently. corticospinal fibers have not yet reached the more caudal levels of the spinal cord in this mid-second trimester fetus.

A   GW19   UPPER THORACIC
Cell body stain

Dorsal funiculus
Lissauer's tract
Lateral corticospinal tract
Lateral funiculus
Ventromedial funiculus
Ventral funiculus
Ventral corticospinal tract

B   MIDDLE THORACIC

Dorsal funiculus
Lissauer's tract
Lateral funiculus
Ventral funiculus
Ventromedial funiculus

0.25 mm

(GW37; *Y117-61*; 310 mm); the other older and bigger (GW44; *Y23-60*; 410 mm). Both the lateral corticospinal tract and the ventral corticospinal tract are clearly delineated in the smaller GW37 neonate by the paucity of reactive glia at middle cervical (Figure 7-32A), low cervical (Figure 7-32B), thoracic (Figure 7-33A), and lumbar (Figure 7-33B) levels of the spinal cord. In this neonate, the ventral corticospinal tract is larger rostrally than the lateral corticospinal tract, and both tracts diminish in size from rostral to caudal. In the older GW44 neonate, the lateral corticospinal tract is large and the ventral corticospinal tract is small in

the upper cervical and middle thoracic cord (Figure 7-34A, B). The lateral corticospinal tract is gradually diminishing in size at upper thoracic, middle thoracic, low thoracic, and lumbar levels (Figures 7-34C-F). In contrast, the ventral corticospinal tract is not recognizable beyond the cervical cord (Figures 7-34C-F). The low concentration of reactive glia in both the lateral and ventral corticospinal tracts indicates that myelination gliosis has not started yet in this late-delivered neonate. The descent of the corticospinal tract as a function of gestational age is schematically summarized in Figure 7-35.

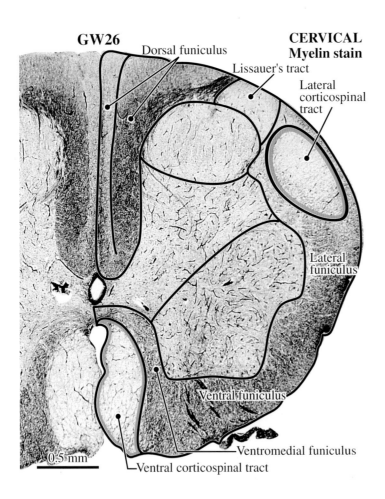

Figure 7-28. The lateral and ventral corticospinal tracts in the cervical spinal cord of a GW26 fetus (*Y60-61*; CR 210 mm). The paucity of reactive glia clearly delineate these two tracts in this myelin-stained section of the late second trimester fetus.

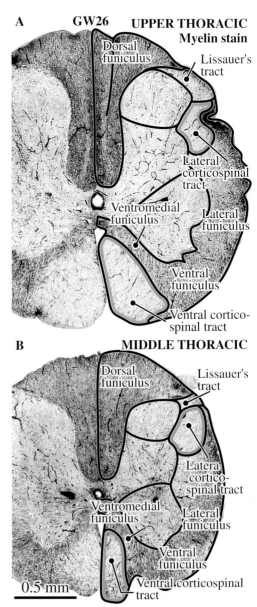

Figure 7-29. The lateral and ventral corticospinal tracts are also outlined by the paucity of reactive glia in the same GW26 fetus as in Figure 7-28, more caudally in the upper thoracic (**A**) and midthoracic (**B**) cord.

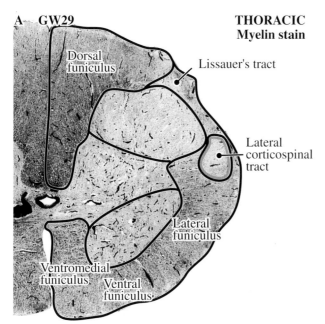

A GW29 **THORACIC**
Myelin stain

Dorsal funiculus

Lissauer's tract

Lateral corticospinal tract

Lateral funiculus

Ventromedial funiculus

Ventral funiculus

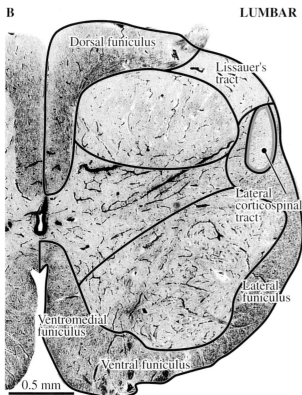

B **LUMBAR**

Dorsal funiculus

Lissauer's tract

Lateral corticospinal tract

Lateral funiculus

Ventromedial funiculus

Ventral funiculus

0.5 mm

Figure 7-30. In this early third trimester fetus (GW29; *Y222-65*; CR 235 mm), the lateral corticospinal tract descends through the thoracic cord (**A**) to the lumbar cord (**B**). A ventral corticospinal tract could not be identified in this fetus at any level of the spinal cord.

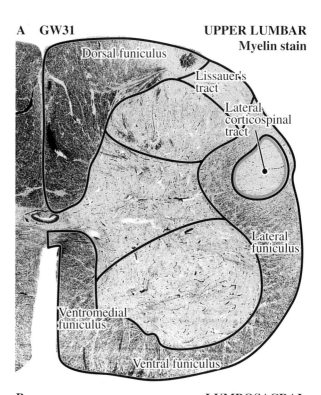

A GW31 **UPPER LUMBAR**
Myelin stain

Dorsal funiculus

Lissauer's tract

Lateral corticospinal tract

Lateral funiculus

Ventromedial funiculus

Ventral funiculus

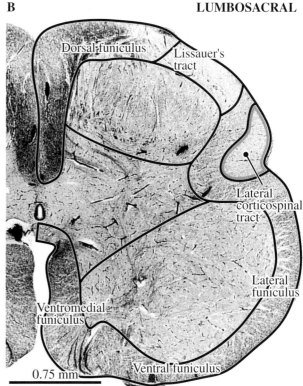

B **LUMBOSACRAL**

Dorsal funiculus

Lissauer's tract

Lateral corticospinal tract

Lateral funiculus

Ventromedial funiculus

Ventral funiculus

0.75 mm

Figure 7-31. The lateral corticospinal tract can be followed from the lumbar spinal cord (**A**) to lumbosacral cord (**B**) in this GW31 fetus (*Y162-61*; CR 270 mm). The ventral corticospinal tract could not be traced in this specimen beyond the midthoracic cord.

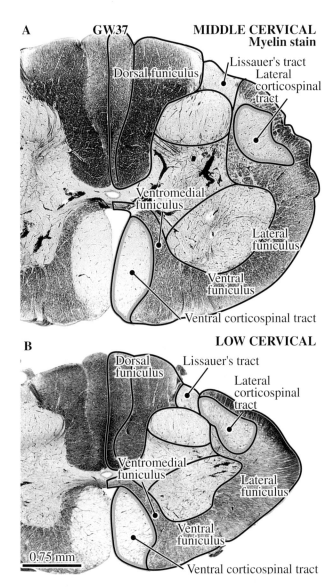

Figure 7-32. The lateral and ventral corticospinal tracts in a GW37 neonate (*Y117-61*; CR 310 mm) at middle cervical (**A**) and low cervical (**B**) levels of the spinal cord.

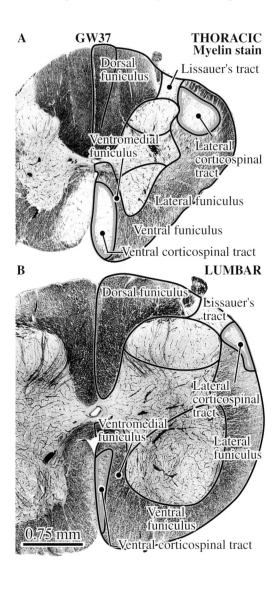

Figure 7-33. The diminishing lateral and ventral corticospinal tracts in the same neonate as in Figure 7-32 at thoracic (**A**) and lumbar (**B**) levels of the spinal cord.

7.2.2 Individual Differences in the Growth of the Lateral and Ventral Corticospinal Tracts.

Figures 7-36 and 7-37 show the differences between the relative size of the lateral corticospinal tract, and the presence or absence of the ventral corticospinal tract, in the cervical spinal cord of two fetuses and two neonates, matched for gestational age and body length. In a GW32 fetus (*Y76-60*; 300 mm; Figure 7-36A), the lateral corticospinal tract is large while the ventral corticospinal tract is small. In a GW33 fetus (*Y36-60*; 315 mm; Figure 7-36B), the lateral corticospinal tract is still larger but the ventral cor-

ticospinal tract is absent. (Differences in these two fetuses in the myelination of the dorsal funiculus are also evident.) In the second comparison, the lateral corticospinal tract is smaller than the ventral corticospinal tract in one of the neonates (GW37; *Y117-61*; 310 mm; Figure 7-37A) while in the other neonate (GW38; *Y163-61*; 320 mm; Figure 7-37B), the lateral corticospinal tract is large but the ventral corticospinal tract is very small. We do not know whether these differences reflect variability in the tempo of development or are indicative of enduring individual differences.

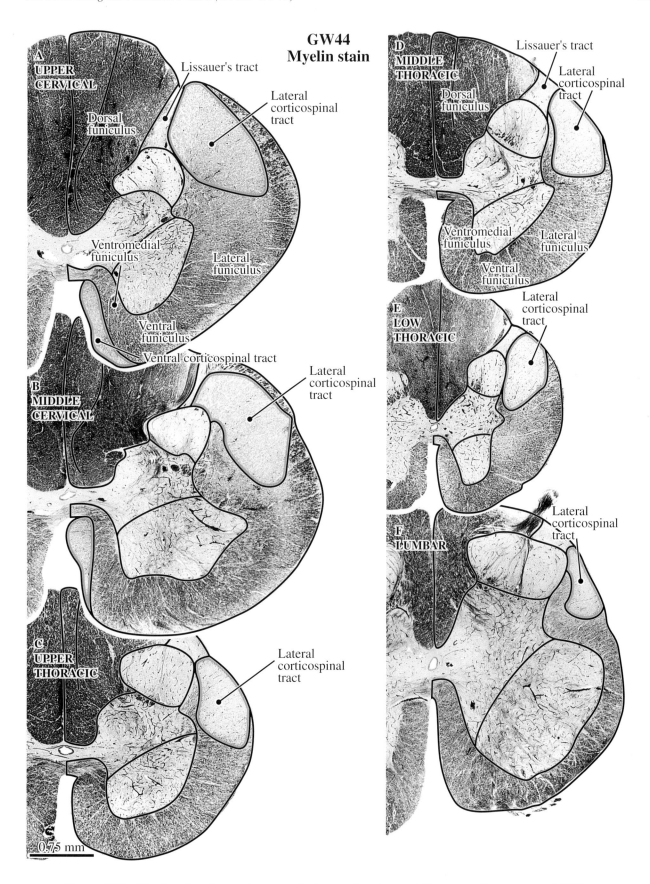

GW44
Myelin stain

Figure 7-34. The lateral and ventral corticospinal tracts in this late-delivered and large neonate (GW44; *Y23-60*; CR 410 mm) from the upper cervical (**A**) to the lumbar (**F**) spinal cord. The ventral corticospinal tract, as judged by the criteria used (paucity of reactive glia), does not reach the thoracic cord in this specimen.

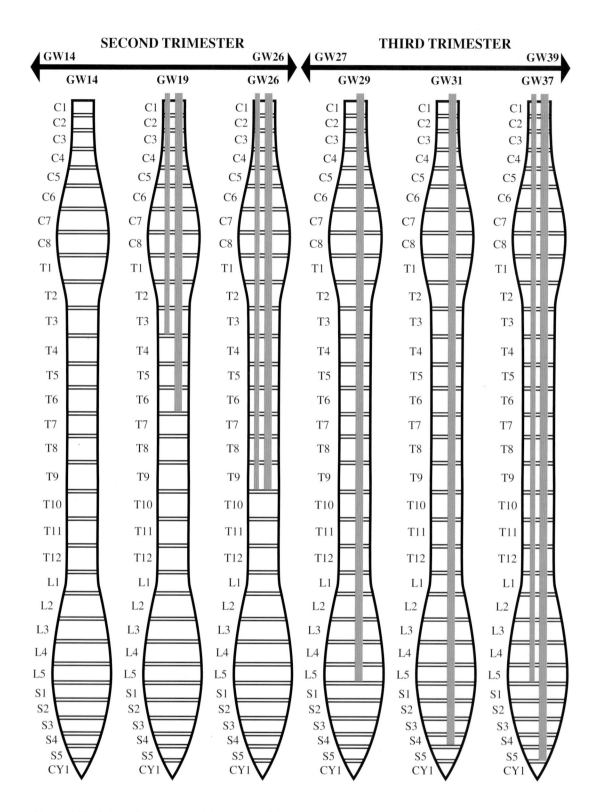

Figure 7-35. Schematic summary of the growth of the descending lateral corticospinal tract and ventral cortico-spinal tract (where present) during the second and third trimesters. Data are based on a limited sample. For the subsequent phase of the reactive gliosis and myelination of the lateral corticospinal tract, see Figure 8-29.

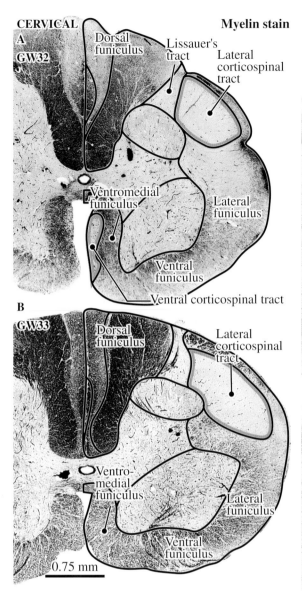

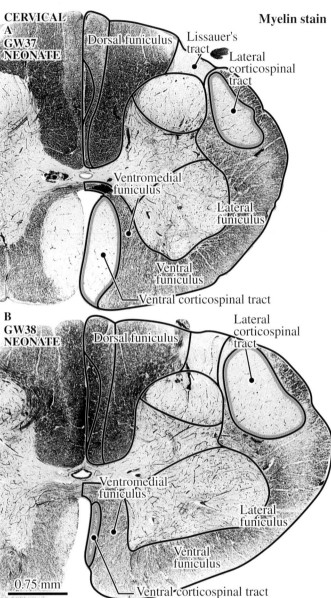

Figure 7-36. The lateral corticospinal tract is smaller in the cervical cord of **A**, the GW32 fetus (*Y76-60*; CR 300 mm), than **B**, in the GW33 fetus (*Y36-60*; CR 315 mm). A small ventral corticospinal tract is present in the GW32 fetus but appears to be absent in the GW33 fetus. Note also the individual differences in the spread of reactive gliosis and myelination in the dorsal funiculus.

Figure 7-37. A. In one neonate (*Y117-61*; GW37; CR 320 mm), the lateral corticospinal tract is smaller than the ventral corticospinal tract. **B.** In the other neonate (*Y163-61*; GW38; CR 320 mm), the lateral corticospinal tract is quite large but the ventral corticospinal tract is very small.

8 MYELINATION OF THE CORTICOSPINAL TRACTS DURING THE FIRST TWO YEARS OF POSTNATAL LIFE

8.1 The Myelinated Subcortical and the Unmyelinated Corticofugal Tracts in the Neonate and the Young Infant

8.1.1 Myelination Pattern in the Brain of a Newborn.
The cerebral cortex, thalamus, hypothalamus, and midbrain tectum are devoid of myelinated fibers in the myelin-stained sagittal section of the brain of a neonate (*Y180-61*; GW37; Figure 8-1A). In contrast, bands of myelinated fibers are present in the midbrain tegmentum, in the medullary layer of the cerebellar cortex, in the core of the pons (but not the pontine gray), and the medulla. The pattern of myelination in the latter regions is shown at higher magnification in Figure 8-1B. The slender myelinated fiber tract starting in the midbrain beneath the central gray and above the red nucleus is the medial longitudinal fasciculus. That tract contains fibers from the interstitial nucleus and the vestibular nuclei, and descends in a dorsal position through the pons and medulla then turns ventrally as it approaches the spinal cord. The core of the pontine gray and of the medulla, perhaps representing the region of the raphe nuclei and the reticular formation, is filled with myelinated fibers, and the inferior olive is surrounded by a mass of densely stained myelinated fibers. Inferior olivary fibers that reach the cerebellum by way of the inferior cerebellar peduncle (the lower transcerebellar loop; Altman and Bayer, 1996) may contribute myelinated fibers to the medullary layer of the cerebellum. In sharp contrast, the corticofugal fibers descending through the pontine gray, the pontocerebellar fibers that reach the cerebellum by way of the middle cerebellar peduncle (the upper transcerebellar loop), and the corticospinal fibers in the pyramids are devoid of myelin.

8.1.2 Myelination Pattern in a 3-Day-Old Infant.
The pattern of myelination in the sagittal section of the brain of a 3-day-old infant (*Y62-61*; GW37) is very similar to that of the newborn. The cerebral cortex is devoid of myelinated fibers (Figure 8-2A) and the corticofugal fibers in the pontine gray are unmyelinated (Figure 8-2B). In contrast, the medial longitudinal fasciculus and inferior cerebellar peduncle in the brain stem, and the fasciculus gracilis and ventral funiculus in the upper cervical spinal cord are myelinated (Figure 8-2C).

8.2 Onset of Myelination in the Cortical Projection Areas and the Corticofugal Tracts During Early Infancy. Age: 6 to 8 Weeks

8.2.1 Early Myelination in the Primary Sensory and Motor Areas.
Myelination of the cerebral cortex begins during the second month of postnatal life and is initially limited, as originally described by Flechsig (1876), to the primary sensory and motor "projection" areas. Myelination of the cortical "association" areas, according to Flechsig, is a later development.

The somatosensory and motor areas, as seen in two parasagittal sections of a 7-week-old infant (*Y130-61;* Figure 8-3), are among the earliest myelinating regions of the cerebral cortex. Laterally, myelinated fibers are confined to the white matter of the convolutions flanking the central sulcus (Figures 8-3A). The cortex of the anterior bank of the central sulcus (the precentral gyrus) is the primary motor projection area, the cortex on the posterior bank (the postcentral gyrus) is the primary somesthetic projection area. Myelination is more dense at the base of the central sulcus than superficially (Figure 8-3B). This raises the possibility that the somatosensory and motor regions representing the upper body begin to myelinate before the regions representing the lower body. Another early myelinating region in the cerebral cortex is the white matter in the primary visual area in the occipital lobe. This is seen in a horizontal section from the same 7-week-old infant (*Y130-61*; Figures 8-4A, B). This band can be followed from the occipital cortex to the basal ganglia, suggesting that at least some of the myelinated fibers are corticofugal rather than thalamocortical fibers (axons of the visual radiation). The white matter in the rest of the occipital lobe shows signs of reactive gliosis

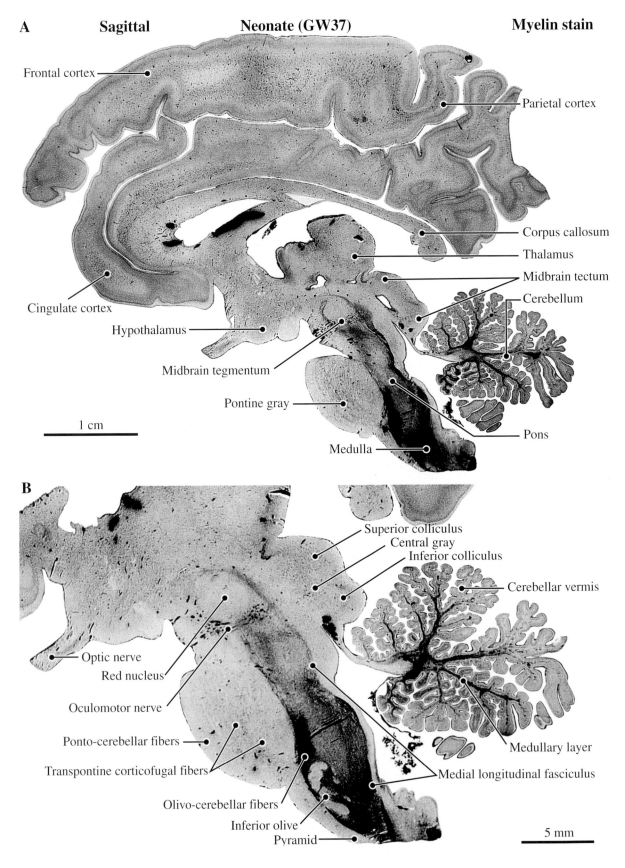

A   **Sagittal**   **Neonate (GW37)**   **Myelin stain**

Frontal cortex

Parietal cortex

Corpus callosum

Thalamus

Midbrain tectum

Cerebellum

Cingulate cortex

Hypothalamus

Midbrain tegmentum

Pontine gray

Pons

Medulla

1 cm

B

Superior colliculus

Central gray

Inferior colliculus

Cerebellar vermis

Optic nerve

Red nucleus

Oculomotor nerve

Ponto-cerebellar fibers

Transpontine corticofugal fibers

Olivo-cerebellar fibers

Inferior olive

Pyramid

Medullary layer

Medial longitudinal fasciculus

5 mm

Figure 8-1. A. The forebrain and brain stem in a myelin-stained sagittal section of a newborn (*Y180-61*; GW37). The cerebral cortex, diencephalon, midbrain tectum, and pontine gray are devoid of myelinated fibers. Myelinated fibers are present in the midbrain tegmentum, the medullary layer of the cerebellum, and in the core of the medulla and pons. **B.** The myelinated components of the brain stem at higher magnification. The transpontine corticofugal tract is unmyelinated.

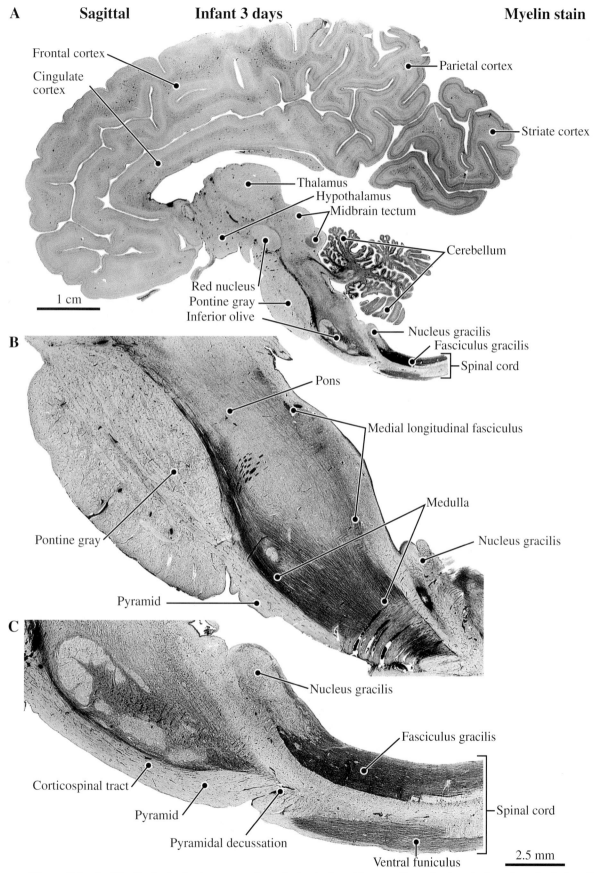

A   **Sagittal**   **Infant 3 days**   **Myelin stain**

Frontal cortex
Cingulate cortex
Parietal cortex
Striate cortex
Thalamus
Hypothalamus
Midbrain tectum
Cerebellum
Red nucleus
Pontine gray
Inferior olive
Nucleus gracilis
Fasciculus gracilis
Spinal cord
1 cm

B

Pons
Medial longitudinal fasciculus
Medulla
Pontine gray
Nucleus gracilis
Pyramid

C

Nucleus gracilis
Fasciculus gracilis
Corticospinal tract
Spinal cord
Pyramid
Pyramidal decussation
Ventral funiculus
2.5 mm

Figure 8-2. A. The forebrain, brain stem, and cervical spinal cord in a myelin-stained sagittal section of a 3-day-old infant (*Y62-61*; GW37). Myelinated fiber tracts are present only in the brain stem and the spinal cord. The myelinated and unmyelinated fiber tracts in the pons, medulla and spinal cord are illustrated at higher magnification in **B** and **C**.

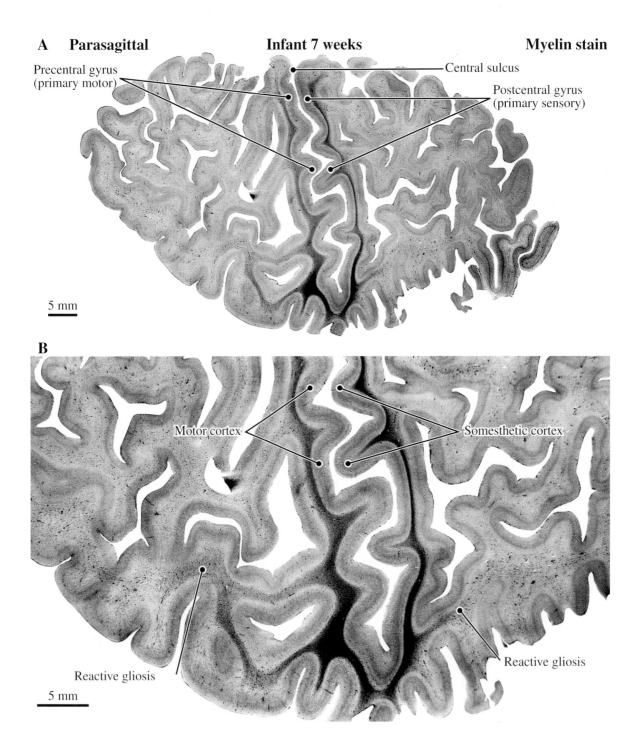

Figure 8-3. Myelinated and unmyelinated areas of the cerebral cortex in a parasagittal section from a 7-week-old infant (*Y130-61*) at lower (**A**) and higher (**B**) magnification. Myelinated fibers are limited to the white matter of the precentral gyrus (primary motor area) and the postcentral gyrus (primary somesthetic area) flanking the central sulcus. At the base of the central sulcus, myelination appears to be more advanced than superficially.

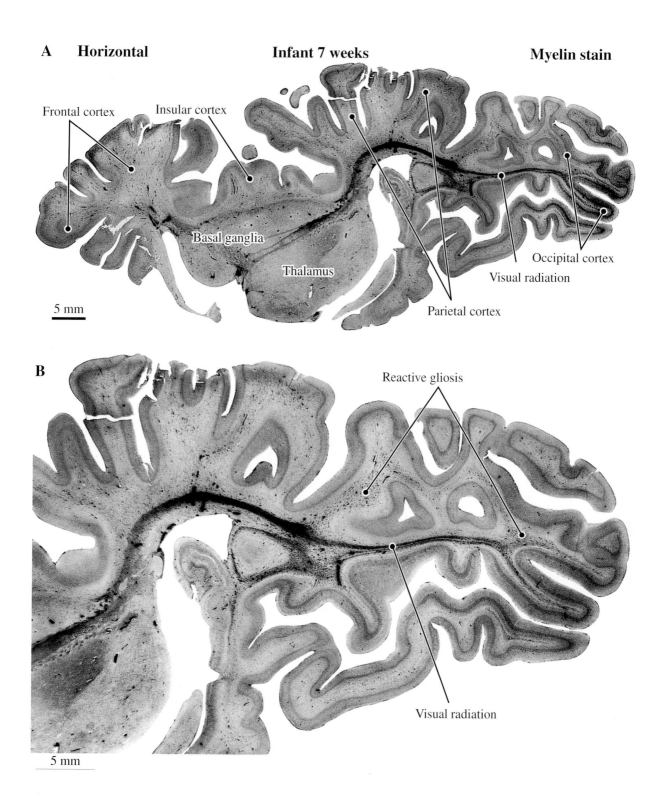

A   **Horizontal**   **Infant 7 weeks**   **Myelin stain**

Frontal cortex   Insular cortex

Basal ganglia

Thalamus

Parietal cortex

Occipital cortex

Visual radiation

5 mm

B

Reactive gliosis

Visual radiation

5 mm

Figure 8-4. Myelination of the fibers of the visual radiation in a horizontal section from the same 7-week-old infant (*Y130-61*) at lower (**A**) and higher (**B**) magnification. The myelinated fibers may be a composite of sensory and motor fibers of the occipital lobe. Reactive gliosis is starting in adjacent areas.

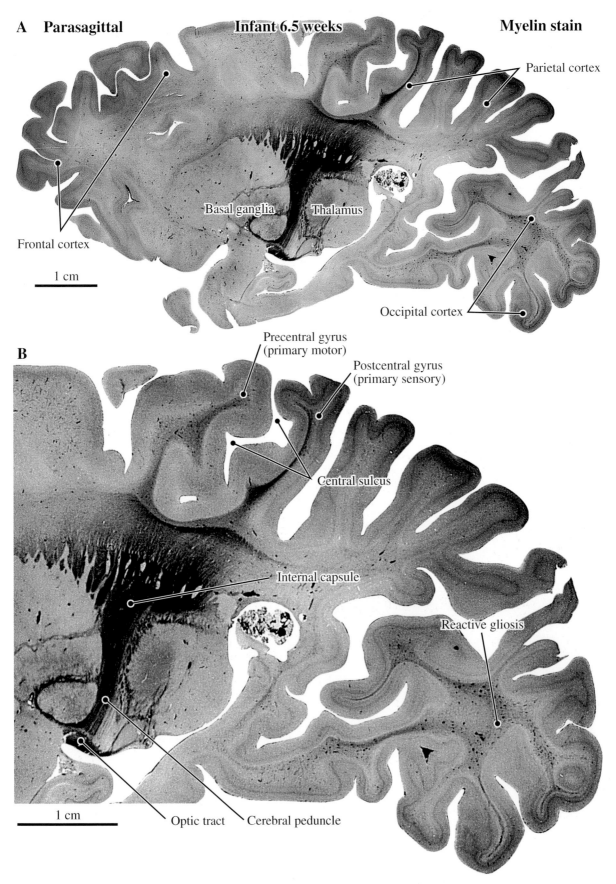

A   Parasagittal   **Infant 6.5 weeks**   **Myelin stain**

Parietal cortex

Frontal cortex

1 cm

Basal ganglia   Thalamus

Occipital cortex

B

Precentral gyrus
(primary motor)

Postcentral gyrus
(primary sensory)

Central sulcus

Internal capsule

Reactive gliosis

1 cm

Optic tract   Cerebral peduncle

Figure 8-5. Myelinated fibers in the white matter of the precentral and postcentral gyri, the internal capsule, and the cerebral peduncle in a 6.5-week-old infant (*Y152-61*) at lower (**A**) and higher (**B**) magnification.

8.2.2 Myelination of the Descending Corticofugal Tract. The onset of myelination is evident in the white matter of the gyri flanking the central sulcus in a parasagittal section of the cerebral cortex in a 6.5-week-old infant (*Y152-61*; Figures 8-5A, B). There is a horizontal band of heavily myelinated fibers beneath this lightly myelinated cortical region and vertically oriented fibers traverse the deep white matter underneath this band and enter the internal capsule. An unknown proportion of these fibers are corticofugal rather than thalamocortical fibers; this is suggested by the presence of myelinated fibers in the pontine gray in this infant (Figure 8-6). The discrepancy between the massive bundle of myelinated fibers in the internal capsule and the paucity of myelinated fibers in the pontine gray reflects two concurrent developments. One is the contribution of early myelinating thalamocortical fibers to the internal capsule. The other is that the myelination of the corticofugal tract proceeds from proximal to distal, just as we saw in the dorsal funiculus of the spinal cord. Indeed, the corticofugal fibers are only myelinated rostrally in the pontine gray of this infant (Figure 8-6).

The trajectory of myelinated fibers between the motor cortex and the cerebral peduncle is seen in a coronal section of the forebrain of an another infant (*Y28-60*; Figure 8-7A). The heavy band of myelinated fibers in the precentral gyrus and the internal capsule appear to fan out laterally (towards the basal ganglia) and medially (particularly towards the subthalamic nucleus and the red nucleus) before a thinner band of myelinated fibers joins the cerebral peduncle distally. It is uncertain what proportion of these fibers are descending cortical efferents but the few myelinated fascicles that traverse the pontine gray (Figure 8-7B) must be corticofugal fibers.

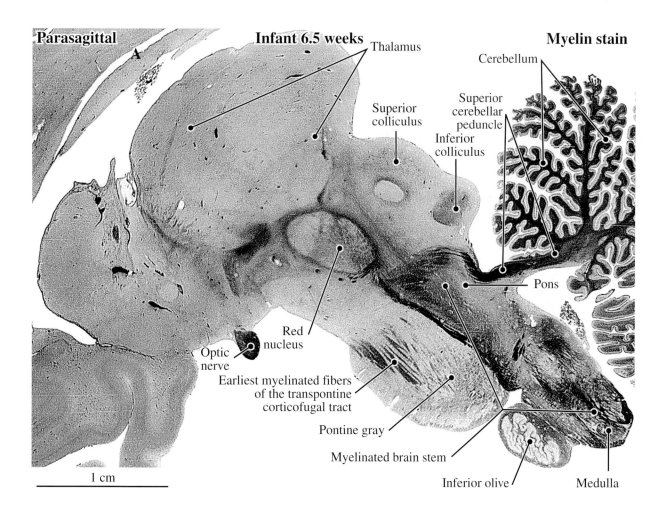

Figure 8-6. Myelinated corticofugal fibers in the pontine gray of the same 6.5-week-old infant (*Y152-61*). Only a small proportion of the transpontine corticofugal fibers are myelinated.

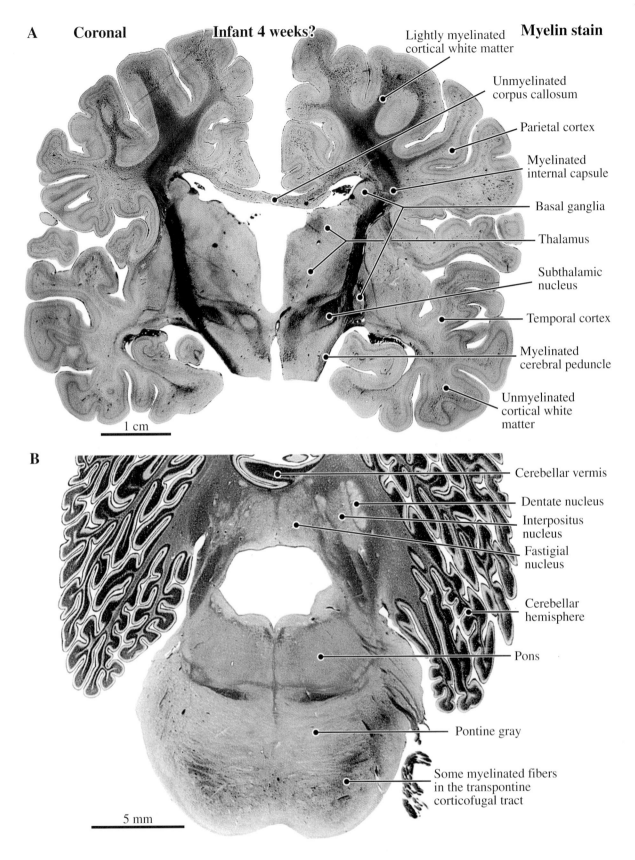

A   **Coronal**   **Infant 4 weeks?**   **Myelin stain**

Lightly myelinated cortical white matter

Unmyelinated corpus callosum

Parietal cortex

Myelinated internal capsule

Basal ganglia

Thalamus

Subthalamic nucleus

Temporal cortex

Myelinated cerebral peduncle

Unmyelinated cortical white matter

1 cm

B

Cerebellar vermis

Dentate nucleus

Interpositus nucleus

Fastigial nucleus

Cerebellar hemisphere

Pons

Pontine gray

Some myelinated fibers in the transpontine corticofugal tract

5 mm

Figure 8-7. A. Myelinated fibers in the cerebral cortex, internal capsule, and cerebral peduncle in a coronal section of the forebrain in a young infant (*Y28-60*; about 4 weeks of age). **B.** Some early myelinating corticofugal fibers in the pontine gray in the same infant.

8.3 Progressive Cortical Myelination and the Growth of the Corticocofugal Tracts During Late Infancy. Age: 4 to 8 Months

8.3.1 Expansion and Intensification of Cortical Myelination. Cortical myelination is far more extensive and dense in a 4-month-old infant (*Y160-61*; Figure 8-8) than in the younger infants. Myelination in the cortical white matter extends from the medial to the lateral gyri, and from the depth to the surface of the gyri. Moreover, a much larger proportion of myelinated fibers of the internal capsule penetrate and traverse the pontine gray (Figure 8-8). There is further increase in the intensity and spread of myelin staining throughout the cortex in the 7-month-old infant (Y123-61) illustrated in Figure 8-9A. There is also an increase in the bulk of myelinated transpontine fibers (Figure 8-9B).

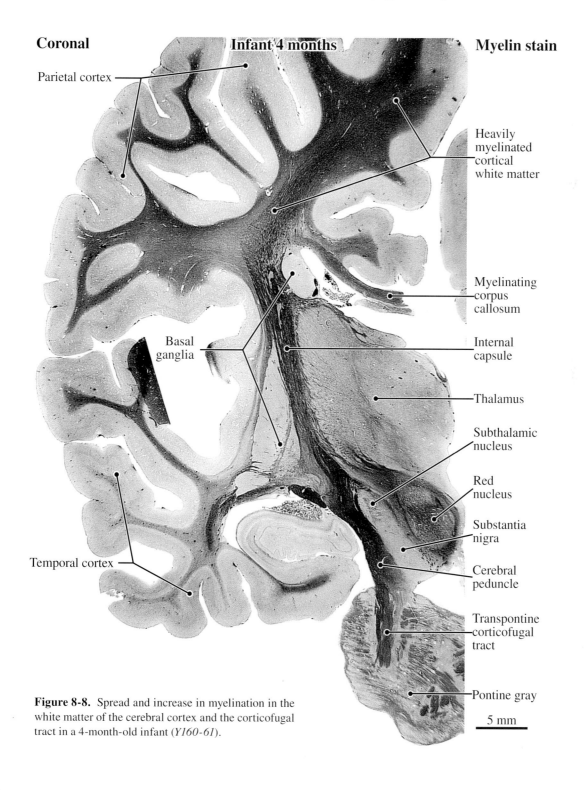

Coronal   **Infant 4 months**   **Myelin stain**

Parietal cortex

Heavily myelinated cortical white matter

Myelinating corpus callosum

Internal capsule

Basal ganglia

Thalamus

Subthalamic nucleus

Red nucleus

Substantia nigra

Temporal cortex

Cerebral peduncle

Transpontine corticofugal tract

Pontine gray

5 mm

Figure 8-8. Spread and increase in myelination in the white matter of the cerebral cortex and the corticofugal tract in a 4-month-old infant (*Y160-61*).

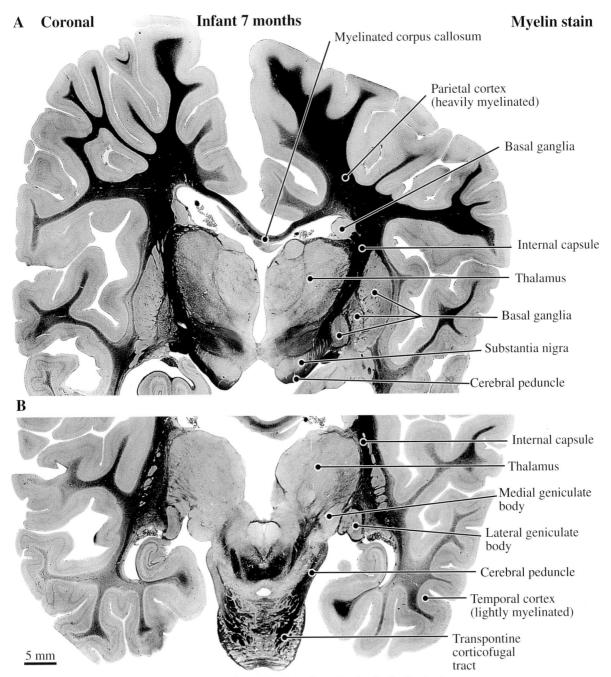

A   Coronal   Infant 7 months   Myelin stain

Myelinated corpus callosum

Parietal cortex
(heavily myelinated)

Basal ganglia

Internal capsule

Thalamus

Basal ganglia

Substantia nigra

Cerebral peduncle

B

Internal capsule

Thalamus

Medial geniculate
body

Lateral geniculate
body

Cerebral peduncle

Temporal cortex
(lightly myelinated)

Transpontine
corticofugal
tract

5 mm

Figure 8-9. Further spread and intensification of myelination in the forebrain
(**A**) and the pontine gray (**B**) in a 7-month-old infant (*Y123-61*).

8.3.2 Progressive Myelination of the Transpontine Corticofugal Tract.

Coronal sections of the pontine gray (Figure 8-10) illustrate the progressive increase in the proportion of myelinated to unmyelinated transpontine corticofugal fibers between the neonatal period and early chidhood. No myelinated transpontine corticofugal fibers are visible in the 2-day-old infant (*Y128-63*; Figure 8-10A). There is a small collection of myelinated fibers in the lower half of the pontine gray in the 1-month-old infant (*Y125-61*; Figure 8-10B). Most of the transpontine corticofugal fibers are myelinated in the 4-month-old infant (*Y160-61*; Figure 8-10C). There is little increase in myelinated transpontine fascicles and their staining intensity in the 7-month-old infant (*Y123-61*; Figure 8-10D).

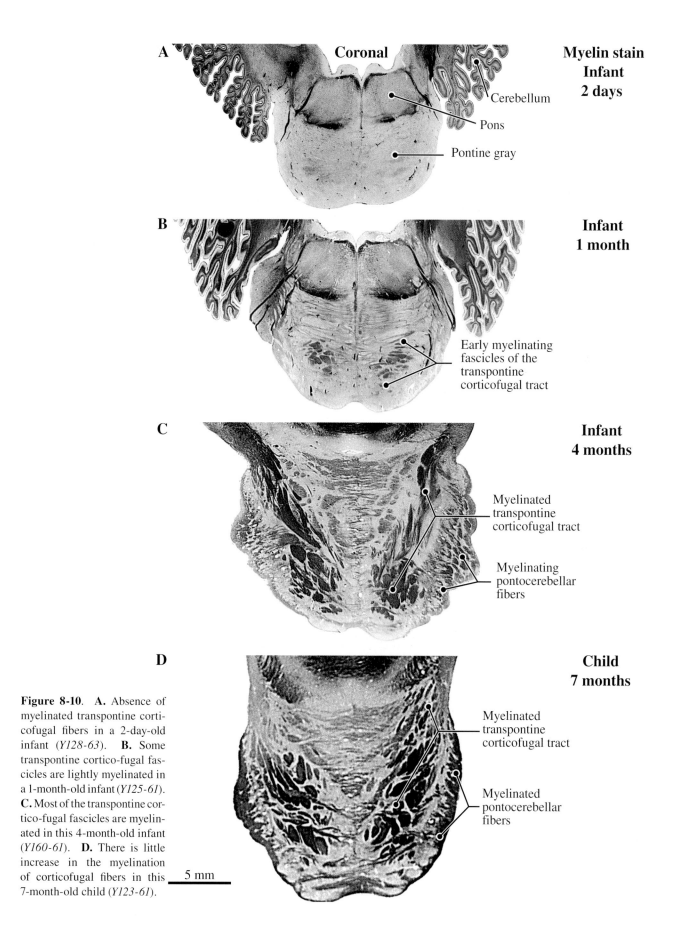

A **Coronal** **Myelin stain Infant 2 days**

Cerebellum

Pons

Pontine gray

B **Infant 1 month**

Early myelinating fascicles of the transpontine corticofugal tract

C **Infant 4 months**

Myelinated transpontine corticofugal tract

Myelinating pontocerebellar fibers

D **Child 7 months**

Myelinated transpontine corticofugal tract

Myelinated pontocerebellar fibers

Figure 8-10. **A.** Absence of myelinated transpontine corticofugal fibers in a 2-day-old infant (*Y128-63*). **B.** Some transpontine cortico-fugal fascicles are lightly myelinated in a 1-month-old infant (*Y125-61*). **C.** Most of the transpontine cortico-fugal fascicles are myelinated in this 4-month-old infant (*Y160-61*). **D.** There is little increase in the myelination of corticofugal fibers in this 7-month-old child (*Y123-61*).

5 mm

The relationship between the myelination of transpontine corticofugal fibers and the myelination of pontocerebellar fibers is illustrated in sagittal sections in Figures 8-11 and 8-12. Unmyelinated longitudinally oriented fascicles of the corticofugal tract occupy the core of the pontine gray in the 1-day-old infant (*Y235-66*; Figure 8-11A). The outer shell of the pontine gray, which contains the transversely oriented pontocerebellar fibers, is also devoid of myelin. Corticofugal fascicles begin to myelinate in the outer half of the core of the pontine gray in the 6-week-old infant (*Y152-61*; Figure 8-11B), while the pontocerebellar fibers are still unmyelinated. Most of the transpontine corticofugal fibers are myelinated in the

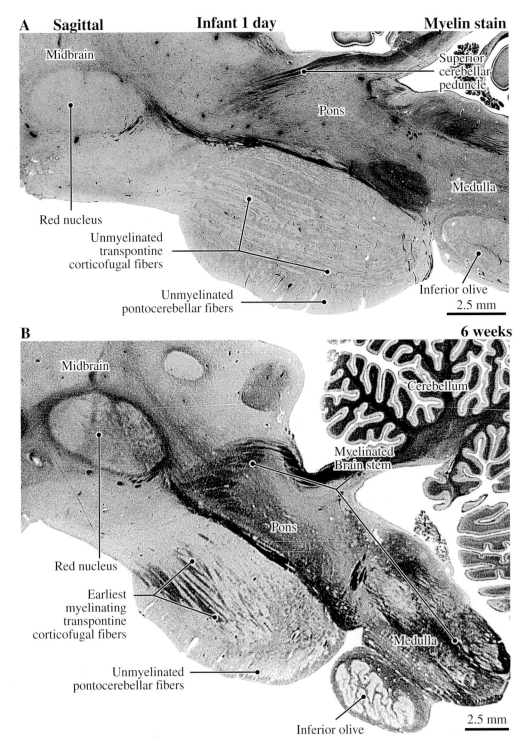

Figure 8-11. A. Absence of myelinated transpontine corticofugal fascicles in a 1-day-old infant (*Y235-66*). The pontocerebellar fibers are also unmyelinated. **B.** The earliest myelinating fascicles of the transpontine corticofugal tract in a 6-week-old infant *(Y152-61)*. The pontocerebellar fibers remain unmyelinated.

8-month-old infant, except for a few fibers in the inner half of the pontine gray (*Y228-61*; Figure 8-12A). Some of the pontocerebellar fibers are also myelinating. All the transpontine fibers are well-myelinated, and myelination of pontocerebellar fibers is in progress in the 2-year-old child (Y425-63; Figure 8-12B). These observations justify the tentative conclusion

that the myelination of the lower corticofugal tract begins at about 1 month of age, is well advanced by about 8 months of age, and precedes the myelination of the pontocerebellar fibers. Our limited data of the progressive myelination of the upper and lower corticofugal tract during infancy is schematically summarized in Figures 8-13 and 8-14.

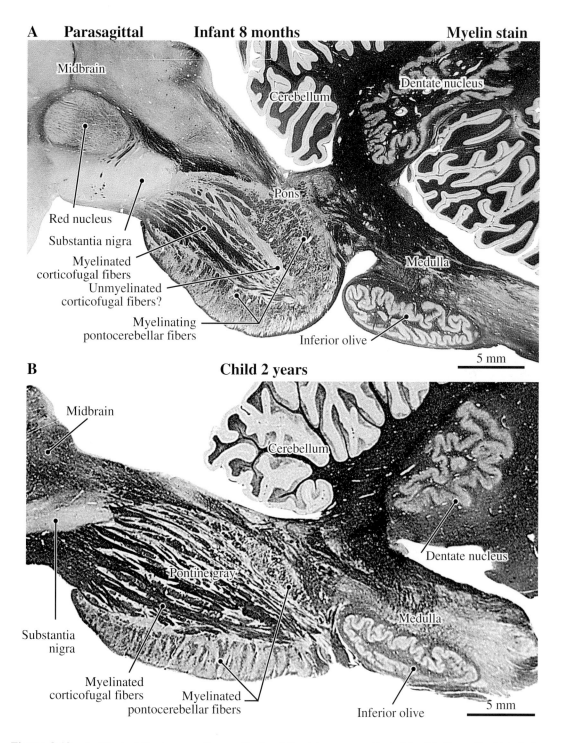

Figure 8-12. A. Most of the transpontine corticofugal fascicles are myelinated in this 8-month-old infant (*Y228-61*). The myelination of the pontocerebellar fibers is in progress. **B.** All the transpontine corticofugal fascicles and the fascicles of the pontocerebellar tract appear to be myelinated in this 2-year-old child (*Y425-63*).

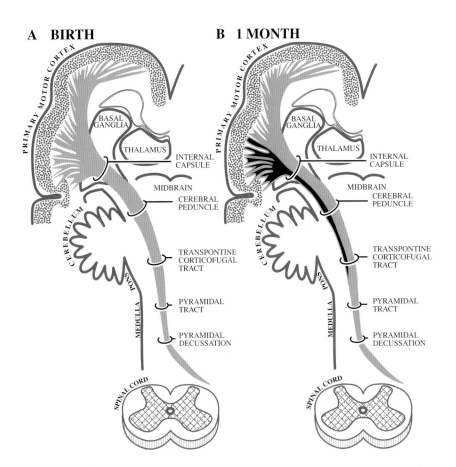

A BIRTH

B 1 MONTH

Figure 8-13. Schematic summary of the myelination of the corticofugal tract. **A.** The corticospinal tract that descends through the internal capsule, the cerebral peduncle, the pontine gray, and crosses in the pyramid is devoid of myelin at birth **B.** Some time about 1 month of age, a small complement of myelinating corticofugal fibers reach the pontine gray. The bulk of the corticofugal tract remains unmyelinated.

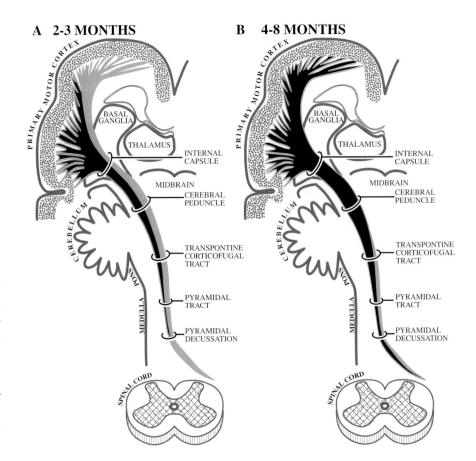

A 2-3 MONTHS

B 4-8 MONTHS

Figure 8-14. Schematic summary of the myelination of the corticofugal tract between 2 and 8 months of age. **A.** There is an increase in the proportion of myelinated fibers in the upper corticofugal tract between 2 and 3 months but few fibers are myelinated caudally in the pontine gray. **B.** The myelination of the bulk of the lower corticospinal tract takes place sometime between 4 and 8 months of age.

8.4 Proliferative Gliosis, Reactive Gliosis, and Myelination of the Lateral Corticospinal Tract. Age: Birth to 2 Years

8.4.1 The Onset of Proliferative Gliosis in the Lateral Corticospinal Tract During the First Month of Life. The lateral corticospinal tract stands out in myelin-stained sections of the fetal and neonatal spinal cord by the absence of any reaction with myelin products (Figures 7-28 to 7-34). Here we examine the relationship between the increase in glial concentration (proliferative gliosis) and the concentration of reactive glia in the lateral corticospinal tract in adjacent cell body-stained sections and myelin-stained sections of the spinal cord of newborns and infants.

Preterm Newborn. In the myelin-stained section of the cervical spinal cord of the premature newborn (*Y36-60*; GW33; CR 315 mm), the lateral corticospinal tract can be distinguished from the neighboring tracts of the white matter by the virtual absence of reactive glia (Figure 8-15A). There are a few scattered glia (by inference, nonreactive glia) in the same location in an adjacent cell body-stained section (Figure 8-15B). However, the concentration of nonreactive glia does not approach the density seen, for instance, in the adjacent tracts of the lateral funiculus and in the two fasciculi of the dorsal funiculus (Figure 8-15B). In this specimen, there is also a few nonreactive glia in the lateral corticospinal tract of the thoracic cord (Figure 8-16A) and the lumbar cord

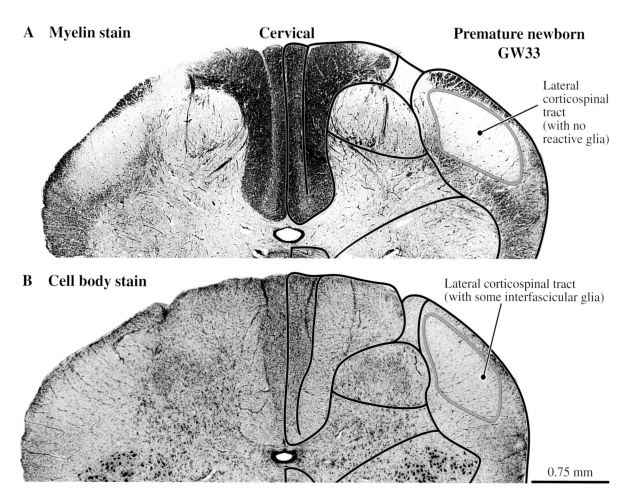

A Myelin stain   **Cervical**   **Premature newborn GW33**

Lateral corticospinal tract (with no reactive glia)

B Cell body stain

Lateral corticospinal tract (with some interfascicular glia)

0.75 mm

Figure 8-15. A. Myelin-stained section of the cervical spinal cord of a premature newborn (*Y36-60*; GW33; CR 315 mm). The lateral corticospinal tract is clearly delineated from the other tracts of the lateral funiculus by the absence of reactive glia. **B.** A nearby cell body-stained section reveals the presence of a small concentration of perifascicular glia in the territory of the corticospinal tract. The presence of these nonreactive glia may signal the onset of proliferative gliosis.

(Figure 8-16B). These observations suggest that the first step in the myelination of the corticospinal tract – proliferative gliosis – does not commence before term.

4-Day-Old Infant. The staining pattern is different in the lateral corticospinal tract of the cervical spinal cord of a 4-day-old infant (*Y299-62*; GW40; CR 350 mm). While reactive glia are still absent in the lateral corticospinal tract in the myelin-stained section (Figure 8-17A), which is clearly distinguishable by its paleness from the neighboring tracts (the nonmyelinating Lissauer's tract excepted), the lateral corticospinal tract contains a high concentration of interfascicular glia in the adjacent cell body-stained

section (Figure 8-17B). Because of this, the boundaries of the lateral corticospinal tract are difficult to delineate in cell body-stained sections. The same differential staining pattern is seen in this specimen in the thoracic and lumbar spinal cord. While reactive glia are virtually absent in myelin-stained sections of the thoracic cord (Figure 8-18A) and the lumbar cord (Figure 8-19A), there is a high concentration of nonreactive glia in the same locations in cell body-stained sections (Figures 8-18B and 8-19B). These observations indicate that while proliferative gliosis is in full swing throughout the lateral corticospinal tract in this infant, the proliferating glia are not yet producing those sudanophilic substances that react with the myelin stain.

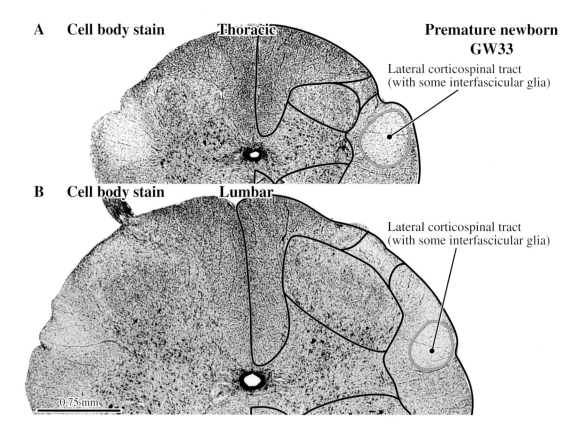

Figure 8-16. In cell body-stained sections of a premature newborn (*Y36-60*; GW33; CR 315 mm), there is a small population of glia in the lateral corticospinal tract in the thoracic (**A**) and lumbar (**B**) spinal cord. This hints at the onset of proliferative gliosis in the lateral corticospinal tract before term.

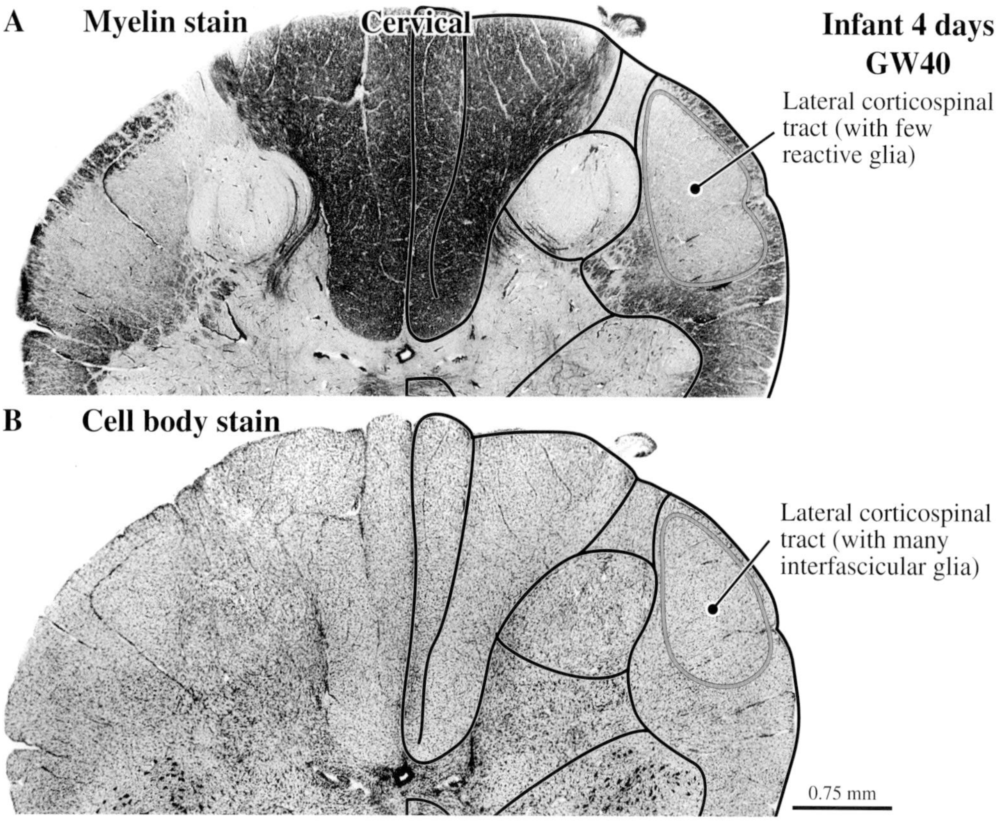

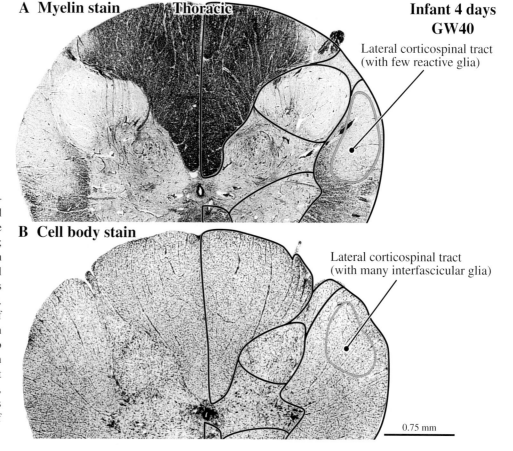

A Myelin stain Cervical Infant 4 days GW40

Lateral corticospinal tract (with few reactive glia)

B Cell body stain

Lateral corticospinal tract (with many interfascicular glia)

0.75 mm

Figure 8-17. A. Myelin-stained section of the cervical spinal cord of a 4-day-old infant (*Y299-62*; GW40; CR 350 mm). Reactive glia are virtually absent in the lateral corticospinal tract. **B.** In contrast, the net concentration of interfascicular glia (by inference, nonreactive glia) is high in the territory of the lateral corticospinal tract in this adjacent cell body-stained section. The growing concentration of interfascicular glia in the lateral corticospinal tract indicates ongoing proliferative gliosis in this infant.

A Myelin stain Thoracic Infant 4 days GW40

Lateral corticospinal tract (with few reactive glia)

B Cell body stain

Lateral corticospinal tract (with many interfascicular glia)

0.75 mm

Figure 8-18. The concentration of glia in the lateral corticospinal tract of the 4-day-old infant (*Y299-62*; GW40; CR 350 mm) in myelin-stained (**A**) and cell body-stained (**B**) sections of the thoracic spinal cord. The low concentration of reactive glia in the myelin stained section relative to the high net concentration of glia indicates that the first stage of myelination gliosis, i.e., proliferative gliosis, is in progress at this level of the spinal cord.

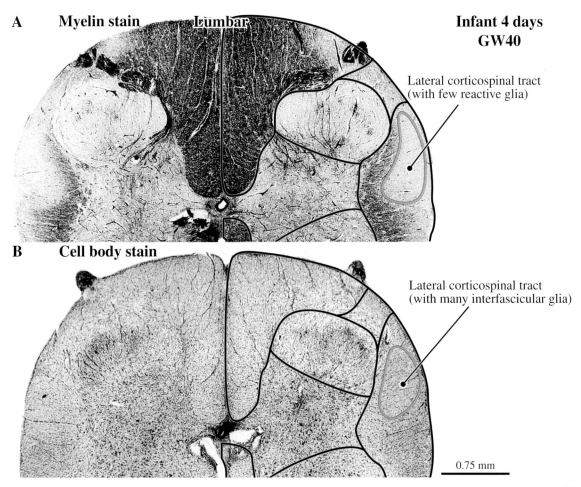

A   **Myelin stain**   **Lumbar**   **Infant 4 days**
                                                             GW40

Lateral corticospinal tract
(with few reactive glia)

B   **Cell body stain**

Lateral corticospinal tract
(with many interfascicular glia)

0.75 mm

Figure 8-19. Concentration of glia in the lateral corticospinal tract in the same 4-day-old infant (*Y299-62*) in myelin-stained (**A**) and cell body-stained (**B**) sections of lumbar spinal cord. The high net concentration of glia in the cell body-stained section but low concentration of reactive glia indicates that proliferative gliosis predominates at this age in the caudal spinal cord.

8.4.2 The Onset of Reactive Gliosis in the Lateral Corticospinal Tract During the Early Months of Infancy. The progress in the lateral corticospinal tract from proliferative gliosis (the first stage in myelination gliosis) to reactive gliosis (its second stage) is a slow and gradual process. That is suggested by a comparison of net glial concentration in cell body-stained sections and reactive glia concentration in myelin-stained sections in the lateral corticospinal tract of 1-, 1½-, and 2-month-old infants at different levels of the spinal cord.

1-Month-Old Infant. In the cervical spinal cord of a 33-day-old infant (*Y125-61*; CR 370 mm), net glial concentration is comparable in the lateral corticospinal tract to that seen in the adjacent tracts of the white matter (Figure 8-20B). However, the concentration of reactive glia (punctate sudanophilic staining) is still very low, with a hint of a medial-to-lateral gradient (Figure 8-20A). Net glial concen-

tration decreases in this infant more caudally in the thoracic spinal cord (Figure 8-20D) and reactive glial concentration appears to be lower here (Figure 8-20C) than in the cervical cord. That suggests a rostral-to-caudal (or orthograde) progression in the steps leading to the myelination of the lateral corticospinal tract.

Figure 8-20. Comparison of the concentration of reactive glia with net glial concentration in the cervical and thoracic cord of a 33-day-old infant (*Y125-61*; CR 370 mm). There is a modest concentration of reactive glia in the myelin-stained section (**A**) and a high net glial concentration in the cell body-stained section (**B**) in the cervical cord. In the thoracic cord reactive glial concentration (**C**) and net glial concentration (**D**) are both lower than more rostrally.

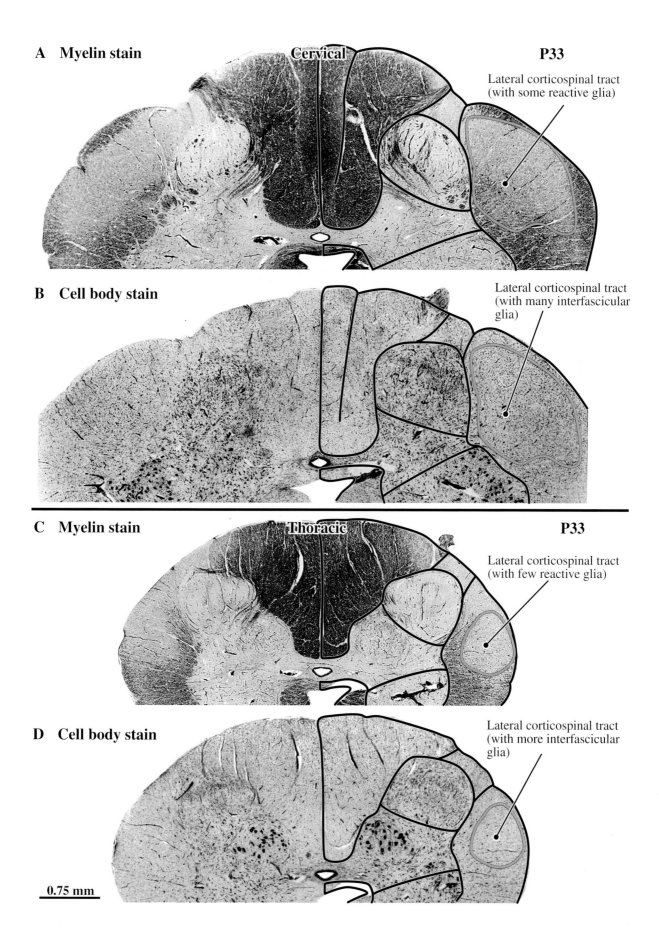

A Myelin stain

Cervical

P33

Lateral corticospinal tract
(with some reactive glia)

B Cell body stain

Lateral corticospinal tract
(with many interfascicular
glia)

C Myelin stain

Thoracic

P33

Lateral corticospinal tract
(with few reactive glia)

D Cell body stain

Lateral corticospinal tract
(with more interfascicular
glia)

0.75 mm

1½-Month-Old Infant. The comparison of a myelin-stained section and a cell body-stained section of the thoracic cord in a 45-day-old infant (*Y162-61*; CR 390 mm) indicates a rostral-to-caudal gradient in the advance of reactive gliosis in the lateral corticospinal tract. Whereas the net concentration of glia is high and comparable to that seen in other tracts of the thoracic cord (Figure 8-21B), the concentration of reactive glia is much lower at this caudal level (Figure 8-21A) than at more rostral levels of the spinal cord (not shown).

53-Day-Old Infant. The scarcity of reactive glia in the lateral corticospinal tract at caudal levels of the spinal cord is illustrated in myelin-stained sections of the upper lumbar (Figure 8-22A), middle lumbar (Figure 8-22B), lumbosacral (Figure 8-22C), and sacral (Figure 8-22D) cord of a 53-day-old infant (*Y130-61*; CR 390 mm). Because reactive gliosis is well advanced at cervical and thoracic levels of the cord in this infant (not shown), we infer a slow spread of reactive gliosis from rostral to caudal in the lateral corticospinal tract.

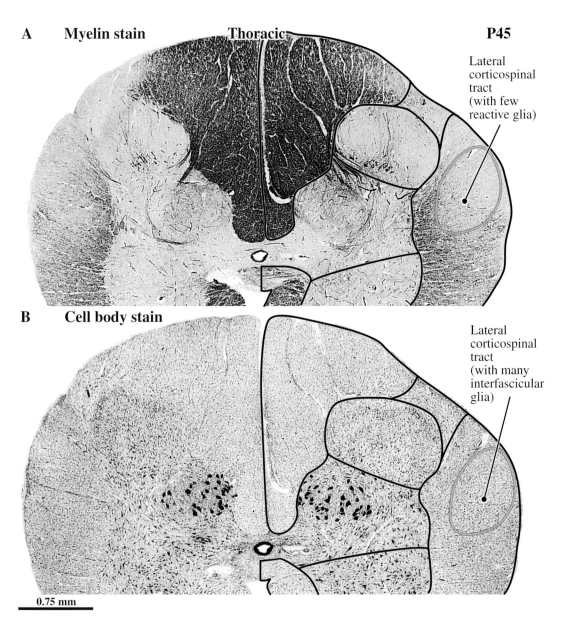

Figure 8-21. A myelin-stained section (**A**) and an adjacent cell body-stained section (**B**) of the thoracic spinal cord from a 45-day-old infant (*Y152-61*; CR 390 mm). The high concentration of glia in the cell body-stained section shows that proliferative gliosis is in full progress in the lateral corticospinal tract . However, the low concentration of reactive glia in the myelin-stained suggests an early stage of reactive gliosis.

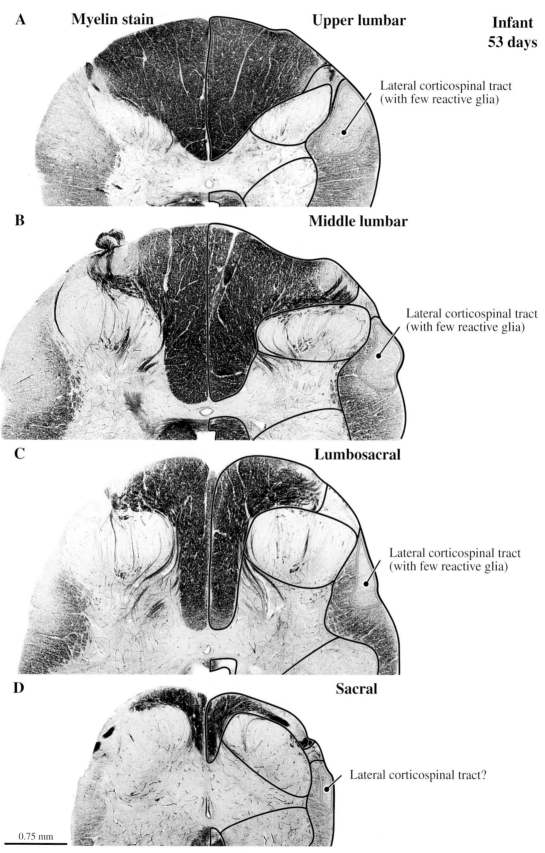

A   **Myelin stain**   **Upper lumbar**   **Infant**
                                                                    53 days

Lateral corticospinal tract
(with few reactive glia)

B   **Middle lumbar**

Lateral corticospinal tract
(with few reactive glia)

C   **Lumbosacral**

Lateral corticospinal tract
(with few reactive glia)

D   **Sacral**

Lateral corticospinal tract?

0.75 mm

Figure 8-22. Myelin-stained sections of the spinal cord from upper cervical to sacral levels in a 53-day-old infant (*Y130-61*; CR 390 mm). The concentration of reactive glia is still very low in the lateral corticospinal tract at these caudal levels .

8.4.3 The Onset of Myelination in the Lateral Corticospinal Tract in a 4-Month-Old Infant.

In sharp contrast to the paucity of reactive glia in the cervical spinal cord of younger infants, myelination of the lateral corticospinal tract is well advanced in the spinal cord of a 4-month-old infant (*Y286-62*; 440 mm) at both the upper cervical (Figure 8-23A) and the lower cervical (Figure 8-23B) levels. Indeed, since the lateral corticospinal tract is no longer distinguishable from the neighboring tracts in myelin-stained sections, we merely infer its location from the evidence seen in younger infants. However, myelination of the lateral corticospinal tract has not yet spread in this 4-month-old infant to the caudal levels of the spinal cord. In the thoracic cord (Figure 8-24A), instead of being myelinated, the lateral corticospinal tract is characterized by advanced reactive gliosis (punctate staining), and farther caudally the lumbosacral cord still stands out by a paucity of reactive glia (Figure 8-24B). These observations in a single specimen suggest that myelination of the corticospinal tract is in progress at about 4 months of age in the cervical cord but has not yet advanced to more caudal levels.

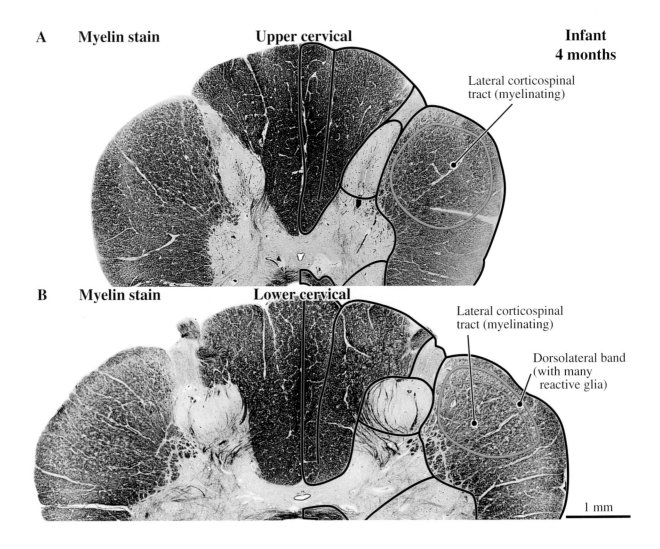

Figure 8-23. Myelin-stained sections of the upper cervical (**A**) and lower cervical (**B**) spinal cord in a 4-month-old infant (*Y286-62;* CR 440 mm). The punctate staining of the lateral corticospinal tract, seen in younger infants, has been replaced by coarse staining in the same location (the inferred site of the lateral corticospinal tract). This indicates that the myelination of the corticospinal tract has begun at the cervical level of the spinal cord.

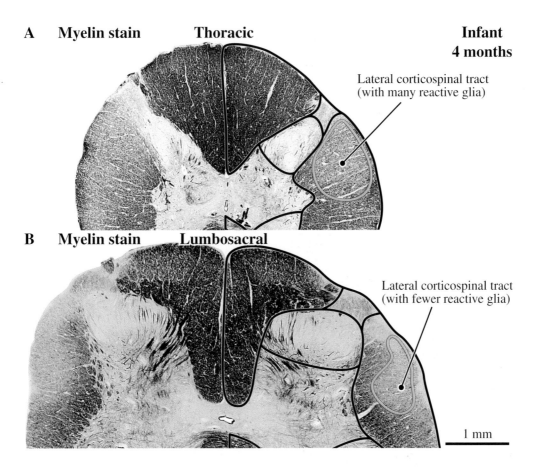

A   Myelin stain   Thoracic   Infant 4 months

Lateral corticospinal tract (with many reactive glia)

B   Myelin stain   Lumbosacral

Lateral corticospinal tract (with fewer reactive glia)

1 mm

Figure 8-24. Myelin-stained sections of the thoracic **(A)** and lumbar **(B)** spinal cord in the same 4-month-old infant (*Y286-62; CR 440 mm*). Instead of coarse staining, the lateral corticospinal tract is characterized by punctate staining in the thoracic cord and the paucity of punctate staining in the lumbosacral cord. This suggests a rostral-to-caudal gradient in the advance of the myelination of the lateral corticospinal tract.

8.4.4   Myelination of the Lateral Corticospinal Tract During Early Childhood. Figure 8-25 illustrates the myelin staining pattern of the lateral corticospinal tract at four levels of the spinal cord, from rostral to caudal, in an 11-month-old child (*Y132-61*). The intensity of myelin staining is uniform throughout much of the lateral funiculus, except for a faint dorsolateral band in the cervical (Figures 8-25A, B) and lumbar (Figure 8-25D) spinal cord This band delineates the dorsolateral border of the lateral corticospinal tract; the other boundaries are inferential. There is a hint that the staining of the lateral corticospinal tract is less intense in the tho-racic and lumbar cord (Figure 8-25C, D) than in the cervical cord (Figure 8-25A, B). (We shall return to the possible significance of this rostral-to-caudal and ventromedial-to-dorsolateral gradient in the myelination of the lateral corticospinal tract in Chapter 9.)

Finally, in the spinal cord of the 2-year-old child (*Y425-63*), as seen in Figures 8-26 and 8-27, the staining intensity of the lateral corticospinal tract is comparable to most other tracts of the lateral funiculus. We assume that by this age the myelination of the corticospinal tract is as advanced as the myelination of the other descending tracts of the spinal cord.

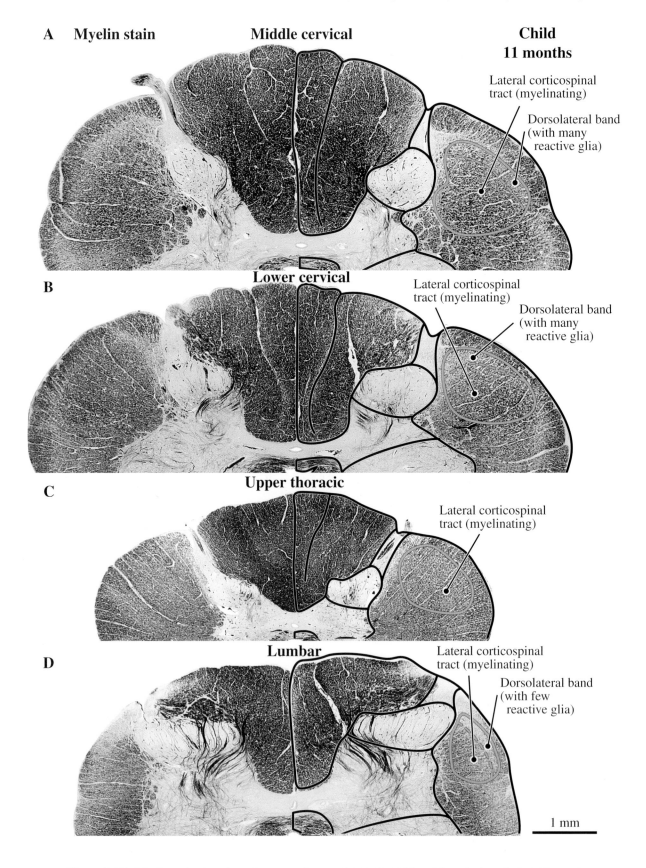

A   Myelin stain   **Middle cervical**   **Child
                                                                     11 months**

Lateral corticospinal
tract (myelinating)

Dorsolateral band
(with many
reactive glia)

B   **Lower cervical**

Lateral corticospinal
tract (myelinating)

Dorsolateral band
(with many
reactive glia)

C   **Upper thoracic**

Lateral corticospinal
tract (myelinating)

D   **Lumbar**

Lateral corticospinal
tract (myelinating)

Dorsolateral band
(with few
reactive glia)

1 mm

Figure 8-25. Myelin-stained sections, from rostral to caudal (**A**, **B**, **C**, **D**), of the spinal cord of an 11-month-old child (*Y132-61*). Because of the great increase in its staining density, the indicated location and boundaries of the lateral corticospinal tract are inferential. There is a hint of less intense staining in the lumbar spinal cord than more rostrally, and of a less densely stained dorsolateral band in both the cervical and the lumbar cord.

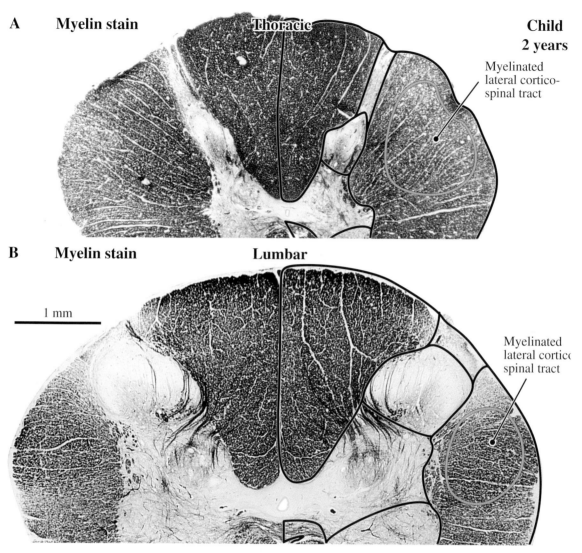

Figure 8-26. Myelin-stained sections of the cervical (**A**) and thoracic (**B**) spinal cord in a 2-year-old child (*Y425-63*). There is great increase in the staining density of the lateral corticospinal tract, indicating the completion of its myelination.

8.4.5 The Orthograde Growth and Myelination of the Lateral Corticospinal Tract. We described and summarized earlier (Figures 7-23 and 7-24) the growth of the corticofugal tract from rostral to caudal between the end of the first trimester and through the second trimester. The descending corticofugal fibers first reach the telencephalon, where they form the internal capsule. The growing corticofugal fibers then reach the midbrain and form the cerebral peduncle. Next, they approach and then traverse the pontine gray. Upon reaching the medulla, where they form the pyramids, the corticofugal tract splits into two components, the lateral and ventral corticospinal tracts. The descent of these two tracts takes place from the middle of the second trimester through the third trimester in a rostral-to-caudal sequence (Figure 7-35). In this chapter we offered some evidence that, in a similar manner, the separate steps in the myelination of the lateral corticospinal tract follow a rostral-to-caudal gradient along the length of the spinal cord. This rostral-to-caudal spread of proliferative gliosis, reactive gliosis, and myelination of the corticospinal tract from birth to 2 years of age is schematically summarized in Figure 8-28.

In contrast to the rostral-to-caudal gradient in the growth and myelination of the corticospinal fibers, in our examination of the growth of the ascending dorsal root fibers, including the dorsal funiculus, we obtained evidence for growth in the opposite direction, i.e., a caudal-to-rostral gradient in both fiber growth and myelination. Thus, the growth and myelination of the local branches (including collaterals) of the dorsal root axons antedate the main branches that proceed rostrally to the dorsal column nuclei (summarized in Figure 6-31). Similarly, the fibers of the gracile funiculus show proliferative gliosis (Figure 6-32) and become myelinated earlier in

the lumbar spinal cord caudally than they do in the cervical cord rostrally (Figure 6-33). The difference between these two systems (the corticofugal and the spinolemniscal) is, of course, that the former originates in the cortex and descends to the spinal cord while the latter originates in the spinal cord and ascends to the brain. Hence, the two systems may be said to follow the same principle of axonal growth, proliferative gliosis, reactive gliosis, and myelination, namely, a proximal-to-distal (orthograde or centrifugal) progression from the site where the neuron cell bodies are located to the terminal targets of their axons and collaterals.

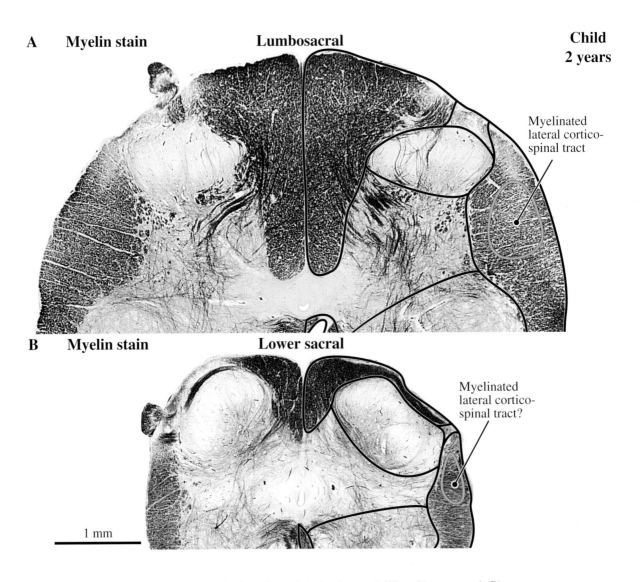

Figure 8-27. Myelin-stained sections of the lumbosacral (**A**) and lower sacral (**B**) spinal cord in the same 2-year-old child (*Y425-63*). Myelination of the entire corticospinal tract appears to be well advanced by this age.

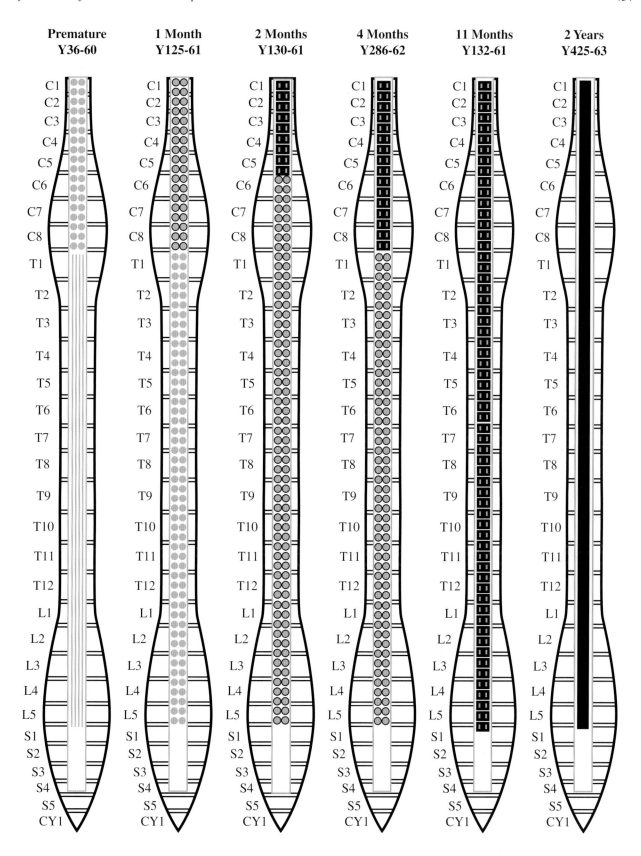

Figure 8-28. Summary diagram of the proximal-to-distal (orthograde) progression of proliferative gliosis (orange spheres), reactive gliosis (black circles), and the spread of myelination (broken lines and heavy lines) in the lateral corticospinal tract in 6 specimens ranging in maturity between birth and 2 years of age.

9 CORRELATIONS BETWEEN THE MORPHOLOGICAL MATURATION OF THE SPINAL CORD AND BEHAVIORAL DEVELOPMENT

9.1 The Early Development of Motility in Relation to Spinal Cord Development

9.1.1 Pioneering Studies of the Development of Motility and Sensorimotor Reflexes in Aborted Embryos.

The study of the embryology of human behavior began with occasional reports by clinicians of spontaneous movements seen in aborted embryos and reflex-like movements triggered by tactile stimulation (e.g., Minkowski, 1923; Bolaffio and Artom, 1924; Fizgerald and Windle, 1942; for a review see, Carmichael, 1970). Thus, for instance, Fitzgerald and Windle observed spontaneous movements in embryos with a crown-rump (CR) length of 20-21 mm; that is, at about the estimated gestational age of 7 weeks. Hooker (1938, 1942, 1954) must be credited with pioneering a large-scale experimental research project of the development of sensorimotor reflexes in human embryos. Hooker immersed aborted fetuses in an isotonic saline of normal body temperature and stimulated selected body parts with graded hair asthesiometers to elicit visible movements. In many instances the responses were recorded cinematographically. Stimulation sites included the face and mouth supplied by the trigeminal nerve; other sites that are of a more direct relevance to us here involved stimulation of the hand, the trunk, the genital area, and the feet. More recently Hooker's findings were described by Humphrey (1964) along with her own observations. In their reports, Hooker and Humphrey most often used the menstrual age of embryos but in some cases also reported their CR length. Where CR length was available, we changed their menstrual age estimates to gestational age in weeks (GW), using the standardized timetable in Figure 5-1. Otherwise, we deducted 2 weeks from the menstrual age to estimate gestational age.

The age of the youngest embryo in which Hooker obtained responses to stimulation was GW6.5.

Brushing the mouth region (supplied by the trigeminal nerve) with a hair triggered rotation of the face contralateral to the stimulus, extension of both arms, and rotation of the pelvis to the contralateral side. That behavior could be elicited more consistently in GW7.5 embryos. Hooker classified these avoidance reflexes as "total pattern" movements rather than "local reflexes" in line with an earlier theoretical dichotomy proposed by Coghill (1929). Rotation of the head without trunk movement (classified as a local reflex) could not be elicited until GW11–GW12. Other writers distinguished between earlier-emerging gross (or holokinetic) movements and later-emerging discrete (or idiokinetic) movements.

With reference to holokinetic reactions mediated by spinal nerves, Hooker reported that stimulation of the palm of the hand triggered discernible gross motor reactions in a few GW8 embryos and in most of the GW10 embryos. Stimulation of the shoulder, the genital and anal regions, and the soles of the feet did not trigger gross movements until GW10.5–GW11. In terms of idiokinetic responses, stimulation of the palm of the hand triggered partial closure of the fingers (but not the thumb) in GW10 embryos (Figure 9-1A). Finger closure was more pronounced in GW15.5 fetuses (Figure 9-1B). That response often included wrist and elbow flexion, medial rotation of the arm and forearm pronation, and it sometimes persisted long enough to produce a grasping reaction. Opponent movement of the thumb was not consistently produced until GW20 (Figure 9-1C), and the thumb did not participate in the grasping response until GW23. By GW25, a fetus can support its weight for a short time by grasping a rod.

Effective grasping requires cutaneous and proprioceptive feedback. A few sensory fibers reach the palm by GW8.5 (Cauna and Mannon, 1961) but they do not contact epithelial cells until about GW10.5

Figure 9-1. A. The first hint of finger closure in response to stroking of the palm of the hand in a GW10.0 embryo (Hooker specimen # 26). **B.** Improved finger closure in response to stimulation of the hand in a GW15.5 fetus (Hooker specimen # 7). The thumb is still not involved in the response. **C.** Effective closure of the hand (grasping response) in a GW20 fetus (Hooker specimen # 15). After Humphrey (1964).

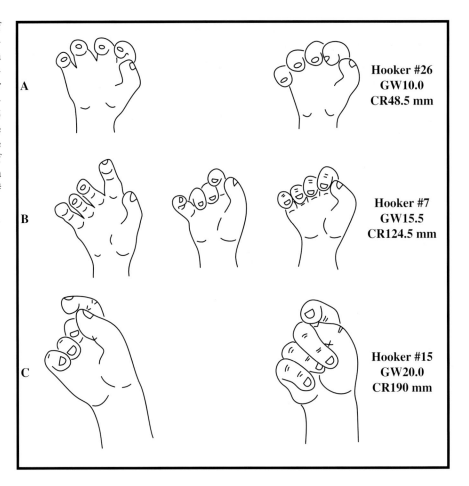

(Hogg, 1941). The little evidence available suggests that innervation of cutaneous sensors starts sometime between GW10.5 and GW14.5. It is also about GW10.5 that immature Pacinian corpuscles begin to form (Cauna and Mannon, 1959). Nerve fibers do not penetrate the epithelium between papillary ridges of the palm until about GW12 (Hogg, 1941), and definite Merkel discs do not form until GW14.5 (Szymonowicz, 1933).

9.1.2   Recent Ultrasonic Studies of the Emergence of Spontaneous Motility During the First Trimester.

In contrast to the stimulus-evoked reflexes studied earlier with aborted embryos, the introduction of ultrasonic recordings in the 1970s has made possible the intrauterine analysis of spontaneous embryonic motility in normal embryos. Furthermore, ultrasound recording has the added advantage of yielding real-time data about the emergence of motility in healthy embryos and permits follow-up (longitudinal) observations. Most of the available

ultrasonic studies have dealt with embryonic motility during the second and third trimesters; only a few reports are currently available about the emergence of motor activity during the first trimester.

In a large-scale study of 1,166 pregnant women, Natsuyama (1991) recorded fetal movements in embryos ranging in length from CR 8–9 mm to CR 22 mm for the standardized duration of 5 minutes (Figure 9-2A). Embryonic motility was difficult to distinguish from maternal movement in the 8-9 mm embryos (GW5.0). Spontaneous movements were recorded in about 20% of the embryos smaller than CR 16 mm (GW6.5), and in 90% of the larger embryos (GW7.0). Natsuyama distinguished between dormant and active periods, and within the active periods between brief, isolated movements, and longer motor phases. The number and duration of motor phases increased greatly, though with considerable variability, in embryos exceeding CR 16 mm, estimated age GW6.5–7.0 (Figure 9-2B).

In an earlier longitudinal study, de Vries and his associates (1982) investigated the emergence of various classes of spontaneous movements in 12 embryos (GW5–GW13). In the summary presented in Figure 9-3, we have omitted some of the movements they observed that are not controlled by the spinal cord (e.g., hiccups, jaw opening, yawning) and modified their postmenstrual age to estimated gestational age. The earliest movements of uncertain nature, called "just discernible movements," were seen at GW5 and GW6. What the authors interpreted as a "startle response" was first observed in GW6 and GW7 embryos. Discrete arm movements were first seen at GW7 and GW8, and isolated leg movements at about the same age or a little thereafter. Head rotation, and hand and face contact was seen in most embryos by GW8 and GW10. Stretching appeared variably between GW8 and G13. Forward flexion of the head was seen in most embryos between GW10 and GW13.

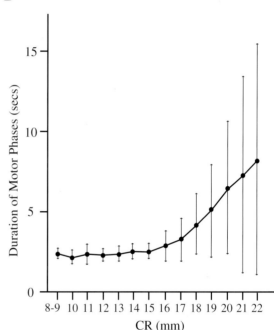

Figure 9-2. Average number of active "motor phases" (**A**) and their duration (**B**) during ultrasonic recording periods of 5-minute duration, in embryos ranging from CR 8-9 to 22 mm (GW5.0–GW7.0). After Natsuyama (1991).

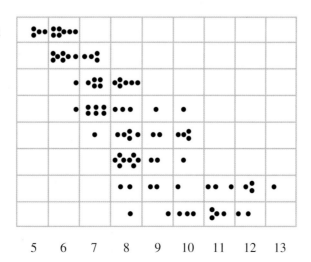

Figure 9-3. A longitudinal study of the first emergence, as determined by ultrasonic recordings, of certain classes of spontaneous movements in 12 human embryos. After de Vries et al. (1982).

9.1.3 Stages of Spinal, Somatic, and Behavioral Development During the First Trimester.
There is little evidence of true spontaneous motility in embryos younger than GW5.0. According to Natsuyama (1991), the occasional brief "motor phases" in some GW5 embryos (CR 8–9 mm or younger) cannot be reliably distinguished from maternal movements. Similarly, the "just discernible movements" that de Vries et al. (1982) observed in a few of their GW5–GW6 embryos (Figure 9-3) are of uncertain identity. The brief spontaneous movement Natsuyama recorded in about 20% of the GW6–GW7 embryos (Figure 9-2) involved both the head and the trunk. The same may apply to the "startle" response in the GW6–GW7 embryos of de Vries et al. (Figure 9-3). These limited observations suggest that the earliest age when spinal cord-mediated holokinetic endogenous motility emerges is some time around GW6-GW7. Ideokinetic spontaneous motility (like isolated arm and leg movements) emerges next, at about GW7-GW8.

The currently available evidence of behavioral development during the first trimester is correlated with the stages of spinal cord maturation in Table 5-1, and with concurrent somatic maturation (as described in Chapter 5). Three epochs of spinal cord development are distinguished, with a total of 10 stages. The first epoch is the period when the stem cells of spinal cord neurons (the spinal NEP cells) are produced en masse in the germinal neuroepithelium surrounding the spinal canal (stages 1-4, roughly embryonic ages GW3.0 to GW4.5). That occurs before the differentiation of spinal cord neurons and before the first emergence of spontaneous embryonic motility (Table 9-1). The highlight of the second epoch is the period of neurogenesis, the time when, in an overlapping sequence, the differentiating (postmitotic) motoneurons, interneurons, and microneurons leave the germinal neuroepithelium and begin to settle in the ventral horn, intermediate gray, and dorsal horn, respectively (stages 5-8; roughly between GW4.5 and GW8.5). We begin our correlations below with the initial stage of the second epoch, stage 5.

Stage 5 (GW4.5–5.5; CR 9-15 mm). An important event during stage 5 of embryonic development is the formation of the arm buds and the leg buds (Figure 5-8C). However, the muscles are still represented by myotomes and the bones are precar-

tilagenous (Figure 5-16C). Spinal cord development in stage 5 embryos is characterized (at the cervical level) by the following features. (a) Motoneuron production is at its peak and the exiting motoneurons assemble as an amorphous mass in the incipient ventral horn (Figures 5-8D, 5-10B). (b) The earliest motor fibers leave the ventral horn to form the ventral root (Figure 5-9). (c) The earliest dorsal root fibers enter the spinal cord and form the bifurcation zone (Figures 5-23A, B; 5-24A). The latter event signals the beginning of the growth of the local ascending and descending branches of primary sensory fibers. If embryonic motility is, in fact, absent during stage 5, the conclusion is warranted that the ingrowth of the earliest sensory fibers into the spinal cord and the outgrowth of the earliest motor fibers toward the periphery are not by themselves sufficient to produce motility. The inability of these afferent and efferent elements to produce overt movements could be due to one or more of the following factors: (i) lack of synaptic contact between the dorsal root fibers and motoneurons; (ii) the absence of local circuits (central pattern generators) that control the discharge of motoneuron pools; (iii) the absence of effective neuromuscular contacts; and (iv) the inability of the undifferentiated muscle masses to contract. The virtual absence of the white matter, except for the ventral commissure, during this stage of spinal cord development (Figure 5-10B) also may be important. The early developing intraspinal (propriospinal) fibers that interconnect the different segments of the spinal cord and produce intersegmental reflexes, are probably still absent at this stage of development.

Stage 6 (GW5.5–6.5; CR 15–20 mm). Stage 6 is the period when spontaneous motility is first displayed by human embryos. By this time the differentiation of the trunk, shoulder and pelvic muscles is in progress (Figure 5-17B). These proximal muscles are presumably able to contract in response to motoneuron firing. The following advances occur in spinal cord development during this stage. (a) Motoneurons begin to segregate into two clusters in the ventral horn: an inferior compartment, the future medial columns, and a superior compartment, the future lateral columns (compare Figures 5-17A, 5-18A). (b) The production of ventral horn interneurons is at its peak and they begin to settle in the intermediate gray during this period (compare Figures 5-17A and 5-18A). (c) The dorsal root bifurcation zone expands greatly (compare Figures 5-24A and 5-24B), attesting to the entry and branching of more and more dorsal root fibers. (d) The ventral and lateral funiculi are beginning to expand (compare Figures 5-5A and 5-5B). That allows the possibility that the earliest intraspinal fibers and some descending bulbospinal efferents are making contact with ventral horn interneurons and/or motoneurons. However, there is as yet no indication of the sprouting of locally terminating dorsal root collaterals. Therefore, the sensorimotor "reflex arcs" are still "open" during stage 6 of spinal cord development.

Although spontaneous motility is displayed by stage 6 embryos (de Vries et al., 1982; Natsuyama, 1991), which suggests that the spinal cord pattern generators are becoming operational, we may recall Hooker's (1938, 1944) failure to elicit reflex movements by stimulating body parts served by spinal afferents (palm of the hand, trunk, sole of the foot) in fetuses younger than GW8–GW11 (stages 8–9). So the motility displayed by stage 6 embryos are not reflexes triggered by spinal afferents. Hooker did obtain body movements in stage 6 embryos following stimulation of the mouth region, but this would be reflexes mediated by trigeminal input. Therefore, the spontaneous movements during stage 6 are either the responses of pattern generators to descending supraspinal (vestibular, trigeminal?) impulses or they are endogenous activities of the maturing pattern generators.

Stage 7 (GW6.5–7.5; CR 20–25 mm). According to Natsuyama (1991), 90% of stage 7 embryos (GW7.0; CR 17–22 mm) display spontaneous motility and the movements tend to be of longer duration. While in the smaller (GW6.0; CR 17–18 mm) embryos the arms tended to move in unison with the trunk (holokinetic movement), in the larger embryos (CR 19–22 mm), one arm often moved independently of the other (ideokinetic movement). That agrees with the emergence of isolated arm and leg movements in many (though not all) of the GW7 embryos (de Vries et al., 1982). Notwithstanding these advances in motor coordination, the evidence we currently have indicates that the spinal "reflex arcs" are still not closed because movements cannot be triggered during this stage by stimulating the trunk or the extremities (Hooker, 1938, 1942).

The highlight of somatic maturation during stage 7 is the differentiation of the distal arm and leg muscles (Figure 5-19B). With reference to spinal cord maturation, we may note the following landmark events. (a) The gelatinosal microneurons of the dorsal horn, the targets of dorsal root cutaneous afferents, are settling in the incipient dorsal horn (Figures 5-12). (b) The collateralization zone, composed of locally terminating branches of dorsal root fibers, has begun to form (compare Figures 5-25A and 5-25B). However, there is no evidence that these collaterals have reached their targets in the gray matter of the spinal cord. (c) The interneuronal fields of the ventral horn and the intermediate gray are expanding (Figure 5-19A). (d) The segregation of motoneurons in the lateral panel of the ventral horn is in progress (Figure 5-19A). (e) There is a sudden increase in the concentration of synapses between GW7 and GW8 in the ventral horn (Figure 5-22). Finally, (f) the ventral and lateral funiculi are expanding (Figures 5-6A, B). The latter suggests an increase in intraspinal fibers and the arrival of the earliest supraspinal efferents (medial longitudinal fasciculus, the medial and lateral vestibulospinal tracts).

These anatomical and behavioral observations allow the following inferences. First, the segregation of motoneurons in the lateral columns of the ventral horn, the expansion of the field of interneurons, and the formation of a small population of ventral horn synapses during (or by the end of) stage 7 reflect the onset of the structural maturation of the spinal cord pattern generators. The pattern generators could coordinate the isolated limb movements during recurrent episodes of spontaneous motility. Second, Hooker's observation that stimulation of the trunk and extremities do not trigger overt responses until about GW7, indicates that the local reflex arcs are still open at this stage. This is probably so because the local collaterals of dorsal root afferents still have not reached the interneurons and motoneurons. Third, the endogenous mechanisms of motor coordination mature before spinal afferents can trigger or modulate that activity. It is not clear whether the pattern generators are activated at this stage by oscillating endogenous mechanisms or by descending commands from the brain stem.

Stage 8 (GW7.5–8.5; CR 25–35 mm). This stage is distinguished by one landmark event with regard to sensorimotor development, namely, the closure of the reflex arc, and by some advances in somatic maturation, in particular the articulation of fingers and toes (Figure 5-13A).

Table 9-1
Behavioral Development in Relation to Somatic and Spinal Cord Development
During the First Trimester (Part 1)

Stage	Gestational Age (in weeks)	Neurogenesis Gliogenesis	Growth of Primary Afferents	Maturation of Motoneurons	Intraspinal and Supraspinal Connections
1	<GW3.0	Proliferation of			
2	<GW3.0	NEP cells			
3	GW3.0 GW3.5	in the pre-exodus			
4	GW3.5 GW4.5	neuroepithelium.			
5	GW4.5 GW5.5	Peak period of motoneuron production and exodus.	Arrival of earlies dorsal root fibers. Onset of dorsal root bifurcation zone (oval bundle of His).	Motoneurons settle as a single mass in incipient ventral horn. Exit of ventral root axons.	Formation of the ventral funiculus. (Arrival of vestibulo-spinal tract?)
6	GW5.5 GW6.5	Peak period of interneuron production and exodus.	Expansion of dorsal root bifurcation zone. (Formation of local ascending and de-scending branches.)	Segregation of inferior and superior motoneuron compartments.	Formation of the lateral funiculus. (Formation of intraspinal tracts?)
7	GW6.5 GW7.5	Onset of gelatinosal neuron production. Microneuronal exodus.	Formation of dorsal root collateralization zone. (Sprouting of local dorsal root collaterals.)	Segregation of medial and lateral motoneuron compartments.	Expansion of the lateral funiculus.
8	GW7.5 GW8.5	Peak period of gelatinosal and visceral interneuron production.	Expansion of dorsal root collateralization zone. (Growth of local dorsal root collaterals.)	Segregation of central and lateral motoneuron compartments.	Expansion of the lateral funiculus. (Formation of spino-cerebellar and spino-cephalic tracts.)
9	GW8.5 GW11	Cessation of neuron production. Onset of neuroepithelial glia production.	Dorsal root collaterals reach intermediate gray and ventral horn.	Onset of segregation of far-lateral and retrodorsal motoneuron compartments.	Formation of cuneate fasciculus. (Ascending spino-lemniscal fibers.)
10	GW10.5 GW13	Cessation of neuroepithelial glia production.	Great increase in the number of dorsal root collaterals distributed in the gray matter.	Continuing seg-regation of far-lateral and retro-dorsal motoneuron compartments.	Formation of gracile fasciculus. Growth of dorsal, lateral, and ventral funiculi.

Table 9-1
Behavioral Development in Relation to Somatic and Spinal Cord Development During the First Trimester (Part 2)

Stage	Gestational Age (in weeks)	Somatic Development	Skeletomuscular Development	Spontaneous Movements	Stimulus-evoked Movements	Neuro-behavioral Landmarks
1	<GW3.0					Absence of physiological motility.
2	<GW3.0					
3	GW3.0 GW3.5					
4	GW3.5 GW4.5					
5	GW4.5 GW5.5	Formation of arm and leg buds.	Axial myotomes. Mesenchymal muscle primordia. Primordia of arm and leg bones.			
6	GW5.5 GW6.5	Formation of hand and foot buds.	Differentiation of trunk, shoulder, and pelvic muscles. Precartilaginous arm and leg bones.			
7	GW6.5 GW7.5	Formation of finger buds.	Beginning of arm and leg muscle differentiation.	Joint head and body movements of short duration.		Earliest organization of central pattern generators.
8	GW7.5 GW8.5	Onset of articulation of fingers and toes.	Onset of arm and leg ossification.	First emergence of independent arm and leg movements.	Stimulation of palm of hand triggers body movements.	Earliest closure of local reflex arcs.
9	GW8.5 GW10.5		Onset of hand and foot ossification.		Stimulation of palm of hand or feet elicits partial finger closure or toe movements.	Increse in the frequency and fine-tuning of spontaneous and stimulus-evoked movements.
10	GW10.5 GW13	Continuing articulation of fingers and toes.		Jerky movements are replaced by graceful movements.	Reduced stereotypy and increased variability of movements.	

Hooker (1938, 1942) reported that GW8 is the earliest age when stimulation of the palm of the hand triggers motor responses. This is the first behavioral indication of the closure of local reflex arcs in the spinal cord. In somewhat older embryos (GW8.5), stimulation of the shoulder, the genital and anal area, and the sole of the foot also triggered discernible overt responses. In addition to this behavioral evidence for the maturation of spinal reflexes, there are also behavioral indications for advances in the maturation of pattern generators during stage 8. Coordinated hand and face contact, as described by de Vries et al. (1982), exemplifies this (Figure 9-3). With regard to the spinal cord maturation, stage 8 is characterized by the following advances. (a) Settling microneurons form the substantia gelatinosa in the dorsal horn (Figures 5-6B, 5-13B). (b) The collateralization zone is expanding (Figures 5-13B; 5-26A). (c) Some dorsal root collaterals reach the intermediate gray and the ventral horn (Figure 5-27A). (d) The segregation of motor columns continues in the ventral, dorsal, and retrodorsal tiers of the lateral panel of the ventral horn (Figures 5-20A, 5-39A, B). Finally, (e) there is a sudden and pronounced increase in the concentration of ventral horn synapses (Figure 5-22). Some of these morphogenetic advances may be correlated with the behavioral evidence of the emergence of some spinal reflexes during stage 8.

Stage 8 ends the second epoch of spinal cord development (Table 5-1), beginning at about GW4.5 and ending at about GW8.5. In terms of spinal cord development, the major event during this epoch is the sequential differentiation of all spinal cord neurons. In terms of physiological development, the major events are the formation of the earliest central pattern generators and the subsequent closure of some reflex arcs. Finally, in terms of behavioral development, it is during this period that the early spontaneous holokinetic movements are gradually replaced by stimulus-evoked, ideokinetic movements. However, these movements are usually jerky in nature and tend to be brief.

Stage 9 (GW8.5–10.5; CR 35–60 mm). An important behavioral achievement during stage 9 is the partial closure of the fingers in response to stroking the palm of the hand (Figure 9-1A). While still ineffective in grasping and holding onto an object, this response is sometimes associated with wrist and elbow flexion, medial rotation of the arm, and forearm pronation (Humphrey, 1964). Occasionally, the

response to stroking the palm of the hand is an extension, rather than flexion of the fingers. The thumb is typically not involved in these movements (Hooker, 1938, 1954). Stimulation of the sole of the foot also produces overt responses. These include plantar flexion, accompanied by dorsiflexion of the great toe and fanning of the other toes. Either type of toe movement may be accompanied by hip and knee flexion, rotation of the thigh inward or outward, abduction of the thigh, and a kick by the extended limb (Humphrey, 1964). Such observations suggest considerable advances in the intersegmental coordination of pattern generators and stimulus-evoked reflexes (perhaps the forerunners of the grasp, plantar, and other fetal reflexes).

The following advances in the morphogenesis of the spinal cord may contribute to these behavioral developments during stage 9. (a) Spinal cord neurogenesis is completed and the persisting neuroepithelium surrounding the central canal (Figure 5-14) starts to generate satellite cells, including neuroglia. (b) The dorsal root bifurcation zone expands greatly (Figure 5-26B), signaling the sprouting of more and more locally arborizing and terminating sensory fibers. (c) The ventral and lateral funiculi are expanding (see the juxtaposed sections of a GW8.5 embryo and a GW10.5 embryo in Figures 5-31 to 5-38). That raises the possibility that messages conveyed by fibers of early forming fiber tracts – the intraspinal tract, the ascending spinocephalic and spinocerebellar tracts, and the descending vestibulospinal and reticulospinal tracts – are increasingly integrated with the spinal pattern generators to organize more complex movements. Finally, (d) it is during stage 9 that the segregating motoneurons begin to form discrete columns in the far-lateral sector of the ventral horn (Figures 5-32B, 5-34A, 5-40B). We may recall that these motoneurons, in particular those occupying the retrodorsal tier, are innervating the distal muscles of the hand and foot.

Stage 10 (GW10.5–13.0; CR 60–90 mm). This lengthy stage ends the first trimester. Unfortunately, our anatomical material is quite limited for this period, and behavioral reports are also scanty. Hooker (1938, 1942) and Humphrey (1964) singled out the following behavioral developments in GW11–13 fetuses. (a) The "total pattern" (holokinetic) responses to sensory stimulation have become rare and the typical behavioral responses are various combinations of "local reflexes" (ideokinetic movements). (b) The responses to repeated stimuli are becoming less stereotyped and more variable. (c) The triggered movements are losing their jerky character and are becoming more steady and graceful. These behavioral developments suggest great strides in the fine-tuning of pattern generator circuits and the development of ever more complex intersegmental and suprasegmental connections. In terms of spinal cord development, a landmark event at the beginning of this stage is the great increase in the number of dorsal root collaterals that reach the intermediate gray and the ventral horn (Figure 5-27B).

In an attempt to reconstruct the development of the spinal cord by the end of this stage, we relied on a single specimen that, strictly speaking, belongs to the first week of the next period, a GW14 fetus (Figures 5-15, 5-20C, 5-43, 5-44). Among landmark development in this fetus are the following. (a) The gray matter appears mature (Figure 5-15). Particularly noteworthy is the expansion of the dorsal horn, and the even greater enlargement of the ventral horn. (b) Although the white matter is still small relative to the gray matter, all the funiculi are present (with the notable exception of the superior lateral funiculus that will be occupied by the descending lateral corticospinal tract). (c) There is great increase in the number of motoneuron columns in the far-lateral and retrodorsal sectors of the ventral horn in the cervical enlargement (Figure 5-43C) and in the lumbosacral enlargement (Figure 5-44C). Finally, (d), there is considerable increase in the concentration of ventral horn synapses (Figure 5-22). However, there are no interfascicular glia in the developing white matter of the spinal cord and no indication anywhere of the onset of myelination. The absence of myelination must greatly hamper impulse conduction along the afferent and efferent pathways that make possible intersegmental integration and supraspinal control.

9.2 Behavioral Development During the Second and Third Trimesters in Relation to Spinal Cord Maturation

9.2.1 Intrauterine Observations of Spontaneous Motility in Normal Fetuses.
Spontaneous fetal movements, referred to by some authors as "general movements" (Roodenburg et al., 1991; Prechtl, 1997), were initially known from the reports of pregnant women. Newbery (1941) classified these subjectively perceived fetal movements into three types: (a) squirming, pushing, stretching, and turning; (b) kicks, thrusts and jerks of the extremities; and (c) rhythmic convulsive movements. Pregnant women first become aware of these fetal movements at about GW16. The perceived fetal movements tend to increase in frequency for a few months, then decline. While the correlation between subjective maternal reports and objective ultrasonic recordings of fetal movements is not perfect (Valentin and Marsal, 1986), the initial increase in fetal motility and its later decline has been confirmed with the ultrasonic technique (Natale et al., 1988; Roodenburg et al., 1991; Kisilevsky et al., 1999). Fetuses tend to be very active between the ages of GW14 and GW19. The dormant periods between bursts of activity usually do not exceed 5-6 minutes. Then, between GW16 and GW32, there is a decrease in the frequency of fetal movements per unit time. As birth approaches, an hour (or more) may elapse between movement episodes (Patrick et al., 1982). After birth, the seemingly aimless (and presumably involuntary) spontaneous movements, like kicking, persist through the early months of infancy (Jensen et al., 1994; Droit et al., 1996; Piek and Gasson, 1999; Vaal et el., 2000) to be replaced by purposive, voluntary movements at 3 months of age or thereafter (Prechtl and Hopkins, 1986; Roodenburg et al., 1991; Hadders-Algra and Prechtl, 1992; Hadders-Algra, 1993).

There have been attempts to classify these spontaneous fetal movements into basic patterns and determine their course of development (Roodenburg et al., 1991; Kozuma et al., 1997). Stretches and "startle" reactions (both reflecting holokinetic movements) tend to decline during the second trimester, while discrete (ideokinetic) movements, such as isolated arm or leg movements, eye movements, and mouth opening, tend to increase. A longitudinal study of 17 fetuses between GW12 and GW27 showed that the number of arm movements increased between GW15 and GW18 but declined rapidly thereafter (McCartney-Hepper, 1999). According to this study, 83% of the fetuses moved their right arm significantly more often than their left arm, suggesting an early origin in the lateralization of hand use.

Studies have also been made of the development of such specific life-support functions as breathing (Kisilevsky et al., 1999). Brief periods of breathing episodes are first displayed by GW10 embryos (de Vries et al., 1982). By GW19, the incidence of breathing episodes increases from 2% to 6% during the sampling time (de Vries et al., 1985). GW24-GW28 fetuses breathe about 14% of the time (Natale et al., 1988), and GW32-GW42 fetuses breathe 30% of the time or longer (Patrick et al., 1988; Roodenburg et al., 1991). The duration of breathing episodes increases from 10 seconds to 30 seconds between GW25 to GW32 (Higuchi et al., 1991). Increases in fetal breathing occur after an excess of carbon dioxide in the maternal blood (Connors et al., 1988), maternal ingestion of coffee (Salvador and Koos, 1989), and heightened maternal blood glucose levels (Adamson et al., 1983). The latter observations suggest that intrauterine breathing is responsive to stimuli and, hence, may have some functional utility.

Recent studies have shown that the episodes of spontaneous movement during the second and third trimesters are cyclical in nature (Robertson, 1985; Nijhuis et al., 1999). These cycles of activity and rest may represent alternating behavioral states rather than responses to external stimuli, reminiscent of the sleeping-waking cycle in terms of heart rate patterns and eye movements (Groome et al., 1997; Kozuma et al., 1997, 1998). Taken together, these observations suggest that overt fetal motility, initially whole body movements and later isolated movements of the head and limbs, are endogenous in origin and serve morphogenetic rather than behavioral functions. Since the sleeping-waking cycle is regulated by supraspinal mechanisms, a descending influence (perhaps from

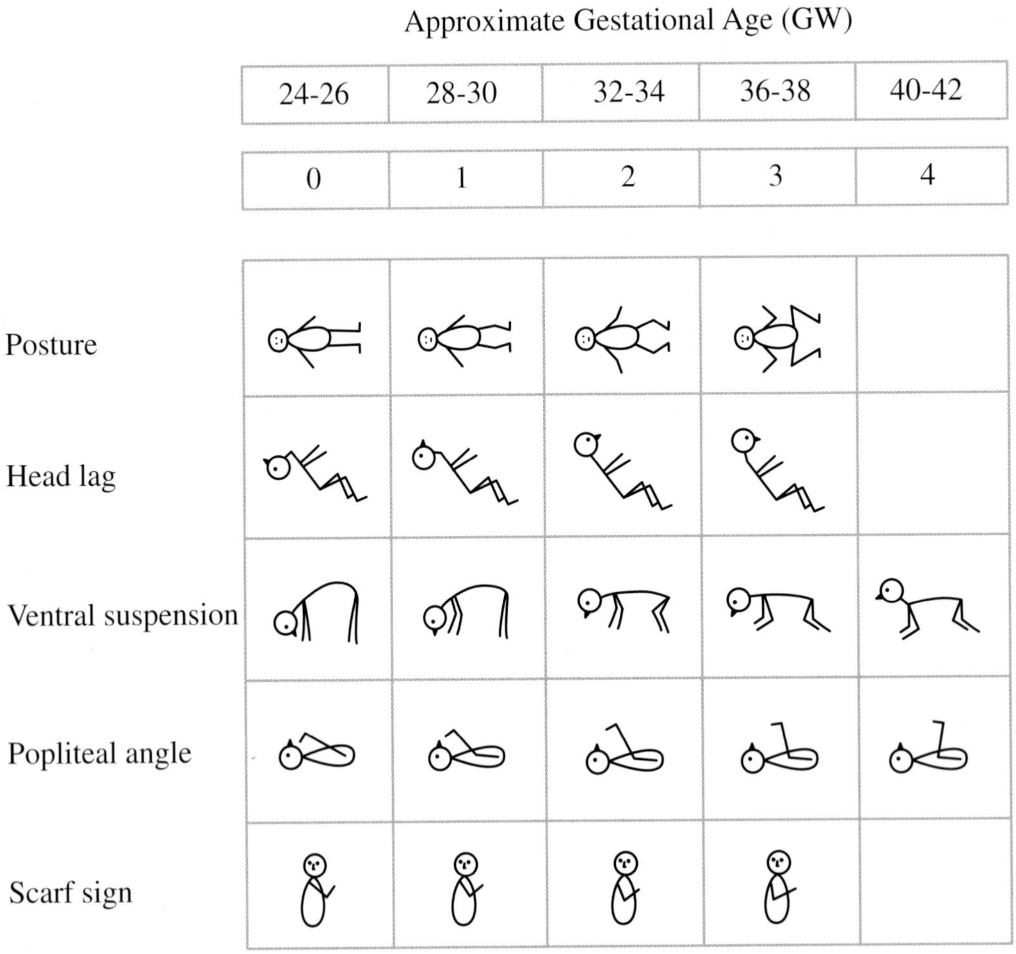

Figure 9-4. A scoring system to assess the postural development of preterm and full-term neonates. Postural hypotonia characterizes premature neonates in the age range of GW24–GW30. Postural reactions with weak flexor and extensor components begin to emerge in GW32 preterm neonates. Strong flexor tonus and mild extensor tonus characterizes the posture of near-term and full-term neonates (GW36–GW42). After Dubowitz et al. (1970) and Ballard et al. (1991).

the reticular formation) is indicated. However, because the execution of head, trunk, and limb movements depend on spinal mechanisms, the changing features of motility are ultimately related to the maturation of the pattern generators within the spinal cord.

9.2.2 Behavioral Development During the Fetal Period: Observations in Preterm Neonates.

An important source of information about the development of fetal behavior has been the study of premature infants, particularly the so-called "extremely premature" infants (GW23–GW25). The survival rate of extremely premature infants has greatly increased recently due to the beneficial effects of assisted ventilation and surfactant therapy (Hack and Fanaroff, 1999). The current survival rate of GW23 infants may be as high as 35%; of GW24 infants, 58%; and of GW25 infants, 85%. Unfortunately, there is a little information about the physiological and behavioral status of these extremely immature neonates.

The early attempts to assess the sensorimotor development of preterm infants were based on bedside tests that concerned muscle tone, postural responses, and responses to cutaneous stimuli (Peiper, 1929; André-Thomas and Dargassis, 1960; Amiel-Tison, 1968). All observers noted a gradual change from the completely flaccid muscles of preterm neonates to the styrongly flexed muscles of full-term neonates (Maekawa and Ochiai, 1975). More recently, neurological scoring systems have been developed (Dubowitz et al., 1981; Fenichel, 1985; Ballard et al., 1991) to gauge the behavioral maturity of premature infants (Figure 9-4).

Postural Reactions. Postural hypotonia is a striking feature of the preterm neonate. When the GW30 neonate is held in a ventral position by the chest, its limp head and limbs fall forward (Figure 9-5A). When placed on its back, the hypotonic legs can be pushed back all the way to the head without any resistance (Figure 9-5B). When suspended upright, the head and legs fall forward without any sign of an antigravity support reaction (Figure 9-5C). The attempt to align the head with the trunk when pulled up from a supine position emerges in GW32 neonates (Figure 9-4). (The mature reaction of raising the head into an upright position, to be described later, develops postnatally.) The assumption of an active quadruped stance, with partially flexed limbs, when suspended in a ventral position does not appear until

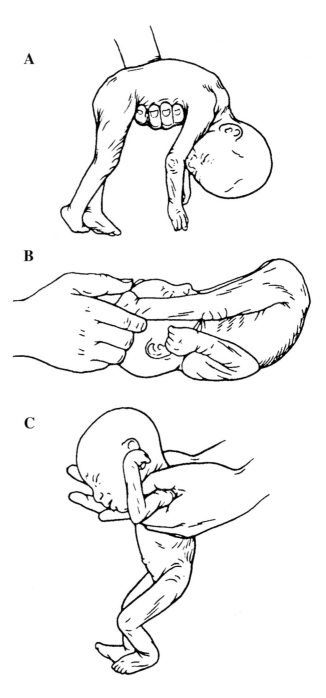

Figure 9-5. Lack of postural reactions in a GW30 preterm neonate. **A.** When suspended in a ventral position, the head and limbs fall downward, displaying no overt signs of any antigravity reactions. **B.** When placed on its back, the neonate's legs offer no resistance when pushed backwards. **C.** When suspended upright, there are no indications of postural supporting reactions to maintain an erect stance. From Swaiman (1999).

about GW36 (Figure 9-4). Deep tendon reflexes are weak in most neonates younger than GW33, but in older infants the achilles, patellar, biceps, thigh adductor and brachioradialis reflexes are reliably evoked (Kuban et al., 1986). Other postural reactions that can be elicited in GW35 to GW36 neonates are the tonic neck reflex and the crossed extensor reflex (Swaiman, 1999).

Sensorimotor Reflexes. Sudden loss of support, abrupt elevation of the body, or jarring of the surface on which the infant rests tend to elicit a startle response, the Moro reflex. This reflex is often interpreted as an atavistic "clamping" reaction, reminiscent of the clinging of young primates to their mother when in need of support (McGraw, 1943). According to clinical observations, the Moro reflex is poorly developed in preterm neonates younger than GW28 and emerges gradually in later delivered or older neonates (Swaiman, 1999). When a rod is pushed against an infant's palm, it automatically grasps it; this grasp reflex may also be a phylogenetic heritage from tree-dwelling ancestors. At GW28, the grasp reflex consists of the closure of the fingers around the rod, without the palm's participation. By GW32, the palm becomes involved, and a little later the shoulder and elbow muscles also participate so that the infant can be lifted from the supine position when it grasps a rod.

Stepping Movements. The GW28 preterm neonate does not support its weight when its feet are brought in contact with a solid surface after it is suspended in a vertical position (Swaiman, 1999). This suggests an absence of the antigravity extensor reflex at this age. During the succeeding weeks that reflex is gradually acquired, and the GW34 neonate displays a good supporting response. Automatic stepping, which can be induced by resting the neonate's feet on a surface, tilting the neonate forward and rocking it from one foot to the other, is first obtained at GW32–GW34. However, the preterm infant usually steps on its toes. By GW37, the stepping response can be more reliably elicited and the full-term infant tends to use both heels and toes in reflex stepping.

Rooting and Sucking. In contrast to the postural reactions, rooting and sucking are early developing reflexes. In a recent study of the development of breast feeding, Nyqvist et al. (1999) found that, irrespective of gestational age at delivery (which ranged from GW26 to GW36) neonates respond by rooting

and sucking when they first contact the mother's breast. Efficient rooting, areolar grasping, and latching on to the nipple appears at GW28, instances of nutritive sucking by GW30.5, and repeated bursts of sucking by GW32. Effective breast feeding was established in a large proportion of the preterm neonates by GW36. (We shall return to the maturation of the sucking reaction during the postnatal period in the next Section.)

The sketchy evidence we currently have about motor development during the second trimester (based mostly on intrauterine ultrasonic recordings) and during the third trimester (which includes also observations and testing of preterm infants) allows the following generalization. The most prevalent intrauterine fetal activity during the second trimester is spontaneous or general motility. These appear first as gross holokinetic movements of the entire body but are then displaced by discrete ideokinetic movements of the head and extremities, either in isolation or in variable combinations. These movements are cyclical in nature and probably reflect alternating interal states rather than responses to environmental contingencies. As such, they are probably controlled by endogenous mechanisms rather than by sensory stimuli. The utility of these spontaneous movements is conjectural. They are more likely to serve morphogenetic organizational functions than effective responses to environmental challenges.

Whatever their triggering mechanism, the exhibition of these organized general movements during fetal development attest to the ongoing maturation of the spinal cord pattern generators that coordinate and execute these movements. In contrast to general motility, the postural support reactions that are essential for the performance of any purposive (goal-seeking, means-end) transaction with the external world are still absent or poorly developed as late as the end of the second trimester. This is indicated by the flaccidity of prematurely delivered infants in the age range of GW24–GW30. Indeed, because of the absence of postural reactions, most of the highly coordinated reactions that can be elicited in the full-term neonate – such as grasping or stepping – are performances in vacuo that are devoid of any behavioral utility. There is no evidence (as discussed later) that these reflexes are the precursors of the later acquired skills of reaching, grasping, or walking. The only exception is the early maturation of the rooting and sucking response, a vital behavioral function that shows progressive improvement with age (see p. 482).

With this sketchy background of fetal behavioral development, we now turn to an assessment of the maturation of the spinal cord during the fetal period in an attempt to show some correlations between the two.

9.2.3 Spinal Cord Development During the Second and Third Trimesters in Relation to Behavioral Development.

The spinal cord is the target of exteroceptive and proprioceptive messages from skin and muscle, of interoceptive signals from the internal organs, and of feedback information and instructions from higher brain stations. After integrating that input, the spinal cord issues spatially and temporally patterned motor commands that result in overt behavior. By the end of the first trimester, the receiving microneurons, the coordinating interneurons, and the executive motoneurons responsible for this integration are all settled in their final locations in the gray matter. These cellular constituents of the spinal cord, of course, cannot operate as integrated circuits until they are appropriately interconnected with one another. Much of that must take place during the second and third trimesters, and some of it continues during infancy.

Unfortunately, we know next to nothing about the "wiring" of the intrinsic spinal circuits during the second and third trimesters. The branching and ramification of the primary afferents; the development of intraspinal and supraspinal fiber connections; the dendritic arborization of different classes of interneurons; the dendritic bundling of motoneurons; and, above all, the development of the various classes of synapses, with their different neurotransmitters and receptors are all unknown. Fortunately, we know a little about the outgrowth and expansion of the different ascending and descending fiber tracts of the spinal cord, and their subsequent myelination in the white matter. That sketchy information allows for some important correlations between spinal cord maturation and behavioral development.

During the second trimester the white matter progressively expands relative to the gray matter. The initial expansion reflects the growth of various ascending and descending fiber tracts responsible for intersegmental and supraspinal connections of the gray matter. The later volumetric expansion is due

to the proliferating interfascicular glia and the deposition of myelin in many of the fiber tracts. Significantly, the different fiber tracts emerge, expand, and become myelinated at different times and at different rates. That temporal difference provides the basis for the sequential development of the interspinal, the ascending, and the descending supraspinal connections of the spinal cord. Accordingly, in an attempt to reconstruct spinal cord maturation in relation to behavioral development, we will first examine when these fiber tracts emerge during the fetal period and, once present, when they mature in terms of the successive phases of myelination.

Table 9-2 summarizes the growth and maturation of 10 fiber tracts or fasciculi in the cervical spinal cord of 6 specimens, ranging in age from the beginning of the second trimester until birth, roughly separated from each other by 5–7 weeks. The following maturational criteria are used for the presumptive fiber tracts: (a) its absence or presence; (b) onset of proliferative gliosis; (c) onset of reactive gliosis; (d) advanced reactive gliosis; (e) onset of myelination, and (f) advanced myelination. The 10 fiber tracts singled out for this purpose are: (i) the collateralization zone; (ii) the cuneate fasciculus; (iii) the gracile fasciculus; (iv) the external portion of the ventromedial funiculus (the location of the medial longitudinal fasciculus, the medial vestibular tract, and the tectospinal tract); (v) the ventral funiculus (the location of the ventral vestibulospinal tract); (vi) the inferior circumferential fasciculus (the putative location of the ventrolateral intraspinal tract); (vii) the marginal fasciculus (the location of the dorsal and ventral spinocerebellar tracts); (viii) the inferior lateral funiculus (the location of the spinocephalic tract); (ix) the superior lateral funiculus (the location of the lateral corticospinal tract); and (x) the internal portion of the ventromedial funiculus (the location of the ventral corticospinal tract). The description below, though not included in Table 9-2, begins with a brief reference to reactive gliosis and myelination of the dorsal and ventral roots.

The Ventral Root and the Dorsal Root. The material used in this study does not provide any information about the growth and myelination of the sensory and motor nerves distally, i.e., near their target structures in skin or muscle. All we have available are proximal dorsal and ventral root fragments that remained attached to the spinal cord during dissection. These fragments reveal the following: Reactive

Table 9-2
Reactive Gliosis and Myelination of Some Fiber Tracts
During the Second and Third Trimesters (Part 1)

Gestational Age (Figure references)	Collateraliza-tion Zone	Cuneate Fasciculus	Gracile Fasciculus	Inferior Circumferential Fasciculus (Intraspinal Tract)	Ventral Funiculus (Ventral Vestibulospinal Tract)
GW14 Fig. 6-16A	Present Few glia	Present Few glia	Present Few glia	---------- ----------	Present Few glia
GW20 Fig. 6-16B	Reactive gliosis	Reactive gliosis (Depth)	Few reactive glia	Advanced reactive gliosis	Reactive gliosis
GW26 Fig. 6-17	Onset of myelination	Onset of reactive gliosis in stalk	Few glia (Reactive gliosis in wedge)	Advanced reactive gliosis	Onset of reactive gliosis
GW33 Fig. 6-18	Advanced myelination	Advanced myelination in stalk	Onset of reactive gliosis (Wedge myelinating)	Myelinating	Myelinating
GW37 Fig. 6-19	Advanced myelination	Advanced myelination in stalk. Reactive gliosis in apex	Advanced myelination in wedge. Reactive gliosis in apex	Myelinating	Myelinating
GW44 Fig 6-20	Advanced myelination	Myelinated throughout	Myelinated throughout	Myelinating	Myelinating

gliosis (punctate myelin staining of Schwann cell peri-karya) begins in the proximal ventral root by GW14 (Figure 6-16A), and myelination (coarse myelin stain-ing) is in progress by GW20 (Figure 6-16B) and well advanced by GW26 (Figure 6-17). Myelinated motor fibers are evident in the ventral horn and are in tran-sit through the white matter at the same age. Evi-dently, some motor fibers are myelinated centrally by GW26 and, at least in the vicinity of the spinal cord, also peripherally. In sharp contrast, the myelination of the dorsal root sensory fibers is delayed consider-ably. The onset of reactive gliosis occurs in the prox-imal dorsal root in the GW20 fetus (Figure 6-16B) with little progress in reactive gliosis on GW26 (Fig-ures 6-17, 6-25, 6-27) or GW29 (Figure 6-13B). By GW32 (Figure 6-33B) and GW33 (Figure 6-29B),

the dorsal root fibers begin to myelinate peripherally. From that age onward, myelination of the dorsal root is evident in the preterm (Figures 6-19, 6-36B), full term (Figure 6-23A), and late term (Figure 6-15B) neonates. The temporal difference in the myelina-tion of the ventral and dorsal roots implies that the motor branch of the reflex arc is functionally mature by GW20 but its sensory branch does not mature until GW33. That parallels the behavioral sequence of the early development of centrally initiated spontaenous motility and the late development of stimulus-trig-gered reflexes.

The Collateralization Zone. A few dorsal root collaterals reach the ventral horn as early as GW8, and many more by GW11 (Figure 5-27). From

Table 9-2
Reactive Gliosis and Myelination of Some Fiber Tracts
During the Second and Third Trimesters (Part 2)

External Ventromedial Fasciculus (Medial Longitudinal Fasciculus, Medial Vestibulospinal Tract, Tectospinal Tract)	Marginal Fasciculus (Spinocerebellar Tract)	Inferior Lateral Fasciculus (Spinocephalic Tract)	Superior Lateral Fasciculus (Lateral Corticospinal Tract)	Internal Ventromedial Funiculus (Ventral Corticospinal Tract)	Gestational Age (Figure references)
Present Few glia	---------- ----------	---------- ----------	---------- ----------	---------- ----------	**GW14** Fig. 6-16A
Few glia	Present Few glia	Present Few glia	Present Few glia	Present Few glia	**GW20** Fig. 6-16B
Onset of reactive gliosis	Onset of reactive gliosis	Few glia	Few glia	Few glia	**GW26** Fig. 6-17
Onset of myelination	Myelinating	Reactive gliosis	Few glia	(Absent)	**GW33** Fig. 6-18
Advanced myelination	Myelinating	Reactive gliosis	Few glia	Few glia	**GW37** Fig. 6-19
Advanced myelination	Myelinating	Myelinating	Few glia	Few glia	**GW44** Fig 6-20

GW8 onward there is a sudden and substantial increase in the number of synapses in the ventral horn (Figure 5-22). Thus, some spinal reflex arcs are "closed" before the end of the first trimester. However, myelination of these circuits is a slow process. The collateralization zone contains few reactive glia at the beginning of the second trimester in the GW14 fetus (Figure 6-16A). Reactive gliosis is in progress in the greatly expanded collateralization zone in the GW20 fetus (Figure 6-16B) but myelination of the collaterals entering the gray matter takes place toward the end of the second trimester and the mid-third trimester, as seen in the GW26 (Figure 6-17), and GW33 (Figure 6-18) fetuses. The collaterals of the central dorsal root myelinate before their parent axons peripherally. That is paradoxical and leaves the functional status of the collaterals uncertain. If the stimulus threshold, speed of conduction, and frequency of impulses conveyed by slow propagating unmyelinated fibers (or discontinuously myelinated fibers) differ drastically from those of fast propagating myelinated fibers, it may be that there are two phases in the closure of the reflex arcs of the spinal cord. In the first phase, sensory information is conveyed at low speed by unmyelinated fibers that have a high threshold and limited resolving power, while in the second phase myelinated fibers convey low threshold sensory messages rapidly and with greater discriminative powers. If that is correct, the sensory control of motor activity must be different at the beginning of the second trimester than toward the end of the third trimester. Furthermore, because the motor fibers are myelinated much earlier (the end of the second trimester), the outflow of coordinated motor commands to the skeletal muscles may antedate by several months the inflow of properly coded exteroceptive messages and proprioceptive feedback. That temporal mismatch in myelination of the peripheral input and output lines of the spinal cord supports the hypothesis that early fetal movements are automatisms controlled either by endogenous mechanisms or descending supraspinal commands rather than sensory input from the periphery. The cyclical motility of the young fetus may serve some morphogeneticfunction.

The Cuneate and Gracile Fasciculi. The cuneate and gracile fasciculi are growing in the cervical cord of the GW14 fetus but they contain few glia (Figure 6-16A). Both fasciculi are larger in the GW20 fetus and contain some reactive glia, but glial concentration is far lower here than in the adjacent collateralization zone (Figure 6-16B). In the GW26 fetus, reactive gliosis is in progress in the superficial portion of the cuneate and gracile fasciculi, and myelination is well advanced in the deep portion of the cuneate fasciculus and in the "wedge" of the gracile fasciculus (Figure 6-17). In the GW33 fetus (Figure 6-18) and the preterm neonate (Figure 6-19) myelination is well advanced throughout the cuneate fasciculus; the wedge region of the gracile fasciculus is myelinating and the rest is in the stage of reactive gliosis. The entire dorsal funiculus is well myelinated in the late term neonate (Figure 6-20). It is noteworthy that as early as GW30, many fibers of the medial lemniscus, the somesthetic relay to the thalamus, are already myelinated in the medulla (Figure 6-37A).

Since the gracile and cuneate fasciculi of the spinolemniscal tract are myelinated by the middle of the third trimester, that pathway may be mature enough to convey adequately coded sensory messages to the thalamus. However, it is doubtful that this is the function of its early myelination. First, the peripheral dorsal root fibers are not yet myelinated at this stage, hence the sensory messages conveyed may have limited discriminative properties. Second, the sensorimotor areas of the cortex, the ultimate target of these fibers, do not start to myelinate until 1-2 months after birth (Figures 8-3 to 8-5). Third, the efferent pathway from the cerebral cortex to the spinal cord, the corticospinal tract, does not become myelinated until about the 2-4 months after birth (Figure 8-29). The fragmentary myelination during the third trimes-

ter and early months of infancy makes it unlikely that this suprasegmental loop can effectively control spinal cord activity. Instead, this fragmentary maturation might play a morphogenetic role in establishing somatotopic maps in the sensory and motor areas of the cerebral cortex.

The Ventrolateral Intraspinal Tract. The inferior circumferential fasciculus that surrounds the ventral horn is composed of the putative intraspinal (propriospinal) fibers of the spinal cord. That fasciculus is present in the GW14 fetus but contains few reactive glia (Figure 6-16A). Reactive gliosis is conspicuous here on GW20 (Figure 6-16B) and GW26 (Figure 6-17). Myelination begins in this fasciculus on GW33 (Figure 6-18), and is well advanced by birth (Figures 6-19 and 6-20). The interneurons of the gray matter that are the source of intraspinal axons provide the interconnections between near and far segments of the spinal cord. The early outgrowth and early myelination of this intraspinal fiber system may reflect the maturation of the circuits that initiate the cyclical smooth and graceful movements of the young fetus. The mechanisms for triggering and modulating these pattern generator circuits by exteroceptive and proprioceptive messages will not become fully functional until some months later when the peripheral sensory nerves become myelinated.

The Ventral and Medial Vestibulospinal Tracts, the Medial Longitudinal Fasciculus, and the Tectospinal Tract. There are several descending pathways from the midbrain and brain stem that control or influence spinal cord activity. The ventromedial funiculus contains descending fibers of the medial longitudinal fasciculus, the medial vestibulospinal tract, and the tectospinal tract. The ventral funiculus is a conduit for the ventral vestibulospinal tract. Although the medial longitudinal fasciculus is usually described as the earliest fiber tract to descend in the spinal cord, the present material indicates that the onset of reactive gliosis and myelination in that tract lags behind the intraspinal tract (Figures 6-2, 6-3B, 6-4B, 6-5B). Myelination of the tectospinal and the medial vestibular tracts also lag behind the intraspinal tract. Reactive gliosis in these supraspinal fiber tracts is first seen in the GW20 fetus (Figure 6-16B) but reactive gliosis is far more advanced at this stage in the intraspinal tract. Reactive gliosis is more prominent in the tectospinal and vestibulospinal tracts in the GW26 fetus (Figure 6-17). Onset of myelination in these tracts is finally evident in the GW33 fetus (Figure 6-18) and progresses slowly in the preterm (Figure 6-19) and late term neonates (Figures 6-19, 6-20). The lag in myelination of these supraspinal fiber tracts relative to the intraspinal tract suggests that general fetal movements are more likely to be triggered by oscillating local pattern generators than by supraspinal commands.

The Spinocerebellar Tracts. The dorsal spinocerebellar tract, situated in the dorsal portion of marginal fasciculus, is absent or poorly developed in the GW14 fetus (Figure 6-16A). It is present above the lateral corticospinal tract in the GW20 fetus but contains few intrafascicular glia (Figure 6-16B). Reactive gliosis of the dorsal spinocerebellar tract is in progress in the GW26 fetus (Figure 6-17), and its myelination is evident from GW33 on (Figures 6-18, 6-19, 6-20). The boundaries of the ventral spinocerebellar tract are poorly defined; its maturation may lag behind that of the dorsal spinocerebellar tract. The relatively late myelination of this proprioceptive afferent system suggests the late maturation of the cerebellar feedback circuit to the spinal cord.

The Spinocephalic (Spinothalamic) Tract. The ascending spinocephalic tract – which is a major conduit of postsynaptic protopathic afferents that terminate widely in the medulla, pons, midbrain, and thalamus – is developing later than the descending supraspinal tracts just considered. It is either absent or very slender in the GW14 fetus (Figure 6-16A). It forms a narrow band lateral to the intraspinal tract in the GW20 (Figure 6-16B) and GW26 (Figure 6-17) fetuses but contains fewer reactive glia than the intraspinal tract. Reactive gliosis is advanced in the spinocephalic tract by GW33 (Figure 6-18) and the perinatal period (Figure 6-19). Myelination of the spinocephalic tract may begin in the late term neonate (Figure 6-20) when a later myelinating tract of unnknown identity surrounds it superficially.

The Lateral and Ventral Corticospinal Tracts. The delayed myelination of the lateral (and ventral) corticospinal tract is unique among the fiber tracts of the spinal cord. The lateral corticospinal tract reaches the spinal cord relatively early in the fetal period: it may be present by GW14 (Figure 6-16A) and is conspicuous and large by GW20 (Figure 6-16B). It is difficult to determine when the areal expansion of the tract ends because of great individual variability in its size (Figures 6-17 to 6-20). What is consistent, however, is that in none of the many specimens examined is there any indication of reactive gliosis during the fetal and perinatal periods. The same applies to the ventral corticospinal tract. The size of the latter is highly variable (and it may be altogether absent in some fetuses) but there is no hint either for the onset of reactive gliosis or its myelination during the fetal or perinatal period. Therefore, to the extent that myelination reflects the functional maturation of a fiber tract, the inference is justified that the cerebral cortex plays little or no role in the supraspinal control of spinal cord during the late fetal and perinatal periods.

9.2.4 Some Correlations with Behavioral Development.

What is the relationship between spinal cord maturation and behavioral development during the second and third trimesters? We begin with a paradox. In contrast to the progressive maturation of the spinal cord, behavioral development slows down during the fetal period. The human embryo exhibits spontaneous motility as early as the middle of the first trimester (about GW6), and the frequency and duration of movements increase in the ensuing weeks. Although the movements become better articulated and more graceful, however, there is a decline in spontaneous motility from GW16 onward. It has been suggested that the decreasing motility is due to the physical constraints imposed by the uterine wall upon the growing fetus. Another contributing factor may be that descending facilitatory and inhibitory influences impose a cyclical alternation of ever longer active and dormant periods of movement. If so, the apparent reduction in spontaneous motility may be a sampling artifact. Another paradox is the contrast between the large repertoire of spontaneous movements but few or no adaptive responses to sensory stimuli. For example, the third trimester fetus periodically stretches, squirms, turns, pushes, kicks, and so forth while in the womb. But if delivered prematurely, it tends to lie with hypotonic muscles when placed on its back, and fails to extend its extremities when suspended in a horizontal or a vertical position. Why does the fetus display coordinated motor activities in its intrauterine environment but becomes immobile once it is delivered?

The discrepancy between intrauterine and extrauterine behavior may be partially due to the different ambient conditions and adaptive demands in the two environments. Inside the uterus the fetus is suspended in a liquid medium. It is well supported and protected irrespective of the position that it occupies relative to gravity. Limited reactivity to external stimuli may also be explained by the circumstance that in the shielded and uniform intrauterine environment, responses to external stimuli, if they reach the fetus, do not serve any useful function. However, if delivered prematurely, or indeed at term, the support of the head and the body becomes a necessity. That is usually provided by caretakers who place the helpless newborn on a supporting surface. In the absence of voluntary postural control (the ability to lift or turn the head, rotate the trunk, use arms or legs for maintaining or changing a desirable position), flaccidity and immobility is the best guarantee that if placed on its stomach, its back, or its side on a horizontal surface, the neonate's body will conform to the surface and will not roll off and hurt itself. This absence of perinatal postural skills is correlated with the relatively late myelination of the spinocerebellar system. But it is also possible that hypotonia and immobility are fostered by active supraspinal inhibition during the third trimester and the perinatal period.

If the foregoing analysis is correct, what requires an explanation from the perspective of behavioral adaptation is why the fetus is so often active within the womb. One possibility is that the periodic bursts of spontaneous motility aids the morphological and physiological maturation of both the spinal cord and the skeletomuscular system. Perhaps, the pattern generator circuits responsible for the coordination of different synergies, routines and subroutines are fine-tuned through cyclical activation of the peripheral motor apparatus, much before the motor system becomes directly linked to peripheral sensory channels.

According to this interpretation, the morphogenesis of the human spinal cord during the fetal period is not geared to facilitate responsiveness to external stimuli. Instead, the developmental thrust during this period is the periodic testing and refinement of the "pre-wired" motor synergies, subroutines, and routines that will be used after birth as the building blocks of behavioral skills that can be modified by exteroceptive information and proprioceptive feedback. The late myelination of the dorsal root is compatible with this hypothesis. Particularly noteworthy is the apparent existence of an unmyelinated gap at the dorsal root entry zone throughout the third trimester (e.g., Figures 6-22B, 6-25B, 6-40). That gap may specifically block transmission of sensory stimuli to the spinal cord. It is not until birth, when exposure to the external world begins, that the myelination

of this gap is completed. Since the central branches and collaterals of dorsal root axons are well myelinated by birth, the system can quickly become operational and transmit sensory messages to the spinal cord and the brain when the last gap in the myelination of the primary afferents is eliminated.

9.3   Reflexes and Automatisms in the Neonate and Young Infant Prior to Myelination of the Corticospinal Tract

9.3.1 Behavioral Development During Early Infancy. There are several classical surveys of motor development from birth through infancy and early childhood (Ames, 1927; Burnside, 1927; Shirley, 1931; Gesell et al., 1938; Gesell and Halverson, 1942; McGraw, 1943; Pratt, 1954). Several older studies are also available concerning the emergence and maturation (and, in some cases, disappearance) of several spinal reflexes. These sensorimotor reflexes include postural adjustments and head turning (McGraw, 1943), rooting and sucking (Kussmaul, 1859; Popper, 1921; Wolff, 1968), the clasping or startle reflex (Stirnimann, 1943; Landis and Hunt, 1943), the plantar reflex (Hogan and Milligan 1971), and grasping (Halverson, 1931, 1937; Richter, 1934). Among coordinated automatisms present at birth are crawling (Bauer, 1926), stepping (Peiper, 1929; Stirnimann, 1938), and swimming (McGraw, 1943) movements. These early surveys relied principally on visual observation and photographic documentation. More recently, experimental tools, such as electromyographic recordings of muscle activity, computerized video recordings of movements in combination with the digitization of anatomic landmarks, and such devices as treadmills, force plates, moving platforms, and simulated moving rooms are used to assess the development of motor skills.

Some of the premises and lines of evidence used in the following discussion regarding the relationship between behavioral development and spinal cord maturation during early infancy are as follows. First, there are two fundamentally different classes of motor behavior: (a) involuntary reflexes and automatisms, and (b) voluntary, goal-directed acts and skills. Second, evidence is presented that most of the overt movements of the newborn are involuntarily triggered reflexes and automatisms rather than voluntary acts. That is, the spinal cord at birth is incapable of executing voluntary movements that are directed to achieve a specific end or goal. (Exceptions to this generalization are some activities controlled by brain stem mechanisms and conveyed by cranial nerves, such as sucking or directed gaze.) Third, the early period of involuntary infantile behavior is relatable to the stage of spinal cord maturation when only the paleospinal descending tracts originating in the brain stem and medulla are myelinated but the neencephalic corticospinal tract is unmyelinated. Fourth, the argument will be made that there is a transitional period of spinal cord development during which many of the automatisms and reflexes disappear and are replaced by goal-directed activities. Finally, evidence will be presented that the emergence and growth of voluntary, goal-directed motor behavior during later infancy and early childhood is correlated with the progressive myelination of the corticospinal tract.

9.3.2 Automatisms and Reflex Activities of the Neonate and Young Infant.

The neonate is endowed with the inborn ability to perform a multitude of complex visceromotor and somatomotor housekeeping functions that are essential for its survival. Most of these may be classified as involuntary reflexes and automatisms.

Visceral Reflexes and Automatisms. From the moment of delivery, spinal cord motoneuron pools under the control of medullary mechanisms can effectively coordinate the rhythmic contraction and relaxation of the muscles of the ribcage and diaphragm to supply the lungs with air. These and several additional muscle groups are also involved in the inborn reflexes that clear the air passages of obstructions, such as coughing, yawning, and sneezing. The newborn sucks and swallows milk effectively upon first exposure to the breast, and the ingested milk is passed through its digestive and gastrointestinal system by a series of well coordinated visceral muscle movements. The newborn burps, vomits, urinates, and defecates to rid its body of wastes. All these reflexes and automatisms, and many more, attest to the effective operation of spinal pattern generators under the guidance of paleospinal control mechanisms in the medulla and brain stem.

Proprioceptive Reflexes and Postural Automatisms. In addition to the reflexes and automatisms concerned with domestic maintenance and protective functions, the neonate is also endowed with an inborn repertoire of responses to specific external stimuli.

These include various postural and protective reactions and some specific motor and locomotor automatisms. The simplest of reflexes are various segmental tendon and muscle reactions – such as the patellar, achilles, biceps, triceps and periosteal reflexes. These, and several cutaneous reflexes – such as the abdominal, cremasteric, and plantar reflexes – can be elicited by appropriate stimuli in the newborn (McGraw, 1943). In addition to local proprioceptive reflexes, the neonate also displays some postural reactions that affect the whole body. Extensor muscles contract when stretched by the pull of gravity or other forces; this antigravity response plays a major role in the maintenance of erect posture. The contraction of antigravity muscles is initiated by the muscle spindles in skeletal muscle, whose afferents trigger the monosynaptic stretch reflex. If not modulated or inhibited, this reflex produces extensor hypertonia, the rigidity of the neck and limbs. An exaggerated form of the stretch reflex, known as decerebrate rigidity (Sherrington, 1906), is seen under certain pathological conditions. The normal newborn never displays extensor hypertonia, which implies either that the stretch reflex is not fully mature or, what is more likely, that it is inhibited by supraspinal mechanisms. However, the full-term newborn and young infant is not flaccid when at rest. Rather, it displays an active posture that may be described as flexor hypertonia. If resting on its back, the full term neonate's legs tend to be bent at the hip and knee and pulled upward, the arms are similarly bent at the elbow and pulled towards the chest, and the fingers are partially closed or clenched (McGraw, 1943). The head is usually turned to one side when in a supine position, typically to the right (Goodwin and Michel, 1981; Rönnqvist and Hopkins, 1998, 2000). If placed on its stomach, the newborn will similarly adopt a flexed posture and remain in that position. Periodically, the infant will flay its arms and legs in a rapid sequence, and in the process may propel itself forwards or backwards (Bauer, 1926). These displays have been termed "writhing movements" and contrasted with the "fidgety movements," "swipes," and "swats" of older infants (Hadders-Algra and Prechtl, 1992). Writhing movements resemble more the aimless spontaneous movements of the fetus than the goal-seeking voluntary acts of the older infant and young child (Prechtl and Hopkins, 1986).

The ability of the newborn to make effective postural adjustments when perturbed is very limited. The neonate or young infant cannot raise its head, use its arms or legs to turn over, or respond adaptively when suspended upside-down in mid-air (McGraw, 1943; Figure 9-6A). When put in such an uncomfortable position, the neonate will instantly start to cry but will not be able to make appropriate adjustments (McGraw, 1943). That changes as development proceeds. The 2-4 months old infant will try to turn its head and trunk when suspended in an inverted position (Figure 9-6B, C), the first hint of a voluntary attempt to rectify an undesired posture. At about 6 months of age, the young child will finally be able to extend its arms toward a supporting surface to effectively support its body from falling (Figure 9-6D).

The Tonic Neck Reflex. Some postural reflexes are present and can be triggered in the newborn but they are without any behavioral utility. One of these is the tonic neck reflex (Gesell, 1954). If the head of an infant lying on its back is turned to one side, the ipsilateral arm extends in the same direction and the contralateral arm becomes flexed (Figure 9-7). This tonic neck reflex can be consistently elicited in decerebrate mammals, and is particularly pronounced when the vestibular apparatus is also destroyed (Magnus, 1924, 1925). That response has been interpreted as an involuntary postural reflex that readies a quadruped animal to turn its limbs in the direction that its head turns. Gesell (1954) found that all infants younger that 20 weeks displayed a tonic neck reflex, indeed, many of them often assumed and maintained this head and forelimb posture spontaneously (Figure 9-7).

The Grasp and Clasp Reflex. In view of the neonate's inability to execute even the simplest of vol-

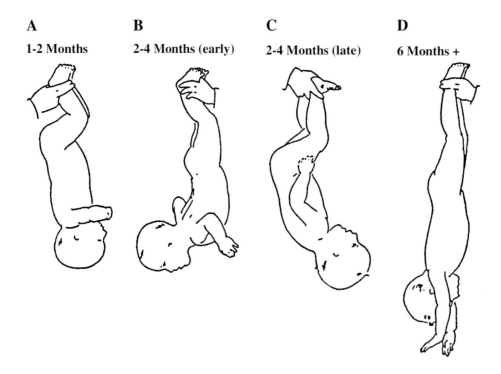

A
1-2 Months

B
2-4 Months (early)

C
2-4 Months (late)

D
6 Months +

Figure 9-6. Four phases in the development of postural control in an infant suspended in an inverted position. **A.** At 1-2 months, the infant shows no evident overt reaction. **B, C.** By 2-4 months, the infant displays abortive attempts to right its head and turn its trunk. The arms do not yet participate in this reaction. **D.** By the age of 6 months (or later) the young child exhibits an effective supporting response by extending its arm towards a solid surface (the placing reaction). After McGraw (1943).

untary postural adjustments, it is surprising that it has an extensive repertoire of highly specific reactions to certain stimuli. An example of these are the reactions known as the grasp reflex and the clamp (or startle) reflex. When a rod is pushed against the palm of the newborn or young infant, its fingers close tightly around the rod (Figure 9-8). Although the thumb does not participate in this response, the grasp may be strong enough so that the infant may be raised upright or suspend in mid-air. Neonates holding on to a rod with two hands may support themselves for as long as 1 to 2 minutes (Richter, 1934). The grasp is firmest when the infant is emotionally disturbed, as when crying (Sherman et al., 1936) or hungry (Hal-

verson, 1937). The grasp reflex has been interpreted as a vestigial simian reaction of holding on to a tree branch when support is lost. We may recall that a grasp reflex with effective gripping may be elicited in fetuses as young as GW16 (Hooker, 1938). In terms of suspension duration, the grasp reflex reaches its peak at about 1 month postnatally, then declines. Goal-directed grasping, which usually follows upon the voluntary effort to reach a distant object, like a dangling ball, reappears by about 4-5 months of age and involves the thumb (Section 9.4.1).

When an infant is dropped, jarred, or exposed to some other sudden or intense stimulus, it responds

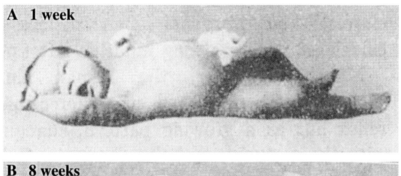

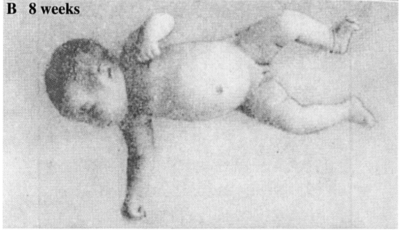

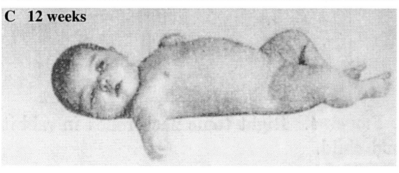

Figure 9-7. The tonic neck reflex in an infant at 1 week (**A**), 8 weeks (**B**) and 12 weeks (**C**) of age. This reaction is often displayed spontaneously by infants younger than 20 weeks. (For the preferred posture of this infant at a later age, see Figure 9-20.) After Gesell (1954).

by a quick extension of both arms and legs, followed by an embrace-like flexion of arms and hands (Figure 9-9). That has been variably known as the Moro reflex (McGraw, 1937), the clasp reflex (Stirnimann, 1943), or the startle response (Landis and Hunt, 1939; Clarke, 1939). According to Stirnimann (1943), this reflex is not accompanied by crying, implying that it is not initiated by fear; however, it is usually followed by crying (McGraw, 1937). The clasp reflex is most easily obtained during the first month of life then it gradually disappears (McGraw, 1943). This complex reflex is best interpreted as a vestigial simian clasping reaction; the young primate holding on to or embracing its mother when frightened or when she moves about.

Creeping, Stepping, and Swimming Reflexes. The newborn cannot turn over when placed on its stomach or its back, and cannot move from one place to another to change its location. However, the infant's position may change as a result of squirming and kicking; a dislocation that has been called creeping (Bauer, 1926; Peiper, 1929; Stirnimann, 1938). Stirnimann (1938) observed creeping in an anencephalic infant; indeed, kicking has been observed in anencephalic fetuses (Visser et al., 1985). Creeping must be a subcortically mediated involuntary behavior.

But even though the neonate cannot voluntarily move from place to place, organized movements resembling stepping and swimming can be evoked under special conditions. Thus, when the newborn or young infant is held upright, tilted slightly forward, and the soles of its feet are brought into contact with a surface, the legs extend and begin to move in a alternating sequence, as if walking (Peiper, 1929, 1963; McGraw, 1932; Zelazo et al., 1972; Gotts, 1972; Thelen and Fisher, 1982). In the absence of its postural control, the infant's stepping movements are, of course, not effective means of ambulation. While it has been argued that these stepping movements represent an early stage in the development of effective, goal-directed locomotion, two observations speak against that. First, the infantile stepping reflex disappears by about 2 months of age. Second, for several months thereafter, and much before the infant begins to crawl, the raised infant no longer extends its legs and feet but, instead, tends to flex and raise them, as if trying to assume a sitting posture (McGraw, 1932).

When a neonate or young infant is placed into a water tank in prone position, it tends to remain prone

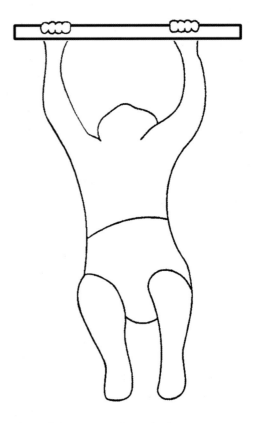

Figure 9-8. The grasping reflex in a neonate.

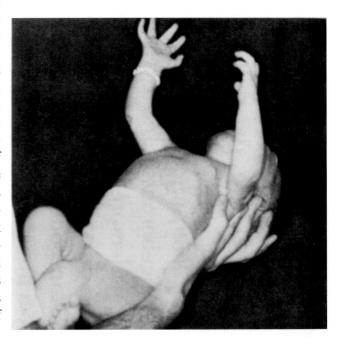

Figure 9-9. The grasping (Moro) reflex in a full-term newborn. After Joppich and Schulte (1968).

and may start to move its arms and legs in a well coordinated quadruped rhythm and effectively swim for a short distance (McGraw, 1939; 1943; Figure 9-10A). The young infant swallows little or no water while swimming. According to McGraw, this reflex swimming is better coordinated than the reflex stepping response. As the infant gets older, the coordinated reflex swimming rhythm disappears and, when placed into a water tank, it tends to struggle in an agitated manner (Figure 9-10B), gasps for air, swallows water, and coughs a lot. The incidence of organized reflex swimming and disorganized struggling as a function of age is plotted in Figure 9-11. Coordinated swimming does not reappear again until about 1 year of age in association with the onset of voluntary walking (McGraw, 1943).

In summary, the newborn's neurobehavioral development is characterized by two apparently mismatched features. One is its inability to make adequate postural adjustments when perturbed. The other is its ability to execute some well-coordinated reflexes and automatisms, such as grasping a rod, stepping when held upright, and swimming. Without the ability to control body posture none of these reflexes serve any useful purpose. Reflex grasping does not involve reaching for something and holding on to a desired object, reflex stepping or reflex swimming do not take the infant from an undesired location to a desired one.

But if these reflexes are devoid of any behavioral utility, what is their function? One possibility is that these reflexes are building blocks (synergies and subroutines) that are later incorporated into the motor patterns of more complex behavioral skills (Thelen and Fisher, 1982; Thelen and Ulrich, 1991). But the traditional evolutionary view that these are ancient synergies that were hard-wired into the spinal cord of man's ancestors but are inhibited or disassembled during human ontogeny is a more likely explanation. There is a temporal discontinuity between reflex stepping and voluntary stepping, and between reflex swimming and voluntary swimming. Both reflexes disappear during early infancy and are not replaced by their voluntary homologues until many months later. The time that elapses between the involuntary and voluntary activities suggests that the early innate synergies are replaced by newly organized learned synergies. In hypothetical neurological terms, the pattern generators responsible for the phylogenetically old, innate reflexes are either disassembled or are

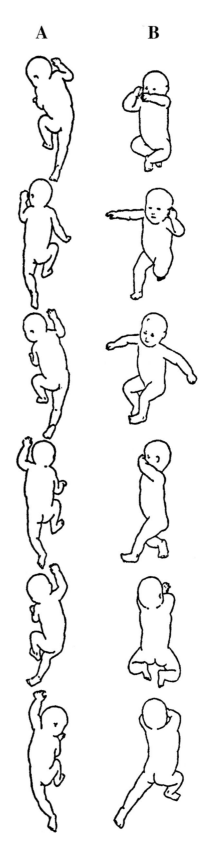

Figure 9-10. **A.** Coordinated and effective reflex swimming in a young infant submerged in the water. **B.** Disorganized struggling of a several-months-old infant under the same conditions. Tracings of successive frames from a 16 mm movie. After McGraw (1943).

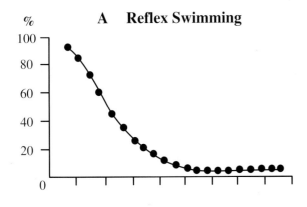

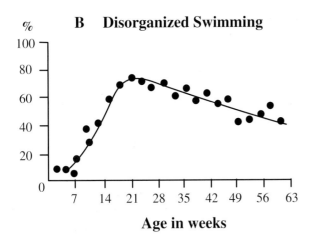

Figure 9-11. The incidence of reflex swimming (**A**) and disorganized struggling (**B**), as a percentage of total activity, plotted as a function of age in weeks. After McGraw (1943).

tive reflex profile," and motor activity level at 3 and 6 months of age, as assessed by an "infant motor scale." This lack of continuity contrasts with the persistence of low or high level of spontaneous motility in the same individuals during the fetal period and after birth (Groome et al., 1999).

Head Movements and Rooting. The foregoing considerations imply that all neonatal sensorimotor activities are involuntary reflexes and automatisms, none bears the features of voluntary goal-seeking behavior. There is at least one exception to this generalization. This is the head turning and rooting that helps the infant to reach the mother's breast and suckle. When a neonate's cheek is touched with a finger, it turns its head toward that side, open its mouth, and latches on to the finger. This was first described by Kussmaul (1859) as the "search reflex" and analyzed in some detail by Popper (1921). If mouth contact is maintained, the infant may shake its head from side to side (Stirnimann, 1937). Gentry and Aldrich (1948) called head turning and mouth opening, the rooting reflex, the first phase of neonatal feeding behavior, and distinguished that from sucking as the second phase. The rooting reflex is most easily elicited when the neonate is awake and hungry. Since head turning and head shaking are ultimately under spinal control, rooting is an instance of a goal-seeking behavior executed by spinal mechanisms at birth.

Sucking and Swallowing. As soon as the newborn is brought into contact with the mother's breast (or an artificial nipple) it begins to suck in a rhythmic fashion (Wolff, 1968). Successful sucking involves the participation of the lips, the cheek, the jaw, and the tongue in a coordinated manner (Eishima, 1991). Sucking begins with the coordinated activity of labial and facial muscles to form an airtight seal around the nipple. Concurrently, the tongue encloses the lateral sides and the bottom of the nipple while the central portion of the tongue caves in to form a hollow. Thereafter, a peristaltic wave of muscular activity is initiated that propels the milk into the mouth. Swallowing of the milk is another complex activity and it has to be coordinated with breathing to prevent choking (Bu'Lock et al., 1990; Mathew, 1991). Rightfully, sucking has been referred to as "perhaps the most precocious purposeful motor skill evident in a newborn infant's movement repertoire" (Craig and Lee, 1999, p. 371). Another important consideration is the evidence of a continuous

actively inhibited by cortical mechanisms that control learned voluntary behavior. That change, as we shall see momentarily, may be related to the progressive myelination of the corticospinal tract during late infancy and early childhood.

Another bit of evidence against the idea that the early reflex synergies are building blocks of later acquired voluntary skills comes from a follow-up (longitudinal) study of motor behavior in a large sample of individual infants. Bartlett (1997) reports the absence of any correlation in 156 infants between reflex activity level at 6 weeks of age, as assessed by a "primi-

improvement in sucking efficiency from the day of birth through the first few weeks of life. This is unlike the discontinuity between reflexive and purposive grasping, stepping, and swimming previously discussed. However, it is significant to note that cranial nerves (the trigeminal, facial, accessory, and hypoglossal) rather than spinal nerves supply the bulk of the afferents and efferents involved in the coordination of sucking. Therefore, these early voluntary movements depend on rostral brain stem coordination rather than the spinal cord. (Voluntary eye movements also belong in this category.)

In summary, the principal features of the behavioral status of the newborn and young infant are the following: The newborn is endowed with a series of innate visceromotor and somatomotor automatisms that ensure some of its vital needs for survival and growth, including breathing, sucking, swallowing, digestion, and the voiding of metabolic wastes. The neonate also exhibits several atavistic reflexes that do not aid its survival and growth – such as its purposeless grasping of a rod or finger, or stepping and swimming under artificial conditions. In sharp contrast to these complex coordinations, the neonate is unable to right itself or turn around, and lacks the motor and locomotor skills that could empower it to move about from place to place and interact with its environment to get what it needs or wants.

9.3.3 Correlations with Neonatal Spinal Cord Development.

What is the maturational status of the neonate's spinal cord that enables it to perform very complex life-support functions but does not allow it to effectively interact with its environment? We do not know enough about the morphological and physiological maturation of the gray matter of the spinal cord – such as its dendritic and synaptic development – to answer that question. However, we can analyze the myelination of the major fiber tracts of the spinal cord and that analysis allows certain inferences about spinal cord maturation.

The operation of visceromotor and somatomotor automatisms in neonates is correlated with advanced myelination of the intraspinal tracts, and with reactive gliosis or myelination of all the ascending tracts and all but one of the descending tracts (i.e., the corticospinal tract; Figure 9-12A). It is inferred that the well-myelinated intraspinal tracts and the descending paleocephalic tracts from the brain stem effectively interconnect the intersegmental pattern generator circuits and brain stem trigger mechanisms to produce hard-wired reflexes and automatisms. At birth and early infancy, the descending corticospinal tract shows no signs even of the commencement of reactive gliosis (Figure 9-12B). Indeed, myelination is absent in the white matter of the cerebral cortex (though not in many subcortical structures) in the young infant (Figure 9-13A). Because the corticospinal tract is unmyelinated, the cortical control of spinal mechanisms is ineffective or absent in the neonate and young infant.

The gradual acquisition of voluntary behavior during late infancy and early childhood is correlated with progressive cortical myelination, beginning proximally in the motor cortex (Figure 9-13B) then spreading to the corticospinal tract (Figures 8-7, 8-8, 8-23). As the cerebral cortex (Figure 8-9) and the corticospinal tract (Figure 8-25) become well myelinated in the ensuing months, voluntary control of spinal cord mechanisms improves and the child is enabled to engage in purposive activities and master ever more complex skills. Support for this interpretation comes from the evidence, described below, of a rostral-to-caudal and proximal-to-distal gradient in the development of the voluntary motor control in correlation with a corresponding gradient in the myelination of the corticospinal tract.

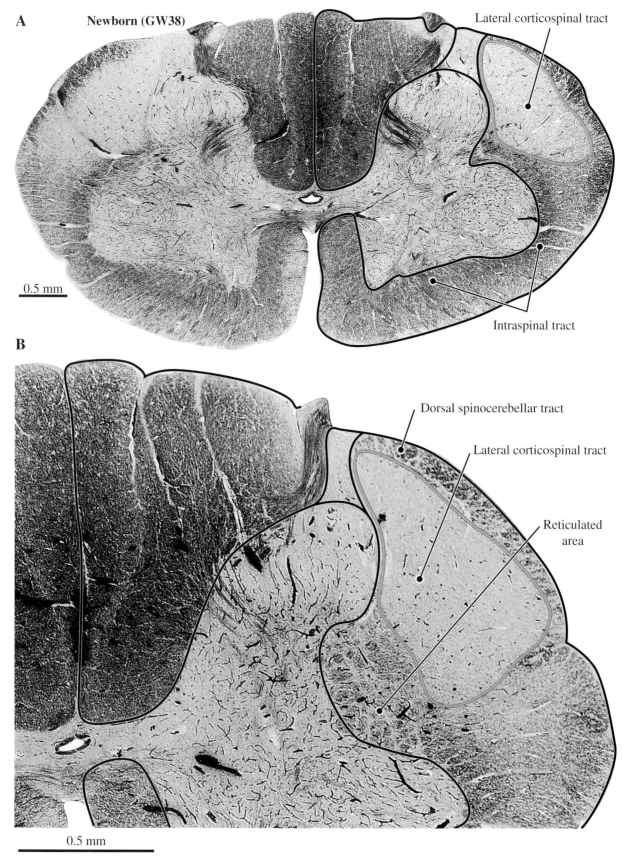

A. Newborn (GW38)

Lateral corticospinal tract

0.5 mm

Intraspinal tract

B.

Dorsal spinocerebellar tract

Lateral corticospinal tract

Reticulated area

0.5 mm

Figure 9-12. A. In the cervical spinal cord of this full term neonate (*Y163-61*), the intraspinal tract of the circumferential fasciculus is myelinated, and myelination or advanced reactive gliosis characterize the other descending tracts, except the lateral corticospinal tract. **B.** The absence of reactive gliosis in the lateral corticospinal tract, as seen at higher magnification, in an adjacent section from the same neonate.

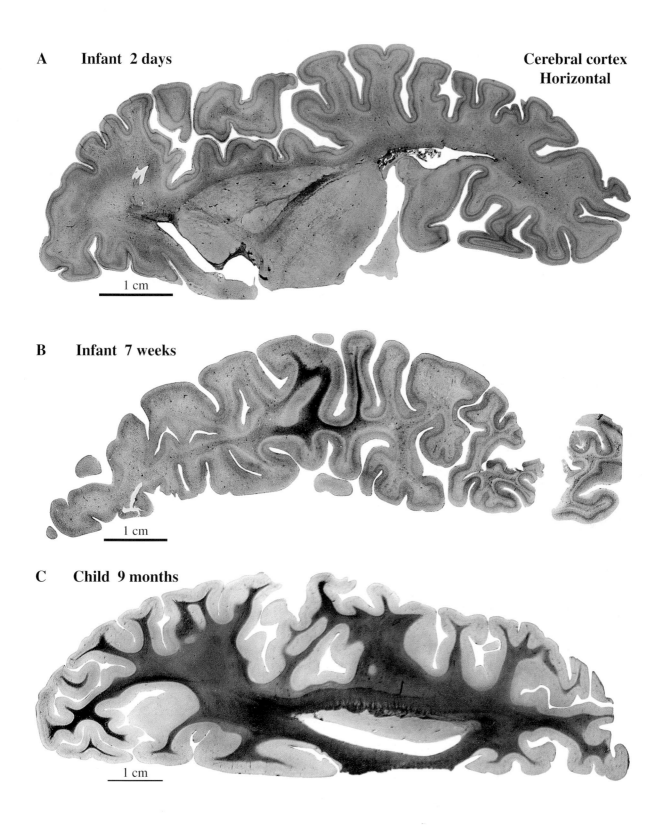

A Infant 2 days

Cerebral cortex Horizontal

1 cm

B Infant 7 weeks

1 cm

C Child 9 months

1 cm

Figure 9-13. A. Absence of myelination in the white matter of the cerebral cortex in a 2-day-old infant (*Y128-63*). **B.** Myelination in the precentral and postcentral gyri (the primary motor and somatosensory cortical areas) in a 7-week-old infant (*Y130-61*). **C.** Advanced myelination through the entire cortical white matter in a 9-month-old child (*Y302-62*).

9.4   Development of Voluntary Behavior During Late Infancy and Early Childhood in Relation to Myelination of the Corticospinal Tract

9.4.1 Beginnings of Voluntary, Goal-Seeking Behavior.   The human neonate's inability to right itself is unique among placental mammals. For instance, the far less mature newborn rat will consistently turn over when placed on its back by engaging in a rocking motion (Altman and Sudarshan, 1975). Newborn and very young babies (1-3 weeks of age) display muscular tension, kick with their legs in a random fashion, and cry when left in an uncomfortable position but they cannot turn their head and use their arms and legs to roll over (Shirley, 1931; Gesell et al. 1938; McGraw, 1943).

The Development of Postural Control.   In Figure 9-14 we reproduce Shirley's (1931) summary of the successive events in the development of motor control in a sample of 16-22 babies through the ages

of 1 to 76 weeks.   The graph provides age ranges and median age in the development of 17 landmark events that are directly controlled by the spinal cord. (We have omitted from the original graph behavioral events that are controlled by supraspinal mechanisms, such as "notice object," "smile at person," "babble when talked to," etc.).   In our brief summary below, the chronological dates refer to the approximate median ages in months.   Supplementing Shirley's descriptive chronology, Figure 9-15 reproduces a few drawings from McGraw's (1943) classic work of some landmark achievements in the development of motor behavior between birth and 14 months of age.

Classical Studies of the Development of Postural Control.   The 2-week-old infant lying on its stomach periodically raises its head for a few seconds (Figure 9-14/1) but cannot maintain that prone posture (Figure 9-15A).   The 4-week-old infant may raise its head and chest for several seconds (Figure 9-14/2) and maintain that posture for several seconds by resting on its elbows with partially extended arms (Figure

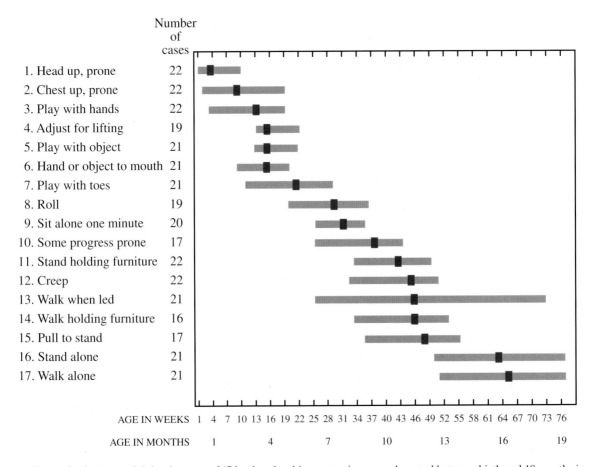

Figure 9-14. Sequential development of 17 landmark achievements in postural control between birth and 18 months in a sample of 17–22 babies. Horizontal lines (gray) indicate the range, vertical bars (red) indicate the median age in the first emergence of a particular accomplishment. After Shirley (1931).

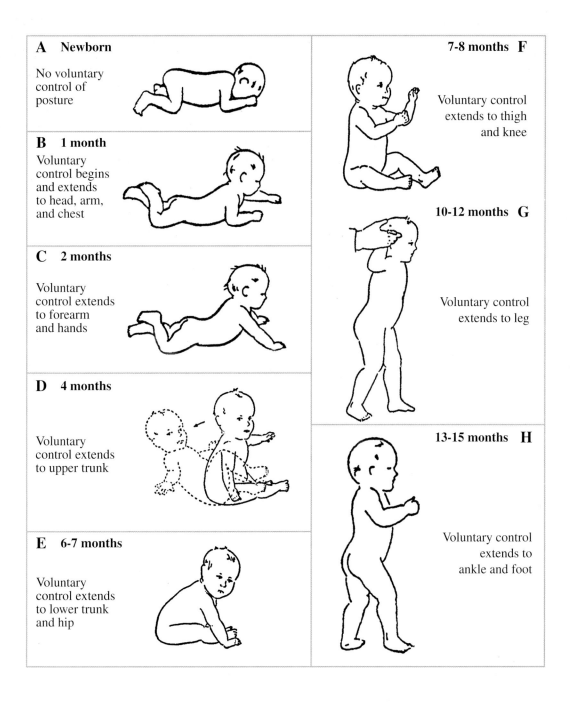

Figure 9-15. The sequential acquisition of postural control between birth and 15 months of age. The newborn tends to maintain a posture of flexor hypertonia (**A**). Voluntary control of body posture begins with raising of the head and resting the lifted shoulder the elbows of the extended arm (**B**). Next follows the elevation of the torso with extended arms and hands (**C**). Next, the can sit upright with support but topples when not supported (**D**). The young child acquires the ability to support its seated posture by extending its arms and leaning on its hands (**E**) and, later, by extending one or both legs for support (**F**). The next achievement is the ability to stand upright with support (**G**) and, then, without support (**H**). Note the rostrocaudal gradient (hands to feet) and proximodistal gradient (chest to hands rostrally, and hip to foot caudally) in the development of the voluntary control of the upright stance. Drawings from McGraw (1943).

9-15B). The 2-month-old infant can lift its head and neck by extending and placing its forearms and hands on the ground (Figure 9-15C). The 3-month-old infant, may play with its hands when on its back (Figure 9-14/3). Great strides are made in voluntary control at about 4 months of age. The 4-month-old infant adjusts its posture when lifted, plays with an object placed into its hands while lying on its back, and brings the hand or object to the mouth (Figures 9-14/4,5,6). The voluntary control of the distal hand is evidently in progress. However, while it can stay in a seated position when held in the arm or confined by a chair, the 4 month-old infant topples over when not supported (Figure 9-15D).

At about 5-6 months of age, the young child may begin to play with its toes (Figure 9-14/7). The next momentous development, at about 6-8 months, is the infant's ability to roll over and sit without outside support for a short period (Figures 9-14/8,9). Independent sitting is initially accomplished by leaning forward and supporting the body with extended arms and hand in contact with the ground (Figure 9-15E). Within a short period that is accomplished more efficiently by supporting the balance of the upper body with an extended leg (Figure 9-15F). These developments reflect the extension of voluntary control to the lower limb. Voluntary control of leg placement to support a sitting posture makes possible the free use of the hands while reaching for and handling objects. That turns babies into independently acting agents. The next development is the gradual acquisition of voluntary control of the legs, and later of the feet. At 10 to 12 months, the young child can crawl on its arms and legs, stand on its toes by holding on to a table or chair, and walk erect when held by the arms (Figures 9-14/11, 12, 13, 14, 15; Figure 9-15G). The ability to support the erect posture independently while standing or walking, which requires the transfer of body weight to the feet and a new balancing skill, is usually acquired by about 13-15 months of age (Figure 9-14/16, 17; Figure 9-15H). In summary, the ontogenetic progression of voluntary motor control follows two gradients: a rostral to caudal gradient – from the head, the chest, the arms, to the legs; and a proximal to distal gradient – from the shoulder to the hands in the upper body, and from the hip to the feet in the lower body.

Some Recent Studies of the Development of Postural Control. Effective goal-directed behavior is difficult without postural control but the acquisition of the ability to sit and stand upright without outside support takes a long time. The ability to maintain the head in an upright position develops first. In standard pediatric examinations, the infant is pulled forward by its arms (traction) to determine what position its head will assume as the body is moved from the horizontal to the vertical position (Swaiman, 1999). Up to 2 months, infants cannot align their head and trunk: the head tends to lag behind the body as the trunk is raised, and it tends to fall forward when the trunk reaches the upright position. The ability to align head and trunk and keep the upper part of the body erect is acquired at about 3-4 months of age but the infant is still unable to maintain a seated posture without outside support (Touwen, 1976; Thelen and Spencer, 1998). According to one experimental study (Woollacott et al., 1987), 3-5 month-old infants propped up in a chair on a mobile platform fail to respond with appropriate compensatory head and trunk swaying if they are suddenly moved forward or backward. The ability to sit upright and maintain that position develops at about 8 months (Van der Fits, 1999). Significantly, independent sitters of that age when placed on a mobile platform, display directionally appropriate neck and trunk responses when the platform is moved forward or backward (Woollacott et al., 1987). These findings are in line with the classical studies of McGraw (1943) and others. The legs play an important role in sitting without support, but the development of voluntary control of the legs lags behind the voluntary control of the arms. Although the young infant's legs are often more active than its arms, this exuberant trashing and kicking has more the character of spontaneous involuntary movements than voluntary goal-directed acts (McGraw (1943).

Classical Studies of the Development of Biped Locomotion. The slow development of postural balance is paralleled by the slow development of locomotor skills. And, again, the arms play an active role in ambulation much before the legs do (Gesell and Ames, 1940; Gesell and Halverson, 1942). The first attempt to get from one place to another takes the form of crawling, and at least two stages have been distinguished in its development. During the first stage (Figure 9-16A), at the age of about 4-6 months, the belly remains in contact with the ground and the body is pulled forward by the arms and hands while the kicking legs are dragged along and provide minimal assistance in ambulation. During the second stage (Figure 9-16B), at about 8 months, the extended arms and the dorsiflexed hands lift the trunk and hips

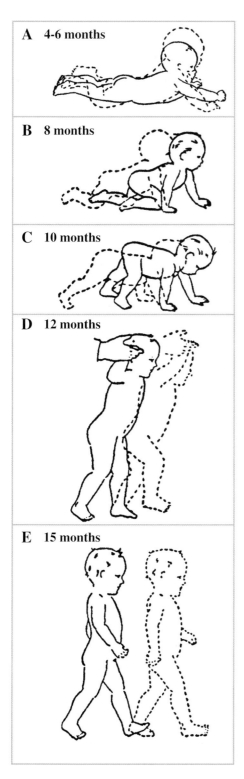

Figure 9-16. Stages in the development of locomotion from belly-crawling (**A**), through the quasi-quadruped crawling on hands and knees (**B**), the quadruped pattern of ambulation on hands and feet (**C**), walking on the toes (digitigrade walking) with outside support (**D**), to walking independently with the feet on the ground (plantigrade walking). The arms and hands that play a major role in early ambulation are gradually replaced by the legs and feet. Drawings from McGraw (1943).

off the ground, and the hands, knees and legs, but not the feet, provide the traction for ambulation. (Some infants skip the belly stage of crawling and proceed directly to the quasi-quadruped crawl with their arms and knees; Adolph, 1997.) During the next phase of locomotor development, the quadruped stage, the extended arms and legs raise the body off the ground and traction is provided by the the hands and the feet (Figure 9-16C). Finally, the use of the arms is abandoned during locomotion and the child begins to walk upright. Biped walking first starts with the toes providing both support and propulsion (Figures 9-16D). This is called digitigrade walking (Gray, 1968). Later, the child learns to make successive use of the toes, the plantar surface of the feet, and the heels for support and propulsion (plantigrade walking) and with that the skill is acquired to walk independently (Figure 9-16E). The different footprints made by a child's feet in digitigrade walking (Figure 9-17A) and plantigrade walking (Figure 9-17B) were recorded by McGraw (1935). This sequence in the development of voluntary ambulation attests to a rostral-to-caudal gradient (from the arms to the legs) and a proximal-to-distal gradient (from the knees to the feet). However, the change from digitigrade to plantigrade use of the feet in walking must obey a different developmental principle.

Some Recent Studies of the Development of Biped Locomotion. Figure 9-18A shows stick diagrams of digitigrade walking in a 10-month-old child who walked with support. Figure 9-18B shows the change toward a smoother and more effective plantigrade propulsion in another, independently walking 10-month-old child (Forssberg, 1985). Stick diagrams of the mature plantigrade walking pattern of an adult is illustrated in Figure 9-18C. In addition to support provided by the flat plantar surface of the foot, the maintenance of upright stance requires compensatory sways both at rest and during ambulation. When the young child begins to walk independently, gait is unstable and lurching, and requires a wide path relative to body dimensions to move about (Bril and Breniere, 1992). During the weeks after the child begins to walk independently, there is an appreciable increase in step length, and a decrease in step width (Adolph, 1997; Figure 9-19). The young child has difficulties in negotiating obstacles in its path but the hurdles that stop the biped progression of the 12- to 18-month-old, are easily negotiated by the 24-month-old (Schmuckler, 1996).

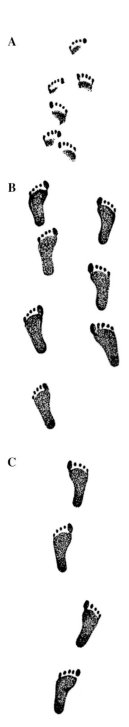

Figure 9-17. Footprints of a child as he progresses from digitigrade walking (**A**), to plantigrade walking (**B**). The subsequent improvement in walking skill is manifested in a decreasing step width and an increasing step length (**C**). From McGraw (1943).

forward in response. When the walls roll backward, they feel as if swaying forward and, in response, they step or shift their weight backward. Infants aged 7-12 months sitting on the stationary floor of a "moving room" move their torsos forwards or backwards in response to the perceived motion of the room (Butterworth and Hicks, 1977). Similar compensatory responses are obtained in 9-month-old infants sitting in a canvas sling (Berthenthal and Bai, 1989). Standing toddlers stagger or fall when tested in simulated moving rooms; however, children 2 years of age or older maintain their upright stance by initiating compensatory swaying movements or steps (Butterworth and Hicks, 1977; Berthenthal and Bai, 1989).

Development of Reaching and Grasping. A 4-6-month-old infant lying on its back will play with its hands and with objects placed into its hands (Figure 9-20). If secured in a retaining chair, infants of the same age will reach for an object suspended in front of them, and may succeed in touching or grasping the object and bring it to their mouths (Gesell, 1954; Hofsten, 1986, 1991; Mathew and Cook, 1990; Thelen et al., 1993). The transition from touching an attractive object and the ability to grasp it is acquired gradually (Figure 9-21). An infant's ability to grasp a target when not supported by a retaining chair, i.e., when tested on a bed with the "long leg posture" (Figure 9-22), develops more slowly. Using electromyographic recordings, Van der Fits et al. (1999) found that postural muscles in 6-month-olds are rarely active when reaching for a target but the postural muscles are active in the same infants at 8 months. By 12-15 months, these infants make anticipatory postural adjustments during reaching.

The arm trajectories during goal-directed reaching are initially circuitous and include multiple movement sequences (Fetters and Todd, 1987). After several months of reaching practice, the same infant develops smoother and straighter arm trajectories (Mathew and Cook, 1990; Konczak et al., 1995; Figure 9-23). Initially, infants rotate the shoulder and torso (i.e., use proximal muscles) to project their arm towards the target; later on, the infants improve the trajectory by using distally acting arm muscles to reach the target (Berthier et al., 1999). According to one study (Konczak et al., 1997), the number of movement sequences during reaching is reduced by the same infant, on the average, from 5 units at 20 weeks to 2 units by 15 months.

While new walkers exhibit poorly coordinated compensatory sway reactions when the platform on which they stand is suddenly moved forward or backward, older toddlers (15-24 months) react with the same kind of compensatory swaying reactions as do adults (Woollacott et al., 1987). "Moving rooms" have been used to study the development of postural control during locomotion (Lee and Lishman, 1975). When the walls roll forward, adults feel as if they are swaying backwards and they step or shift their weight

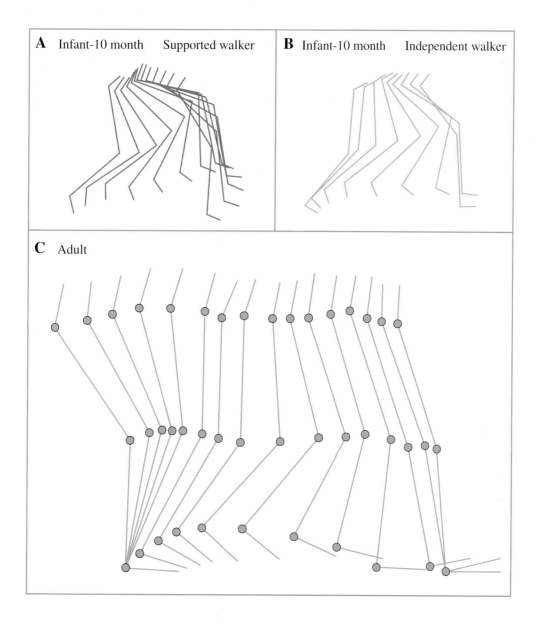

Figure 9-18. A. Stick diagrams showing the transition from the digitigrade stepping of a 10-month-old child that walked with support to the tentative plantigrade stepping of another independently walking 10-month-old child. **B.** Stick diagram of the plantigrade stepping of an adult. After Forssberg (1985).

When handling an object, infants first use a palmar grasp, next a scissors grasp, and finally a pincer grasp (Halverson , 1937; Figure 9-24). The ability to use a precision grip, in which the thumb and index finger are adjusted to fit the shape of the object, does not develop until the beginning of the second year (White et al., 1964; van der Fits et al., 1999). Reaching and grasping are integrated acts in adults,

the fist opens during the deceleration phase of reaching to fit the object to be grasped (Jakobson and Goodale, 1991; Chieffi and Gentilucci, 1993). In infants, reaching and grasping are two separate acts (Mathew and Cook, 1990). A well-coordinated anticipatory adjustment of grip force to the features of the grasped object does not develop until much after 2 years (Forssberg et al., 1992, 1995; Eliasson et al., 1995).

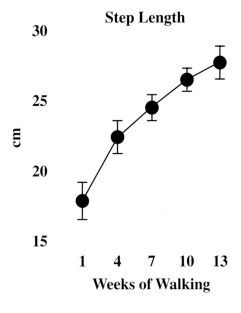

Step Length

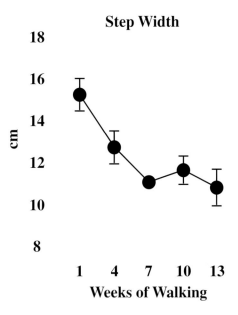

Step Width

Figure 9-19. Increasing step length (**A**) and decreasing step width (**B**) in a small sample of young children as a function of the length of time (in weeks) they have been walking. Bars indicate standard errors. After Adolph (1997).

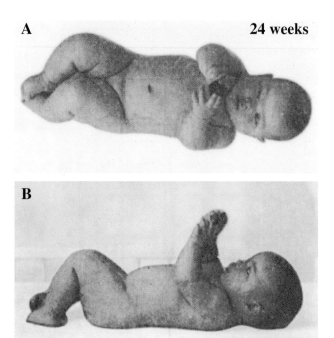

Figure 9-20. A 24-week-old infant lying on its back and playing with an object. Photographs taken concurrently from above (**A**) and the side (**B**). Compare the voluntary behavior displayed by this infant at 24 months of age with its reflex posture at 1, 8, and 12 weeks (Figure 9-7). From Gesell (1954).

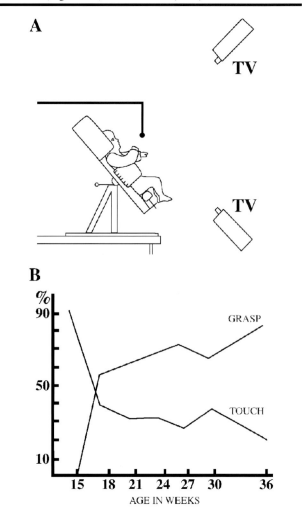

Figure 9-21. A. Experimental setting to record the development of reaching and grasping of a suspended ball. **B.** 15-week-old infants succeeded in touching the ball in 90% of the trials but the ability to grasp the ball does not develop in most infants until several weeks later. After Hofsten (1986).

Figure 9-22. Testing of compensatory postural reactions during reaching and grasping in an infant chair that provides postural support ("upright sitting") and in an unsupported position ("long leg sitting"). From Van der Fits et al. (1999).

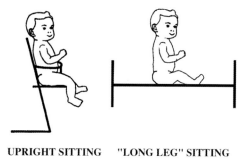

UPRIGHT SITTING   "LONG LEG" SITTING

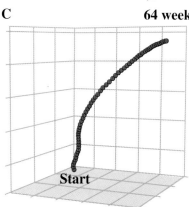

A   20 weeks

B   36 weeks

C   64 weeks

Figure 9-23. Arm trajectory and movement sequences in the goal-directed reaching of an infant at 20 (**A**), 36 (**B**), and 64 (**C**) weeks of age. Time interval between successive data points (circles) is 10 ms. After Konczak et al. (1995).

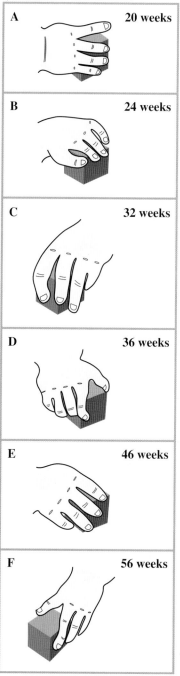

A 20 weeks
B 24 weeks
C 32 weeks
D 36 weeks
E 46 weeks
F 56 weeks

Figure 9-24. Changing pattern of grasping a cube between 20 and 56 weeks of age. The initial palmar grasp (**A**, **B**, **C**) changes to scissors grasp, with palm and opposed thumb (**D**, **E**), then to the precision pincer grip, with opposed index finger and thumb (**F**). After Halverson (1937).

9.4.2 Correlations with the Myelination of the Lateral Corticospinal Tract. The massive lateral corticospinal tract stands out in myelin-stained sections of the cervical spinal cord of the 4-day-old infant by its faintness (Figure 9-25). Reactive gliosis (punctate staining) may have started in the medial tip of the corticospinal tract adjacent to the myelinated reticulated area but its bulk contains very few reactive glia. Provisionally, the medial tip of the lateral corticospinal tract where reactive gliosis may have started is called fascicle 1. Reactive gliosis is definitely in progress in fascicle 1 in the cervical cord of the 33-day-old infant lateral to the reticulated area (Figure 9-26). The pattern of myelin staining is similar in the 53-day-old infant, with a hint of reactive gliosis (darker staining) spreading to the rest of the lateral corticospinal tract (Figure 9-27). Profound change in the myelin staining pattern of the lateral corticospinal tract is evident in the 4-month-old infant. In the middle cervical cord (Figures 9-28), three fascicles can be distinguished in terms of staining intensity. Sudanophilic staining is most intense medially in fascicle 1, suggesting the onset of myelination in this region. The middle portion of the lateral corticospinal tract shows advanced reactive gliosis; that is fascicle 2. The thin outer shell (underneath the myelinated dorsal spinocerebellar tract) shows less advanced reactive gliosis; that is fascicle 3.

Rostral-to-Caudal Gradient in Corticospinal Tract Myelination. There may also be a rostral-to-caudal gradient in myelination of the lateral corticospinal tract from the cervical to the lumbosacral levels. A series of descending spinal cord sections from the same 4-month-old infant illustrate that. At a low cervical level (Figure 9-29A), fascicle is myelinated, reactive gliosis is advanced in fascicle 2, and is less advanced in fascicle 3. At a thoracic level (Figure 9-29B), the three fascicles are still distinguishable in the greatly diminished lateral corticospinal tract. However, the intensity of myelin staining is reduced here relative to the cervical level. The small medial fascicle with the strongest staining may be a remnant of the myelinating fascicle 1. If so, fascicle 1 is composed mostly of corticocervical fibers, and a few corticothoracic fibers. The adjacent two bands with reactive glia, constitute fascicles 2 and 3. At lumbar level (Figure 9-30A), the size of the corticospinal tract is somewhat reduced and the staining pattern suggests the presence of fascicles 2 and 3. These two fascicles, by definition, must be composed of corticolumbar and corticosacral fibers and they contain a greatly reduced

population of reactive glia. Finally, at the lumbosacral level, the greatly diminished lateral corticospinal tract contains virtually no reactive glia (Figure 9-30B). This remnant of the lateral corticospinal tract, presumably composed of fibers of fascicle 3, represents the corticosacral tract. We do not know how fast reactive gliosis and myelination advance from the rostral to the caudal levels of the spinal cord but the process appears be quite slow. In the lumbar spinal cord of an 11-month-old infant that was available for examination (Figure 9-31A), fascicle 2 may be just beginning to myelinate, and fascicle 3 still appears to be at an early stage of reactive gliosis. However, in the spinal cord of a 2-year-old child (Figure 9-31B) myelination of the lateral corticospinal tract is as advanced in the lumbar spinal cord as it is more rostrally. The myelination of the entire corticospinal tract may be completed, undoubtedly with individual variability, some time between 1 and 2 years of age.

Somatotopic Order in the Myelination of the Corticospinal Tract. The limited foregoing evidence indicates that there is a medial-to-lateral gradient and a rostral-to-caudal gradient in the progression of reactive gliosis and subsequent myelination within the lateral corticospinal tract. If subsequent research confirm that, what could be the behavioral significance of those gradients? A possibility is that these gradients are related to the somatotopic organization of the corticospinal tract. Somatotopy in the precentral and postcentral gyri of the human cerebral cortex (with sensory and motor homunculi) has been known for a long time and is well established (e.g., Penfield and Rasmussen, 1950). There is also good evidence for the somatotoic arrangement of the corticofugal fascicles descending in the internal capsule and the cerebral peduncle (reviewed by Brodal, 1981). Foerster (1936), relying on clinical evidence, described a precise segmental organization of corticospinal tract fibers in the cervical spinal cord (Figure 9-32; left side). According to that schema, corticospinal fibers terminating in the upper cervical cord are located most medially, and fibers that successively terminate at lower cervical, thoracic, lumbar, and sacral levels form shells in a medial-to-lateral sequence. It must be pointed out that this schema, which is reproduced in several modern textbooks (e.g., Williams and Warwick, 1980), is controversial (Brodal, 1981).

The preceding evidence of a medial-to-lateral and a rostral-to-caudal gradient in reactive gliosis and myelination of the lateral corticospinal tract does not directly bear on the claim that it is topographically organized. However, somatotopic organization is indirectly supported. First, the medial fascicle of the corticospinal tract myelinates earlier in the cervical cord than the lateral fascicles. Second, the bulk of the earlier myelinating medial fascicle terminates in the cervical cord and only a small complement reaches the thoracic cord. Hence, the medial fascicle must contain mostly corticocervical fibers. Third, the later myelinating laterally situated fascicles extend beyond the thoracic cord. Hence, the lateral fascicles must contain a large complement of corticolumbar and perhaps a small complement of corticosacral fibers.

The somatotopic organization of the corticospinal tract at the cervical level of the human spinal cord, may be roughly like that shown in Figure 9-32 opposite Foerster's segmental map. According to this tentative scheme, the medially situated corticocervical fibers (C1–C8) act upon motoneuron pools that control the neck, shoulder, arm, wrist, and hand muscles in a rostral-to-caudal sequence. The intermediate corticothoracic fibers (T1–T12) act upon motoneurons of the thoracic cord that control the trunk muscles. Finally, the laterally situated corticolumbar and corticosacral fibers (L1–S4) successively act upon motoneuron pools that control the hip, thigh, leg, ankle, and foot muscles. If the illustrated schema is correct,

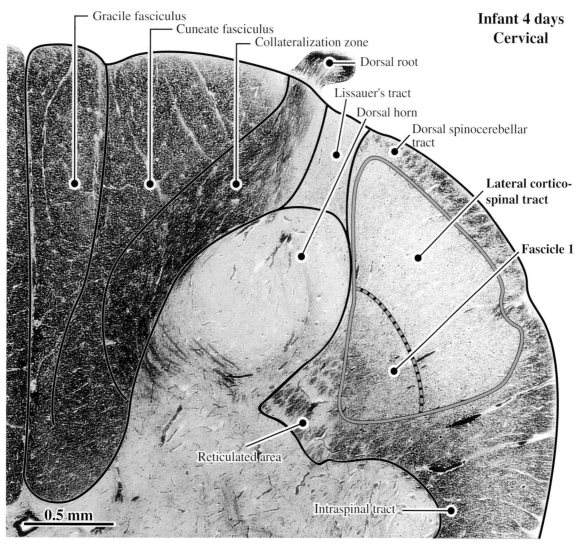

Figure 9-25. The unmyelinated lateral corticospinal tract of the cervical spinal cord in a 4-day-old infant (*Y299-62*). There is a hint of the onset of reactive gliosis (punctate staining) in the medial tip of the tract, provisionally designated as fascicle 1. The bulk of the corticospinal tract is devoid of reactive glia.

**Infant 33 days
Cervical**

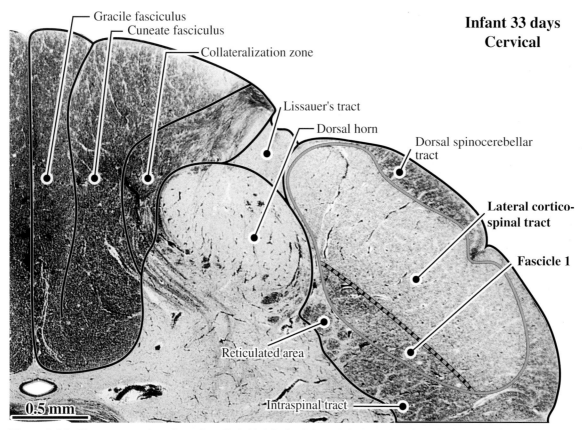

Figure 9-26. The concentration of reactive glia is high in fascicle 1 of the lateral corticospinal tract in the cervical spinal cord of this 33-day-old infant (*Y125-61*), with a hint of the onset of light myelination (some coarse staining). There are few reactive glia in the rest of the lateral corticospinal tract.

**Infant 53 days
Upper Cervical**

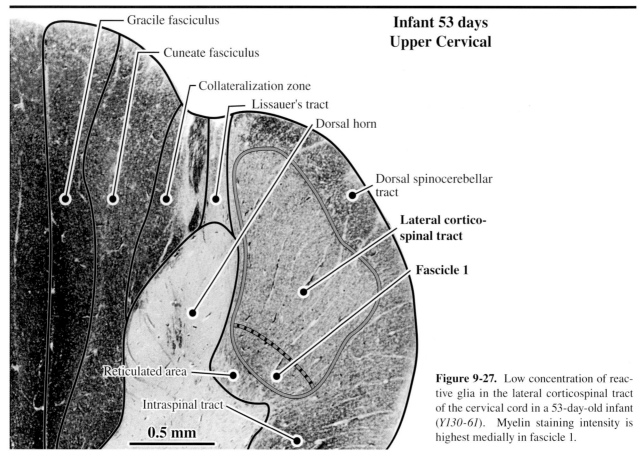

Figure 9-27. Low concentration of reactive glia in the lateral corticospinal tract of the cervical cord in a 53-day-old infant (*Y130-61*). Myelin staining intensity is highest medially in fascicle 1.

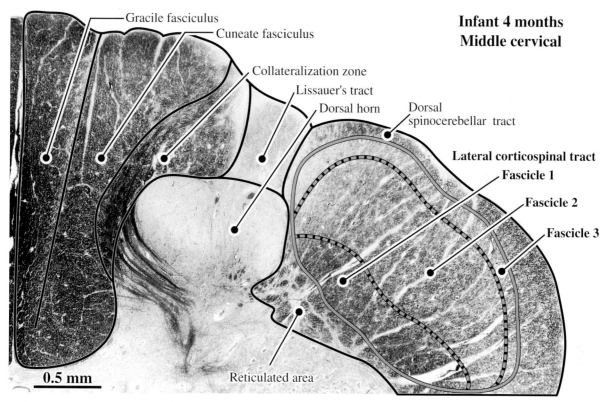

Figure 9-28. Myelination is well advanced in fascicle 1 of the lateral corticospinal tract in this 4-month-old infant (*Y286-62*). The staining pattern indicates that reactive gliosis is high in fascicle 2, and is in progress in fascicle 3.

the existing myelination gradients imply a rostral-to-caudal gradient in the functional maturation of corticospinal fibers acting upon spinal cord pattern generators and motoneuron pools. Hence, as effective cortical control advances from the cervical to the thoracic cord, there ought to be corresponding gradient in the advance of voluntary control, starting at the head and the neck, and ending with the leg and the foot. That is exactly what the sequence of behavioral development indicates.

Parallels in Corticospinal Tract Myelination and in the Development of Voluntary Control. Figure 9-33 summarizes schematically the hypothetical relationship between the rostral-to-caudal gradient in the myelination of the corticospinal tract during the first postnatal year, and the correlated progressive advance of voluntary motor control of parts of the body from rostral-to-caudal and from proximal-to-distal. The hypothesis is based on three assumptions. First, the somatic motoneurons and the central pattern generators of the spinal cord are under the control of two different efferent pathways from the brain: the

paleospinal tracts (roughly the subcortical extrapyramidal pathway of classical neurology) and the corticospinal tract (a component of the pyramidal pathway). Second, the paleospinal pathway is responsible for triggering and coordinating inborn reflexes and automatisms, whereas the corticospinal tract makes possible the voluntary initiation and coordination of acquired skills and purposive acts. Third, effective control of the spinal cord motoneurons and pattern generators either by fibers of the paleospinal tracts or of the corticospinal tract requires that they are myelinated. The great difference between the two tracts is that while the paleospinal tracts are myelinated by birth, the myelination of the corticospinal tract begins after birth and progeses slowly from the rostral to the caudal levels of the spinal cord.

The extremely premature infant can be kept alive only with the aid of artificial life-support devices and intensive care. In contrast, the viable premature infant and the full-term infant carries out a host of bodily functions that ensure its survival and growth. However, since the neonate has very limited behav-

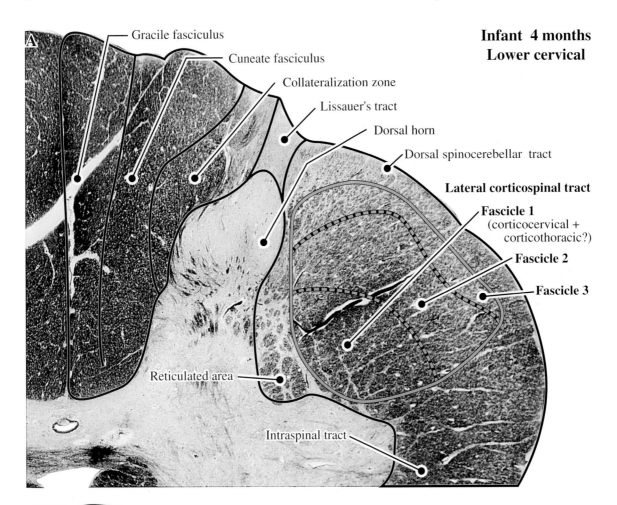

Infant 4 months
Lower cervical

Gracile fasciculus

Cuneate fasciculus

Collateralization zone

Lissauer's tract

Dorsal horn

Dorsal spinocerebellar tract

Lateral corticospinal tract

Fascicle 1
(corticocervical +
corticothoracic?)

Fascicle 2

Fascicle 3

Reticulated area

Intraspinal tract

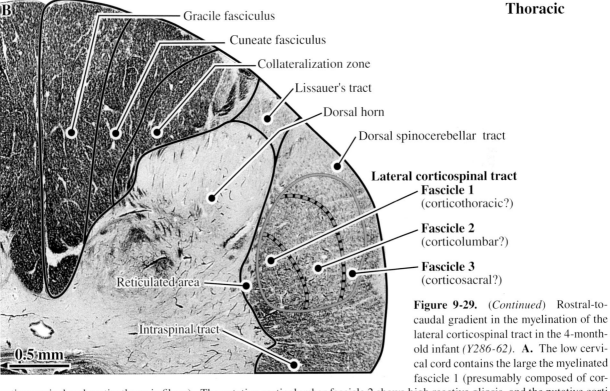

Thoracic

Gracile fasciculus

Cuneate fasciculus

Collateralization zone

Lissauer's tract

Dorsal horn

Dorsal spinocerebellar tract

Lateral corticospinal tract
Fascicle 1
(corticothoracic?)

Fascicle 2
(corticolumbar?)

Fascicle 3
(corticosacral?)

Reticulated area

Intraspinal tract

0.5 mm

Figure 9-29. (*Continued*) Rostral-to-caudal gradient in the myelination of the lateral corticospinal tract in the 4-month-old infant *(Y286-62)*. **A.** The low cervical cord contains the large the myelinated fascicle 1 (presumably composed of corticocervical and corticothoracic fibers). The putative corticolumbar fascicle 2 shows high reactive gliosis, and the putative corticosacral fascicle 3 shows low reactive gliosis. **B.** In the thoracic cord, the myelinated fascicle 1 is small, indicating that most of these fibers terminated in the cervical cord. Reactive gliosis is lower at this level in fascicles 2 and 3 than more rostrally.

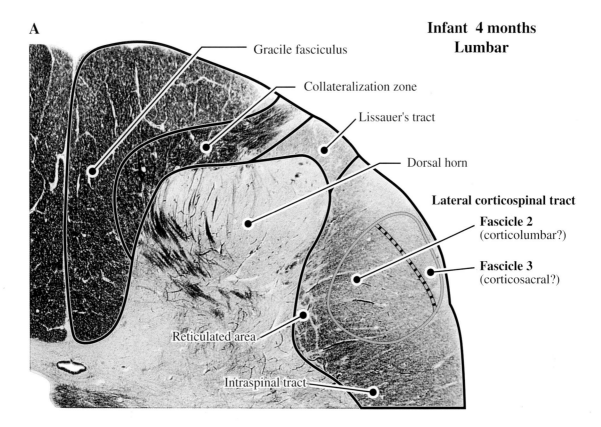

A   **Infant 4 months**
                                                     Lumbar

Gracile fasciculus

Collateralization zone

Lissauer's tract

Dorsal horn

Lateral corticospinal tract

Fascicle 2
(corticolumbar?)

Fascicle 3
(corticosacral?)

Reticulated area

Intraspinal tract

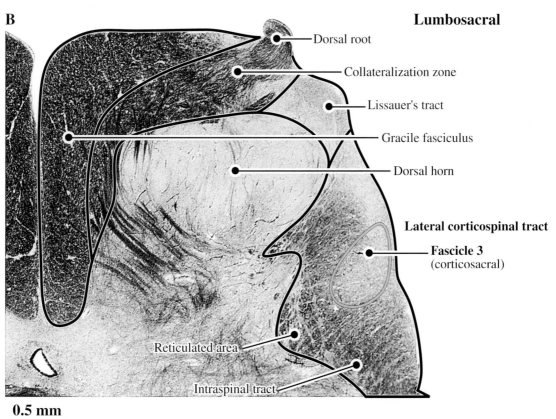

B   **Lumbosacral**

Dorsal root

Collateralization zone

Lissauer's tract

Gracile fasciculus

Dorsal horn

Lateral corticospinal tract

Fascicle 3
(corticosacral)

Reticulated area

Intraspinal tract

0.5 mm

Figure 9-30. Rostral-to-caudal gradient in the myelination of the lateral corticospinal tract in the 4-month-old infant. **A.** Two regions are distinguished: the larger medial region with many reactive glia (the putative corticolumbar fascicle 2) and a smaller lateral shell with fewer reactive glia (the putative corticosacral fascicle 3). **B.** The diminutive lateral corticospinal tract of the lumbosacral cord (the putative corticosacral fascicle) contains few reactive glia.

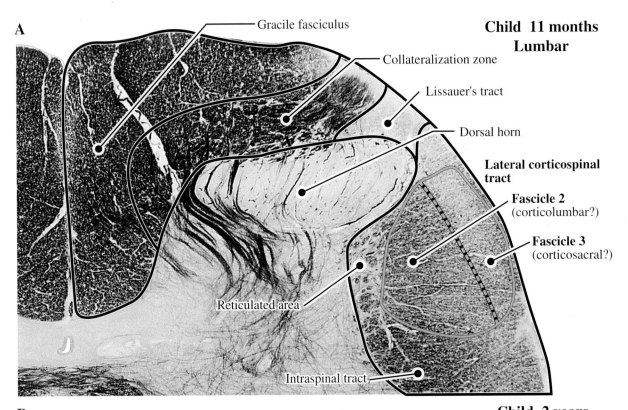

**Child 11 months
Lumbar**

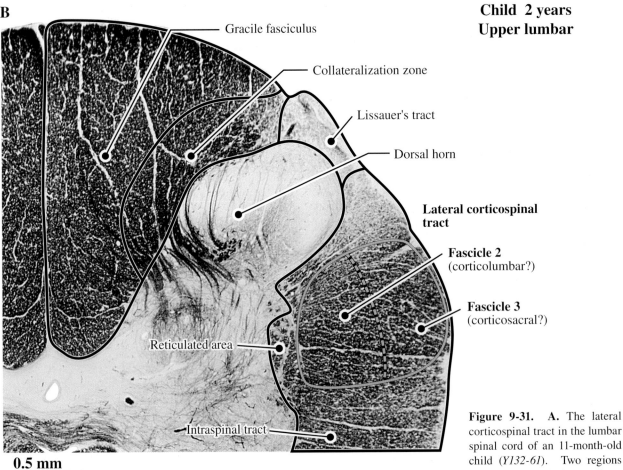

**Child 2 years
Upper lumbar**

0.5 mm

Figure 9-31.   A. The lateral corticospinal tract in the lumbar spinal cord of an 11-month-old child (*Y132-61*).   Two regions are distinguished: the myelinating presumptive corticolumbar fascicle 2, and the unmyelinated presumptive corticosacral fascicle 3 with a fair concentration of reactive glia. **B.** The lateral corticospinal tract in the lumbar spinal cord of a 2-year-old child (*Y425-63*). Both the presumptive corticolumbar and corticosacral fascicles are well myelinated by this age.

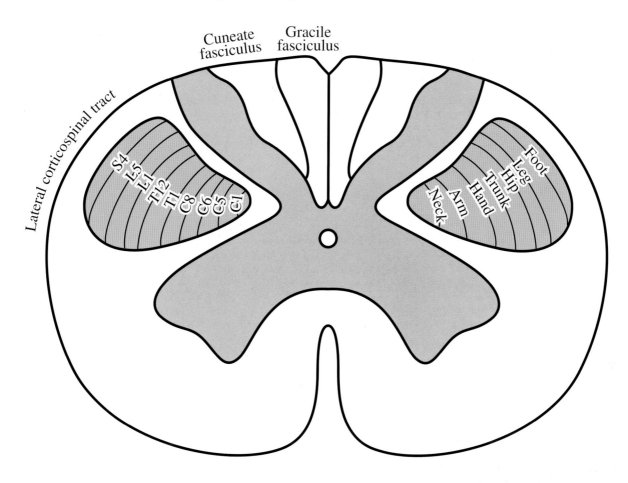

Figure 9-32. Segmental organization in the lateral corticospinal tract of the human cervical spinal cord (**left**), according to the clinical studies of Foerster (1936), and inferred somatotopic organization(**right**).

ioral capacities, it cannot fend for itself; it has to be fed, kept clean, and protected from the hazards of the environment by caretakers. The ability of the newborn to autonomously perform a host of vital functions is attributed to the early myelination of most of the paleospinal tracts that interconnect the spinal cord with the lower brain stem. In Figure 9-33A, the black border along the paleospinal tract of the newborn (green column) indicates that this pathway is myelinated over its entire length. The absence of any black border along the corticospinal tract (red column) indicates that this tract is unmyelinated. The green outline over the entire body surface indicates that the entire body is, at this stage of development, under paleospinal control. Reflexes and automatisms are operational along the entire body but the newborn cannot engage its spinal motor mechanisms for voluntary behavior because the corticospinal tract is unmyelinated.

The short black border at the top of corticospinal pathway (red column) in infants 1-2 months of age (Figure 9-33B) indicates the onset of myelination at upper cervical levels of the spinal cord. The concurrent acquisition of voluntary control over the muscles of the neck and shoulders (red outline over body) is correlated with the myelination of the upper corticospinal tract. The 1-month-old infant can voluntarily turn its head while tracking a moving target with its eyes, or lift its head and shoulder, and support itself with outstretched arms while lying on its stomach. Other parts of the body, like the randomly kicking legs, remain under involuntary paleospinal control.

Myelination spreads along the entire cervical spinal cord by 3-4 months (extended black border along the red column in Figure 9-33C). By that age an infant seated in a supporting chair will voluntarily reach for a suspended ball nearby and try to touch it. However, the infant cannot grasp the ball, indicating the absence of voluntary control of the distal hand and finger muscles. Since the infant cannot sit without outside support, voluntary control of the distal muscles of the wrist and hand, and the caudal muscles of the pelvic girdle and legs have not developed either. In the available material we could not trace the spread of myelination in the corticospinal tract during the crucial period between 5 and 9 months. The reconstruction of the spread of myelination along the corticospinal tract (black border along the red column) in Figures 9-33D and 9-33E is inferred from the behavioral evidence. Behavioral observations indicate that most 5-7-month-old infants will grasp a ball suspended in front of them. Grasping at this age takes the form of a primitive palmar grip. Infants of this age can roll over, sit momentarily by themselves, and crawl on their hands and knees. The acquisition of gross voluntary control over the hands (but not the distal individual fingers) and the thigh muscles (but not the distal feet and toes) suggests the spread of myelination in the corticospinal tract to the thoracic and upper lumbar cord. However, the lower cervical cord may still have unmyelinated components because there is no discrete voluntary control of the fingers. The next landmark in behavioral development, beginning at about 8-9 months, is the infant's ability to sit up and maintain that posture with leg support, play with toys while sitting, walk in a quadruped style on hands and feet, and, if given outside support, stand momentarily on its feet or walk. We infer that myelination of the corticospinal tract has spread far-

ther along the lumbar cord and it is completed in the cervical cord.

At 10-11 months (Figure 9-33F), myelination of the corticospinal tract is in progress in the lumbar spinal cord but the lateral fascicle, which is presumed to contain descending fibers to the sacral cord, is still unmyelinated. Myelination of the corticospinal tract in the lumbar cord is behaviorally correlated with the ability of the 10-11-month-old child to raise itself upright when holding on to a chair or table, and walk on its toes when supported by an adult. Most children cannot walk upright independently until about 12-14 months. We infer that the myelination of the corticospinal tract is nearing completion by that age (Figure 9-33G). Effective biped posture and plantigrade locomotion, which allows the child to run, hop, jump, and climb over obstacles, to throw and catch a ball, and begin to master other skills, is usually not acquired until the end of the second year. In a single case we illustrated the advanced myelination of the corticospinal tract in the lumbar spinal cord of a 2-year-old child (Figure 9-31B). The most difficult task that awaits the child of this age is the acquisition of voluntary control of micturition and defecation. Successful toilet training may have to wait until the latest maturing corticosacral fibers reach and arborize in the sacral cord.

Figure 9-33. A. The development by birth of involuntary control of the entire body (life-supporting reflexes and automatisms) is indicated by the green outline over the body surface. The green column symbolizes the paleospinal pathway and the black border indicates that it is myelinated at birth. The rostral-to-caudal and proximal-to-distal advance in the development of voluntary control of different body parts (spreading red outline over body surface) is traced from 1-2 months of age up to 2 years of age (**B-G**) in relation to the rostral-to-caudal spread of myelination (black border) along the corticospinal tract (red columns).

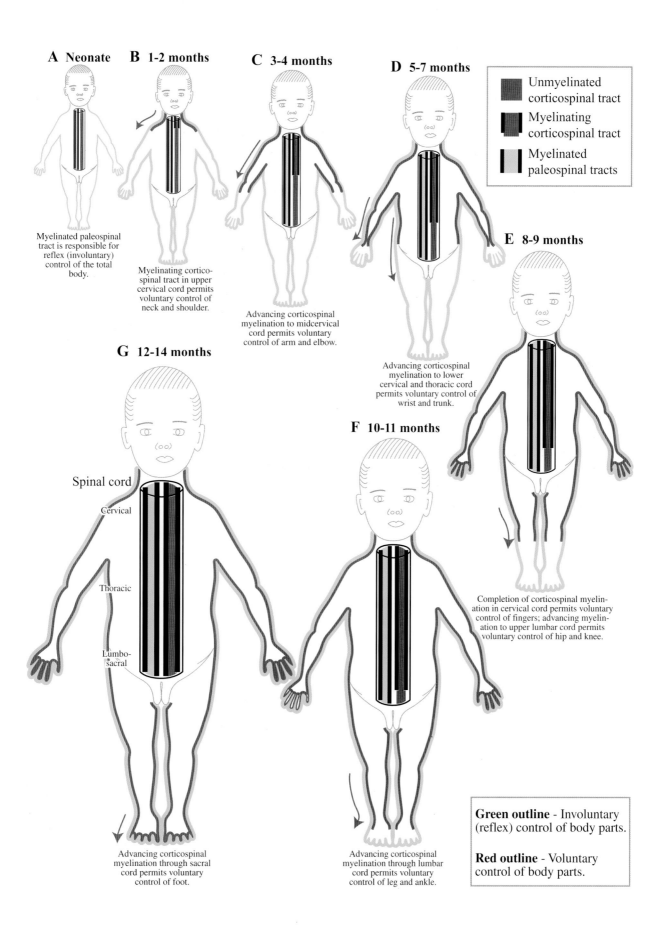

A Neonate

Myelinated paleospinal tract is responsible for reflex (involuntary) control of the total body.

B 1-2 months

Myelinating cortico-spinal tract in upper cervical cord permits voluntary control of neck and shoulder.

C 3-4 months

Advancing corticospinal myelination to midcervical cord permits voluntary control of arm and elbow.

D 5-7 months

Advancing corticospinal myelination to lower cervical and thoracic cord permits voluntary control of wrist and trunk.

Unmyelinated corticospinal tract

Myelinating corticospinal tract

Myelinated paleospinal tracts

E 8-9 months

Completion of corticospinal myelin-ation in cervical cord permits voluntary control of fingers; advancing myelin-ation to upper lumbar cord permits voluntary control of hip and knee.

F 10-11 months

Advancing corticospinal myelination through lumbar cord permits voluntary control of leg and ankle.

G 12-14 months

Spinal cord

Cervical

Thoracic

Lumbo-sacral

Advancing corticospinal myelination through sacral cord permits voluntary control of foot.

Green outline - Involuntary (reflex) control of body parts.

Red outline - Voluntary control of body parts.

REFERENCES

Adamson, S. L., A. Bocking, A. J. Cousin, I. Rapoport and J. E. Patrick. 1983. Ultrasonic measurement of rate and depth of human fetal breathing: Effect of glucose. *American Journal of Obstetrics and Gynecology*, 147:288-295.

Adolph, K. E. 1997. Learning in the development of infant locomotion. *Monographs of the Society for Research in Child Development*, 62, No. 3 (Serial No. 251).

Adrian, E. D. and Y. Zotterman. 1926. The impulses produced by sensory nerve endings. Part 3: Impulses set up by touch and pressure. *Journal of Physiology*, 61:151-171.

Agduhr, E. 1920. Studien über die postembryonale Entwicklung der Neurone und die Verteilung der Neuriten in den Wurzeln der Spinalnerven. *Journal für Psychologie und Neurologie*, 25:463-626.

Aidar, O., W. A. Geohegan and L. H. Ungewitter. 1952. Splanchnic afferent pathways in the central nervous system. *Journal of Neurophysiology*, 15:131-138.

Aitken, J. T. and J. E. Bridger. 1961. Neuron size and neuron population density in the lumbosacral region of the cat's spinal cord. *Journal of Anatomy*, 95:38-53.

Akil, H. and J. C. Liebeskind. 1975. Monoaminergic mechanisms of stimulation-produced analgesia. *Brain Research*, 94:279-296.

Albers, R. W. and R. O. Brady. 1969. The distribution of glutamic decarbolylase in the nervous system of the rhesus monkey. *Journal of Biological Chemistry*, 234:926-928.

Al-Chaer, E. D., N. B. Lawand, K. N. Westlund and W. D. Willis. 1996a. Pelvic visceral input into the nucleus gracilis is largely mediated by the postsynaptic dorsal column pathway. *Journal of Neurophysiology*, 76:2675-2690.

Al-Chaer, E. D., N. B. Lawand, K. N. Westlund and W. D. Willis. 1996b. Visceral nociceptive input into the ventral posterolateral nucleus of the thalamus: A new function for the dorsal column pathway. *Journal of Neurophysiology*, 76:2661-2674.

Alisky, J. M., T. D. Swink and D. L. Tolbert. 1992. The postnatal spatial and temporal development of corticospinal projections in cats. *Experimental Brain Research*, 88:265-276.

Alstermark, B. , A. Lundberg and S. Sasaki. 1984. Integration in descending motor pathways controlling the forelimb in the cat. 12. Interneurones which may mediate descending feed-forward inhibition and feed-back inhibition from the forelimb to C3–C4 propriospinal neurones. *Experimental Brain Research*, 56:308-322.

Altman, J. 1966. Proliferation and migration of undifferentiated precursor cells in the rat during postnatal gliogenesis. *Experimental Neurology*, 16:263-278.

Altman, J. 1969. DNA metabolism and cell proliferation. In: A. Lajtha (ed.), *Handbook of Neurochemistry*, vol. 2, *Structural Neurochemistry*, pp. 137-182. New York: Plenum Press.

Altman, J., W. J. Anderson and K. A. Wright. 1968. Differential radiosensitivity of stationary and migratory primitive cells in the brains of infant rats. *Experimental Neurology*, 22:52-74.

Altman, J. and S. A. Bayer. 1980a. Development of the brain stem in the rat: I. Thymidine-radiographic study of the time of origin of neurons in the lower medulla. *Journal of Comparative Neurology*, 194:1-35.

Altman, J. and S. A. Bayer. 1980b. Development of the brain stem in the rat. II. Thymidine-radiographic study of the time of origin of neurons in the upper medulla, excluding the vestibular and auditory nuclei. *Journal of Comparative Neurology*, 194:37-56.

Altman, J. and S. A. Bayer. 1980c. Development of the brain stem in the rat. IV. Thymidine-radiographic study of the time of origin of neurons in the pontine region. *Journal of Comparative Neurology*, 194:905-929.

Altman, J. and S. A. Bayer. 1981. Development of the brain stem in the rat. V. Thymidine-radiographic study of the time of origin of neurons in the midbrain tegmentum. *Journal of Comparative Neurology*, 198:677-716.

Altman, J. and S. A. Bayer. 1982. *Development of the Cranial Nerve Ganglia and Related Nuclei in the Rat.* (Advances in Anatomy, Embryology and Cell Biology, vol. 74.) Berlin: Springer-Verlag.

Altman, J. and S. A. Bayer. 1984. *The Development of the Rat Spinal Cord.* (Advances in Anatomy, Embryology and Cell Biology, vol. 85.) Berlin: Springer-Verlag.

Altman, J. and S. A. Bayer. 1990. Mosaic organization of the hippocampal neuroepithelium and the multiple germinal sources of dentate granule cells. *Journal of Comparative Neurology*, 301:325-342.

Altman, J. and S. A. Bayer. 1996. *Development of the Cerebellar System in Relation to its Evolution, Structure, and Functions.* Boca Raton, FL: CRC Press.

Altman, J. and M. B. Carpenter. 1961. Fiber projections of the superior colliculus in the cat. *Journal of Comparative Neurology*, 116:157-177.

Altman, J. and K. Sudarshan. 1975. Postnatal development of locomotion in the laboratory rat. *Animal Behavior*, 23:896-920.

Amendt, K., J. Czachurski, K. Dembowsky and H. Seller. 1979. Bulbospinal projections to the intermediolateral cell column: A neuroanatomical study. *Journal of the Autonomic Nervous System*, 1:103-117.

Ames, L. B. 1937. The sequential patterning of prone progression in the human infant. *Genetic Psychology Monographs*, 19:409-460.

Amiel-Tison, C. 1968. Neurological evaluation of the maturity of newborn infants. *Archives of the Diseases of Childhood*, 43:89-93.

Andersen, P., S. A. Andersson and S. Landgren. 1966. Some properties of the thalamic relay cells in the spino-cervico-lemniscal path. *Acta Physiologica Scandinavica*, 68:72-83.

Anderson, F. D. 1963. The structure of chronically isolated segment of the cat spinal cord. *Journal of Comparative Neurology*, 120:297-316.

Anderson, F. D. and C. M. Berry. 1959. Degeneration studies of long ascending fiber systems in the cat brain stem. *Journal of Comparative Neurology*, 111:195-229.

Anderson, W. J., D. L. Bellinger and D. Lorton. 1988. Morphology of dendrite bundles in the cervical spinal cord of the rat: A light microscopic study. *Experimental Neurology*, 100:121-138.

Anderson, W. J., M. W. Stromberg and E. J. Hinsman. 1976. Morphological characteristics of dendritic bundles in the lumbar spinal cord of the rat. *Brain Research*, 110:215-227.

André-Thomas, A. and S. St. Anne Dargassis. 1960. *The Neurological Examination of Infants*. London: Spastic International Medical Pulications.

Andres, K. H. 1961. Untersuchungen über den Feinbau von Spinalganglien. *Zeitschrift für Zellforschung*, 55:1-48.

Angaut-Petit, D. 1975. The dorsal column system. I. Existence of long ascending postsynaptic fibres in the cat's funiculus gracilis. *Experimental Brain Research*, 22:457-470.

Angulo y Gonzalez, A. W. 1932. The prenatal development of behavior in the albino rat. *Journal of Comparative Neurology*, 55:395-442.

Anthony, J. 1970. Le neuraxe des reptiles. *Traité de Zoologie*, 14:202-232.

Apkarian, A. V., R. T. Stevens and C. J. Hodge. 1985. Funicular location of ascending axons of lamina I cells in the cat spinal cord. *Brain Research*, 334:160-164.

Applebaum, A. E., J. E. Beall, R. D. Foreman and W. D. Willis. 1975. Organization and receptive fields of primate spinothalamic tract neurons. *Journal of Neurophysiology*, 38:572-586.

Ariens-Kappers, C. U., G. C. Huber and E. C. Crosby. (1936) 1967. *The Comparative Anatomy of the Nervous System of Vertebrates, Including Man*. Vol. 1. New York: Hafner (reprint).

Armand, J., S. A. Edgley, R. N. Lemon and E. Olivier. 1994. Protracted postnatal development of corticospinal projections from the primary motor cortex to hand motoneurones in the macaque monkey. *Experimental Brain Research*, 101:178-182.

Armand, J., E. Olivier, S. A. Edgkey and R. N. Lemon. 1997. Postnatal development of corticospinal projections from motor cortex to the cervical enlargement in the macaque monkey. *Journal of Neuroscience*, 17:251-266.

Armand, J., Y. Padel and A. M. Smith. 1974. Somatotopic organization of the corticospinal tract in cat motor cortex. *Brain Research*, 74:209-227.

Atlas, M. and V. P. Bond. 1965. The cell generation cycle of the eleven-day mouse embryo. *Journal of Cell Biology*, 26:19-24.

Auclair, F., M.-C. Bélanger and R. Marchand. 1993. Ontogenetic study of early brain stem projections to the spinal cord in the rat. *Brain Research Bulletin*, 30:281-289.

Azulay, A. and A. S. Schwartz. 1975. The role of the dorsal funiculus of the primate in tactile discrimination. *Experimental Neurology*, 46:315-332.

Baddeley, A. D. 1976. *The Psychology of Memory*. New York: Harper and Row.

Bain, W. A., J. T. Irving and B. A. McSwiney. 1935. The afferent fibres from the abdomen in the splanchnic nerve. *Journal of Physiology*, 84:323-333.

Ballard, J. L., J. C. Khoury, K. Wedig, L. Wang, B. L. Eilers-Walsman and R. Lipp. 1991. New Ballard score, expanded to include extremely premature infants. *Journal of Pediatrics*, 119:417-423.

Ballerini, L., M. Galante, M. Grandolfo and A. Nistri. 1999. Generation of rhythmic patterns of activity by ventral interneurones in rat organotypic slice culture. *Journal of Physiology*, 517:459-475.

Barber, R. P., P. E. Phelps, C. R. Houser, G. D. Crawford, P. M. Salvaterra and J. E. Vaughn. 1984. The morphology and distribution of neurons containing choline acetyltransferase in the adult rat spinal cord: An immunocytochemical study. *Journal of Comparative Neurology*, 229:329-346.

Barber, R. P., P. E. Phelps and J. E. Vaughn. 1991. Generation patterns of immunocytochemically identified cholinergic neurons at autonomic levels of the rat spinal cord. *Journal of Comparative Neurology*, 311:509-519.

Barber, R. P. and J. E. Vaughn. 1986. Differentiation of dorsal root ganglion cells with processes in their synaptic target zone of embryonic mouse spinal cord: A retrograde tracer study. *Journal of Neurocytology*, 207-218.

Bardeen, C. R. and W. H. Lewis. 1901. The development of the limbs, body wall, and back. *American Journal of Anatomy*, 1:1-37.

Barilari, M. G. and H. G. J. M. Kuypers. 1969. Propriospinal fibers interconnecting the spinal enlargements in the cat. *Brain Research*, 14:321-330.

Baron, W., J. C. DeJonge, H. De Vries and D. Hoekstra. 1998. Regulation of oligodendrocyte differentiation: Protein kinase C activation prevents differentiation of O2A progenitor cells toward oligodendrocytes. *Glia*, 22:121-129.

Barr, M. L., L. F. Bertram and H. A. Lindsay. 1950. The morphology of nerve cell nucleus according to sex. *Anatomical Record*, 107:283-297.

Barrett, J. N. and W. E. Crill. 1974. Specific membrane properties of cat motoneurones. *Journal of Physiology*, 239:301-324.

Bartlett, D. 1997. Primitive reflexes and early motor development. *Journal of Developmental and Behavioral Pediatrics*, 18:151-157.

Basbaum, A. I., C. H. Clanton and H. L. Fields. 1978. Three bulbospinal pathways from the rostral medulla of the cat: An autoradiographic study of pain modulating systems. *Journal of Comparative Neurology*, 178:209-224.

Basbaum, A. I. and H. L. Fields. 1978. Endogenous pain control mechanisms: Review and hypothesis. *Annals of Neurology*, 4:451-462.

Basbaum, A. I. and H. L. Fields. 1979. The origin of descending pathways in the dorsolateral funiculus of the spinal cord of the cat and the rat: Further studies of the anatomy of pain modulation. *Journal of Comparative Neurology*, 187:513-532.

Bauer, J. 1926. Das Kriechphänomen des Neugeborenen. *Klinische Wochenschrift*, 5:1468-1469.

Bayer, S. A. and J. Altman. 1974. Hippocampal development in the rat: Cytogenesis and morphogenesis examined with autoradiography and low-level X-irradiation. *Journal of Comparative Neurology*, 158:55-80.

Bayer, S. A. and J. Altman. 1991. *Neocortical Development*. New York: Raven Press.

Beal, J. and T. N. Bice. 1994. Neurogenesis of spinothalamic and spinocerebellar tract neurons in the lumbar spinal cord of the rat. *Developmental Brain Research*, 78:49-56.

Beal, J. A. and M. H. Cooper. 1978. The neurons of the gelatinosal complex (laminae II and III) of the monkey (*Macaca mulatta*): A Golgi study. *Journal of Comparative Neurology*, 179:89-122.

Beal, J. A., J. E. Penny and H. R. Bicknell. 1981. Structural diversity of marginal (lamina I) neurons in the adult monkey (*Macaca mulatta*) lumbosacral spinal cord: A Golgi study. *Journal of Comparative Neurology*, 202:237-254.

Beall, J. E., A. E. Applebaum, R. D. Foreman and W. D. Willis. 1977. Spinal cord potentials evoked by cutaneous afferents in the monkey. *Journal of Neurophysiology*, 40:199-211.

Beall, J. E., R. F. Martin, A. E. Applebaum and W. D. Willis. 1976. Inhibition of primate spinothalamic tract neurons by stimulation in the region of the nucleus raphe magnus. *Brain Research*, 114:328-333.

Beattie, M. S., Q. Li, M. G. Leedy and J. C. Breshnahan. 1990. Motoneurons innervating the external anal and urethral sphincters of the female cat have different patterns of dendritic arborization. *Neuroscience Letters*, 111:69-74.

Beck, C. H. and W. W. Chambers. 1970. Speed, accuracy and strength of forelimb movement after unilateral pyramidotomy in rhesus monkeys. *Journal of Comparative and Physiological Psychology*, 70:1-22.

Belcher, G., R. W. Ryall and R. Schaffner. 1978. The differential effects of 5-hydroxytryptamine, noradrenaline and raphe stimulation on nociceptive and non-nociceptive dorsal horn interneurons in the cat. *Brain Research*, 151:307-321.

Belford, G. R. and H. P. Killackey. 1980. The sensitive period in the development of the trigeminal system of the neonatal rat. *Journal of Comparative Neurology*, 193:335-350.

Belford, G. R. and H. P. Killackey. 1979. Vibrissae representation in subcortical trigeminal centers of the neonatal rat. *Journal of Comparative Neurology*, 183:305-322.

Bellinger, D. L. and W. J. Anderson. 1987a. Postnatal development of cell columns and their associated dendritic bundles in the lumbosacral spinal cord of the rat. I. The ventrolateral cell column. *Developmental Brain Research*, 35:55-67.

Bellinger, D. L. and W. J. Anderson. 1987b. Postnatal development of cell columns and their associated dendritic bundles in the lumbosacral spinal cord

of the rat. II. The ventromedial cell column. *Developmental Brain Research*, 35:69-82.

Bennett, G. J., M. Abdelmoumene, H. Hayashi and R. Dubner. 1980. Physiology and morphology of substantia gelatinosa neurons intracellularly stained with horseradish peroxidase. *Journal of Comparative Neurology*, 194:809-827.

Bennett, G. J., M. Abdelmoumene, H. Hayashi, M. J. Hoffert and R. Dubner. 1981. Spinal cord layer I neurons with axon collaterals that generate local arbors. *Brain Research*, 209:421-426.

Berkley, K. J. and C. H. Hubscher. 1995. Are there separate central nervous system pathways for touch and pain? *Nature Medicine*, 1:766-773.

Bernhard, C. G., E. Bohm and I. Petersen. 1953. Investigations on the organization of the corticospinal system in monkeys. *Acta Physiologica Scandinavica*, 29:79-103.

Berthenthal, B. I. and D. L. Bai. 1989. Infants' sensitivity to optical flow for controlling posture. *Developmental Psychology*, 25:936-945.

Berthier, N. E., R. K. Clifton, D. D. McCall and D. J. Robin. 1999. Proximodistal structure of early reaching in human infants. *Experimental Brain Research*, 127:259-269.

Berthold, C.-H. and T. Carlstedt. 1982. Myelination of the S1 dorsal root axons in the cat. *Journal of Comparative Neurology*, 209:225-232..

Besson, J. M. and A. Chaouch. 1987. Peripheral and spinal mechanisms of nociception. *Physiological Reviews*, 67:67-186.

Biber, M. P., L. W. Kneisly and J. H. LeVail. 1978. Cortical neurons projecting to the cervical and lumbar enlargements of the spinal cord in young and adult rhesus monkeys. *Experimental Neurology*, 59:492-508.

Bice, T. N. and J. A. Beal 1997. Quantitative and neurogenic analysis of the total population and subpopulations of neurons defined by axon projection in the superficial dorsal horn of the rat lumbar spinal cord. *Journal of Comparative Neurology*, 388:550-564.

Bidder, H. F. and C. Kupffer. 1857. *Untersuchungen über die Textur des Rückenmarks*. Leipzig: Hirzel.

Bikeles, G. 1905. Zur Lokalisation im Rückenmark. *Deutsche Zeitschrift für Nervenheilkunde*, 29:180-207.

Bing, Z., L. Villanueva and D. Le Bars. 1990. Ascending pathways in the spinal cord involved in the activation of subnucleus reticularis dorsalis neurons in the medulla of the rat. *Journal of Neurophysiology*, 63:424-438.

Björkeland, M. and J. Boivie. 1984. The termination of spinomesencephalic fibers in cat: An experimental anatomical study. *Anatomy and Embryology*, 170:265-277.

Blinkov, S. M. and I. I. Glezer. 1968. *The Human Brain in Figures and Tables: A Quantitative Handbook*. New York: Basic Books.

Blix, M. 1884. Experimentelle Beiträge zur Lösung der Frage über die spezifische Energie der Hautnerven. *Zeitschrift für Biologie*, 20:140-156.

Bodian, D. 1966. Synaptic types on spinal motoneurons: An electron microscopic study. *Bulletin of the Johns Hopkins Hospital*, 119:16-45.

Boehme, C. C. 1968. The neural structure of Clarke's nucleus of the spinal cord. *Journal of Comparative Neurology*, 132:445-462.

Böhme, G. 1988. Formation of the central canal and dorsal glial septum in the spinal cord of the domestic cat. *Journal of Anatomy*, 159:37-47.

Boivie, J. 1970. The termination of the cervicothalamic tract in the cat: An experimental study with silver impregnation methods. *Brain Research*, 19:333-360.

Boivie, J. 1971. The termination of the spinothalamic tract in the cat: An experimental study with silver impregnation methods. *Experimental Brain Research*, 12:331-333.

Boivie, J. 1980. Thalamic projections from lateral cervical nucleus in monkey: A degeneration study. *Brain Research*, 198:13-26.

Boivie, J. J. G. and E. R. Perl. 1975. Neural substrates of somatic sensation. In: C. C. Hunt (ed.), *MTP Physiology*, Series One, vol. 3, *Neurophysiology*, pp. 303-411. London: Butterworths.

Bok, S. T. 1928. Das Rückenmark. In: W. von Möllendorf (ed.), *Handbuch der mikroskopischen Anatomie des Menschen*. Vol. 4. *Das Nervensystem*, Teil 1, pp. 478-578. Berlin: Springer.

Bolaffio, M. and G. Artom. 1924. Richerche sulla fisiologia del sistema nervosa del feto umano. *Archivio di Scienze Biologiche*, 5:457-487.

Bone, Q. 1960. The central nervous system in Amphioxus. *Journal of Comparative Neurology*, 115:27-64.

Boshes, B. and F. Padberg. 1953. Studies on the cervical spinal cord of man: Sensory pattern after interruption of the posterior columns. *Neurology*, 3:90-101.

Bossy, J. G. and R. Ferratier. 1968. Studies of the spinal cord of *Galago senegalensis* compared to that in man. *Journal of Comparative Neurology*, 132:485-498.

Bovolenta, P. and J. Dodd. 1990. Guidance of commissural growth cones at the floor plate in embryonic spinal cord. *Development*, 109:435-477.

Bovolenta, P. and J. Dodd. 1991. Perturbation of neuronal differentiation and axon guidance in the spinal cord of mouse embryos lacking a floor plate: Analysis of Danforth's short-tail mutation. *Development*, 113:625-639.

Bowker, R. M., H. W. M Steinbusch and J. D. Coulter. 1981. Serotonergic and peptidergic projections to the spinal cord demonstrated by a combined retrograde HRP histochemical and immunocytochemical staining method. *Brain Research*, 211:412-417.

Bowsher, D. 1957. Termination of the central pain pathway in man: The conscious appreciation of pain. *Brain*, 80:606-622.

Bowsher, D. 1976. Role of reticular formation in responses to noxious stimulation. *Pain*, 2:361-378.

Breedlove, S. M. and A. P. Arnold. 1981. Sexually dimorphic motor nucleus in the rat lumbar spinal cord: Response to adult hormone manipulation, absence in androgen-insensitive rats. *Brain Research*, 225:297-307.

Breedlove, S. M. and A. P. Arnold. 1983. Hormonal control of a developing neuromuscular system: I. Complete demasculinization of the male rat spinal nucleus of the bulbocavernosus using anti-androgen Flutamide. *Journal of Neuroscience*, 3:417-423.

Bril, B. and Y. Breniere. 1992. Postural requirements and progression velocity in young walkers. *Journal of Motor Behavior*, 24:105-116.

Brinley, F. J. 1974. Excitation and conduction in nerve fibers. In: V. B. Mountcastle (ed.), *Medical Physiology*, vol. 1, pp. 34-76. St. Louis: Mosby.

Brodal, A. 1981. *Neurological Anatomy in Relation to Clinical Medicine*, (3rd edition). New York: Oxford University Press.

Brodal, A. and B. Rexed. 1953. Spinal afferents to the lateral cervical nucleus in the cat. *Journal of Comparative Neurology*, 98:179-211.

Brodal, A., F. Walberg and T. Blackstad. 1950. Termination of spinal afferents to inferior olive in cat. *Journal of Neurophysiology*, 13:431-454.

Broman, J., S. Anderson and O. P. Ottersen. 1993. Enrichment of glutamate-like immunoreactivity in primary afferent terminals throughout the spinal cord dorsal horn. *European Journal of Neuroscience*, 8:1050-1061.

Brosamle, C. and M. E. Schwab. 1997. Cells of origin, course, and termination patterns of the ventral, uncrossed component of the mature rat corticospinal tract. *Journal of Comparative Neurology*, 386:293-303.

Brown, A. G. 1981. *Organization in the Spinal Cord: The Anatomy and Physiology of Identified Neurones*. Berlin: Springer-Verlag.

Brown, A. G. and D. N. Franz. 1969. Responses of spinocervical tract neurons to natural stimulation of identified cutaneous receptors. *Brain Research*, 7:231-249.

Brown, A. G., R. Noble and J. S. Riddell. 1986. Relations between spinocervical and post-synaptic dorsal column neurones in the cat. *Journal of Physiology*, 381:333-349.

Brown, A. G., P. K. Rose and P. J. Snow. 1977. The morphology of spinocervical tract neurones revealed by intracellular injection of horseradish peroxidase. *Journal of Physiology*, 270:747-764.

Brown, P. B. and J. L. Culberson. 1981. Somatotopic organization of hind limb cutaneous dorsal root projections to cat dorsal horn. *Journal of Neurophysiology*, 45:137-143.

Brown, P. B. and J. L. Fuchs. 1975. Somatotopic representation of hind limb skin in cat dorsal horn. *Journal of Neurophysiology*, 38:1-9.

Brown, P. B., W. E. Gladfelter, J. C. Culberson, D. Covalt-Dunning, R. V. Sonty, L. M. Pubols and R. J. Millechia. 1991. Somatotopic organization of single primary afferent axon projections to cat spinal cord dorsal horn. *Journal of Neuroscience*, 11:298-309.

Bruce, A. 1901. *A Topographical Atlas of the Spinal Cord*. London: Williams.

Buchanan, J. T. 1996. Lamprey spinal interneurons and their roles in swimming activity. *Brain, Behavior and Evolution*, 48:287-296.

Buchanan, J. T. 1999. Commissural interneurons in rhythm generation and intersegmental coupling in the lamprey spinal cord. *Journal of Neurophysiology*, 81:2037-2045.

Bucy, P. C., R. Ladpli and A. Ehrlich. 1966. Destruction of the pyramidal tract in monkeys: The effects of bilateral section of the cerebral peduncles. *Journal of Neurosurgery*, 25:1-23.

Buijs, R. M. 1978. Intra- and extrahypothalamic vasopressin and oxytocin pathways in the rat: Pathways to the limbic system, medulla oblongata and spinal cord. *Cell and Tissue Research*, 192:423-435.

Bu'Lock, F., M. W. Woolridge and J. D. Baum. 1990. Development of coordination of sucking, swallowing, and breathing: Ultrasound study of term and preterm infants. *Developmental Medicine and Child Neurology*, 32:699-678.

Burke, R. E., P. L. Strick, K. Kanda, C. C. Kim and B. Walmsley. 1977. Anatomy of medial gastrocnemius and soleus motor nuclei in cat spinal cord. *Journal of Neurophysiology*, 40:667-680.

Burnside, L. H. 1927. Coordination in the locomotion of infants. *Genetic Psychology Monographs*, 2:284-372.

Burstein, R., K. D. Cliffer and G. J. Giesler. 1987. Direct somatosensory projections from the spinal cord to the hypothalamus and telencephalon. *Journal of Neuroscience*, 7:4159-4164.

Burstein, R., R. J. Dado, K. D. Cliffer and G. J. Giesler. 1991. Physiological characterization of spinohypothalamic tract neurons in the lumbar enlargement of the rat. *Journal of Neurophysiology*, 66:261-284.

Burstein, R., R. J. Dado and G. J. Giesler. 1990. The cells of origin of the spinothalamic tract of the rat: A quantitative reexamination. *Brain Research*, 511:329-337.

Burstein, R. and G. J. Giesler. 1989. Retrograde labeling of neurons in the spinal cord that project directly to the nucleus accumbens or the septal nuclei in the rat. *Brain Research*, 497:149-154.

Burstein, R. and S. Potrebic. 1993. Retrograde labeling of neurons in the spinal cord that project directly to the amygdala or the orbital cortex in the rat. *Journal of Comparative Neurology*, 35:469-485.

Burton, H. and A. D. Loewy. 1976. Descending projections from the marginal cell layer and other regions of monkey spinal cord. *Brain Research*, 116:485-491.

Butterworth, G. and L. Hicks. 1977. Visual proprioception and postural stability in infancy: A developmental study. *Perception*, 6:255-262.

Cabana, T. and G. F. Martin. 1984. Developmental sequence in the origin of descending spinal pathways: Studies using retrograde transport techniques in the North American opossum (*Didelphis virginiana*). *Developmental Brain Research*, 15:247-263.

Cabana, T. and G. F. Martin. 1985. Corticospinal development in the North-American opossum: Evidence for a sequence in the growth of cortical axons in the spinal cord and for transient projections. *Developmental Brain Research*, 23:69-80.

Calvillo, O., J. L. Henry and R. S. Newman. 1974. Effects of morphine and naloxone on dorsal horn neurons in the cat. *Canadian Journal of Physiology and Pharmacology*, 52:1207-1211.

Cameron, W. E., D. B. Averill and A. J. Berger. 1983. Morphology of cat phrenic motoneurons as revealed by intracellular injection of horseradish peroxidase. *Journal of Comparative Neurology*, 219:70-80.

Cameron-Curry, P. and N. M. Le Douarin. 1995. Oligodendrocyte precursors originate from both the dorsal and the ventral parts of the spinal cord. *Neuron*, 15:1299-1310.

Campbell, C. B. G., D. Yashon and J. A. Jane. 1966. The origin, course and termination of corticospinal fibers in the slow loris, *Nycticebus coucang* (Boddaert). *Journal of Comparative Neurology*, 127:101-112.

Carlen, P. L., D. A. McCrea and D. Durand. 1984. Dendrites and motoneuronal integration. In: R. A. Davidoff (ed.), *Handbook of the Spinal Cord*, vols. 2 and 3: *Anatomy and Physiology*, pp. 243-267. New York: Dekker.

Carmichael, L. 1970. The onset and early development of behavior. In: P. H. Mussen (ed.), *Carmichael's Manual of Child Psychology*, vol. 1, pp. 447-563. New York: Wiley.

Carstens, E. and D. L. Trevino. 1978. Laminar origins of spinothalamic projections in the cat determined by the retrograde transport of horseradish peroxidase. *Journal of Comparative Neurology*, 182:151-166.

Casey, K. L. 1969. Somatic stimuli, spinal pathways, and the size of cutaneous fibers influencing unit activity in the medial reticular formation. *Experimental Neurology*, 25:35-56.

Cassidy, G. and T. Cabana. 1993. The development of long descending propriospinal projections in the opossum, Monodelphis domestica. *Developmental Brain Research*, 72: 291-299.

Castro, A. J. 1972. Motor performance in rats: The effects of pyramidal tract section. *Brain Research*, 44:313-323.

Cauna, N. and G. Mannon. 1959. Development and postnatal changes of digital Pacinian corpuscles (corpuscula lamellosa) in the human hand. *Journal of Anatomy*, 93:271-286.

Cauna, N. and G. Mannon. 1961. Organization and development of the preterminal nerve pattern in the palmar digital tissues of man. *Journal of Comparative Neurology*, 117:309-328

Caverson, M. M., J. Ciriello and F. R. Calaresu. 1984. Paraventricular nucleus of the hypothalamus: An electrophysiological investigation of neurons projecting directly to the intermediolateral nucleus in the cat. *Brain Research*, 305:380-383.

Cayaffa, J. 1981. Anatomy and vascular supply of the spinal cord. In: L. Calenoff (ed.), *Radiology of Spinal Cord Injury*, pp. 3-22. St. Louis: Mosby.

Cechetto, D. F. and C. B. Saper. 1988. Neurochemical organization of the hypothalamic projection to the spinal cord in the rat. *Journal of Comparative Neurology*, 272:579-604.

Cervero, F., A. Iggo and V. Molony. 1977. Responses of spinocervical tract neurones to noxious stimulation of the skin. *Journal of Physiology*, 267:537-558.

Cervero, F., A. Iggo and V. Molony. 1979. Ascending projections of nociceptor-driven lamina I neurones in the cat. *Experimental Brain Research*, 35:135-149.

Chambers, W. W. and C. N. Liu. 1957. Corticospinal tract of the cat: An attempt to correlate the pattern of degeneration with deficits in reflex activity following neocortical lesions. *Journal of Comparative Neurology*, 108:23-55.

Chan-Palay, V. and S. L. Palay. 1977. Ultrastructural identification of substance P cells and their processes in rat sensory ganglia and their terminals in spinal cord by immunocytochemistry. *Proceedings of the National Academy of Sciences*, 74:4050-4054.

Chang, H. T. and T. C. Ruch. 1947. Topographical distribution of spinothalamic tract fibres in the thalamus of the spider monkey. *Journal of Anatomy*, 81:150-164.

Chaouch, A., D. Menétrey, D. Binder and J. M. Besson. 1983. Neurons at the origin of the medial component of the bulbopontine spinoreticular tract in the rat: An anatomical study using horseradish peroxidase retrograde transport. *Journal of Comparative Neurology*, 214:309-320.

Cheema, S. S., A. Rustioni and B. L. Whitsel. 1984. Light and electron microscopic evidence for a direct corticospinal projection to superficial laminae of the dorsal horn in cats and monkeys. *Journal of Comparative Neurology*, 225:276-290.

Chen, E. W. and A. Y. Chiu. 1992. Early stages in the development of spinal motor neurons. *Journal of Comparative Neurology*, 320:291-303.

Chi, J., F. Gilles, C. Kerr and Hare. 1976. Sudanophilic material in the developing nervous system. *Journal of Neuropathology and Experimental Neurology*, 35:119-120.

Chieffi, S. and M. Gentilucci, 1993. Coordination between the transport and grasp components during prehension movements. *Experimental Brain Research*, 94:471-477.

Choi, J. Y. and J. E. Hoover. 1996. The organization of the acromiodeltoid and spinodeltoid motor nuclei in rat spinal cord. *Brain Research*, 738:146-149.

Christensen, B. N. and E. R. Perl. 1970. Spinal neurons specifically excited by noxious or thermal stimuli: Marginal zone of the dorsal horn. *Journal of Neurophysiology*, 33:293-307.

Chung, K., J. M. Chung, F. W. LaVelle and R. D. Wurster. 1979b. Sympathetic neurons in the cat spinal cord projecting to the stellate ganglion. *Journal of Comparative Neurology*, 185:23-30.

Chung, K. and R. E. Coggeshall. 1987. Postnatal development of the rat dorsal funiculus. *Journal of Neuroscience*, 7:972-977.

Chung, J. M., D. R. Kenshalo, K. D. Gerhart and W. D. Willis. 1979a. Excitation of primate spinothalamic neurons by cutaneous C-fiber volleys. *Journal of Neurophysiology*, 42:1354-1369.

Chung, K., L. A. Langford, A. E. Applebaum and R. E. Coggeshall. 1979c. Primary afferent fibers in the tract of Lissauer in the rat. *Journal of Comparative Neurology*, 184:587-598.

Ciriello, J. and F. R. Calaresu. 1983. Central projections of afferent renal fibers in the rat: An anterograde transport study of horseradish peroxidase. *Journal of the Autonomic Nervous System*, 8:273-285.

Clark, D. A. 1931. Muscle counts of motor units: A study in innervation ratios. *American Journal of Physiology*, 96:296-304.

Clark, R. 1984. Anatomy of the mammalian cord. In: R. A. Davidoff (ed.), *Handbook of the Spinal Cord*, vols. 2 and 3: *Anatomy and Physiology*, pp. 1-45. New York: Dekker.

Clarke, F. M. 1939. A developmental study of the bodily reaction of infants to an auditory startle stimulus. *Journal of Genetic Psychology*, 55:415-427.

Clarke, J. L. 1851. Researches into the structure of the spinal cord. *Philosophical Transactions of the Royal Society*, Series B, part 1:607-621.

Clarke, J. L. 1859. Further researches on the gray substance of the spinal cord. *Philosophical Transactions of the Royal Society*, 149:437-467.

Cliffer, K. D., R. Burstein and G. J. Giesler. 1991. Distributions of spinothalamic, spinohypothalamic and spinotelencephalic fibers revealed by anterograde transport of PHA-L in rats. *Journal of Neuroscience*, 11:852-868.

Coghill, G. E. 1929. *Anatomy and the Problem of Behaviour*. Cambridge: Cambridge University Press.

Cohen, A. H. and R. M. Harris-Warrick. 1984. Strychnine eliminates alternating motor output during fictive locomotion in the lamprey. *Brain Research*, 293:164-167.

Collins, W. F., A. W. Seymour and S. W. Klugewicz. 1992. Differential effect of castration on the somal size of pudendal motoneurons in the adult male rat. *Brain Research*, 577:326-330.

Collinson, J. M., D. Marshall, C. S. Gillespie and P. J. Brophy. 1998. Transient expression of neurofascin by oligodendrocytes at the onset of myelogenesis: Implications for mechanisms of axon-glial interaction. *Glia*, 23:11-23.

Connors, G., C. Hunse, L. Carmichael, R. Natale and B. Richardson. 1988. The role of carbon dioxide in the generation of human fetal breathing movements. *American Journal of Obstetrics and Gynecology*, 158:322-327.

Conradi, S. 1969. On motoneuron synaptology in adult cats. *Acta Physiologica Scandinavica*, Suppl. 332:1-76.

Conradi, S., S. Cullheim, L. Gollvik and J.-O. Kellerth. 1983. Electron microscopic observations on the synaptic contacts of group Ia muscle spindle afferents in the cat lumbosacral spinal cord. *Brain Research*, 265:31-39.

Cook, A. W. and E. J. Browder. 1965. Functions of the posterior columns in man. *Archives of Neurology*, 12:72-92.

Corner, G. W. 1929. A well-preserved human embryo of 10 somites. *Carnegie Institution of Washington, Contributions to Embryology*, 20:81-102.

Coulter, J. D., L. Ewing and C. Carter. 1976. Origin of primary sensorimotor cortical projection to lumbar spinal cord of cat and monkey. *Brain Research*, 103:366-372.

Coulter, J. D. and E. G. Jones. 1977. Differential distribution of corticospinal projections from individual cytoarchitectonic fields in the monkey. *Brain Research*, 123:335-340.

Craig, A. D. 1976. Spinocervical tract cells in cat and dog, labeled by the retrograde transport of horseradish peroxidase. *Neuroscience Letters*, 3:173-177.

Craig, A. D. 1978. Spinal and medullary input to the lateral cervical nucleus. *Journal of Comparative Neurology*, 181:729-744.

Craig, A. D. 1995. Distribution of brainstem projections from spinal lamina I neurons in the cat and the monkey. *Journal of Comparative Neurology*, 361:225-248.

Craig, C. M. and D. N. Lee. 1999. Neonatal control of nutritive sucking pressure: Evidence for an intrinsic τ-guide . *Experimental Brain Research*, 124:371-382.

Crosby, E. C., T. Humphrey and E. W. Lauer. 1962. *Correlative Anatomy of the Nervous System*. New York: Macmillan.

Cruce, W. L. R. 1974a. The anatomical organization of hindlimb motoneurons in the lumbar spinal cord of the frog, *Rana catesbeiana*. *Journal of Comparative Neurology*, 153:59-76.

Cruce, W. L. R. 1974b. A supraspinal monosynaptic input to hindlimb motoneurons in lumbar spinal cord of the frog, *Rana catesbeiana*. *Journal of Neurophysiology*, 37:691-704.

Cuello, A. C., J. M. Polak and A. G. E. Pearse. 1976. Substance P: A naturally occurring transmitter in human spinal cord. *Lancet*, II:1054-1056.

Curfs, M. H. J. M., A. A. M. Gribnau and P. J. W. C. Dederen. 1993. Postnatal maturation of the dendritic fields of motoneurons supplying flexor and extensor muscles in the distal forelimb in the rat. *Development*, 117:535-541.

Curfs, M. H. J. M., A. A. M. Gribnau and P. J. W. C. Dederen. 1994. Selective elimination of transient corticospinal projections in the rat cervical spinal cord gray matter. *Developmental Brain Research*, 78:182-190.

Curtis, D. R. and G. A. R. Johnston. 1974. Amino acid transmitters in the mammalian central nervous system. *Ergebnisse der Physiologie*, 69:97-188.

Curtis, D. R. and J. C. Watkins. 1960. The excitation and depression of spinal neurons by structurally related amino acids. *Journal of Neurochemistry*, 6:117-141.

Dado, R. J., J. T. Katter and G. J. Giesler. 1994a. Spinothalamic and spinohypothalamic tract neurons in the cervical enlargement of rats. II. Responses to innocuous and noxious mechanical or thermal stimuli. *Journal of Neurophysiology*, 71:981-1002.

Dado, R. J., J. T. Katter and G. J. Giesler. 1994b. Spinothalamic and spinohypothalamic tract neurons in the cervical enlargement of rats. III. Locations of antidromically identified axons in the cervical white matter. *Journal of Neurophysiology*, 71:1003-1021.

Dahlström, A. and K. Fuxe. 1965. Evidence for the existence of monoamine neurons in the central nervous system: II. Experimentally induced changes in the intraneuronal amine levels of bulbospinal neuron systems. *Acta Physiologica Scandinavica*, 64 (Suppl. 247):1-36.

Dallenbach, K. M. 1927. The temperature spots and end-organs. *American Journal of Psychology*, 39:402-427.

Dalsgaard, C.-J. and L.-G. Elfvin. 1979. Spinal origin of preganglionic fibers projecting onto the superior cervical ganglion and inferior mesenteric ganglion of the guinea pig, as demonstrated by the horseradish peroxidase technique. *Brain Research*, 172:139-143.

Davenport, H. and R. T. Bothe. 1934. Cells and fibers in spinal nerves. II. A study of C_2, C_6, T_4, T_9, L_3, S_2 and S_5 in man. *Journal of Comparative Neurology*, 59:167-174.

De Biasi, S. and A. Rustioni. 1988. Glutamate and substance P coexist in primary afferent terminals in the superficial laminae of spinal cord. *Proceedings of the National Academy of Sciences*, 85:820-824.

De Biasi, S. and A. Rustioni. 1990. Ultrastructural immunocytochemical localization of excitatory amino acids in the somatosensory system. *Journal of Histochemistry and Cytochemistry*, 38:1745-1754.

De Groat, W. C., I. Nadelhaft, C. Morgan and T. Schauble. 1978. Horseradish peroxidase tracing of visceral efferent and primary afferent pathways in the cat's sacral spinal cord using benzidine processing. *Neuroscience Letters*, 10:103-108.

Dejerine, J. 1914. *Semeiologie des Affections du Systéme Nerveux*. Paris: Masson.

Dekker, J. J., D. G. Lawrence and H. G. J. M. Kuypers. 1973. The location of longitudinally running dendrites in the ventral horn of the cat spinal cord. *Brain Research*, 51:319-325.

Dembowsky, K., J. Czachurski and H. Seller. 1985. Morphology of sympathetic neurons in the thoracic spinal cord of the cat: An intracellular horseradish peroxidase study. *Journal of Comparative Neurology*, 238:453-465.

DeKort, E. J. M., A. A. M. Gribnau, H. T. H. van Aanholt, and R. Nieuwehuys. 1985. On the development of the pyramidal tract in the rat. I. The morphology of the growth zone. *Anatomy and Embryology*, 172:195-204.

DeMyer, W. Number of axons and myelin sheaths in adult human medullary pyramids: Study with silver impregnation and iron hematoxylin staining methods. *Neurology*, 9:42-47.

Denham, S. 1967. A cell proliferation study of the neural retina in the two-day rat. *Journal of Embryology and Experimental Morphology*, 18:53-66.

Denny-Brown, D. 1966. *The Cerebral Control of Movement*. Liverpool: Liverpool University Press.

Desmedt, J. E. and E. Godaux. 1977. Ballistic contractions in man: Characteristic recruitment pattern of single motor units of the tibialis anterior muscle. *Journal of Physiology*, 264:673-693.

de Vries, J. I. P., G. H. A. Visser and H. F. R. Prechtl. 1982. The emergence of fetal behavior. I. Qualitative aspects. *Early Human Development*, 7:302-322.

de Vries, J. I. P., G. H. A. Visser and H. F. R. Prechtl. 1985. The emergence of fetal behavior. II. Quantitative aspects. *Early Human Development*, 12:99-120.

Dickinson, P. J., M. L. Fanarraga, I. R. Griffiths, J. M. Barrie, E. Kyriakides and P. Montague. 1996. Oligodendrocyte progenitors in the embryonic spinal cord express DM-20. *Neuropathology and Applied Neurobiology*, 22:188-198.

Djouhri, L., A. G. Brown and A. D. Short. 1995. Effects of upper cervical spinal cord stimulation on neurones in the lumbosacral enlargement of the cat: Spinothalamic tract neurones. *Neuroscience*, 68:1237-1246.

Djouhri, L. and E. Jankowska. 1998. Indications of coupling between feline spinocervical tract neurones and midlumbar interneurones. *Experimental Brain Research*, 119:39-46.

Djouhri, L.,., Z. Meng, A. G. Brown and A. D. Short. 1997. Electrophysiological evidence that spinomesencephalic neurons in the cat may be excited via spinocervical tract collaterals. *Experimental Brain Research*, 116:477-484.

Dobry, P. J. K. and K. L. Casey. 1972. Roughness discrimination in cats with dorsal column lesions. *Brain Research*, 44:385-397.

Donatelle, J. M. 1977. Growth of the corticospinal tract and the development of placing reactions in the postnatal rat. *Journal of Comparative Neurology*,175:207-232.

Droit, S., A. Boldrini and G. Cioni. 1996. Rhythmical leg movements in low-risk and brain-damaged preterm infants. *Early Human Development*, 44:201-213.

Dubowitz, L. M. S. and V. Dubowitz and C. Goldberg. 1970. Clinical assessment of gestational age in the newborn infant. *Journal of Pediatrics*, 77:1-10.

Dubrovsky, B., E. Davelaar and E. Garcia-Rill. 1971. The role of dorsal columns in serial order acts. *Experimental Neurology*, 33:93-102.

Duce, I. R. and P. Keen. 1977. An ultrastructural classification of the neuronal cell bodies of the rat dorsal root ganglion, using zinc iodine-osmium impregnation. *Cell and Tissue Research*, 185:362-377.

Duggan, A. W., J. G. Hall and P. M. Heady. 1976. Morphine, enkephalin and the substantia gelatinosa. *Nature*, 264:456-458.

Earle, K. M. 1952. The tract of Lissauer and its possible relation to the pain pathway. *Journal of Comparative Neurology*, 96:93-109.

Ebbeson, S. O. E. 1967. Ascending fiber degeneration following hemisection of the spinal cord in the tegu lizard (*Tupinambis nigropunctatus*). *Brain Research*, 5:178-206.

Ebbeson, S. O. E. 1976. Morphology of the spinal cord. In: R. Llinás and W. Precht (eds.), *Frog Neurobiology: A Handbook*, pp. 679-706. Berlin: Springer-Verlag.

Eccles, J. C. 1964. *The Physiology of Synapses*. Berlin: Springer.

Eccles, J. C., R. M. Eccles and A. Lundberg. 1958. The action potentials of the alpha motoneurones supplying fast and slow muscles. *Journal of Physiology*, 142:275-291.

Eccles, J. C., R. Schmidt and W. D. Willis. 1963. Pharmacological studies on presynaptic inhibition. *Journal of Physiology*, 168:500-530.

Eccles, J. C. and C. S. Sherrington. 1930. Numbers and contraction-values of individual motor-units examined in some muscles of the limb. *Proceedings of the Royal Society*, B106:326-357.

Edwards, F. R., S. J. Redman and B. Walmsley. 1976. The effects of polarizing currents on unitary Ia excitatory post-synaptic potentials evoked in spinal motoneurones. *Journal of Physiology*, 259:705-723.

Edwards, S. B. 1972. The ascending and descending projections of the red nucleus in the cat: An experimental study using an autoradiographic tracing method. *Brain Research*, 48:45-63.

Edwards, S. B. 1975. Autoradiographic studies of the midbrain reticular formation: Descending projections of nucleus cuneiformis. *Journal of Comparative Neurology*, 161:341-358.

Eide, A. L., J. Glover, O. Kjaeulff and O. Kiehn. 1999. Characterization of commissural interneurons in the lumbar region of the neonatal rat spinal cord. *Journal of Comparative Neurology*, 403:332-345.

Eishima, K. 1991. The analysis of sucking behavior in newborn infants. *Early Human Development*, 27: 163-171.

Elders, C. 1910. Die motorischen Centren und die Form des Vorderhorns in den fünf letzten Segmenten des Cervicalmarkes und dem ersten Dorsalsegmente einer Mannes, der ohne linken Vorderarm geboren ist. *Monatschrift für Psychiatrie und Neurologie*, 28:491.

Eliasson, A.-C., H. Forssberg, K. Ikuta, I. Apel, G. Westling and R. Johansson. 1995. Development of human precision grip. V. Anticipatory and triggered grip actions during sudden loading. *Experimental Brain Research*, 106:425-433.

Elliott, H. C. 1942. Studies on the motor cells of the spinal cord. I. Distribution in the normal human cord. *American Journal of Anatomy*, 7:95-117.

Elliott, H. C. 1944. Studies on the motor cells of the spinal cord. IV. Distribution in experimental animals. *Journal of Comparative Neurology*, 81:97-103.

Elliott, K. A. 1945. Cross sectional diameters and areas of the human spinal cord. *Anatomical Record*, 93:287-293.

Enevoldson, T. P. and G. Gordon. 1989. Spinocervical neurons and dorsal horn neurons projecting to the dorsal column nuclei through the dorsolateral fascicle: A retrograde HRP study in the cat. *Experimental Brain Research*, 75:621-630

Engberg, I., J. A. Flatman and J. D. Lambert. 1979. The actions of excitatory amino acids on motoneurons in the feline spinal cord. *Journal of Physiology*, 288:227-261.

Erlanger, J. and H. S. Gasser. 1937. *Electrical Signs of Nervous Activity*. Philadelphia: University of Pennsylvania Press.

Espenschade, A. S. and H. M. Eckert. 1967. *Motor Development*. Columbus, OH: Merrill.

Evans, M. H. 1963. Alterations in activity of gamma efferents during distension of the bladder in the cat. *Journal of Physiology*, 165:358-367.

Fawcett, J. W. and R. J. Keynes. 1990. Peripheral nerve regeneration. *Annual Review of Neuroscience*, 13:43-60.

Feinstein, B., B. Lindegard, E. Nyman and G. Wohlfart. 1955. Morphologic studies of motor units in normal human muscles. *Acta Anatomica*, 23:127-142.

Feldman, W. M. 1920. *Principles of Antenatal and Postnatal Child Psychology: Pure and Applied.* New York: Longmans, Green.

Fenichel, G. M. (ed.) 1985. *Neonatal Neurology.* (2nd ed.) New York: Churchill, Livingstone.

Ferraro, A. and S. E. Barrera. 1935. Posterior column fibers and their termination in *Macacus rhesus. Journal of Comparative Neurology,* 62:507-530.

Fetters, L. and J. Todd. 1987. Quantitative assessment of infant reaching movements. *Journal of Motor Behavior,* 19:147-166.

Fields, H. L., A. I. Basbaum, C. H. Clanton and S. D. Anderson. 1977. Nucleus raphe magnus inhibition of spinal cord dorsal horn neurons. *Brain Research,* 126:441-453.

Fields, H. L., G. M. Wagner and S. D. Anderson. 1975. Some properties of spinal neurons projecting to the medial brain-stem reticular formation. *Experimental Neurology,* 47:118-134.

Fitzgerald, G. E. and W. Windle. 1942. Some observations on early human fetal movements. *Journal of Comparative Neurology,* 76:159-167.

Fitzgerald, M. 1987. Prenatal growth of fine-diameter primary afferents into the rat spinal cord: A transganglionic tracer study. *Journal of Comparative Neurology,* 261:98-104 .

Flechsig, P. 1876. *Die Leitungsbahnen im Gehirn und Rückenmark des Menschen auf Grund entwicklungsgeschichtlicher Untersuchungen.* Leipzig: Engelmann.

Fleischauer, K. and H. Hillebrand. 1966. Über die Vermehrung der Gliazellen bei der Markscheidenbildung. *Zeitschrift für Zellforschung,* 69:61-68.

Florence, S. L., J. T. Wall and J. H. Kaas. 1989. Somatotopic organization of inputs from the hand of the spinal grey and cuneate nucleus of monkeys with observations on the cuneate nucleus of humans. *Journal of Comparative Neurology,* 286:48-70.

Florence, S. L., J. T. Wall and J. H. Kaas. 1991. Central projections from the skin of the hand in squirrel monkeys. *Journal of Comparative Neurology,* 311:563-578.

Foerster, O. 1936. Motorische Felder und Bahne. In O. Bumke and O. Foerster (eds.), *Handbuch der Neurologie.* Vol. 6, pp. 1-357. Berlin: Springer.

Foerster, O. and O. Gagel. 1932. Die Vorderseitenstrang-durchschneidung beim Menschen: Eine klinisch-patho-physiologisch-anatomische Studie. *Zeitschrift für die gesammte Neurologie und Psychiatrie,* 138:1-92.

Forssberg, H. 1985. Ontogeny of human locomotor control. I. Infant stepping, supported locomotion and transition to independent locomotion. *Experimental Brain Research,* 57:480-493.

Forssberg, H., A. C. Eliasson, H. Kinoshita, G. Westling and R. S. Johansson. 1995. Development of human precision grip. IV. Tactile adaptation of isometric finger forces to the frictional condition. *Experimental Brain Research,*104:323-330.

Forssberg, H., H. Kinoshita, A. C. Eliasson, R. S. Johansson, G. Westling and A. M. Gordon. 1992. Development of human precision grip. II. Anticipatory control of isometric forces targeted for object's weight. *Experimental Brain Research,* 90:393-398.

Fox, M. W., O. R. Inman and W. A. Himwich. 1967. The postnatal development of the spinal cord of the dog. *Journal of Comparative Neurology,* 130:233-240.

Fraher, J. P. 1976. The growth and myelination of the central and peripheral segments of ventral motoneuron axons: A quantitative ultrastructural study. *Brain Research,* 105:193-211.

Frey, M. von. 1894. Beiträge zur Physiologie des Schmerzsinns. *Berichte der sächsische Gesellschaft für die Wissenschaften; Mathematisch-physikalische Classe,* 46:186-196, 283-296.

Friede, R. L. 1961. A histochemical study of DNP-diaphorase in human white matter, with some notes on myelination. *Journal of Neurochemistry,* 8:17-30.

Fritz, N., M. Illert and P. Saggau. 1986a. Location of motoneurones projecting to the cat distal forelimb. I. Deep radial motor nuclei. *Journal of Comparative Neurology,* 244:286-301.

Fritz, N., M. Illert and P. Reeh. 1986b. Location of motoneurones projecting to the cat distal forelimb. II. Median and ulnar motor nuclei. *Journal of Comparative Neurology,* 244:302-312.

Fuller, P. M. 1974. Projections of the vestibular nuclear complex in the bullfrog (*Rana catesbeiana*). *Brain, Behavior and Evolution,* 10:157-169.

Furicchia, J. V. and H. G. Goshgarian. 1987. Dendritic organization of phrenic motoneurons in the adult rat. *Experimental Neurology,* 96:621-634.

Fyffe, R. E. W. 1992. Laminar organization of primary afferent terminations in the mammalian spinal cord. In: S. A. Scott (ed.), *Sensory Neurons: Diversity, Development, and Plasticity,* pp. 131-139. New York: Oxford University Press.

Gamse, R. and A. Saria. 1986. Nociceptive behavior after intrathecal injections of substance P, neurokinin A, and calcitonin gene-related peptide in mice. *Neuroscience Letters,* 70:143-147.

Gao, W. C. and J. T. Qiao. Nitric oxide contributes to both spinal nociceptive transmission and its descending inhibition in rats: An immunocytochemical study. *Neuroscience Letters,* 240:143-146.

Gardner, E. 1968. *Fundamentals of Neurology.* (5th ed.) Philadelphia: Saunders.

Gardner, E. and H. Cuneo. 1945. Lateral spinothalamic tract and associated tracts in man. *Archives of Neurology and Psychiatry,* 53:423-430.

Gaskell, W. H. 1916. *The Involuntary Nervous System.* London: Longmans, Green.

Gasser, H. S. 1943. Pain producing impulses in peripheral nerves. *Association for Research in Nervous and Mental Disease,* 23:44-62.

Gaze, R. M. and G. Gordon. 1954. The representation of cutaneous sense in the thalamus of the cat and monkey. *Quarterly Journal of Experimental Physiology,* 39:279-304.

Geldard, F. A. 1972. *The Human Senses.* New York: Wiley.

Gelfan, S., G. Kao and D. S. Ruchkin. 1970. The dendritic tree of spinal neurons. *Journal of Comparative Neurology,* 139:385-412.

Gentry, E. F. and C. A. Aldrich. 1948. Rooting reflex in the newborn infant: Incidence and effect on it of sleep. *American Journal of Diseases of Childhood*, 75:528-539.

Gesell, A. 1954. The ontogenesis of infant behavior. In: L. Carmicheal (ed.), *Manual of Child Psychology*, pp. 335-373. 2nd ed. New York: Wiley.

Gesell, A. and L. B. Ames. 1940. The ontogenetic organization of prone behavior in human infancy. *Journal of Genetic Psychology*, 56:247-263.

Gesell, A. and H. M. Halverson. 1942. The daily maturation of infant behavior: A cinema study of postures, movements, and laterality. *Journal of Genetic Psychology*, 61:3-32.

Gesell, A., H. Thompson and C. Amatruda. 1938. *The Psychology of Early Growth*. New York: Macmillan.

Getz, B. 1952. The termination of spinothalamic fibres in the cat as studied by the method of terminal degeneration. *Acta Anatomica*, 16:271-290.

Gibson, S. J., J. M. Polak, S. R. Bloom and P. D. Wall. 1981. The distribution of nine peptides in rat spinal cord with special emphasis on the substantia gelatinosa and on the area around the central canal (lamina X). *Journal of Comparative Neurology*, 201:65-79.

Giesler, G. J., R. L. Nahin and A. M. Madsen. 1984. Postsynaptic dorsal column pathway of the rat. I. Anatomical studies. *Journal of Neurophysiology*, 51:260-275.

Giesler, G. J., G. Urca, J. T. Cannon and J. C. Liebeskind. 1979. Response properties of neurons of the lateral cervical nucleus in the rat. *Journal of Comparative Neurology*, 186:65-78.

Giesler, G. J., R. P. Yezierski, K. D. Gerhart and W. D. Willis. 1981. Spinothalamic tract neurons that project to medial and/or lateral thalamic nuclei: Evidence for a physiologically novel population of spinal cord neurons. *Journal of Neurophysiology*, 46:1285-1308.

Gilles, F. H., W. Shankle and E. C. Dooling. 1983. Myelinated tracts: Growth patterns. In: F. H. Gilles, A. Leviton and E. C. Dooling (eds.), *The Developing Human Brain*, pp. 117-183. Boston: Wright.

Gilman, S. and D. Denny-Brown. 1966. Disorders of movement and behavior following dorsal column lesions. *Brain*, 89:397-417.

Giuffrida, R. and A. Rustioni. 1992. Dorsal root ganglion neurons projecting to the dorsal column nuclei of rats. *Journal of Comparative Neurology*, 316:206-220.

Glazer, E. J. and A. I. Basbaum. 1981. Immunohistochemical localization of leucine-enkephalin in the spinal cord of the cat: Enkephalin-containing marginal neurons and pain modulation. *Journal of Comparative Neurology*, 196:377-389.

Glover, J. C. 1993. The development of brain stem projections to the spinal cord in the chicken embryo. *Brain Research Bulletin*, 30:265-271.

Gobel, S., W. M. Falls, G. J. Bennett, M Abdelmoumene, H. Hayashi and E. Humphrey. 1980. An EM analysis of the synaptic connections of horseradish peroxidase-filled stalked cells and islet cells in the substantia gelatinosa of adult cat spinal cord. *Journal of Comparative Neurology*, 194:781-807.

Goering, J. H. 1928. An experimental analysis of the motor-cell columns in the cervical enlargement of the spinal cord of the albino rat. *Journal of Comparative Neurology*, 46:125-152.

Golden, J. P., J. A. Demaro and M. F. Jacquin. 1997. Postnatal development of terminals and synapses in laminae I and II of the rat medullary dorsal horn. *Journal of Comparative Neurology*, 383:326-338.

Golding, J. P. and J. Cohen. 1997. Border controls at the mammalian spinal cord: Late-surviving neural crest boundary cap cells at dorsal root entry sites may regulate sensory afferent ingrowth and entry zone morphogenesis. *Molecular and Cellular Neurosciences*, 9:381-396.

Goldstein, L. A. and D. R. Sengelaub. 1993. Motoneuron morphology in the dorsolateral nucleus of the rat spinal cord: Normal development and androgenic regulation. *Journal of Comparative Neurology*, 338:588-600.

Goodwin, R. S. and G. F. Michel. 1981. Head orientation position during birth and infant neonatal period and hand preference at nineteen weeks. *Child Development*, 52:819-826.

Gordon, D. C., G. E. Loeb and F. J. R. Richmond. 1991. Distribution of motoneurons supplying cat sartorius and tensor fasciae latae, demonstrated by retrograde multiple-labeling methods. *Journal of Comparative Neurology*, 304:357-372.

Gordon, D. C. and F. J. R. Richmond. 1991. Distribution of motoneurons supplying dorsal suboccipital and intervertebral muscles in the cat neck. *Journal of Comparative Neurology*, 304:343-356.

Gordon, G. and M. G. M. Jukes. 1964. Dual organization of the exteroceptive components of the cat's gracile nucleus. *Journal of Physiology*, 173:263-290.

Gordon, G. and C. H. Paine. Functional organization in nucleus of gracilis of the cat. *Journal of Physiology*, 153:331-349.

Gorgels, T. G. M. F. 1990. A quantitative analysis of axon outgrowth, axon loss, and myelination in the rat pyramidal tract. *Developmental Brain Research*, 54:51-61.

Gorgels, T. G. M. F., E. J. M. DeKort, H. T. H van Aanhalt and R. Nieuwenhuys. 1989. A quantitative analysis of the development of the pyramidal tract in the cervical spinal cord in the rat. *Anatomy and Embryology*, 179:377-385.

Gorgels, T. G. M. F, A. M. Oestreicher, E. J. M. De Kort and W. H. Gosepn. 1987. Immunocytochemical distribution of the protein kinase C substrate B-50 (GAP43) in developing rat pyramidal tract. *Neuroscience Letters*, 83:59-64.,

Gotts, E. E. 1972. Nerwborn walking. *Science*, 177:1057-1058.

Granit, R., H. D. Henatsch and G. Steg. 1956. Tonic and phasic ventral horn cells differentiated by posttetanic potentiation in cat extensors. *Acta Physiologica Scandinavica*, 37:114-126..

Grant, G. and J. Ygge. 1981. Somatotopic organization of the thoracic spinal nerve in the dorsal horn demonstrated with transganglionic degeneration. *Journal of Comparative Neurology*, 202:357-364.

Grant, G., J. Ygge and C. Molander. 1981. Projection patterns of peripheral sensory nerves in the dorsal horn. In: A. G. Brown and M. Réthelyi (eds.), *Spinal Cord Sensations*, pp. 33-44. Edinburgh: Scottish Academic Press.

Gray, E. G. 1969. Electron microscopy of excitatory and inhibitory synapses: A brief review. *Progress in Brain Research*, 31:141-155.

Gray, J. 1968. *Animal Locomotion*. London: Weidenfeld and Nicolson.

Greving, R. 1928. Die zentralen Anteile des vegetativen Nervensystems. In: W. von Möllendorf (ed.), *Handbuch der mikroskopischen Anatomie des Menschen*, vol. 4. *Das Nervensystem*, Teil 1. Berlin: Springer.

Gribnau, A. A. M., E. J. M. DeKort, P. J. W. C. Dederen and R. Nieuwenhuys. 1986. On the development of the pyramidal tract in the rat. II. An anterograde tracer study of the outgrowth of the corticospinal fibres. *Anatomy and Embryology*, 175:1101-110.

Grillner, S. 1975. Locomotion in vertebrates: Central mechanisms and reflex interaction. *Physiological Reviews*, 55:247-304.

Grillner, S. T. Hongo and S. Lund. 1970. The vestibulospinal tract: Effects on alpha-motoneurons in the lumbosacral spinal cord in the cat. *Experimental Brain Research,* 10:94-120.

Groome, L. J., M. J. Swiber, J. L. Atterbury, L. S. Bentz and S. B. Holland. 1997. Similarities and differences in behavioral state organization during sleep periods in the perinatal infant before and after birth. *Child Development*, 68:1-11.

Groome, L. J., M. J. Swiber, S. B. Holland, L. S. Bentz, J. L. Atterbury and R. F. Trimm. 1999. Spontaneous motor activity in the perinatal infant before and after birth: Stability of individual differences. *Developmental Psychobiology*, 35:15-24.

Groos, W. P., L. K. Ewing, C. M. Carter and J. D. Coulter. 1978. Organization of corticospinal neurons in the cat. *Brain Research*, 143:393-419.

Gross, D. 1974. Pain and the autonomic system. In: J. J. Bonica (ed.), *Advances in Neurology,* vol. 4: *Pain*, pp. 93-103. New York: Raven Press.

Grottel, K., P. Krutki and W. Mrowczynski. 1999. Bidirectional neurones in the cervical enlargement of the cat spinal cord with axons descending to sacral segments and ascending to the cerebellum and the lateral reticular nucleus. *Experimental Physiology*, 84:1059-1071.

Ha, H. 1971. Cervicothalamic tract in the rhesus monkey. *Experimental Neurology*, 33:205-212.

Ha, H. and C.-N. Liu. 1966. Organization of the spino-cervico-thalamic system. *Journal of Comparative Neurology*, 127:445-470.

Haber, L. H., B. D. Moore and W. D. Willis. 1982. Electrophysiological response properties of spinoreticular neurons in the monkey. *Journal of Comparative Neurology*, 207:75-84.

Hack, M. and A. A. Fanaroff. 1999. Changes in the delivery room care of extremely small infant (<750 gm): Effects on morbidity and mortality. *New England Journal of Medicine*, 308:1330-1336.

Hadders-Algra, M. 1993. General movements in early infancy: What do they tell us about the nervous system? *Early Human Development*, 34:29-37.

Hadders-Algra, M. and H. F. R. Prechtl. 1992. Developmental course of general movements in early infancy. I. Descriptive analysis of change in form. *Early Human Development*, 28:201-213.

Hagevik, A. and A. D. McClellan. 1999. Coordination of locomotor activity in the lamprey: Role of descending drive to oscillators along the spinal cord. *Experimental Brain Research*, 128:481-490.

Haggar, R. A. and M. L. Barr. 1950. Quantitative data on the size of synaptic bulbs in the cat's spinal cord. *Journal of Comparative Neurology*, 93:13-37.

Haleem, M. 1990. *Diagnostic Categories of the Yakovlev Collection of Normal and Pathological Anatomy and Development of the Brain*. Washington, DC: Armed Forces Institute of Pathology.

Hall, A., N. A. Giese and W. D. Richardson. 1996. Spinal cord oligodendrocytes develop from ventrally derived progenitor cells that express PDGF alpha-receptors. *Development*, 122:4085-4094.

Halverson, H. M. 1931. Study of prehension in infants. *Genetic Psychology Monographs*, 10:110-286.

Halverson, H. M. 1937. Studies of grasping responses of early infancy. I, II, III. *Journal of Genetic Psychology*, 51:371-449.

Hamann, W. C., S. K. Hong, K. D. Kniffki and R. F. Schmidt. 1978. Projections of primary afferent fibres from muscle to neurones of the spinocervical tract in the cat. *Journal of Physiology*, 283:369-378.

Hamburger, V. 1963. Some aspects of the embryology of behavior. *Quarterly Review of Biology*, 38:342-365.

Hamilton, T. C. and J. I. Johnson. 1973. Somatotopic organization related to nuclear morphology in the cuneate-gracile complex of opossums *Didelphis marsupialis virginiana*. *Brain Research* , 51:125-140.

Hamilton, W. J., J. D. Boyd and H. W. Mossman. 1964. *Human Embryology*, 3rd ed. Baltimore: Williams and Wilkins.

Hammar, I., Z. S. Läckberg and E. Jankowska. 1994. New observations on input to spino-cervical tract neurons from muscle afferents. *Experimental Brain Research*, 100:1-6.

Hancock, M. B. and C. A. Peveto. 1979. A preganglionic autonomic nucleus in the dorsal gray commissure of the lumbar spinal cord of the rat. *Journal of Comparative Neurology*, 183:65-72.

Hankey, G. J. and R. H. Edis. 1989. The utility of testing tactile perception of direction of scratch as a sensitive clinical sign of posterior column dysfunction in spinal cord disorders. *Journal of Neurology, Neurosurgery and Neuropsychiatry*, 52:395-398.

Hannover, A. 1844. *Recherches Microscopiques sur le Système Nerveus*. Copenhagen: Brockhaus.

Hartman, B. K., H. C. Agrawal, S. Kalmbach and W. T. Shearer. 1979. A comparative study of the immunohistochemical localization of basic protein to myelin and oligodendrocytes in rat and chicken brain. *Journal of Comparative Neurology*, 188:273-290.

Hartman, C. G. 1936. *Time of Ovulation in Women*. Baltimore: Williams and Wilkins.

Hatai, S. 1901. The finer structure of the spinal ganglion cells in the white rat. *Journal of Comparative Neurology*, 11:1-24.

Hayes, A. G. and M. B. Tyers. 1980. Effects of capsaicin on nociceptive heat, pressure and chemical thresholds and on substance P levels in the rat. *Brain Research,* 189:561-564.

Hayes, N. L. and A. Rustioni. 1981. Descending projections from brain stem and sensorimotor cortex to spinal enlargements in the cat: Single and double retrograde tracer studies. *Experimental Brain Research,* 41:89-107.

Haymaker, W. and B. Woodhall. 1953. *Peripheral Nerve Injuries: Principles and Diagnosis..* Philadelphia: Saunders.

Head, H. 1920. *Studies in Neurology.* Vol. 1. London: Oxford University Press.

Heinbecker, P., G. H. Bishop and J. O'Leary. 1933. Pain and touch fibers in peripheral nerves. *Archives of Neurology and Psychiatry,* 29:771-789.

Henry, J. L. 1976. Effects of substance P on functionally identified units in cat spinal cord. *Brain Research,* 114:439-451.

Heuser, C. H. 1930. A human embryo with 14 pairs of somites. *Carnegie Institution of Washington, Contributions to Embryology,* 22:135-154.

Hicks, S. P. and C. J. D'Amato. 1977. Locating corticospinal neurons by retrograde axonal transport of horseradish peroxidase. *Experimental Neurology,* 56:410-420.

Higuchi, M., H. Hirano, K. Gotoh, K. Otomo and M. Maki. 1991. Relationship between the duration of fetal breathing movements and gestational age, and the development of the central nervous system at 25-32 weeks of gestation of normal pregnancy. *Gynecologic and Obstetric Investigations, 31:136-140.*

Hinman, A. and M. B. Carpenter. 1959. Efferent fiber projections of the red nucleus in the cat. *Journal of Comparative Neurology,* 113:61-82.

Hirakawa, M., J. T. McCabe and M. Kawata. 1992. Time-related changes in the labeling pattern of motor and sensory neurons innervating gastrocnemius muscle, as revealed by the retrograde transport of the cholera toxin B subunit. *Cell Tissue Research,* 267:419-427.

His, W. 1886. Zur Geschichte des menschlichen Rückenmarkes und der Nervenwurzeln. *Abhandlungen der königlisches Gesellschaft der Wissenschaften, mathematisch-physikalische Klasse,* 13:479-513.

His, W. 1889. Die Neuroblasten und deren Entstehung im embryonalen Mark. *Abhandlungen der königlisches Gesellschaft der Wissenschaften, mathematisch-physikalische Klasse,* 15:313-372.

Hobson, J. A. and M. A. B. Brazier. 1980. *The Reticular Formation Revisited: Specifying Function for a Nonspecific System.* New York: Raven Press.

Hodges, L. L., C. L. Jordan and S. M. Breedlove. 1993. Hormone-sensitive periods for the control of motoneuron number and soma size in the dorsolateral nucleus of the rat spinal cord. *Journal of Comparative Neurology,* 602:187-190.

Hofsten, C. von. 1986. The emergence of manual skills. In: M. G. Wade and H. T. A. Whiting (eds.), *Motor Development in Children: Aspects of Coordination and Control,* pp. 167-186. Dordrecht: Nijhoff.

Hofsten, C. von. 1991. Structuring of early reaching movements: A longitudinal study. *Journal of Motor Behavior,* 23:280-292.

Hogan, G. R. and J. E. Milligan. 1971. The plantar reflex of the newborn. *New England Journal of Medicine,* 285:502-503.

Hogg, I. D. 1941. Sensory nerves and associated structures in the skin of human fetuses of 8 to 14 weeks of menstrual age correlated with functional capability. *Journal of Comparative Neurology,* 75:371-410.

Hogg, I. D. 1944. The development of the nucleus dorsalis (Clarke's column). *Journal of Comparative Neurology,* 81:69-95.

Hökfelt, T., R. Elde, L. Johansson, L. Terenius and L. Stein. 1977. The distribution of enkephalin-immunoreactive cell bodies in the rat central nervous system. *Neuroscience Letters,* 5:25-31.

Hökfelt, T., J.-O. Kellerth, G. Nilsson, and B. Pernow. 1975. Experimental immunohistochemical studies on the localization and distribution of substance P in cat primary sensory neurons. *Brain Research,* 100:235-252.

Holstege, J. C. 1991. Ultrastructural evidence for GABAergic brainstem projections to spinal motoneurons in the rat. *Journal of Neuroscience,* 11:159-167.

Holstege, J. C., H. van Dijken, R. M. Buijs, H. Goedknegt, T. Gosens and C. M. H. Bongers. 1996. Distribution of dopamine immunoreactivity in the rat, cat, and monkey spinal cord. *Journal of Comparative Neurology,* 376:631-652.

Hong, S. K., K. D. Kniffki, S. Mense, R. F. Schmidt and M. Wendisch. 1979. Descending influences on the responses of spinocervical tract neurones to chemical stimulation of fine muscle afferents. *Journal of Physiology,* 290:129-140.

Hongo, T., E. Jankowska and A. Lundberg. 1966. Convergence of excitatory and inhibitory action on interneurones in the lumbosacral cord. *Experimental Brain Research,* 1:338-358.

Hongo, T., E. Jankowska and A. Lundberg. 1969. The rubrospinal tract. I. Effects on alpha-motoneurons innervating hindlimb muscles in cats. *Experimental Brain Research,* 7:344-364.

Hongo, T., E. Jankowska and A. Lundberg. 1972. The rubrospinal tract. IV. Effects on interneurons. *Experimental Brain Research,* 15:54-78.

Hongo, T., S. Kitazawa, Y. Ohki, M. Sasaki and M.-C. Xi. 1989. A physiological and morphological study of premotor interneurons in the cutaneous reflex pathway in cats. *Brain Research,* 505:163-166.

Hongo, T., S. Kitazawa, Y. Ohki and M.-C. Xi. 1989. Functional identification of last-order interneurons of skin reflex pathways in the cat forelimb segments. *Brain Research,* 505:167-170.

Hooker, D. 1938. The origin of the grasping movement in man. *Proceedings of the Philosophical Society,* 79:597-606.

Hooker, D. 1942. *The Origin of Overt Behavior.* Ann Arbor: University of Michigan Press.

Hooker, D. 1954. Early human fetal behavior, with a preliminary note on double simultaneous fetal stimulation. *Research Publication of the Association of Nervous and Mental Disease,* 33:98-113.

Hoover, J. E. and R. G. Durkovic. 1991. Morphological relationships among extensor digitorum longus, tibialis anterior, and semitendinosus motor nuclei of the cat: An investigation employing the retrograde transport of multiple fluorescent tracers. *Journal of Comparative Neurology*, 303:255-266.

Horcholle-Bossavit, G., L. Jami, D. Thiesson and D. Zytnicki. 1988. Motor nuclei of peroneal muscles in the cat spinal cord. *Journal of Comparative Neurology*, 277:430-440.

Hore, J., Phillips and R. Porter. 1973. The effects of pyramidotomy on motor performance in the bush-tailed possum (*Trichosurus vulpecula*). *Brain Research*, 49:181-184.

Hörner, M. and H. Kümmel. 1993. Topographical representation of shoulder motor nuclei in the cat spinal cord as revealed by retrograde fluorochrome tracers. *Journal of Comparative Neurology*, 335:309-319.

Hoshino, K., T. Matsuzawa and U. Murakami. 1973. Characteristics of the cell cycle of matrix cells in the mouse embryo during histogenesis of telencephalon. *Experimental Cell Research*, 77:89-94.

Hosoya, Y. 1980. The distribution of spinal projection neurons in the hypothalamus of the rat, studied with the HRP method. *Experimental Brain Research*, 40:79-87.

Houghton, A. K., S. Kadura and K. N. Westlund. 1997. Dorsal column lesions reverse the reduction of homecage activity in rats with pancreatitis. *Neuroreport*, 8:3795-3800.

Hubbard, J. L. and O. Oscarsson. 1962. Localization of the cell bodies of the ventral spinocerebellar tract in lumbar segments of the cat. *Journal of Comparative Neurology*, 118:199-204.

Hultborn, H. and M. Udo. 1972. Convergence in the reciprocal Ia inhibitory pathway of excitation from descending pathways and inhibition from motor axon collaterals. *Acta Physiologica Scandinavica*, 84:95-108.

Humphrey, T. 1964. Some correlations between the appearance of human fetal reflexes and the development of the nervous system. *Progress in Brain Research*, 4:93-135.

Hunt, C. C. and A. K. McIntyre. 1960. An analysis of fibre diameter and receptor characteristics of myelinated cutaneous afferent fibres in cat. *Journal of Physiology*, 153:99-112.

Hunt, S. P. 1983. Cytochemistry of the spinal cord. In: P. C. Emson (ed.), *Chemical Neuroanatomy*, pp. 53-84. New York: Raven Press.

Hylden, J. L., H. Hayashi, R. Dubner and G. J. Bennett. 1986. Physiology and morphology of the lamina I spinomesencephalic projection. *Journal of Comparative Neurology*, 247:505-515.

Hyndman, O. R. and C. Van Epps. 1939. Possibility of differential section of the spinothalamic tract. *Archives of Surgery*, 38:1036-1053.

Illert, M., A. Lundberg, Y. Padel and R. Tanaka. 1978. Integration of descending motor pathways controlling the forelimb in the cat. V. Properties of monosynaptic excitatory convergence on C3–C4 propriospinal neurones. *Experimental Brain Research*, 33:101-130.

Illert, M. and R. Tanaka. 1976. Transmission of corticospinal IPSP's to cat forelimb motoneurones via high cervical propriospinal neurones and Ia inhibitory interneurones. *Brain Research*, 103:143-146.

Ingalls, N. W. 1918. A human embryo before the appearance of the myotomes. *Carnegie Institution of Washington, Contributions to Embryology*, 7:111-134.

Ishizuka, N., H. Mannen, T. Hongo and S. Sasaki. 1979. Trajectory of Ia afferent fibers stained with horseradish peroxidase in the lumbosacral spinal cord of the cat: Three dimensional reconstruction from serial sections. *Journal of Comparative Neurology*, 186:189-212.

Jacobsohn, L. 1908. Über die Kerne des menschlishen Rückenmarks. *Neurologische Zentralblatt*, 27:617-626.

Jacobson, M. 1978. *Developmental Neurobiology*. 2nd ed. New York: Plenum.

Jakobson, L. S. and M. A. Goodale. 1991. Factors affecting higher-order movement planning: A kinematic analysis of human prehension. *Experimental Brain Research*, 86:199-208.

Jancsó, G. and A. Jancsó-Gábor. 1959. Dauerausschaltung der chemischen Schmerzempfindlichkeit durch Capasicin. *Naunyn-Schmiedeberg's Archiv für experimentelle Pathologie und Pharmakologie*, 236:142.

Jankowska, E. and S. Lindström. 1972. Morphology of interneurones mediating Ia reciprocal inhibition of motoneurones in the spinal cord of the cat. *Journal of Physiology*, 226:805-823.

Jankowska, E., S. Lund, A. Lundberg and O. Pompeiano. 1968. Inhibitory effects evoked through ventral reticulospinal pathways. *Archives Italiennes de Biologie*, 106:124-140.

Jankowska, E., A. Lundberg, W. J. Roberts and D. Stuart. 1974. A long propriospinal system with direct effects on motoneurones in the cat lumbosacral cord. *Experimental Brain Research*, 21:169-194.

Jankowska, E., A. Lundberg and D. Stuart. 1973. Propriospinal control of last order interneurones of spinal reflex pathways in the cat. *Brain Research*, 53:227-231.

Jankowska, E., J. Rastad and P. Zarzecki. 1979. Segmental and supraspinal input to cells of origin of nonprimary fibres in the feline dorsal columns. *Journal of Physiology*, 290:185-200.

Jankowska, E. and W. J. Roberts. 1972. Synaptic actions of single interneurones mediating reciprocal Ia inhibition of motoneurones. *Journal of Physiology*, 222:623-642.

Jenny, A. B. and J. Inukai. 1983. Principles of motor organization of the monkey cervical spinal cord. *Journal of Neuroscience*, 3:567-575.

Jensen, J. L., B. D. Ulrich, E. Thelen, K. Schneider and R. F. Zernicke. 1994. Adaptive dynamics of the leg movement patterns of human infants. I. The effect of posture on spontaneous kicking. *Journal of Motor Behavior*, 26:303-312.

Jensen, K. F. and H. P. Killackey. 1987. Terminal arbors of axons projecting to the somatosensory cortex of the adult rat. I. The normal morphology of specific thalamocortical afferents. *Journal of Neuroscience*, 7:3529-3543.

Jessell, T. M., P. Bovolenta, M. Placzek, M. Tessier-Lavigne and J. Dodd. 1988. Polarity and patterning in the neural tube: The origin and role of the floor plate. *Ciba Foundation Symposium*, 144:255-280.

Jessell, T. M., L. L. Iversen and A. C. Cuello. 1978. Capsaicin-induced depletion of substance P from primary sensory neurones. *Brain Research*, 152:183-188.

Jessell, T. M., K. Yoshika and C. E. Jahr. 1986. Amino acid receptor mediated transmission at primary afferent synapses in rat spinal cord. *Journal of Experimental Biology*, 124:239-258.

Johnson, J. I., W. I. Welker and B. H. Pubols. 1968. Somatotopic organization of raccoon dorsal column nuclei. *Journal of Comparative Neurology*, 132:1-44.

Jones, E. G. and H. Burton. 1974. Cytoarchitecture and somatic sensory connectivity of thalamic nuclei other than the ventrobasal complex in the cat. *Journal of Comparative Neurology*, 154:395-432.

Jones, M. W., C. J. Hodge, A. V. Apkarian and R. T. Stevens. 1985. A dorsolateral spinothalamic pathway in cat. *Brain Research*, 335:188-193.

Joosten, E. A. J., P. R. Bär and W.-H. Gispen. 1994. Corticospinal axons and mechanisms of target innervation in rat lumbar spinal cord. *Developmental Brain Research*, 79:122-127.

Joosten, E. A. J., A. A. M. Gribnau and P. J. W. C. Dederen. 1987. An anterograde tracer study of the developing corticospinal tract in the rat: Three components. *Developmental BrainResearch*, 36:121-130.

Joosten, E. A. J., A. A. M. Gribnau and P. J. W. C. Dederen. 1989. Postnatal development of the corticospinal tract in the rat: An ultratructural anterograde HRP study. *Anatomy and Embryology*, 179:449-456.

Joosten, E. A. J., R. L. Schuitman, M. E. J. Vermelis and P. J. W. C. Dederen. 1992. Postnatal development of the ipsilateral corticospinal component in rat spinal cord: A light and electron microscopic anterograde HRP study. *Journal of Comparative Neurology*, 326:133-146.

Joppich, G. and F. J. Schulte. 1968. *Neurologie des Neugeborenen*. Berlin: Springer-Verlag.

Jordan, C. L., S. M. Breedlove and A. P. Arnold. 1982. Sexual dimorphism and the influence of neonatal androgen in the dorsolateral motor nucleus of the rat lumbar spinal cord. *Brain Research*, 249:309-314.

Joseph, B. S. and D. G. Whitlock. 1968a. The morphology of spinal afferent-efferent relationships in vertebrates. *Brain, Behavior and Evolution*, 1:2-18.

Joseph, B. S. and D. G. Whitlock. 1968b. Central projections of selected spinal dorsal roots in anuran amphibians. *Anatomical Record*, 160:279-288.

Kaiser, O. 1891. *Die Funktionen der Ganglienzellen des Halsmarkes auf Grund einer anatomischen Untersuchung*. Haag: Nijhoff.

Kalb, R. G. 1994. Regulation of motor neuron dendrite growth by NMDA receptor activation. *Development*, 120:3063-3071.

Kalil, K. and M. Perdew. 1988. Expression of two developmentally regulated brain-specific proteins is correlated with late outgrowth of the pyramidal tract. *Journal of Neuroscience*, 8:4797-4808.

Kalil, K. and J. H. P. Skene. 1986. Elevated synthesis of an axonally transported protein correlates with axonal outgrowth in normal and injured pyramidal tracts. *Journal of Neuroscience*, 6:2563-2570.

Kalyani, A., K. Hobson and M. S. Rao. 1997. Neuroepithelial stem cells from embryonic spinal cord: Isolation, characterization, and clonal analysis. *Developmental Biology*, 186:202-223.

Kameyama, M. D., Y. Hashizume and G. Sobue. 1996. Morphologic features of the normal human cadaveric spinal cord. *Spine*, 11:1285-1290.

Kangrga, I. and M. Randic. 1990. Tachykinins and calcitonin gene related peptide enhance release of endogenous glutamate and aspartate from the rat dorsal horn slice. *Journal of Neuroscience*, 10:2026-2038.

Katter, J. T., R. J. Dado, E. Kostarczyk and G. J. Giesler 1996a. Spinothalamic and spinohypothalamic tract neurons in the sacral spinal cord of rats. I. Locations of antidromically identified axons in the cervical cord and diencephalon. *Journal of Neurophysiology*, 75:2581-2605.

Katter, J. T., R. J. Dado, E. Kostarczyk and G. J. Giesler 1996b. Spinothalamic and spinohypothalamic tract neurons in the sacral spinal cord of rats. II. Responses to cutaneous and visceral stimuli. *Journal of Neurophysiology*, 75:2606-2628.

Kaufman, S. L. 1968. Lengthening of the generation cycle during embryonic differentiation of the mouse neural tube. *Experimental Cell Research*, 49:420-424.

Kawatani, M., J. Nagel and W. C. de Groat. 1986. Identification of neuropeptides in pelvic and pudendal nerve afferent pathways to the sacral spinal cord of the cat. *Journal of Comparative Neurology*, 249:117-132.

Keegan, J. J. and F. D. Garrett. 1948. The segmental distribution of the cutaneous nerves in the limbs of man. *Anatomical Record*, 102:409-437.

Keibel, F. and C. Elze. 1908. *Normaltafel zur Entwicklungsgeschichte des Menschen*. Jena: Fischer.

Keirstead, S. A. and P. K. Rose. 1983. Dendritic distribution of splenius motoneurons in the cat: Comparison of motoneurons innervating different regions of the muscle. *Journal of Comparative Neurology*, 219:273-284.

Keller, J. H. and P. J. Hand. 1970. Dorsal root projections to nucleus cuneatus of the cat. *Brain Research*, 20:1-17.

Kelly, J. S., Z. Gottesfeld and F. Schon. 1973. Reduction in GAD I activity from the dorsal lateral region of the deafferented rat spinal cord. *Brain Research*, 62:581-586.

Kennard, M. A. 1954. The course of ascending fibers in the spinal cord of the cat essential to the recognition of painful stimuli. *Journal of Comparative Neurology*, 100:511-524.

Kennedy, T. E., T. Serafini, J. R. de la Torre and M. Tessier-Lavigne. 1994. Netrins are diffusible chemotropic factors for commissural axons in the embryonic spinal cord. *Cell*, 78:425-435.

Kenshalo, D. R., R. B. Leonard, J. M. Chung and W. D. Willis. 1979. Responses of primate spinothalamic neurons to graded and to repeated noxious heat stimuli. *Journal of Neurophysiology*, 42:1370-1389.

Kerr, F. W. L. 1975. The ventral spinothalamic tract and other ascending systems of the ventral funiculus of the spinal cord. *Journal of Comparative Neurology*, 159:335-356.

Kevetter, G. A., L. H. Haber, R. P. Yezierski, J. M. Chung, R. F. Martin and W. D. Willis. 1982. Cells of origin of the spinoreticular tract in the monkey. *Journal of Comparative Neurology*, 207:61-74.

Kevetter, G. A. and W. D. Willis. 1982. Spinothalamic cells in the rat lumbar cord with collaterals to the medullary reticular formation. *Brain Research*, 238:181-185.

King, J. L. 1910. The corticospinal tract of the rat. *Anatomical Record*, 4:245-252.

Kingsbury, B. F. 1930. The developmental significance of the floor-plate of the brain and spinal cord. *Journal of Comparative Neurology*, 50:177-207.

Kircher, C. and H. Ha. 1968. The nucleus cervicalis lateralis in primates, including the human. *Anatomical Record*, 160:376.

Kisilevsky, B. S., S. M. J. Hains and J. A. Low. 1999. Maturation of body and breathing movements in 24-33 week-old fetuses threatening to deliver prematurely. *Early Human Development*, 55:25-38.

Kitai, S. T., H. Ha and F. Morin. 1965. Lateral cervical nucleus of the dog. *American Journal of Physiology*, 209:307-312.

Kitamura, S. and F. J. R. Richmond. 1994. Distribution of motoneurons supplying dorsal and ventral suboccipital muscles in the feline neck. *Journal of Comparative Neurology*, 347:25-35.

Kitazawa, S., Y. Ohki, M. Sasaki, M. Xi and T. Hongo. 1993. Candidate premotor neurones of skin reflex pathways to T1 forelimb motoneurones of the cat. *Experimental Brain Research*, 95:291-307.

Klockgether, T. 1987. Excitatory amino acid receptor-mediated transmission of somatosensory evoked potentials in the rat thalamus. *Journal of Physiology*, 394:445-461.

Knape, E. 1901. Über die Veränderungen im Rückenmark nach Resection einiger spinaler Nerven der vorderen Extremität. *Beiträge zur pathologischen Anatomie und allgemeine Pathologie*, 29:257-298.

Knyihar-Csillik, E., B. Csillik and P. Rakic. 1982. Ultrastructure of normal and degenerating glomerular terminals of dorsal root axons in the substantia gelatinosa of the rhesus monkey. *Journal of Comparative Neurology*, 210:357-375.

Knyihar-Csillik, E., B. Csillik and P. Rakic. 1995. Structure of the embryonic primate spinal cord at the closure of the first reflex arc. *Anatomy and Embryology*, 191:519-540.

Koerber, H. R. and P. B. Brown. 1982. Somatotopic organization of hindlimb cutaneous nerve projections to cat dorsal horn. *Journal of Neurophysiology*, 48:481-489.

Konstantinidou, A. D., I. Silos-Santiago, N. Flaris and W. D. Snider. 1995. Development of the primary afferent projection in human spinal cord. *Journal of Comparative Neurology*, 354:1-12.

Konczak, J., M. Borutta and J. Dichgans. 1997. Development of goal-directed reaching in infants. II. Learning to produce task-adequate patterns of joint torque. *Experimental Brain Research*, 113:465-474.

Konczak, J., M. Borutta, H. Topka, and J. Dichgans. 1995. Development of goal-directed reaching in infants: Hand trajectory formation and joint force control. *Experimental Brain Research*, 106:156-168.

Kostarczyk, E., X. Zhang and G. J. Giesler. 1997. Spinohypothalamic tract neurons in the cervical enlargement of rats: Locations of antidromically identified ascending axons and their collateral branches in the contralateral brain. *Journal of Neurophysiology*, 77:435-451.

Kozuma, S., T. Okai, A. Nemoto, H. Kagawa, M. Sakai, H. Nishina and Y. Taketani. 1997. Developmental sequence of human fetal body movements in the second half of pregnancy. *American Journal of Perinatolgy*, 14:165-169.

Kozuma, S., T. Okai, E. Ryo, H. Nishina, A, Nemoto, H. Kagawa, M. Sakai and Y. Taketani. 1998. Differential developmental process of respective behavioral states in human fetuses. *American Journal of Perinatology*, 15:203-208.

Kuban, K. C. K., H. N. Skouteli, D. K. Urion and G. A. Lawhon. 1986. Deep tendon reflexes in premature infants. *Pediatric Neurology*, 2:266-271.

Kudo, N., F. Furukawa and N. Okado. 1993. Development of descending fibers to the rat embryonic spinal cord. *Neuroscience Research*, 16:131-141.

Kudo, N. and T. Yamada. 1987. Morphological and physiological studies of the development of the monosynaptic reflex pathway in the rat lumbar spinal cord. *Journal of Physiology*, 389:441-459.

Kuno, M. 1959. Excitability following antidromic activation in spinal motoneurones supplying red muscles. *Journal of Physiology*, 149:374-393.

Kuno, M., E. J. Muñoz-Martinez and M. Randic. 1973. Sensory inputs to neurones in Clarke's column from muscle, cutaneous and joint receptors. *Journal of Physiology*, 228:327-342,

Kuo, D. C. and W. C. de Groat. 1985. Primary afferent projections of the major splanchnic nerve to the spinal cord and gracile nucleus of the cat. *Journal of Comparative Neurology*, 231:421-434.

Kuo, D. C., I. Nadelhaft, T. Hisamitsu and W. C. de Groat. 1983. Segmental distribution and central projections of renal afferent fibers in the cat studied by transganglionic transport of horseradish peroxidase. *Journal of Comparative Neurology*, 216:162-174.

Kussmaul, A. 1859. *Untersuchungen über das Seelenleben des neugeborenen Menschen*. Tübingen: Moser.

Kuzuhara, S., I. Kanayawa and T. Nakanishi. 1980. Topographical localization of the Onuf's nuclear neurons innervating the rectal and vesical striated sphincter muscles: A retrograde fluorescent double labeling in cat and dog. *Neuroscience Letters*, 16:125-130.

Kuypers, H. G. J. M. 1960. Central cortical projections to motor and somatosensory cell groups. *Brain*, 83:161-184.

Kuypers, H. G. J. M. 1964. The descending pathways to the spinal cord: Their anatomy and function. *Progress in Brain Research*, 11:178-202.

Kuypers, H. G. J. M. and J. Brinkman. 1970. Precentral projections to different parts of the spinal intermediate zone in the rhesus monkey. *Brain Research*, 24:29-48.

Kuypers, H. G. J. M., W. R. Fleming and J. W. Farinholt. 1962. Subcorticospinal projections in the rhesus monkey. *Journal of Comparative Neurology*, 118:107-137.

Kuypers, H. G. J. M. and V. A. Maisky. 1975. Retrograde axonal transport of horseradish peroxidase from spinal cord to brain stem cell groups in the cat. *Neuroscience Letters*, 1:9-14.

Laird, J. M., C. Roza and F. Cervero. 1996. Spinal dorsal horn neurons responding to noxious distension of the ureter in anesthetized rats. *Journal of Neurophysiology*, 76:3239-3248.

Lakke, E. A. 1997. The projections of the spinal cord of the rat during development: A timetable of descent. *Advances in Anatomy Embryology and Cell Biology*, 135:1-143.

Lakke, E. A. J. F. and E. Marani. 1991. Prenatal descent of rubrospinal fibers through the spinal cord of the rat. *Journal of Comparative Neurology*, 314:67-78.

LaMotte, C. 1977. Distribution of the tract of Lissauer and the dorsal root fibers in the primate spinal cord. *Journal of Comparative Neurology*, 172:529-562.

LaMotte, C., C. B. Pert and S. H. Snyder. 1976. Opiate receptor binding in primate spinal cord: Distribution and changes after dorsal root section. *Brain Research*, 112:407-412.

Landgren, S., A. Nordwall and C. Wengström. 1965. The location of the thalamic relay in the spino-cervico-lemniscal path. *Acta Physiologica Scandinavica*, 65:164-175.

Landis C. and W. A. Hunt. 1939. *The Startle Pattern*, New York: Farrar and Rinehart.

Langley, J. N. and H. K. Anderson. 1896. The innervation of the pelvic and adjoining viscera. VI. Histological and physiological observations upon the effects of the section of the sacral nerves. *Journal of Physiology*, 20:372-384.

Langman, J., R. L. Guerrant and B. G. Freeman. 1966. Behavior of neuroepithelial cells during closure of the neural tube. *Journal of Comparative Neurology*, 131:15-26.

Langman, J. and G. W. Welch. 1967. Excess vitamin A and development of the cerebral cortex. *Journal of Comparative Neurology*,131: 15-26.

Langworthy, O. R. 1929. A correlated study of the development of reflex action in fetal and young kittens and the myelinization of tracts in the nervous system. *Carnegie Institution of Washington, Contributions to Embryology*, 20:127-171.

Laruelle, L. 1937. La structure de la moelle épinière en coupes longitudinales. *Revue Neurologique*, 67:695-725.

Laruelle, L. 1948. Etude de l'anatomie microscopique du névraxe sur coupes longitudinales. *Acta Neurologica et Psychiatrica Belgica*, 48:138-180.

Lassek, A. M. 1954. *The Pyramidal Tract: Its Status in Medicine*. Springfield, IL: Thomas.

Lassek, A. M. and G. L. Rasmussen. 1938. A quantitative study of newborn and adult spinal cords of man. *Journal of Comparative Neurology*, 69:371-379.

Lawrence, D. G. and D. A. Hopkins. 1976. The development of motor control in the rhesus monkey: Evidence concerning the role of corticomotoneuronal connections. *Brain*, 99:235-254.

Lawrence, D. G. and H. G. J. M. Kuypers. 1968. The functional organization of the motor system in the monkey. I. The effects of bilateral pyramidal lesions. *Brain*, 91:1-14.

Lawrence, D. G., R. Porter and S. J. Redman. 1985. Corticomotoneuronal synapses in the monkey: Light microscopic localization upon motoneurons of intrinsic muscles of the hand. *Journal of Comparative Neurology*, 232:499-510.

Lawson, S. N. 1979. The postnatal development of large light and small dark neurons in mouse dorsal root ganglia: A statistical analysis of cell numbers and size. *Journal of Neurocytology*, 8:275-294.

Lawson, S. N. and T. J. Biscoe. 1979. Development of mouse dorsal root ganglia: An autoradiographic and quantitative study. *Jounal of Neurocytology*, 8:265-274.

Lawson, S. N., K. W. T. Caddy and T. J. Biscoe. 1974. Development of the rat dorsal root ganglion neurones: Studies of cell birthdays and changes in mean cell diameter. *Cell and Tissue Research*, 153:399-413.

Lawson, S. N. and A. A. Harper 1985. Cell types in rat dorsal root ganglia: Morphological, immunocytochemical, and electrophysiological analyses. In: M. Rowe and W. D. Willis (eds.), *Development, Organization, and Processing in Somatosensory Pathways*, pp. 97-103. New York: Liss.

Le Gros Clark, W. E. 1936. The termination of ascending tracts in the thalamus of the macaque monkey. *Journal of Anatomy*, 71:7-40.

Leblond, H. and T. Cabana. 1997. Myelination of the ventral and dorsal roots of the C8 and L4 segments of the spinal cord at different stages of development in the gray opossum, *Monodelphis domestica*. *Journal of Comparative Neurology*, 386:203-216.

Lee, D. N. and J. R. Lishman. 1975. Visual proprioceptive control of stance. *Journal of Human Movement Studies*, 1:87-95.

Lembeck, F. 1953. Zur Frage der zentralen Übertragung afferenter Impulse. III. Das Vorkommen und die Bedeutung der Substanz P in den dorsalen Wurzeln des Rückenmarks. *Naunyn-Schmiedeberg's Archiv für experimentelle Pathologie und Pharmakologie*, 219:197-213.

Lenhossék, M. von. 1889. Untersuchungen über die Entwicklung des markscheiden und den Faserverlauf in Rückenmark der Maus. *Archiv für mikroskopische Anatomie und Entwicklungsgeschichte*, 33:71.

Lenhossék, M. von. 1895. *Der feinere Bau des Nervensystems im Lichte neuerster Forschungen.* (2nd ed.) Berlin: Kornfeld.

Leontovich, T. A. and G. P. Zhukova. 1963. The specificity of the neuronal structure and topography of the reticular formation in the brain and spinal cord of carnivora. *Journal of Comparative Neurology*, 121:347-379.

Levante, A., Y. Lamour, G. Guilbaud and J. M. Besson. 1975. Spinothalamic cell activity in the monkey during intense nociceptive stimulation: Intra-arterial injection of bradykinin into the limbs. *Brain Research*, 88:560-564.

Levi-Montalcini, R. 1950. The origin and development of the visceral system in the spinal cord of the chick embryo. *Journal of Morphology*, 86:253-283.

Levin, P. M. and F. K. Bradford. 1938. The exact origin of the cortico-spinal tract in the monkey. *Journal of Comparative Neurology*, 68:411-422.

Li, Y. and G. Raisman. 1994. Schwann cells induce sprouting in motor and sensory axons in the adult rat spinal cord. *Journal of Neuroscience*, 14:4050-4063.

Liddell, E. G. T. and C. G. Phillips. 1944. Pyramidal section in the cat. *Brain*, 67:1-9.

Liddell, E. G. T. and C. S. Sherrington. 1925. Recruitment and some other factors of reflex inhibition. *Proceedings of the Royal Society*, B97: 488-518.

Lieberman, A. R. 1976. Sensory ganglia. In: D. N. Landon (ed.), *The Peripheral Nerve*, pp. 188-278. London: Chapman and Hall.

Liebeskind, J. C., G. Guilbaud, J.-M. Besson and J.-L. Oliveras. 1973. Analgesia from electrical stimulation of the periaqueductal gray matter in the cat: Behavioral observations and inhibitory effects on spinal cord interneurons. *Brain Research*, 50:441-446.

Light, A. R. and C. B. Metz. 1978. The morphology of the spinal cord efferent and afferent neurons contributing to the ventral roots of the cat. *Journal of Comparative Neurology*, 179:501-516.

Light, A. R. and E. R. Perl. 1979a. Reexamination of the dorsal root projection to the spinal dorsal horn, including observations on the differential termination of coarse and fine fibers. *Journal of Comparative Neurology*, 186:117-132.

Light, A. R. and E. R. Perl. 1979b. Spinal termination of functionally identified primary afferent neurons with slowly conducting myelinated fibers. *Journal of Comparative Neurology*, 186:133-150.

Light, A. R., D. L. Trevino and E. R. Perl. 1979. Morphological features of functionally defined neurons in the marginal zone and substantia gelatinosa of the spinal dorsal horn. *Journal of Comparative Neurology*, 186:151-172.

Liinamaa, T. L., J. Keane and F. J. R. Richmond. 1997. Distribution of motoneurons supplying feline neck muscles taking origin from the shoulder girdle. *Journal of Comparative Neurology*, 377:298-312.

Lima, D. 1990. A spinomedullary projection terminating in the dorsal reticular nucleus of the rat. *Neuroscience*, 34:577-589.

Lima, D. and A. Coimbra. 1986. A Golgi study of the neuronal population of the marginal zone (lamina I) of the rat spinal cord. *Journal of Comparative Neurology*, 244:53-71.

Lissauer, H. 1885. Beitrag zur pathologischen Anatomie de Tabes dorsalis und zum Faserverlauf in menschlichen Rückenmark. *Neurologische Zentralblatt*, 4:245-246.

Liu, C. N. 1956. Afferent nerves to Clarke's and the lateral cuneate nuclei in the cat. *Archives of Neurology and Psychiatry*, 75:67-77.

Liu, C. N. and W. W. Chambers. 1964. An experimental study of the cortico-spinal system in the monkey (*Macaca mulatta*). The spinal pathways and preterminal distribution of degenerating fibers following discrete lesions of the pre- and postcentral gyri and bulbar pyramid. *Journal of Comparative Neurology*, 123:257-284.

Liu, R. P. C. 1983. Laminar origins of spinal projection neurons to the periaqeductal gray of the rat. *Brain Research*, 264:118-122.

Ljungdahl, A. and T. Hökfelt. 1973. Autoradiographic uptake patterns of [³H] GABA and [³H] glycine in central nervous tissues with special reference to the cat spinal cord. *Brain Research*, 62:587-595.

Ljungdahl, A., T. Hökfelt and G. Nilsson. 1978. Distribution of substance P-like immunoreactivity in the central nervous system of the rat. I. Cell bodies and nerve terminals. *Neuroscience*, 3:861-943.

Lloyd, D. P. C. 1941. The spinal mechanisms of the pyramidal system in cats. *Journal of Neurophysiology*, 4:525-546.

Lloyd, D. P. C. 1942. Mediation of descending long spinal reflex activity. *Journal of Neurophysiology*, 5:435-458.

Lloyd, D. P. C. 1944. Functional organization of the spinal cord. *Physiological Reviews*, 24:1-17.

Lloyd, D. P. C. and A. K. McIntyre. 1950. Dorsal column conduction of group I muscle afferent impulses and their relay through Clarke's column. *Journal of Neurophysiology*, 13:39-54.

Loeb, J. A. and G. D. Fischbach. 1997. Neurotrophic factors increase neuregulin expression in embryonic ventral spinal cord neurons. *Journal of Neuroscience*, 17:1416-1424.

Loewy, A. D. 1970. A study of neuronal types in Clarke's column in the adult cat. *Journal of Comparative Neurology*, 139:53-80.

Loewy, A. D. and S. McKellar. 1981. Serotonergic projections from the ventral medulla to the intermediolateral cell column in the rat. *Brain Research*, 211:146-152.

Loewy, A. D., S. McKellar and C. B. Saper. 1979. Direct projection from the A5 catecholamine cell group to the intermediolateral cell column. *Brain Research*, 174:309-314.

Lorente de Nó, R. Architectonics and structure of the cerebral cortex. In: J. F. Fulton, *Physiology of the Nervous System* (2ⁿᵈ ed.), pp. 291-327. London: Oxford University Press.

Lu, Y., Y. J. Du, B. Z. Qin and J. S. Li. 1993. The subdivisions of the intermediolateral nucleus in the sacral spinal cord of the cat. *Brain Research*, 632:351-355.

Luiten, P. G. M., G. J. ter Horst and A. B. Steffens. 1985. The course of paraventricular hypothalamic efferents to autonomic structures in medulla and spinal cord. *Brain Research*, 329:374-378.

Lund, R. D. and K. E. Webster. 1967. Thalamic afferents from the spinal cord and trigeminal nuclei: An experimental anatomical study in the rat. *Journal of Comparative Neurology*, 130:313-328.

Lund, S. and O. Pompeiano. 1965. Descending pathways with monosynaptic action on motoneurones. *Experientia*, 21:602-603.

Lundberg, A. 1975. Control of spinal mechanisms from the brain. In: D. B. Tower (ed.), *The Nervous System*, pp. 253-265. New York: Raven.

Lundberg, A. 1979. Multisensory control of spinal reflex pathways. In: R. Granit and O. Pompeiano (eds.), *Reflex Control of Posture and Movement*, pp. 11-28. Amsterdam: Elsevier.

Ma, W., M. Peschanski and H. J. Ralston. 1987. Fine structure of the spinothalamic projections to the central lateral nucleus of the rat thalamus. *Brain Research*, 414:187-191.

Ma, W., A. Ribeiro-da-Silva, Y. De Koninck, V. Radhakrishnan, A. C. Cuello and J. L. Henry. 1997. Substance P and enkephalin immunoreactivities in axonal boutons presynaptic to physiologically identified dorsal horn neurons: An ultrastructural multiple-labeling study in the cat. *Neuroscience*, 77:793-811.

Maekawa, K. and Y. Ochiai. 1975. Electromyographic studies on flexor hypertonia of the extremities of newborn infants. *Developmental Medicine and Child Neurology*, 17:440-446.

Magnus, R. 1924. *Körperstellung.* Berlin: Springer.

Magnus, R. 1925. Animal posture. *Proceedings of the Royal Society*, 89B:339-353.

Magoun, H. W. and R, Rhines. 1946. An inhibitory mechanism in the bulbar reticular formation. *Journal of Physiology*, 9:165-171.

Makous, J. C., R. M. Friedman and C. J. Vierck. 1996. Effects of dorsal column lesion on temporal processing within the somatosensory system of primates. *Experimental Brain Research*, 112:253-267.

Mall, F. P. 1910. Determination of the age of human embryos and fetuses. In: F. Keibel and F. P. Mall (eds.), *Human Embryology*, vol. 1, pp. 202-242. Philadelphia: Lippincott.

Mall, F. P. 1914. On stages in the development of human embryos from 2 to 25 mm. long. *Anatomische Anzeiger*, 46:78-84.

Mall, F. P. 1918. On the age of human embryos. *American Journal of Anatomy*, 23:397-422.

Mantyh, P. W. 1982. The ascending input to the midbrain periaqueductal gray in the primate. *Journal of Comparative Neurology*, 211:50-64.

Marinesco, G. 1898. Contribution a l'étude des localisations des noyaux moteurs dans la moelle épinière. *Revue Neurologie*, 6:463-470.

Markham, J. A. and J. E. Vaughn. 1991. Migration patterns of sympathetic preganglionic neurons in embryonic rat spinal cord. *Journal of Neurobiology*, 22:811-822.

Marson, L. 1997. Identification of central nervous system neurons that innervate the bladder body, bladder base, or external urethral sphincter of female rats: A transneuronal tracing study using pseudorabies virus. *Journal of Comparative Neurology*, 389:584-602.

Martin, G. F., R. R. Pindzola and X. M. Xu. 1993. The origins of descending projections to the lumbar spinal cord at different stages of development in the North American opossum. *Brain Research Bulletin*, 30:303-317.

Massazza, A. 1922-1924. La citoarchitettonica del midullo spinale umano. I, II, III. *Archiv d'Anatomie, d'Histologie et d'Embryologie*, 1:323-410; 2:1-56; 3:115-189.

Massion, J. 1967. The mammalian red nucleus. *Physiological Reviews, 47:383-436.*

Mathew, A. and M. Cook. 1990. The control of reaching movements by young infants. *Child Development*, 61:1238-1257.

Mathew, O. P. 1991. Breathing patterns of preterm infants during bottle feeding: Role of milk flow. *Journal of Pediatrics*, 119:960-965.

Matsumoto, A. 1997. Hormonally induced neuronal plasticity in the adult motoneurons. *Brain Research Bulletin*, 44:539-547.

Matsushita, M. 1998. Ascending propriospinal afferents to area X (substantia gelatinosa centralis) of the spinal cord in the rat. *Experimental Brain Research*, 119:356-366.

Matsushita, M. and X. Gao. 1997. Projections from the thoracic cord to the cerebellar nuclei in the rat, studied by anterograde axonal tracing. *Journal of Comparative Neurology*, 386:409-421.

Matsushita, M. and M. Ikeda. 1973. Propriospinal fiber connections of the cervical motor nuclei in the cat: A light and electon microscopic study. *Journal of Comparative Neurology*, 150:1-32.

Matsushita, M. and M. Ikeda. 1975. The central cervical nucleus as cell origin of a spinocerebellar tract arising from the cervical cord: A study in the cat using horseradish peroxidase. *Brain Research*, 100:412-417.

Matsushita, M., M. Ikeda and Y. Hosoya. 1979. The location of spinal neurons with long descending axons (long descending propriospinal tract neurons) in the cat: A study with the horseradish peroxidase technique. *Journal of Comparative Neurology*, 184:63-80.

Matthews, B. H. C. 1933. Nerve endings in mammalian muscles. *Journal of Physiology*, 18:1-53.

Matthews, M. A. and D. Duncan. 1971. A quantitative study of morphological changes accompanying the initiation and progress of myelin production in the dorsal funiculus of the rat spinal cord. *Journal of Comparative Neurology*, 142:1-22.

Matthews, P. B. C. 1972. *Mammalian Muscle Spindles and their Central Action.* London: Arnold.

Maunz, R. A., N. G. Pitts and B. W. Peterson. 1978. Cat spinoreticular neurons: Location, responses and changes in responses during repetitive stimulation. *Brain Research*, 148:365-379.

Maxwell, D. J. and H. R. Koerber. 1986. Fine structure of collateral axons originating from feline spinocervical tract neurons. *Brain Research*, 363:199-203.

Mayer, D. J. and D. D. Price. 1976. Central nervous system mechanisms of analgesia. *Pain*, 2:379-404.

Mayer, D. J., D. D. Price and D. P. Becker. 1975. Neurophysiological characterization of the anterolateral spinal cord neurons contributing to pain perception in man. *Pain*, 1:51-58.

McCartney, G. and P. Hepper. 1999. Development of lateralized behaviour in the human fetus from 12 to 27 weeks' gestation. *Developmental Medicine and Child Neurology*, 41:83-86.

McCotter, R. E. 1916. Regarding the length and extent of the human medulla spinalis. *Anatomical Record*, 10:559-564.

McHanwell, S. and T. J. Biscoe. 1981. The localisation of motoneurons supplying the hindlimb muscles of the mouse. *Philosophical Transactions of the Royal Society*, B293:477-508.

McGraw, M. B. 1932. From reflex to muscular control in the assumption of an erect posture and ambulation in the human infant. *Child Development*, 3:291-297.

McGraw, M. B. 1935. *Growth: A Study of Johnny and Jimmy.* New York: Appleton-Century.

McGraw, M. B. 1937. The Moro reflex. *Anerican Journal of Diseases of Children*, 54:240-251.

McGraw, M. B. 1939. Swimming behavior of the human infant. *Journal of Pediatrics*, 15:485-490.

McGraw, M. B. 1943. *The Neuromuscular Maturation of the Human Infant.* New York: Columbia University Press. (Reprinted, New York: Hafner, 1963)

McKanna. J. A. 1993. Primitive glial compartments in the floor plate of mammalian embryos: Distinct progenitors of adult astrocytes and microglia support the notoplate hypothesis. *Perspectives on Developmental Neurobiology*, 1:245-255.

McKenna, K. E. and I. Nadelhaft. 1986. The organization of the pudendal nerve in the male and female rat. *Journal of Comparative Neurology*, 248:532-549.

McLaughlin, B. J. 1972. The fine structure of neurons and synapses in the motor nuclei of the cat spinal cord. *Journal of Comparative Neurology*, 144:429-460.

McLaughlin, B. J., R. Barber, K. Saito, E. Roberts and J. Y Wu. 1975. Immunocytochemical localization of glutamate decarboxylase in rat spinal cord. *Journal of Comparative Neurology*, 164:305-322.

Melzack, R. and J. A. Bridges. 1971. Dorsal column contributions to motor behavior. *Experimental Neurology*, 33:53-68.

Melzack, R. and S. E. Southmayd. 1974. Dorsal column contributions to anticipatory motor behavior. *Experimental Neurology*, 42:274-281.

Mehler, W. R. 1962. The anatomy of the so-called "pain tract" in man: An analysis of the course and distribution of the ascending fibers of the fasciculus anterolateralis. In: J. D. French and R. W. Porter (eds.), *Basic Research in Paraplegia*, pp. 26-55. Springfield, IL: Thomas.

Mehler, W. R. 1974. Central pain and the spinothalamic tract. In: J. J. Bonica (ed.), *Advances in Neurology,* vol. 4, *International Symposium on Pain*, pp. 127-146. New York: Raven.

Mehler, W. R., M. E. Feferman and W. J. H. Nauta. 1960. Ascending axon degeneration following anterolateral cordotomy: An experimental study in the monkey. *Brain*, 83:718-750.

Meissirel, C., C. Dehay and H. Kennedy. 1993. Transient cortical pathways in the pyramidal tract of the neonatal ferret. *Journal of Comparative Neurology*, 338:193-213.

Menétrey, D., A. Chaouch, D. Binder and J. M. Besson. 1982. The origin of spinomesencephalic tract in the rat: An anatomical study using the retrograde transport of horseradish peroxidase. *Journal of Comparative Neurology*, 206:193-207.

Menétrey, D., de Pommery and J. M. Besson. 1984. Electrophysiological characteristics of lumbar spinal cord neurons backfired from lateral reticular nucleus in the rat. *Journal of Neurophysiology*, 52:595-611.

Menétrey, D., G. J. Giesler and J. M. Besson. 1977. An analysis of response properties of spinal cord dorsal horn neurones to nonnoxious and noxious stimuli in the spinal rat. *Experimental Brain Research*, 27:15-33.

Menétrey, D., F. Roudier and J. M. Besson. 1983. Spinal neurons reaching the lateral reticular nucleus as studied in the rat by retrograde transport of horseradish peroxidase. *Journal of Comparative Neurology*, 220:439-452.

Mense, S. and A. D. Craig. 1988. Spinal and supraspinal terminations of primary afferent fibers from the gastrocnemius-soleus muscle in the cat. *Neuroscience*, 26:1023-1035.

Metzger, F., S. Wiese and M. Sendtner. 1998. Effect of glutamate on dendritic growth in embryonic rat motoneurons. *Journal of Neuroscience*, 18:1735-1742.

Michaelis, P. 1906. Alterbestimmung menschlicher Embryonen und Föten auf Grund von Messungen und von Daten der Anamnese. *Archiv für Gynäkologie*, 78:267-288.

Mickel, H. S. and F. H. Gilles. 1970. Changes in glial cells during human telencephalic myelinogenesis. *Brain*, 93:337-346.

Miki, A. 1995. Developmental changes in the expression of alpha-, beta- and gamma-subspecies of protein kinase C at synapses in the ventral horn of the embryonic and postnatal rat spinal cord. *Developmental Brain Research*, 87:46-54.

Miletic, V., M. J. Hoffert, M. A. Ruda, R. Dubner and Y. Shigenaga. 1984. Serotoninergic axonal contacts on identified cat spinal dorsal horn neurons and their correlation with nucleus raphe magnus stimulation. *Journal of Comparative Neurology*, 228:129-141.

Millar, J. and A. I. Basbaum. 1975. Topography of the projection of the body surface of the cat to cuneate and gracile nuclei. *Experimental Neurology*, 49:281-290.

Miller, K. E., J. R. Clements, A. A. Larson and A. J. Beitz. 1988. Organization of glutamate-like immunoreactivity in the rat superficial dorsal horn: Light and electron microscopic observations. *Synapse*, 2:28-36.

Miller, R. A. and N. L. Strominger. 1973. Efferent connections of the red nucleus in the brainstem and spinal cord of the rhesus monkey. *Journal of Comparative Neurology*, 152:327-346.

Milne, R. J., R. D. Foreman, G. J. Giesler and W. D. Willis. 1981. Convergence of cutaneous and pelvic nociceptive inputs onto primate spinothalamic neurons. *Pain*, 11:163-183.

Milner-Brown, H. S., R. B. Stein and R. Yemm. 1973. The orderly recruitment of human motor units during voluntary isometric contractions. *Journal of Physiology*, 230:359-370..

Minckler, J., R. M. Klemme and D. Minckler. 1944. The course of efferent fibers from the human premotor cortex. *Journal of Comparative Neurology*, 81:259-277.

Minkowski, M. 1923. Zur Entwicklungsgeschichte, Lokalisation und Klinik des Fussohlenreflexes. *Schweizerische Archiv für Neurologie und Psychiatrie*, 13:475-514.

Minot, C. S. 1903. *A Laboratory Text-Book of Embryology*. Philadelphia: Blakiston.

Mirnics, K. and H. R. Koerber. 1995a. Prenatal development of rat primary afferent fibers: I. Peripheral projections. *Journal of Comparative Neurology*, 355:589-600.

Mirnics, K. and H. R. Koerber. 1995b. Prenatal development of rat primary afferent fibers: II. Central projections. *Journal of Comparative Neurology*, 355:601-614.

Mizuno, N. 1966. Experimental study of the spino-olivary fibers in the rabbit and the cat. *Journal of Comparative Neurology*, 127:267-292.

Mizuno, N., K. Nakano, M. Imaizumi and M. Okamoto. 1967. The lateral cervical nucleus of the Japanese monkey (*Macaca fuscata*). *Journal of Comparative Neurology*, 129:375-384.

Miyata, Y. and M. Otsuka. 1972. Distribution of γ-aminobutyric acid in cat spinal cord and the alteration produced by local ischemia. *Journal of Neurochemistry*, 19:1833-1834.

Molenaar, I. and H. G. J. M. Kuypers. 1978. Cells of origin of propriospinal fibers and of fibers ascending to supraspinal levels: A HRP study in cat and rhesus monkey. *Brain Research*, 152:429-450.

Monuki, E. S. and G. Lemke. 1995. Molecular biology of myelination. In: S. G. Waxman, J. D. Kocsis and P. K. Stys (eds.), *The Axon: Structure, Function, and Pathophysiology*, pp. 144-163. New York: Oxford University Press.

Moore, R. M. 1938. Some experimental observations relating to visceral pain. *Surgery*, 3:534-555.

Morgan, C., I. Nadelhaft, and W. C. de Groat. 1981. The distribution of visceral primary afferents from the pelvic nerve to Lissauer's tract and the spinal gray matter and its relationship to sacral parasympathetic nucleus. *Journal of Comparative Neurology*, 201:415-440.

Morin, F. 1955. A new spinal pathway for cutaneous impulses. *American Journal of Physiology*, 183:245-252.

Morin, F. and J. Catalano. 1955. Central connections of a cervical nucleus (nucleus cervicalis lateralis) of the cat. *Journal of Comparative Neurology*, 103:17-32.

Morin, F., S. T. Kitai, H. Portnoy and C. Demirjian. 1963. Afferent projection to the NCL: A microelectrode study. *American Journal of Physiology*, 204:667-672.

Morin, F., H. G. Schwartz and J. L. O'Leary. 1951. Experimental study of spinothalamic and related tracts. *Acta Psychiatrica et Neurologica*, 26:371-396.

Moruzzi G. and H. W. Magoun. 1949. Brain stem reticular formation and activation of the EEG. *Electroencephalography and Clinical Neurophysiology*, 1:455-473.

Mott, F. W. 1895. Experimental enquiry upon the afferent tracts of the central nervous system of the monkey. *Brain*, 18:1-20.

Mouncastle, V. B. 1957. Modality and topographic properties of single neurons in cat's somatic sensory cortex. *Journal of Neurophysiology*, 20:408-434.

Mountcastle, V. B. and E. Henneman. 1952. The representation of tactile sensibility in the thalamus of the monkey. *Journal of Comparative Neurology*, 97:409-440.

Mouton, L. J. and G. Holstege. 1998. Three times as many lamina I neurons project to the periaqueductal gray than to the thalamus: A retrograde tracing study in the cat. *Neuroscience Letters*, 255:107-110.

Muir, R. B. and R. N. Lemon. 1983. Corticospinal neurons with a special role in precision grip. *Brain Research*, 261:312-316.

Münzer, E. and H. Wiener. 1910. Experimentelle Beiträge zur Lehre von endogenen Fasersystemen des Rückenmarkes. *Monatschrift für Psychiatrie und Neurologie*, 28:1-25.

Murray, E. A. and J. D. Coulter. 1981. Organization of corticospinal neurons in the monkey. *Journal of Comparative Neurology*, 195:339-365.

Murray, H. M. and D. E. Haines. 1975. The rubrospinal tract in a prosimian primate (*Galago senegalensis*). *Brain, Behavior and Evolution*, 12:311-333.

Nadelhaft, I. and A. M. Booth. 1984. The location and morphology of preganglionic neurons and the distribution of visceral afferents from the rat pelvic nerve: A horseradish peroxidase study. *Journal of Comparative Neurology*, 226:238-245.

Nadelhaft, I., W. C. de Groat and C. Morgan. 1980. Location and morphology of parasympathetic preganglionic neurons in the sacral spinal cord of the cat revealed by retrograde transport of horseradish peroxidase. *Journal of Comparative Neurology*, 193:265-281.

Nafe, J. P. 1929. A quantitative theory of feeling. *Journal of General Psychology*, 2:199-210.

Nahin, R. L., A. M. Madsen and G. J. Giesler. 1983. Anatomical and physiological studies of the gray matter surrounding the spinal cord central canal. *Journal of Comparative Neurology*, 220:321-335.

Nahin, R. L. and P. E. Micevych. 1986. A long ascending pathway of enkephalin-like immunoreactive spinoreticular neurons in the rat. *Neuroscience Letters*, 65:271-276.

Nandi, K. N., D. S. Knight and J. A. Beal. 1991. Neurogenesis of ascending supraspinal projection neurons: Ipsi- versus contralateral projections. *Neuroscience Letters*, 131:8-12.

Nandi, K. N., D. S. Knight and J. A. Beal. 1993. Spinal neurogenesis and axon projection: A correlative study in the rat. *Journal of Comparative Neurology*, 328:252-262.

Napier, J. 1970. *The Roots of Mankind*. Wahington, DC: Smithsonian Institution Press.

Natale, R., C. Nasello-Paterson and G. Connors. 1988. Patterns of fetal breathing activity in human fetus at 24 and 28 week's gestation. *American Journal of Obstetrics and Gynecology*, 158:317-321.

Nathan, P. W. and M. C. Smith. 1959. Fasciculi proprii of the spinal cord in man: Review of present knowledge. *Brain*, 82:610-668.

Nathan, P. W. and M. C. Smith. 1982. The rubrospinal and central tegmental tracts in man. *Brain*, 105:223-269.

Nathan, P. W., M. C. Smith and A. W. Cook. 1986. Sensory effects in man of lesions of the posterior columns and of some other afferent pathways. *Brain*, 109:1003-1041.

Nathan, P. W., M. C. Smith and P. Deacon. 1996. Vestibulospinal, reticulospinal and descending propriospinal nerve fibres in man. *Brain*, 119:1809-1833.

Natsuyama, E. 1991. In utero behavior of human embryos at the spinal-cord stage of development. *Biology of the Neonate*, 60 (Suppl. 1):11-29.

Nauta, H. J., E. Hewitt, K. N. Westlund and W. D. Willis. Surgical interruption of a midline dorsal column visceral pain pathway. *Journal of Neurosurgery*, 86:538-542.

Nemec, H. 1951. Über die Ausbildung der grauen Substanz im Frosch-Rückenmark. *Acta Anatomica*, 13:101-118.

Neuhuber, W. 1982. The central projections of visceral primary afferent neurons of the inferior mesenteric plexus and hypogastric nerve and the locations of the related sensory and preganglionic sympathetic cell bodies in the rat. *Anatomy and Embryology*, 164:413-425.

Newbery, H. 1941. Studies of fetal behavior. IV. The measurement of three types of fetal activity. *Journal of Comparative Psychology*, 32:521-530.

Nicholas, A. P., V. A. Pieribone, U. Arvidsson and T Hökfelt. 1992. Serotonin-, substance P- and glutamate/aspartate-like immunoreactivities in medullo-spinal pathways of rat and primate. *Neuroscience*, 48:545-559.

Nicolopoulos-Stournaras, S. and J. F. Iles. 1983. Motor neuron columns in the lumbar spinal cord of the rat. *Journal of Comparative Neurology*, 217:75-85.

Nieuwenhuys, R. 1964. Comparative anatomy of the spinal cord. *Progress in Brain Research,* 11:1-57.

Nijhuis, I. J., J. ten Hof, J. G. Nijhuis, E. J. Mulder, H. Narayan, D. J. Taylor and G. H. Visser. 1999. Temporal organization of fetal behavior from 24-weeks gestation onwards in normal and complicated pregnacies. *Developmental Psychobiology, 34:257-268.*

Noll, E. and R. H. Miller. 1993. Oligodendrocyte precursors originate at the ventral ventricular zone dorsal to the ventral midline region in the embryonic rat spinal cord. *Development*, 118:563-573.

Nornes, H. O. and M. Carry. 1978. Neurogenesis in spinal cord of mouse: An autoradiographic analysis. *Brain Research*, 159:1-16.

Nornes, H. O. and G. D. Das. 1974. Temporal pattern of neurogenesis in the spinal cord of rat. I. An autoradiographic study. Time and sites of origin and settling patterns of neuroblasts. *Brain Research*, 73:121:138.

Nuding, S. C. and I. Nadelhaft. 1998. Bilateral projections of the pontine micturition center to the sacral parasympathetic nucleus in the rat. *Brain Research*, 785:185-194.

Nyberg, G. and A. Blomqvist. 1985. The somatotopic organization of forelimb cutaneous nerves in the brachial dorsal horn: An anatomical study in the cat. *Journal of Comparative Neurology*, 242:28-39.

Nyberg-Hansen, R. 1964a. The location and termination of tectospinal fibers in the cat. *Experimental Neurology*, 9:212-227.

Nyberg-Hansen, R. 1964b. Origin and termination of fibers from the vestibular nuclei descending in the medial longitudinal fasciculus: An experimental study with silver impregnation methods in the cat. *Journal of Comparative Neurology*, 122:355-367.

Nyberg-Hansen, R. 1965. Sites and mode of termination of reticulo-spinal fibers in the cat: An experimental study with silver impregnation methods. *Journal of Comparative Neurology*, 124:71-100.

Nyberg-Hansen, R. 1966a. Functional organisation of descending supraspinal fibre systems to the spinal cord: Anatomical observations and physiological correlations. *Ergebnisse der Anatomie und Entwicklungsgeschichte*, 39:1-48.

Nyberg-Hansen, R. 1966b. Sites of termination of interstitiospinal fibers in the cat: An experimental study with silver impregnation methods. *Archives Italiennes de Biologie*, 104:98-111.

Nyberg-Hansen, R. 1969. Further studies on the origin of corticospinal fibres in the cat: An experimental study with the Nauta method. *Brain Research*, 16:39-54.

Nyberg-Hansen, R. and A. Brodal. 1964. Sites and mode of termination of rubrospinal fibres in the cat: An experimental study with silver impregnation methods. *Journal of Anatomy*, 98:235-253.

Nyberg-Hansen, R. and T. A. Mascitti. 1964. Sites and mode of termination of fibers of the vestibulospinal tract in the cat: An experimental study with silver impregnation methods. *Journal of Comparative Neurology*, 122:369-387.

Nyqvist, K. H., P. O. Sjoden and U. Ewald. 1999. The development of preterm infants' breastfeeding behavior. *Early Human Development*, 55:247-264.

O'Hanlon, G. M. and M. B. Lowrie. 1994a. Dendritic development in normal lumbar motoneurons and following neonatal nerve crush in the rat. *Developmental Neuroscience*, 16:17-24.

O'Hanlon, G. M. and M. B. Lowrie. 1994b. Both afferent and efferent connections influence postnatal growth of motoneuron dendrites in the rat. *Developmental Neuroscience*, 16:100-107.

Ohyama, K., H. Kawano and K. Kawamura. 1997. Localization of extracellular matrix molecules, integrins and their regulators, TGF betas, is correlated with axon pathfinding in the spinal cord of normal and Danforth's short tail mice. *Developmental Brain Research*, 103:143-154.

Okado, N. 1980. Development of the human spinal cord with reference to synapse formation in the motor nucleus. *Journal of Comparative Neurology*, 191:495-513.

Okado, N. 1981. Onset of synapse formation in the human spinal cord. *Journal of Comparative Neurology*, 201:211-219.

Okado, N., S. Kakimi and T. Kojima. 1979. Synaptogenesis in the cervical cord of the human embryo: Sequence of synapse formation in a spinal reflex pathway. *Journal of Comparative Neurology*, 184:491-518.

Oldfield, B. J. and E. M. McLachlan. 1981. An analysis of the sympathetic preganglionic neurons projecting from the upper thoracic spinal roots of the cat. *Journal of Comparative Neurology*, 196:329-345.

Oliveras, J.-L., J.-M. Besson, G, Guilbaud and J. C. Liebeskind. 1974. Behavioral and electrophysiological evidence of pain inhibition from midbrain stimulation in the cat. *Experimental Brain Research*, 20:32-44.

Oliveras, J.-L., F. Redjemi, G. Guilbaud and J. M.-Besson. 1975. Analgesia induced by electrical stimulation of the inferior centralis nucleus of the raphé in the cat. *Pain*, 1:139-145.

Ono, K., R. Bansal, J. Payne, U. Rutishauser and R. H. Miller. 1995. Early development and dispersal of oligodendrocyte precursors in the embryonic chick spinal cord. *Development*, 121:1743-1754.

Onuf, B. 1900. On the arrangement and function of the cell groups of the sacral region of the spinal cord in man. *Archives of Neurology and Psychopathology*, 3:387-412.

O'Rahilly, R. and F. Müller. 1987. *Developmental Stages in Human Embryos*. Washington, DC: Carnegie Institution of Washington.

O'Rahilly, R. and F. Müller. 1994. *The Embryonic Human Brain: An Atlas of Developmental Stages*. New York: Wiley.

Orentas. D. M. and R. H. Miller. 1996. The origin of spinal cord oligodendrocytes is dependent on local influences from the notochord. *Developmental Biology*, 177:43-53.

Örnung, G., O. P. Ottersen, S. Cullheim and B. Ulfhake. 1998. Distribution of glutamate-, glycine-, and GABA-immunoreactive nerve terminals on dendrites in the cat spinal motor nucleus. *Experimental Brain Research*, 118:517-532.

Oscarsson, O. 1965. Functional organization of the spino- and cuneocerebellar tracts. *Physiological Reviews*, 45:495-522.

Oswaldo-Cruz, E. and C. Kidd. 1964. Functional properties of neurons in the lateral cervical nucleus of the cat. *Journal of Neurophysiology*, 27:1-14.

Otsuka, M. and S. Konishi. 1976. Release of substance P-like immunoreactivity from isolated spinal cord of newborn rat. *Nature*, 264:83-84.

Ottoson, D. 1983. *Physiology of the Nervous System*. New York: Oxford University Press.

Ozaki, S. and W. D. Snider. 1997. Initial trajectories of sensory axons toward laminar targets in the developing mouse spinal cord. *Journal of Comparative Neurology*, 380:215-229.

Papez, J. W. and G. L. Freeman. 1930. Superior colliculi and their fiber connections in the rat. *Journal of Comparative Neurology*, 51:409-439.

Patrick, J., K. Campbell, L. Carmichael, R. Natale and B. Richardson. 1982. Patterns of gross fetal body movements over 24-hour observation intervals during the last 10 weeks of pregnancy. *American Journal of Obstetrics and Gynecology*, 142:363-371.

Patrick, J., K. Campbell, L. Carmichael, R. Natale and B. Richardson. 1988. Patterns of human fetal breathing during the last 10 weeks of pregnancy. *Obstetrics and Gynecology*, 56:24-30.

Patten, B. M. 1953. *Human Embryology*, 2nd ed. New York: McGraw-Hill

Patterson, J. T., P. A. Head, D. L. McNeill, K. Chung and R. E. Coggeshall. 1989. Ascending unmyelinated primary afferents fibers in the dorsal funiculus. *Journal of Comparative Neurology*, 290:384-390.

Paxinos, G. and C. Watson. 1986. *The Rat Brain in Stereotaxic Coordinates*, 2nd ed. San Diego, CA: Academic Press.

Pearce, G. W. and P. Glees. 1956. The termination of the crossed tecto-spinal tract in the spinal cord of the cat. *Journal of Anatomy*, 90:565-566.

Pearson, A. A. 1952. Role of gelatinous substance of spinal cord in conduction of pain. *Archives of Neurology and Psychiatry*, 68:515-529.

Pearson, R. and L. Pearson. 1976. *The Vertebrate Brain*. New York: Academic Press.

Peele, T. L. 1942. Cytoarchitecture of individual parietal areas in the monkey (*Macaca mulatta*) and the distribution of the efferent fibers. *Journal of Comparative Neurology*, 77:693-737.

Pehl, U. and H. A. Schmid. 1997. Electrophysiological responses of neurons in the rat spinal cord to nitric oxide. *Neuroscience*, 77:563-573.

Peiper, A. 1929. Die Schreitbewegungen des Neugeborenen. *Monatsschrift für Kinderheilkunde*, 45:444-448.

Peiper, A. 1963. *Cerebral Function in Infancy and Childhood*. New York: Consultants Bureau.

Penfield, W. and T. Rasmussen. 1950. *The Cerebral Cortex of Man: A Clinical Study of Localization of Function*. New York: Macmillan. (Reprinted by Hafner, New York, 1968)

Perese, D. M. and J. E. Fracasso. 1959. Anatomical considerations in surgery of the spinal cord: A study of vessels and measurements of the cord. *Journal of Neurosurgery*, 16:314-325.

Perl, E. R. 1992. Function of dorsal root ganglion neurons: An overview. In: S. A. Scott (ed.), *Sensory Neurons: Diversity, Development, and Plasticity*, pp. 3-23. New York: Oxford University Press.

Perl, E. R., D. G. Whitlock and J. R. Gentry. 1962. Cutaneous projection to second order neurons of the dorsal column system. *Journal of Neurophysiology*, 25:337-358.

Persson, J. K. E., B. Lindh, R. Elde, B. Robertson, C. Rivero-Melián, N. P. Eriksson, T. Hökfelt and H. Aldskogius. 1995. The expression of different cytochemical markers in normal and axotomised dorsal root ganglion cells projecting to the nucleus gracilis in the adult rat. *Experimental Brain Research*, 105:331-344.

Pert, C., M. Kuhar and S. H. Snyder. 1975. Autoradiographic localization of the opiate receptor in rat brain. *Life Science*, 16:1849-1854.

Peshori, K. R., J. T. Erichsen and W. F. Collins. 1995. Differences in the connectivity of rat pudendal motor nuclei as revealed by retrograde transneuronal transport of wheat germ agglutinin. *Journal of Comparative Neurology*, 353:119-128.

Peterson, B. W., R. A. Maunz, N. G. Pitts and R. G. Mackel. 1975. Patterns of projection and branching of reticulospinal neurons. *Experimental Brain Research*, 23:333-351.

Peterson, B. W., N. G. Pitts, K. Fukushima and R. Mackel. 1978. Reticulospinal excitation and inhibition of neck motoneurons. *Experimental Brain Research*, 32:417-489.

Petit, D. 1972. Postsynaptic fibres in the dorsal columns and their relay in the nucleus gracilis. *Brain Research*, 48:380-384.

Petras, J. M. 1967. Cortical, tectal and tegmental fiber connections in the spinal cord of the cat. *Brain Research*, 6:275-324.

Petras, J. M. and J. F. Cummings. 1972. Autonomic neurons in the spinal cord of the rhesus monkey: A correlation of the findings of cytoarchitectonics and sympathectomy with fiber degeneration following dorsal rhizotomy. *Journal of Comparative Neurology*, 146:189-218.

Petras, J. M. and A. I. Faden. 1978. The origin of sympathetic preganglionic neurons in the dog. *Brain Research*, 144:353-357.

Petrén, K. 1910. Über die Bahnen der Sensibilität im Rückenmarke, besonders nach den Fällen von Stichverletzung studiert. *Archiv für Psychiatrie*, 47:495-557.

Pfeiffer, S. E., A. E. Warrington and R. Bansal. 1993. The oligodendrocyte and its many cellular processes. *Trends in Cell Biology*, 3:191-197.

Phelps, P. E., R. P. Barber, L. A. Brennan, V. M. Maines, P. M. Salvaterra and J. E. Vaughn. 1990. Embryonic development of four different subsets of cholinergic neurons in rat cervical spinal cord. *Journal of Comparative Neurology*, 291:9-26.

Phillips, C. G. and R. Porter. 1977. *Corticospinal Neurones: Their Role in Movement*. London: Academic Press.

Pick, J. 1970. *The Autonomic Nervous System: Morphological, Comparative, Clinical and Surgical Aspects*. Philadelphia: Lippincott.

Pickel, V. M., D. J. Reis and S. E. Leeman. 1977. Ultrastructural localization of substance P in neurons of rat spinal cord. *Brain Research*, 122:534-540.

Piek, J. and N. Gasson. 1999. Spontaneous kicking in full-term and preterm infants: Are there leg asymmetries? *Human Movement Science*, 18:377-395.

Placzek, M. M. Tessier-Lavigne, T. M. Jessell and J. Dodd. 1990. Orientation of commissural axons in vitro in response to a floor-plate-derived chemoattractant. *Development*, 110:19-30.

Poirier, L. J. and C. Bertrand. 1955. Experimental and anatomical investigation of the lateral spino-thalamic and spino-tectal tracts. *Journal of Comparative Neurology*, 102:745-747.

Poirier, L. J. and G. Bouvier. 1966. The red nucleus and its efferent nervous pathways in the monkey. *Journal of Comparative Neurology*, 128:223-244.

Poljak, S. 1924. Die Struktureigentümlichkeiten des Rückenmarkes bei den Chiropteren. Zugleich ein Beitrag zu der Frage über die spinalen Zentren der Sympatheticus. *Zeitschrift für die Anatomie und Entwicklungsgeschichte*, 74:509-576.

Pompeiano, O. and A. Brodal. 1957. Spino-vestibular fibers in the cat. *Journal of Comparative Neurology*, 108:353-382.

Popper, E. Studien über Saugphänomene. *Archiv für Psychiatrie und Nervenkrankheiten*, 63:231-246.

Pratt, K. C. 1954. The neonate. In: L. Carmichael (ed.), *Manual of Child Psychology*, 2ⁿᵈ ed. New York: Wiley.

Precht, W., A. Richter, S. Ozawa and H. Shimazu. 1974. Intracellular study of frog's vestibular neurons in relation to the labyrinth and the spinal cord. *Experimental Brain Research*, 19:377-393.

Prechtl, H. F. R. 1997. State of the art of a new functional assessment of the young nervous system: An early predictor of cerebral palsy. *Early Human Development*, 50:1-11.

Prechtl, H. F. R. and B. Hopkins. 1986. Developmental transformations of spontaneous movements in early infancy. *Early Human Development*, 14:233-238.

Price, D. D. 1984. Dorsal horn mechanisms of pain. In: R. A. Davidoff (ed.), *Handbook of the Spinal Cord*, vols. 2 and 3: *Anatomy and Physiology*, pp. 751-777. New York: Dekker.

Price, D. D., H. Hayashi, R. Dubner and M. A. Ruda. 1979. Functional relationships between neurons of the marginal and substantia gelatinosa layers of the primate dorsal horn. *Journal of Neurophysiology*, 42:1590-1608.

Prochazka, A., F. Clarac, G. E. Loeb, J. C. Rothwell and J. R. Wolpaw. 2000. What do *reflex* and *voluntary* mean? Modern views on an ancient debate. *Experimental Brain Research*, 130:417-432.

Pringle, N. P., S. Guthrie, A. Lumsden and W. D. Richardson. 1998. Dorsal spinal cord neuroepithelium generates astrocytes but not oligodendrocytes. *Neuron*, 20:883-893.

Proshansky, E. and M. D. Egger. 1977. Dendritic spread of dorsal horn neurons in cats. *Experimental Brain Research*, 28:153-166.

Pullen, A. H., D. Tucker and J. E. Martin. 1997. Morphological and morphometric characterisation of Onuf's nucleus in the spinal cord in man. *Journal of Anatomy*, 191:201-213.

Puskár, Z. and M. Antal. 1997. Localization of last-order premotor interneurons in the lumbar spinal cords of rats. *Journal of Comparative Neurology*, 389:377-389.

Pyner, S. and J. H. Coote. 1994. Evidence that sympathetic preganglionic neurones are arranged in target-specific columns in the thoracic spinal cord of the rat. *Journal of Comparative Neurology*, 342:15-22.

Rajaofetra, N., J.-G. Passagia, L. Marlier, P. Poulat, F. Pellas, F. Sandillon, B. Verschuere, D. Gouy, M. Geffard and A. Privat. 1992. Serotoninergic, noradrenergic, and peptidergic innervation of Onuf's nucleus of normal and transected spinal cords of baboons *(Papio papio)*. *Journal of Comparative Neurology*, 318:1-17.

Ralston, D. D. and H. J. Ralston. 1985. The terminations of corticospinal tract axons in the macaque monkey. *Journal of Comparative Neurology*, 242:325-337.

Ralston, H. J. 1968. The fine structure of neurons in the dorsal horn of the cat spinal cord. *Journal of Comparative Neurology*, 132:275-302.

Ralston, H. J. 1979. The fine structure of laminae I, II and III of the macaque spinal cord. *Journal of Comparative Neurology*, 184:619-642.

Ralston, H. J. and D. D. Ralston. 1979. The distribution of dorsal root axons in laminae I, II and III of the macaque spinal cord: A quantitative electron microscope study. *Journal of Comparative Neurology*, 184:643-684..

Ralston, H. J. and D, D. Ralston. 1994. Medial lemniscal and spinal projections to the macaque thalamus: An electron microscopic study of differing GABAergic circuitry serving thalamic somatosensory mechanisms. *Journal of Neuroscience*, 14:2485-2502.

Ramón y Cajal, S. (1909) 1995. *Histology of the Nervous System of Man and Vertebrates*, vol. 1. (Trans. by N. Swanson and L. W. Swanson). New York: Oxford University Press.

Ramón-Moliner, E. and W. J. H. Nauta. 1966. The isodendritic core of the brain stem. *Journal of Comparative Neurology*, 126:311-336.

Randic, M. and V. Miletic. 1977. Effect of substance P in cat dorsal horn neurones activated by noxious stimuli. *Brain Research*, 128:164-169.

Randic, M., V. Miletic and A. D. Loewy. 1981. A morphological study of cat dorsal spinocerebellar tract neurons after intracellular injection of horseradish peroxidase. *Journal of Comparative Neurology*, 198:453-466.

Rando, T. A., C. W. Bowers and R. E. Zigmond. 1981. Localization of neurons in the rat spinal cord which project to the superior cervical ganglion. *Journal of Comparative Neurology*, 196:73-83.

Ranson, S. W. 1913a. The course within the spinal cord of the non-medullated fibers of the dorsal root: A study of Lissauer's tract in the cat. *Journal of Comparative Neurology*, 23:259-281.

Ranson, S. W. 1913b. The fasciculus cerebro-spinalis in the albino rat. *American Journal of Anatomy*, 14:411-424.

Ranson, S. W. and P. R. Billingsly. 1916. The conduction of painful afferent impulses in the spinal nerves: Studies in vasomotor reflex arcs. *American Journal of Physiology*, 40:571-584.

Ranson, S. W. and S. L. Clark. 1959. *The Anatomy of the Nervous System: Its Development and Function*, 10th ed. Philadelphia: Saunders.

Rao. M. S., M. Noble and M. Mayer-Proschel. 1998. A tripotential glial precursor cell is present in the developing spinal cord. *Proceedings of the National Academy of Sciences (USA)*, 95:3996-4001.

Rapoport, S. 1978. Location of sternocleidomastoid and trapezius motoneurons in the cat. *Brain Research*, 156:339-344.

Rasmussen, A. T. 1936. Tractus tecto-spinalis in the cat. *Journal of Comparative Neurology*, 63:501-526.

Rastad, J., E. Jankowska and J. Westman. 1977. Arborization of initial axon collaterals of spinocervical tract cells stained intracellularly with horseradish peroxidase. *Brain Research*, 135:1-10.

Reh,T. and K. Kalil. 1981. Development of the pyramidal tract in the hamster. I. A light microscope study. *Journal of Comparative Neurology*, 200:55-67.

Réthelyi, M. 1970. Ultrastructural synaptology of Clarke's column. *Experimental Brain Research*, 11:159-174.

Réthelyi, M. 1977. Preterminal and terminal axon arborizations in the substantia gelatinosa of cat's spinal cord. *Journal of Comparative Neurology*, 172:511-528.

Réthelyi, M. 1984. Types of synaptic connections in the core of the spinal gray matter. In: R. A. Davidoff (ed.), *Handbook of the Spinal Cord*, vols. 2 and 3: *Anatomy and Physiology*, pp.179-198. New York: Dekker.

Réthelyi, M. and J. Szentágothai. 1969. The large synaptic complexes of the substantia gelatinosa. *Experimental Brain Research*, 7:258-274.

Retzius, G. 1898. Zur Frage von der Endigungsweise der peripherischen sensiblen Nerven. *Biologische Untersuchungen*, 8:114.

Rexed, B. 1952. The cytoarchitectonic organization of the spinal cord in the cat. *Journal of Comparative Neurology*, 96:415-419.

Rexed, B. 1954. The cytoarchitectonic atlas of the spinal cord in the cat. *Journal of Comparative Neurology*. 100:297-379.

Rexed, B. 1964. Some aspects of the cytoarchitectonics and synaptology of the spinal cord. *Progress in Brain Research*, 11:58-92.

Rhines, R. and W. F. Windle. 1941. The early development of the fasciculus longitudinalis medialis and associated secondary neurons in the rat, cat and man. *Journal of Comparative Neurology*, 75:165-183.

Ribeiro-da-Silva, A. and A. Coimbra. 1980. Neuronal uptake of [³H]GABA and [³H]glycine in laminae I–III (substantia gelatinosa Rolandi) of the rat spinal cord: An autoradiographic study. *Brain Research*, 188:449-464.

Ribeiro-da-Silva, A. and A. Coimbra. 1982. Two types of synaptic glomeruli and their distribution in laminae I–II of the rat spinal cord. *Journal of Comparative Neurology*, 209:176-186.

Richardson, W. D., N. P. Pringle, W.-P. Yu and A. C. Hall. 1996. Origins of spinal cord oligodendrocytes: Possible developmental and evolutionary relationships with motor neurons. *Developmental Neuroscience*, 19:58-68.

Richmond, F. J. R., D. A. Scott and V. C. Abrahams. 1978. Distribution of motoneurons of the neck muscles, biventer cervicis, splenius and complexus in the cat. *Journal of Comparative Neurology*, 181:451-464.

Richter, C. P. 1934. The grasp reflex of the newborn infants. *American Journal of Dieases of Childhood*, 48:327-332.

Rigamonti, D. D. and M. B. Hancock. 1974. Analysis of field potentials elicited in the dorsal column nuclei by splanchnic nerve A-beta afferents. *Brain Research*, 77:326-329.

Rikard-Bell, G. C. and E. Bystrzycka. 1980. Localization of phrenic motor nucleus in the cat and rabbit studied with horseradish peroxidase. *Brain Research*, 194:479-483.

Ritchie, T. C. and R. B. Leonard. 1983. Immunohistochenical studies of the distribution and origin of candidate peptidergic primary afferent neurotransmitters in the spinal cord of an elasmobranch fish, the Atlantic stingray (*Dasyatis sabina*). *Journal of Comparative Neurology*, 213:414-425.

Ritter, A., P. Wenner, S. Ho, P. J. Whelan and M. J. O'Donovan. 1999. Activity patterns and synaptic organization of ventrally located interneurons in the embryonic chick spinal cord. *Journal of Neuroscience*, 19:3457-3471.

Ritz, L. A., S. M. Bailey, C. R. Murray and M. L. Sparkes. 1992. Organizational and morphological features of cat sacrocaudal motoneurons. *Journal of Comparative Neurology*, 318:209-221.

Rivero-Mélian, C. and G. Grant. Distribution of lumbar dorsal root fibers in the lower thoracic and lumbosacral spinal cord of the rat studied with choleragenoid horseradish peroxidase conjugate. *Journal of Comparative Neurology*, 299:470-481.

Rivot, J. P., J. Barraud, C. Montecot, B. Jost and J. M. Besson. 1997. Nitric oxide (NO): In vivo electrochemical monitoring in the dorsal horn of the spinal cord of the rat. *Brain Research*, 773:66-75.

Roback, H. N. and H. J Scherer. 1935. Über die feinere Morphologie des frühkindlichen Hirner under besonderer Berücksichtigung der Glia entwicklung. *Virchov's Archiv für pathologische Anatomie*, 294:365-413.

RoBards, M. J., D. W. Watkins and R. B. Masterton. 1976. An anatomical study of some somesthetic afferents to the intercollicular terminal zone of the midbrain of the opossum. *Journal of Comparative Neurology*, 170:499-524.

Robertson, S. S. 1985. Cyclic motor activity in the human fetus after midgestation. *Developmental Psychobiology*, 18:411-419.

Rodriguez-Moldes, I., M. J. Manso, M. Becerra, P. Molist and R. Anadon. 1993. Distribution of substance P-like immunoreactivity in the brain of the elasmobranch, *Scyliorhinus canicula*. *Journal of Comparative Neurology*, 335:228-244.

Romanes, G. J. 1951. The motor cell columns of the lumbo-sacral spinal cord of the cat. *Journal of Comparative Neurology*, 94:313-363.

Romanes, G. J. 1964. The motor pools of the spinal cord. *Progress in Brain Research*, 11: 93-119.

Rönnqvist, L. and B. Hopkins. 1998. Head position preference in the human newborn: A new look. *Child Development*, 69:13-23.

Rönnqvist, L. and B. Hopkins. 2000. Motor asymmetries in the human newborn are state dependent, but independent of position in space. *Experimental Brain Research*, 134:378-384.

Roodenburg, P. J., J. W. Wlamidiroff, A. van Es and H. F. R. Prechtl. 1991. Classification and quantitative aspects of fetal movements during the second half of normal pregnancy. *Early Human Development*, 25:19-35.

Roppolo, J. R., I. Nadelhaft and W. C. de Groat. 1985. The organization of pudendal motoneurons and primary afferent projections in the spinal cord of the rhesus monkey revealed by horseradish peroxidase. *Journal of Comparative Neurology*, 234:475-488.

Rose, J. E. and V. B. Mountcastle. 1959. Touch and kinesthesis. In: H. W. Magoun (ed.), *Handbook of Physiology*, vol.1, *Neurophysiology*, pp. 387-429. Baltimore: Williams and Wilkins.

Rose, P. K. 1981. Distribution of dendrites from biventer cervicis and complexus motoneurons stained intracellularly with horseradish peroxidase in the

adult cat. *Journal of Comparative Neurology*, 197:395-409.

Ross, C. A., D. A. Ruggiero, T. Joh, D. H. Park and D. J. Reis. 1984. Rostral ventrolateral medulla: Selective projections to the thoracic autonomic cell column from the region containing C1 adrenergic neurons. *Journal of Comparative Neurology*, 228:168-185.

Rossi, G. F. and A. Brodal. 1957. Terminal distribution of spinoreticular fibers in the cat. *Archives of Neurology and Psychiatry*, 78:439-453.

Rothmann, M. 1899. Über die secundären Degenerationen nach Ausschaltung des Sacral- und Lendenmarkgrav durch Rückenmarks embolie beim Hunde. *Archiv für Anatomie und Physiologie*, 110-157.

Rotto-Percelay, D. M., J. G. Wheeler. F. A. Osorio, K. B. Platt and A. D. Loewy. 1992. Transneuronal labeling of spinal interneurons and sympathetic preganglionic neurons after pseudorabies virus injections in the rat medial gastrocnemius muscle. *Brain Research*, 574:291-306.

Ruda, M. A. and S. Gobel. 1980. Ultrastructural characterization of axonal endings in the substantia gelatinosa which take up [^{3}H] serotonin. *Brain Research*, 184:57-83.

Russell, J. R. and W. DeMyer. 1961. The quantitative cortical origin of pyramidal axons of *Macaca rhesus*: With some remarks on the slow rate of axolysis. *Neurology*, 11:96-108.

Rustioni, A. 1973. Non-primary afferents to the nucleus gracilis from the lumbar cord of the cat. *Brain Research*, 51:81-95.

Rustioni, A. and M. Cuénod. 1982. Selective retrograde transport of D-aspartate in spinal interneurons and cortical neurons of rats. *Brain Research*, 236:143-155.

Rustioni, A. and A. B. Kaufman. 1977. Identification of cells of origin of non-primary afferents to the dorsal column nuclei of the cat. *Experimental Brain Research*, 27:1-14.

Rustioni, A., H. G. J. M. Kuypers and G. Holstege. 1971. Propriospinal projections from the ventral and lateral funiculi to the motoneurons in the lumbosacral cord of the cat. *Brain Research*, 34:255-275.

Ryan, J. M., J. Cushman, B. Jordan, A. Samuels, H. Frazer and C. Baier. 1998. Topographic position of forelimb motoneuron pools is conserved in vertebrate evolution. *Brain, Behavior and Evolution*, 51:90-98.

Salvador, H. S. and B. J. Koos. 1989. Effects of regular and decaffeinated coffee on fetal breathing and heart rate. *American Journal of Obstetrics and Gynecology*, 160:1043-1047.

Samorajski, T. and R. L. Friede. 1968. A quantitative electron microscopic study of myelination in the pyramidal tract of rat. *Journal of Comparative Neurology*, 134:323-338.

Saper, C. B., A. D. Loewy, L. W. Swanson and W. M. Cowan. 1976. Direct hypothalamo-autonomic connections. *Brain Research*, 117:305-312.

Sato, M., N. Mizuno and A. Konishi. 1978. Localization of motoneurons innervating perineal muscles: A HRP study in cat. *Brain Research,* 140:149-154.

Satomi, H., K. Takahashi, I. Kosaka and M. Aoki. 1989. Reappraisal of projection levels of the corticospinal fibers in the cat, with special reference to the fibers descending through the dorsal funiculus. *Brain Research*, 492:255-260.

Sauer, F. C. 1935. Mitosis in the neural tube. *Journal of Comparative Neurology*, 62:377-405.

Scammon, R. E. 1927. The literature on the growth and physical development of the fetus, infant, and child: A quantitative sumary. *Anatomical Record*, 35:241-267

Scheibel, A. B. 1984. Organization of the spinal cord. In: R. A. Davidoff (ed.), *Handbook of the Spinal Cord*, vols. 2 and 3: *Anatomy and Physiology*, pp. 47-77. New York: Dekker.

Scheibel, M. E. and A. B. Scheibel. 1966. Terminal axonal patterns in cat spinal cord. I. The lateral corticospinal tract. *Brain Research*, 2:330-350.

Scheibel, M. E. and A. B. Scheibel. 1968. Terminal axonal patterns in cat spinal cord: II. The dorsal horn. *Brain Research*, 9:32-58.

Scheibel, M. E. and A. B. Scheibel. 1969. Terminal patterns in cat spinal cord. III. Primary afferent collaterals. *Brain Research*, 13:417-443.

Scheibel, M. E. and A. B. Scheibel. 1970a. Organization of spinal motoneuron dendrites in bundles. *Experimental Neurology*, 28:106-112.

Scheibel, M. E. and A. B. Scheibel. 1970b. Developmental relationship between spinal motoneuron dendrite bundles and patterned activity in the hind limb of cats. *Experimental Neurology*, 29:328-335.

Schmuckler, M. A. 1996. Development of visually guided locomotion: Barrier crossing by toddlers. *Ecological Psychology*, 8:209-236.

Schoen, J. H. R. 1964. Comparative aspects of the descending fiber systems in the spinal cord. *Progress in Brain Research*, 11:203-222.

Schoenen, J. 1982. The dendritic organization of the human spinal cord: The dorsal horn. *Neuroscience*, 7:2057-2087.

Schonbach, J., K. H. Hu and R. L. Friede. 1968. Cellular and chemical changes during myelination: Histologic, autoradiographic, histochemical, and biochemical data on myelination of the pyramidal tract and the corpus callosum. *Journal of Comparative Neurology*, 134:21-38.

Schramm, L. P., J. R. Adair, J. M. Stribling and L. P. Gray. 1975. Preganglionic innervation of the adrenal gland of the rat: A study using horseradish peroxidase. *Experimental Neurology*, 49:540-553.

Schreyer, D. L. and E. G. Jones. 1982. Growth and target finding by axons of the corticospinal tract in prenatal and postnatal rats. *Neuroscience*, 7:1837-1853.

Schreyer, D. L. and E. G. Jones. 1988. Axon elimination in the developing corticospinal tract of the rat. *Developmental Brain Research*, 38:103-119.

Schröder, H. D. 1980. Organization of the motoneurons innervating the pelvic muscles of the male rat. *Journal of Comparative Neurology*, 192:567-587.

Schröder, H. D. 1981. Onuf's nucleus X: A morphological study of a human spinal nucleus. *Anatomy and Embryology*, 162:443-453.

Schwab, M. E. and L. Schnell. 1989. Region-specific appearance of myelin constituents in the developing rat spinal cord. *Journal of Neurocytology*, 18:161-169.

Sengelaub, D. R. and A. P. Arnold. 1989. Hormonal control of neuron number in sexually dimorphic spinal nuclei of the rat. I. Testosterone-regulated death in the dorsolateral nucleus. *Journal of Comparative Neurology*, 328:622-629.

Sermasi, E., J. Howl, M. Wheatley and J. H. Coote. 1998. Localisation of arginine vasopressin V1a receptors on sympatho-adrenal preganglionic neurons. *Experimental Brain Research*, 119:85-91.

Shapovalov, A. I., O. A. Karamjan, G. G. Kurchavyi and Z. A. Repina. 1971. Synaptic actions evoked from the red nucleus on the spinal alpha-motoneurons in the rhesus monkey. *Brain Research*, 32:325-348.

Sharrard, W. J. W. 1955. The distribution of the permanent paralysis in the lower limb in poliomyelitis. *Journal of Bone and Joint Surgery*, 37:540-558.

Sheehan, D. 1933. The afferent nerve supply of the mesentery and its significance in the causation of abdominal pain. *Journal of Anatomy*, 67:233-249.

Sherman, M., I. C. Sherman and C. D. Flory. 1936. Infant behavior. *Comparative Psychology Monographs*, 12, No. 4.

Sherrington, C. S. 1906. *The Integrative Action of the Nervous System*. New Haven: Yale University Press.

Sherrington, C. S. and E. E. Laslett. 1903. Remarks on the dorsal spino-cerebellar tract. *Journal of Physiology*, 29:188-194.

Shik, M. L. and G. N. Orlovsky. 1976. Neurophysiology of locomotor automatisms. *Physiological Reviews*, 56:465-501.

Shinoda, Y., A. P. Arnold and H. Asanuma. 1976. Spinal branching of corticospinal axons in the cat. *Experimental Brain Research*, 26:215-234.

Shinoda, Y., T. Ohgaki and T. Futami. 1986. The morphology of single lateral vestibulospinal tract axons in the lower cervical spinal cord of the cat. *Journal of Comparative Neurology*, 249:226-241.

Shinoda, Y., T. Ohgaki, Y. Sugiuchi and T. Futami. 1992. Morphology of single medial vestibulospinal tract axons in the upper cervical spinal cord of the cat. *Journal of Comparative Neurology*, 316:151-172.

Shinoda, Y., P. Zarzecki and H. Asanuma. 1979. Spinal branching of pyramidal tract neurons in the monkey. *Experimental Brain Research*, 34:59-72.

Shinoda, Y., J. Yokota and T. Futami. 1986. Multiple axon collaterals of single corticospinal axons in the cat spinal cord. *Journal of Neurophysiology*, 55:425-448.

Shirley, M. M. 1931. *The First Two Years, a Study of Twenty-five Babies*. Vol. 1, *Postural and Locomotor Development*. Minneapolis: University of Minnesota Press.

Shortland, P., C. J. Wool and M. Fitzgerald. 1989. Morphology and somatotopic organization of the central terminals of hindlimb hair follicle afferents in the rat lumbar spinal cord. *Journal of Comparative Neurology*, 289:416-433.

Shriver, J. E. and C. R. Noback. 1967. Cortical projections to the lower brain stem and spinal cord in the tree shrew (*Tupaia glis*). *Journal of Comparative Neurology*, 130:25-54.

Shupliakov, O., G. Örnung, L. Brodin, B. Ulfhake, O. P. Ottersen, J. Storm-Mathisen and S. Cullheim. 1993. Immunocytochemical localization of amino acid neurotransmitter candidates in the ventral horn of the cat spinal cord: A light microscopic study. *Experimental Brain Research*, 96:404-418.

Sidman, R. L., I. L. Miale and N. Feder. 1959. Cell proliferation and migration in the primitive ependymal zone: An autoradiographic study of histogenesis in the nervous system. *Experimental Neurology*, 1:322-333.

Silos-Santiago, I. and W. D. Snider. 1992. Development of commissural neurons in the embryonic rat spinal cord. *Journal of Comparative Neurology*, 325:514-526.

Silver, A. and J. H. Wolstencroft. The distribution of cholinesterases in relation to the structure of the spinal cord in the cat. *Brain Research*, 34:205-227.

Silver, M. L. 1942. The motoneurons of the spinal cord of the frog. *Journal of Comparative Neurology*, 77:1-40

Sims, T. J. and J. E. Vaughn. 1979. The generation of neurons involved in an early reflex pathway of embryonic mouse spinal cord. *Journal of Comparative Neurology*, 183:707-719.

Sinclair, D. 1981. *Mechanisms of Cutaneous Sensation*. Oxford: Oxford University Press.

Sindou, M., C. Quoex and C. Baledier. 1974. Fiber organization at the posterior spinal cord-rootlet junction in man. *Journal of Comparative Neurology*, 153:15-26.

Skinner, R. D., J. D. Coulter, R. J. Adams and R. S. Remmel. 1979. Cells of origin of long descending propriospinal fibers connecting the spinal enlargements in cat and monkey, determined by horseradish peroxidase and electrophysiological techniques. *Journal of Comparative Neurology*, 188:443-454.

Smith, C. L. 1983. The development and postnatal organization of primary afferent projections to the rat thoracic spinal cord. *Journal of Comparative Neurology*, 220:29-43.

Smith, C. L. and M. Hollyday. 1983. The development and postnatal organization of motor nuclei in the rat thoracic spinal cord. *Journal of Comparative Neurology*, 220:16-28.

Smith, K. J. and B. J. Bennett. 1987. Topographic and quantitative description of rat dorsal column fibres arising from the lumbar dorsal roots. *Journal of Anatomy*, 153: 203-215.

Smith, M. C. 1970. Retrograde changes in human spinal cord after anterolateral cordotomies: Location and identification after different periods of survival. In: J. J. Bonica and D. Albe-Fessard (eds.), *Advances in Pain Research and Therapy*, vol. 1, pp. 91-98.

Snider, W. D. and S. B. McMahon. 1998. Tackling pain at the source: New ideas about nociceptors. *Neuron*, 20:629-632.

Snider, W. D., L. Zhang, S. Yusoof, N. Gorukanti and C. Tsering. 1992. Interactions between dorsal root axons and their target motor neurons in developing mammalian spinal cord. *Journal of Neuroscience*, 3494-3508.

Snyder, R. 1977. The organization of the dorsal root entry zone in cats and monkeys. *Journal of Comparative Neurology*, 174:47-70.

Snyder, R. L., R. L. M. Faull and W. R. Mehler. 1978. Comparative study of the neurons of origin of the spinocerebellar afferents in the rat, cat and squirrel monkey based on retrograde transport of horseradish peroxidase. *Journal of Comparative Neurology*, 181:833-852.

Sperry, D. G. and P. Grobstein. 1983. Postmetamorphic changes in the lumbar lateral motor column in relation to muscle growth in the toad *Bufo Americanus*. *Journal of Comparative Neurology*, 216:104-114.

Spike, R. C., A. J. Todd and H. M. Johnston. 1993. Coexistence of NADH diaphorase with GABA, glycine, and acetylcholine in rat spinal cord. *Journal of Comparative Neurology*, 335:320-333.

Spiller W. G. and E. Martin. 1912. The treatment of persistent pain of organic origin in the lower part of the body by division of the anterolateral column of the spinal cord. *Journal of the American Medical Association*, 63:1489-1490.

Spivy, D. F. and J. S. Metcalf. 1959. Differential effects of medial and lateral dorsal root sections upon subcortical evoked potentials. *Journal of Neurophysiology*, 22:367-373.

Sprague, J. M. 1948. A study of motor cell localization in the spinal cord of the rhesus monkey. *American Journal of Anatomy*, 82:1-26.

Stanfield, B. B. and D. D. M. O'Leary. 1985. The transient corticospinal projection from the occipital cortex during the postnatal development of the rat. *Journal of Comparative Neurology*, 238:236-248.

Stanfield, B. B., D. M. M. O'Leary and C. Fricks. 1982. Selective collateral elimination in early postnatal development restricts cortical distribution of pyramidal tract axons. *Nature*, 298:371-373.

Stein, P. S. G. 1984. Central pattern generators in the spinal cord. In: R. A. Davidoff (ed.), *Handbook of the Spinal Cord*. Vols. 2 and 3, *Anatomy and Physiology*, pp. 647-672. New York: Dekker.

Stensaas, L. J. and S. E. Stensaas. 1971. Light and electron microscopy of motoneurons and neuropile in the amphibian spinal cord. *Brain Research*, 31:67-84.

Sterling, P. and H. G. J. M. Kuypers. 1968. The anatomical organization of the brachial spinal cord of the cat. III. The propriospinal connections. *Brain Research*, 7:419-443.

Stern, K. 1938. Note on the nucleus ruber magnocellularis and its efferent pathway in man. *Brain*, 61:284-289.

Stirnimann, F. 1937. Die Einstellreaktion beim Neugeborenen. *Jahrbuch der Kinderheilkunde*, 149:326-329.

Stirnimann, F. 1938. Das Kriech- und Schreitphänomen der Neugeborenen. *Schweizer medizinische Wochenschrift*, 19:1374-1376.

Stirnimann, F. 1943. Über dem Moroschen Umklammerungsreflex beim Neugeborenen. *Annales Paediatrica*, 160:1-10.

Stoeckli, E. T., P. Sonderegger, G. E. Pollerberg and L. T. Landmesser. 1997. Interference with axonin-1 and NrCAM interactions unmasks a floor plate activity inhibitory for commissural axons. *Neuron*, 18:209-221.

Streeter, G. L. 1920. Weight, sitting height, head size, foot length, and menstrual age of the human embryo. *Carnegie Institution of Washington, Contributions to Embryology*, 11:143-170.

Streeter, G. L. 1942. Developmental horizons in human embryos: Description of age groups XI, 13to 20 somites, and age group XII, 21 to 29 somites. *Carnegie Institution of Washington, Contributions to Embryology*, 30:211-245.

Streeter, G. L. 1945. Developmental horizons in human embryos: Description of age group XIII, embryos of about 4 or 5 millimeters long, and age group XIV, period of indentation of the lens vesicle. *Carnegie Institution of Washington, Contributions to Embryology*, 31:27-63.

Streeter, G. L. 1948. Developmental horizons in human embryos: Description of age groups XV, XVI, XVII, and XVIII, being the third issue of a survey of the Carnegie Collection. *Carnegie Institution of Washington, Contributions to Embryology*, 32:133-203.

Streeter, G. L., C. H. Heuser and G. W. Corner. 1951. Developmental horizons in human embryos: Description of age groups XIX, XX, XXI, XXII, and XXIII, being the fifth issue of a survey of the Carnegie Collection. *Carnegie Institution of Washington, Contributions to Embryology*, 34:165-196.

Strong, O. S. 1936. Some observations on the course of the fibers from Clarke's column in the human spinal cord. *Bulletin of the Neurological Institute, New York*, 5:378-386.

Sugitani, M., J. Yano, T. Sugai and H. Ooyama. 1990. Somatotopic organization and columnar structure of vibrissae representation in the rat ventrobasal complex. *Experimental Brain Research*, 81:346-352.

Swaiman, K. F. 1999. Neurologic examination of the term and preterm infant. In: K. F. Swaiman and S. Ashwal (eds.), *Pediatric Neurology: Principles and Practice*, pp. 39-53. St. Louis: Mosby.

Swanson, L. W. and S. McKellar. 1979. The distribution of oxytocin- and neurophysin-stained fibers in the spinal cord of the rat and monkey. *Journal of Comparative Neurology*, 188:87-106.

Swett, J. E. and C. J. Woolf. 1985. The somatotopic organization of primary afferent terminals in the superficial laminae of the dorsal horn of the rat spinal cord. *Journal of Comparative Neurology*, 231:66-77.

Sypert G. W. and J. B. Munson. 1984. Excitatory synapses. In: R. A. Davidoff (ed.), *Handbook of the Spinal Cord*, vols. 2 and 3: *Anatomy and Physiology*, pp.315-384. New York: Dekker.

Székely , G. and G. Czéh. 1976. Organization of locomotion. In: R. Llinás and W. Precht (eds.), *Frog Neurobiology: A Handbook*, pp. 765-792. Berlin: Springer-Verlag.

Szentágothai, J. 1964. Neuronal and synaptic arrangement in the substantia gelatinosa Rolandi. *Journal of Comparative Neurology*, 122:219-239.

Szentágothai, J. and T. Kiss. 1949. Projection of dermatomes on the substantia gelatinosa. *Archives of Neurology and Psychiatry*, 62:734-744.

Szymonowicz, W. 1933. Über die Entwicklung der Nervenendigungen in der Haut des Menschen. *Zeitschrift für Zellforschung*, 19:356-382.

Takahashi, T. and M. Otsuka. 1975. Regional distribution of substance P in the spinal cord and nerve roots of the cat and the effects of dorsal root section. *Brain Research*, 87:1-11.

Tamatani, M., E. Senba and M. Tohyama. 1989. Calcitonin gene-related peptide and substance P-containing primary afferents in the dorsal column of the rat. *Brain Research*, 495:122-130.

Tang, F. R., C. K. Tang and E. A. Ling. 1995. The distribution of NADH-d in the central gray region (lamina X) of rat upper thoracic spinal cord. *Journal of Neurocytology*, 24:735-743.

Tasiro, S. 1940. Experimentell-anatomische Untersuchung über die efferenten Bahnen aus den Vierhügeln der Katze. *Zeitschrift für mikroskopische und anatomische Forschung*, 47:1-32.

Terni, T. 1924. Ricerche anatomiche sul sistema nervoso autonomo degli uccelli. *Archivio Italiano di Anatomia e di Embriologia*, 20:433-510.

Tessier-Lavigne, M., M. Placzek, A. G. S. Lumsden, J. Dodd and T. M. Jessell. 1988. Chemotropic guidance of developing axons in the mammalian central nervous system. *Nature*: 336:775-778.

Thelen, E., D. Corbetta, K. Kamm, J. P. Spencer, K. Schneider and R. F. Zernicke. 1993. The transition to reaching: Mapping intention and intrinsic dynamics. *Child Development*, 64:1058-1098.

Thelen, E. and D. M. Fisher. 1982. Newborn stepping: An explanation for a "disappearing" reflex. *Developmental Psychology*, 18:760-775.

Thelen, E. and J. P. Spencer. 1998. Postural control during reaching in young infants: A dynamic systems approach. *Neuroscience and Biobehavioral Reviews*, 22:507-514.

Thelen, E. and B. D. Ulrich. 1991. Hidden skills: A dynamic systems anaysis of treadmill stepping during the first year. *Monographsof the Society for Research in Child Development*, 56, Serial #223.

Theriault, E., M. Otsuka and T. Jessell. 1979. Capsaicin-evoked release of substance P from primary sensory neurons. *Brain Research*, 170:209-213.

Tigges, J., S. Nakagawa and M. Tigges. 1979. Efferents of area 4 in a South American monkey (Saimiri). I. Terminations in the spinal cord. *Brain Research*, 171:1-10.

Tilney, F. and L. Casamajor. 1924. Myelogeny as applied to the study of behavior. *Archives of Neurology and Psychiatry*, 12:1-66.

Todd, J. K. 1964. Afferent impulses in pudendal nerves of the cat. *Quarterly Journal of Experimental Physiology*, 49:258-267.

Tomasulo, K. C. and R. Emmers. 1972. Activation of neurons in the gracile nucleus by two afferent pathways in the rat. *Experimental Neurology*, 36:197-206.

Touwen, B. C. L. 1976. *Neurological Development in Infancy.* London: Heinemann Medical Books.

Tower, S. S. 1940. Pyramidal lesion in the monkey. *Brain*, 63:36-90.

Tower, S. S. 1949. The pyramidal tract. In: P. C. Bucy (ed.), *The Precentral Motor Cortex*, pp. 149-172 2nd ed. Urbana, IL: University of Illinois Press.

Tracey, D. J., S. De Biasi, K. Phend and A. Rustioni. 1991. Aspartate-like immunoreactivity in primary afferent neurons. *Neuroscience*, 40:673-686.

Tracey, D. J. and P. M. E. Waite. 1995. Somatosensory system. In: G. Paxinos (ed.), *The Rat Nervous System* (2nd ed.), pp. 689-704. San Diego, CA: Academic Press.

Trevino, D. L. and E. Carstens. 1975. Confirmation of the location of spinothalamic neurons in the cat and monkey by the retrograde transport of horseradish peroxidase. *Brain Research*, 98:177-182.

Tribollet, E., C. Barberis and Y. Arsenijevic. 1997. Distribution of vasopressin and oxytocin receptors in the rat spinal cord: Sex-related differences and effect of castration in pudendal motor nuclei. *Neuroscience*, 78:499-509.

Trousse, F., M. C. Giess, C. Soula, S. Ghandour, A. M. Duprat and P. Cochard. 1995. Notochord and floor plate stimulate oligodendrocyte differentiation in cultures of the chick dorsal neural tube. *Journal of Neuroscience Research*, 41:552-560.

Truex, R.C., M. J. Taylor and M. Q. Smythe. 1968. The lateral cervical nucleus of the human spinal cord. *Anatomical Record*, 160:443.

Tsering, C. 1992. Demonstration of segmental arrangement of thoracic spinal motor neurons using lipophilic dyes. *Developmental Neuroscience*, 14:308-311.

Uchizono, K. 1966. Excitatory and inhibitory synapses in the cat spinal cord. *Japanese Journal of Physiology*, 16:570-575

Uddenberg, N. 1968. Functional organization of long, second-order afferents in the dorsal funiculus. *Experimental Brain Research*, 4:377-382.

Ueyama, T., N. Mizumo, S. Nomura, A. Konishi, K. Itoh and H. Arakawa. 1984. Central distribution of afferent and efferent components of the pudendal nerve in cat. *Journal of Comparative Neurology*, 222:38-46.

Ulfhake, B. and S. Cullheim. 1988. Postnatal development of cat hind limb motoneurons. III. Changes in size of motoneurons supplying the triceps surae muscle. *Journal of Comparative Neurology*, 278:103-120.

Vaal, J., A. J. van Soest and B. Hopkins. 2000. Spontaneous kicking behavior in infants: Age-related effects of unilateral weighting. *Developmental Psychobiology*, 36:111-122.

Valentin, L. and K. Marsal. 1986. Fetal movement in the third trimester of normal pregnancy. *Early Human Development*, 14:295-306.

Van der Fits, I. B. M., E. Otten, A. W. J. Klip, L. A. van Eykern and M. Hadders-Algra. 1999. The development of postural adjustments during reaching in 6- to 8-month-old infants: Evidence for two transitions. *Experimental Brain Research*, 126:517-528.

VanderHorst, V. G. J. M. and G. Holstege. 1997. Organization of lumbosacral motoneuronal cell groups innervating hindlimb, pelvic floor, and axial muscles in the cat. *Journal of Comparative Neurology*, 382:46-76.

Van der Loos, H. and T. Woolsey. 1973. Somatosensory cortex: Structural alterations following early injury to sense organs. *Science*, 179:395-398.

Van Gehuchten, A. and C. de Neef. 1900. Les noyaux moteurs de la moelle lombo-sacree chez l'homme. *Nevraxe*, 1:201.

Vanner, S. J. and P. K. Rose. 1984. Dendritic distribution of motoneurons innervating the three heads of the trapezius muscle of the cat. *Journal of Comparative Neurology*, 226:96-110.

Vaughn, J. and J. A. Grieshaber. 1973. A morphological investigation of an early reflex pathway in developing rat spinal cord. *Journal of Comparative Neurology*, 148:177-210.

Vereijken, B. and E. Thelen. 1997. Training infant treadmill stepping: The role of individual pattern stability. *Developmental Psychobiology*, 30:89-102.

Vierck, C. J. 1974. Tactile movement detection and discrimination following dorsal column lesions in monkeys. *Experimental Brain Research*, 20:331-346.

Vierck, C. J. 1977. Absolute and differential sensitivities to touch stimuli after spinal cord lesions in monkeys. *Brain Research*, 134:529-539.

Vierck, C. J. 1978. Comparison of forelimb and hindlimb motor deficits following dorsal column section in monkeys. *Brain Research*, 146:279-294.

Vierck, C. J., R. H. Cohen and B. Y. Cooper. 1985. Effects of spinal lesions on temporal resolution of cutaneous sensations. *Somatosensory Research*, 3:45-56.

Vierck, C. J. and M. M. Luck. 1979. Loss and recovery of reactivity to noxious stimuli in monkeys with primary spinothalamic cordotomies followed by secondary or tertiary lesions of other cord sectors. *Brain*, 102:233-248.

Villanueva, L., J. de Pommery, D. Menétrey and D. Le Bars. 1991. Spinal afferent projections to subnucleus reticularis dorsalis in the rat. *Neuroscience Letters*, 134:98-102.

Visser, G. H. A., R. N. Laurini, J. I. P. de Vries, D. J. Bekedam and H. F. R. Prechtl. 1985. Abnormal motor behaviour in anencephalic fetuses. *Early Human Development*, 12:173-182.

Waldeyer, H. 1888. Das Gorilla-Rückenmark. *Abhandlungen der preussischen Akademie der Wissenschaften*, 3:1-147.

Waite, P. M. E. and D. J. Tracey. 1995. Trigeminal sensory system. In: G. Paxinos (ed.), *The Rat Nervous System*, pp. 705-724, (2nd ed.) New York: Academic Press,

Walker, A. E. 1940. The spinothalamic tract in man. *Archives of Neurology and Psychiatry*, 43:284-298.

Wall, P. D. 1970. The sensory and motor role of impulses travelling in the dorsal columns towards the cerebral cortex. *Brain,* 93:505-524.

Wallén, P. and T. L. Williams. 1984. Fictive locomotion in the lamprey spinal cord in vitro compared with swimming in the intact and spinal lamprey. *Journal of Physiology*, 347:225-239.

Wang, X. M., X. M. Xu, Y. Q. Quin and G. F. Martin. 1992. The origins of spuraspinal projections to the cervical and lumbar spinal cord at different stages of development in the gray short-tailed Brazilian opossum, *Monodelphis domestica*. *Developmental Brain Research*, 68:203-216.

Warf, B. C., J. Fok-Seang and R. H. Miller. 1991. Evidence for the ventral origin of oligodendrocyte precursors in the rat spinal cord. *Journal of Neuroscience*, 11:2477-2488.

Wartenberg, R. 1939. A "numeral" test in transverse lesions of the spinal cord. *American Journal of the Medical Sciences*, 198:393-396.

Weaver, T. A. and A. E. Walker. 1941. Topical arrangement within the spinothalamic tract of the monkey. *Archives of Neurology and Psychiatry*, 46:877-883.

Webber, C. L., R. D. Wurster and J. M. Chung. 1979. Cat phrenic nucleus architecture as revealed by horseradish peroxidase mapping. *Experimental Brain Research*, 35:395-406.

Webster, H. deF. 1974. Peripheral nerve structure. In: J. I. Hubbard (ed.), *The Peripheral Nervous System*, pp. 3-26. New York: Plenum Press.

Weeks, O. I. and A. W. English. 1987. Cat triceps surae motor nuclei are organized topologically. *Experimental Neurology*, 96:163-177.

Weil, A. and A. Lassek. 1929. A quantitative distribution of the pyramidal tract in man. *Archives of Neurology and Psychiatry*, 22:495-510.

Weinberg, R. J., F. Conti, S. L. Van Eyck, P. Petrusz and A. Rustioni. 1987. Glutamate immunoreactivity in the superficial laminae of rat dorsal horn and spinal trigeminal nucleus. In: T. P. Hicks, D. Lodge and H. McLennan (eds.), *Excitatory Amino Acid Transmission: Neurology and Neurobiology*, pp. 126-133. New York: Liss.

Welker, C. and T. A. Woolsey. 1974. Structure of layer IV in the somatosensory neocortex of the rat: Description and comparison with the mouse. *Journal of Comparative Neurology*, 158:437-454.

Wentworth, L. E. 1984. The development of the cervical spinal cord of the mouse embryo: I. A Golgi analysis of ventral root neuron differentiation. *Journal of Comparative Neurology*, 222:81-95.

Werman, R., R. A. Davidoff and M. H. Aprison. 1967. Inhibition of motoneurons by iontophoresis of glycine. *Nature*, 214:680-683.

Westerga, J. and A Gramsbergen. 1992. Structural changes of the soleus and the tibialis anterior motoneuron pool during development in the rat. *Journal of Comparative Neurology*, 319:406-416.

Westman, J. 1989. Light and electron microscopical studies of the substance P innervation of the dorsal column nuclei and the lateral cervical nucleus in the primate. *Upsala Journal of Medical Science*, 94:123-128.

White, B., P. Castle and R. Held. 1964. Observations on the development of visually directed reaching. *Child Development*, 35:349-364.

White, J. C. 1974. Sympathectomy for relief of pain. In: J. J. Bonica (ed.), *Advances in Neurology,* vol. 4: *Pain*, pp. 629-638. New York: Raven Press.

White, J. C. and W. H. Sweet. 1969. *Pain and the Neurosurgeon*. Springfield, IL: Thomas.

Whitsel, B. L., L. M. Petrucelli and G. Sapiro. 1969. Modality representation in the lumbar and cervical fasciculus gracilis of squirrel monkeys. *Brain Research*, 15:67-78.

Whitsel, B. L., L. M. Petrucelli, G. Sapiro and H. Ha. 1970. Fiber sorting in the fasciculus gracilis of squirrel monkeys. *Experimental Neurology*, 29:227-242.

Wiberg, M. and A. Blomquist. 1984. The spinomesencephalic tract in the cat: Its cells of origin and termination pattern as demonstrated by the intraaxonal transport method. *Brain Research*, 291:1-18.

Wiesenfeld-Hallin, Z., T. Hökfelt, J. M. Lundberg, W. G. Firssmann, M. Reuneche, F. A. Tschopp and J. A. Fischer. 1984. Immunoreactive calcitonin related-gene peptide and substance P coexist in sensory neurons to the spinal cord and interact in spinal behavioral responses in the rat. *Neuroscience Letters*, 52:199-204.

Williams, J. W. *Obstetrics*. 1931. New York: Appleton-Centurry-Crofts.

Williams, P. L. and R. Warwick (eds.). 1980. *Gray's Anatomy*, 36th ed. Edinburgh: Churchill, Livingstone.

Willis, W. D. 1985. *The Pain System: The Neural Basis of Nociceptive Transmission in the Mammalian Nervous System*. Basel: Karger.

Willis, W. D. and R. E. Coggeshall. 1978. *Sensory Mechanisms of the Spinal Cord*. New York: Plenum Press.

Willis, W. D., D. R. Kenshalo and R. B. Leonard. 1979. The cells of origin of the primate spinothalamic tract. *Journal of Comparative Neurology*, 188:543-574.

Willis, W. D., D. L. Trevino, J. D.Coulter and R. N. Maunz. 1974. Responses of primate spinothalamic tract neurons to natural stimulation of hind limb. *Journal of Neurophysiology*, 37:358-372.

Willis, W. D. and K. N. Westlund. 1997. Neuroanatomy of the pain system and of the pathways that modulate pain. *Journal of Clinical Neurophysiology*, 14:2-31.

Wilson, D. B. 1973. Chronological changes in the cell cycle of chick neuroepithelial cells. *Journal of Embryology and Experimental Morphology*, 29:745-751.

Wilson, V. J. and M. Yoshida. 1969. Comparison of effects of stimulation of Deiters' nucleus and medial longitudinal fasciculus on neck, forelimb, and hindlimb motoneurons. *Journal of Neurophysiology*, 32:743-758.

Wilson, V. J., M. Yoshida and R. H. Schor. 1970. Supraspinal monosynaptic excitation and inhibition of thoracic back motoneurons. *Experimental Brain Research*, 11:282-295.

Windle, W. F. 1944. Genesis of somatic motor functions in mammalian embryos: A synthesizing article. *Physiological Zoology*, 17:247-260.

Windle, W. F. 1970. Development of neural elements in human embryos of four to seven weeks gestation. *Experimental Neurology*, Supplement 5:44-83.

Windle, W. F. and R. E. Baxter. 1936. The first neurofibrillar development in albino rat embryos. *Journal of Comparative Neurology*, 63:173-187.

Windle, W. F., M. W. Fish and J. E. O'Donnell. 1934. Myeologeny of the cat as related to the development of fiber tracts and prenatal behavior patterns. *Journal of Comparative Neurology*, 59:139-165.

Windle, W. F. and J. E. Fitzgerald. 1937. Development of spinal reflex mechanism in human embryos. *Journal of Comparative Neurology*, 67:493-509.

Windle, W. F. and D. W. Orr. 1934. The development of behavior in chick embryos: Spinal cord structure correlated with early somatic motility. *Journal of Comparative Neurology*, 60:287-307.

Winter, D. L. 1965. Nucleus gracilis of cat: Functional organization and corticofugal effects. *Journal of Neurophysiology*, 28:48-70.

Wise, S. P. and E. G. Jones. 1977. Cells of origin and terminal distribution of descending projections of the rat somatic sensory cortex. *Journal of Comparative Neurology*, 175:129-158.

Wise, S. P., E. A. Murray and J. D. Coulter. 1979. Somatotopic organization of corticospinal and corticotrigeminal neurons in the rat. *Neuroscience*, 4:65-78.

Wolff, P. H. 1968. The serial organization of sucking in the young infant. *Pediatrics*, 42:943-956.

Wong, V., C. P. Barrett, E. J. Donati, L. F. Eng and L. Guth. 1983. Carbonic anhydrase activity in first order sensory neurons of the rat. *Journal of Histochemistry and Cytochemistry*, 31:293-300.

Woolf, C. J. and M. Fitzgerald. 1986. Somatotopic organization of cutaneous afferent terminals and dorsal horn neuronal receptive fields in the superficial and deep laminae of the rat lumbar spinal cord. *Journal of Comparative Neurology*, 251:517-531.

Woollacott, M. M., M. Debu and M. Mowatt. 1987. Neuromuscular control of posture in the infant and the child: Is vision dominant? *Journal of Motor Behavior*, 19:167-186.

Woolsey, T. A., J. R. Anderson, J. R. Wann and B. B. Stanfield. 1979. Effects of early vibrissae damage on neurons in the ventrobasal thalamus of the mouse. *Journal of Comparative Neurology*, 184:363-380.

Woolsey, T. A. and H. van der Loos. 1970. The structural organization of layer IV in the somatosensory region (SI) of mouse cerebral cortex. *Brain Research*, 17:205-242.

Woolsey, T. A., C. Welker and R. H. Schwartz. 1975. Comparative anatomical studies of the SmI face cortex with special reference to the occurrence of "barrels" in layer IV. *Journal of Comparative Neurology*, 164:79-94.

Wu, W., L. Ziskind-Conhaim and M. A. Sweet. 1992. Early development of glycine- and GABA-mediated synapses in rat spinal cord. *Journal of Neuroscience*, 12:3935-3945.

Xu, Q. and G. Grant. 1994. Course of spinocerebellar axons in the ventral and lateral funiculi of the spinal cord with projections to the anterior lobe: An experimental study in the cat with retrograde tracing techniques. *Journal of Comparative Neurology*, 345:288-302.

Yaginuma, H., S. Homma, R. Kunzi and R. W. Oppenheim. 1991. Pathfinding by growth cones of commissural interneurons in the chick embryo spinal cord: A light and electron microscopic study. *Journal of Comparative Neurology*, 304:78-102.

Yaginuma, H. and M. Matsushita. 1987. Spinocerebellar projections from the thoracic cord in the cat, as studied by anterograde transport of wheat germ agglutinin-horseradish peroxidase. *Journal of Comparative Neurology*, 258:1-27.

Yaksh, T. L. and P. R. Wilson. 1979. Spinal serotonin terminal system mediates antinocipeption. *Journal of Pharmacology and Experimental Therapy*, 208:446-453.

Yamadori, T. 1971. A light and electron microscopic study of the post-natal development of spinal ganglia. *Acta Anatomica Nipponica*, 45:191-205.

Yezierski, R. P. and R. H. Schwartz. 1986. Response and receptive-field properties of spinomesencephalic tract cells in the cat. *Journal of Neurophysiology*, 55:79-96.

Yezierski, R. P., L. S. Sorkin and W. D. Willis. 1987. Response properties of spinal neurons projecting to midbrain or midbrain-thalamus in the monkey. *Brain Research*, 437:165-170.

Young, M. R., S. M. Fleetwood-Walker, T. Dickinson, G. Blackburn-Munro, H. Sparrow, P. J. Birch and C. Bountra. 1997. Behavioural and electrophysiological evidence supporting a role for group I metabotropic glutamate receptors in the mediation of nociceptive inputs to the rat spinal cord. *Brain Research*, 777:161-169.

Yu, W.-P., E. J. Collarini, N. P. Pringle and W. D. Richardson. 1994. Embryonic expression of myelin genes: Evidence for a focal source of oligodendrocyte precursors in the ventricular zone of the neural tube. *Neuron*, 12:1353-1362.

Zelazo, P. R., N. Zelazo and S. Kolb. 1972. "Walking" in the newborn. *Science*, 176:314-315.

Zhang, X., V. Verge, Z. Wiesenfeld-Hallin, G. Ju, D. Bredt, S. H. Snyder and T. Hökfelt. 1993. Nitric oxide synthase-like immunoreactivity in lumbar dorsal root ganglia and spinal cord of rat and monkey and effect of peripheral axotomy. *Journal of Comparative Neurology*, 335:563-575.

Zhu, Q., E. Runko, R. Imondi, T. Milligan, D. Kapitula and Z. Kaprielian. 1998. New cell surface marker of the rat floor plate and notochord. *Developmental Dynamics*, 211:314-326.

Ziskind-Conhaim, L. 1990. NMDA receptors mediate poly- and monosynaptic potentials in motoneurons of rat embryos. *Journal of Neuroscience*, 110:125-135.

INDEX